Clare Collins and Sharon Kirkpatrick (Eds.)

# Assessment of Nutrient Intakes

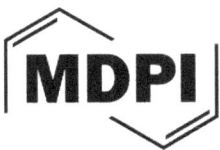

**MDPI**

This book is a reprint of the Special Issue that appeared in the online, open access journal, *Nutrients* (ISSN 2072-6643) from 2014–2016, available at:

http://www.mdpi.com/journal/nutrients/special_issues/assessment-nutrient-intakes

*Guest Editors*
Clare Collins
Priority Research Centre in Physical Activity and Nutrition, Faculty of Health, School of Health Sciences, University of Newcastle
Australia

Sharon Kirkpatrick
School of Public Health and Health Systems, University of Waterloo
Canada

| *Editorial Office* | *Publisher* | *Senior Assistant Editor* |
| --- | --- | --- |
| MDPI AG | Shu-Kun Lin | Xiaocen Zhang |
| St. Alban-Anlage 66 | | |
| Basel, Switzerland | | |

**1. Edition 2017**

MDPI • Basel • Beijing • Wuhan • Barcelona • Belgrade

ISBN 978-3-03842-288-4 (Hbk)
ISBN 978-3-03842-289-1 (PDF)

# Table of Contents

## Section 1: Development and Evaluation of Measures to Collect Dietary Data from Populations across the Lifecycle and across Contexts

## Section 2: Advances in Biomarkers and Metabolomics

## Section 3: Comparisons of Food Consumption Data and Statistical Methods

## Section 4: Application of Dietary Assessment Methods to Enhance Our Understanding of Dietary Intakes among Populations

## Section 5: Assessment of Dietary Patterns and Dietary Quality

## Section 6: Evaluation of a Dietary Intervention

# List of Contributors

**Tanisha F. Aflague** Human Nutrition, Food, and Animal Sciences University of Hawaii at Mānoa, Honolulu, HI96822, USA.

**Samuel Aguiar Jr.** Department of Pelvic Surgery, A.C. Camargo Cancer Center, Rua Professor Antônio Prudente, 211, Liberdade, São Paulo (SP) CEP 01509-010, Brazil.

**Ziad Ahmad** Video and Image Processing Laboratory, School of Electrical and Computer Engineering, Purdue University, West Lafayette, IN 47907-2035, USA.

**Hiroshi Akasaka** School of Medicine, Sapporo Medical University, Sapporo 060-8556, Japan.

**Salwa A. Albar** Nutritional Epidemiology Group, School of Food Science and Nutrition, University of Leeds, Leeds LS2 9JT, UK.

**Nisreen A. Alwan** Nutritional Epidemiology Group, School of Food Science and Nutrition, University of Leeds, Leeds LS2 9JT, UK; Academic Unit of Primary Care and Population Sciences, Faculty of Medicine, University of Southampton, Southampton General Hospital, Southampton SO16 6YD, UK.

**Kaarin J. Anstey** Centre for Research on Ageing, Health & Wellbeing, The Australian National University, Florey, Building 54, Mills Road, Acton, ACT 2601, Australia.

**Ghada Asaad** Department of Agricultural, Food and Nutritional Science, University of Alberta, Edmonton, AB T6G 2R3, Canada.

**Susan Ash** School of Exercise and Nutrition Sciences, Faculty of Health, and Institute of Health and Biomedical Innovation, Queensland University of Technology, Kelvin Grove, Queensland 4059, Australia.

**Kimberly Ashby-Mitchell** Centre for Research on Ageing, Health & Wellbeing, The Australian National University, Florey, Building 54, Mills Road, Acton, ACT 2601, Australia.

**John Attia** School of Medicine and Public Health, University of Newcastle, New South Wales 2308, Australia; Hunter Medical Research Institute, New Lambton Heights, New South Wales 2305, Australia.

**Rhonda C. Bell** Department of Agricultural, Food and Nutritional Science, 4-002 Li Ka Shing Centre for Health Research Innovation, University of Alberta, Edmonton, AB T6G 2E1, Canada.

**Casey Berglund** Department of Agricultural, Food and Nutritional Science, 4-002 Li Ka Shing Centre for Health Research Innovation, University of Alberta, Edmonton, AB T6G 2E1, Canada.

**Hanne C. Bertram** Department of Food Science, Aarhus University, Kirstinebjergvej 10, Aarslev DK-5792, Denmark.

**Colin W. Binns** School of Public Health, Curtin University, Kent Street, Perth 6845, Australia.

**May M. Boggess** Occupational Health and Safety, School of Health Sciences, Faculty of Health and Medicine, University of Newcastle, Newcastle 2300, Australia; School of Mathematical and Statistical Sciences, College of Liberal Arts and Science, Arizona State University, Tempe, AZ 85287, USA.

**Carol J. Boushey** Epidemiology Program, University of Hawaii Cancer Centre, Honolulu, HI 96844, USA; Video and Image Processing Laboratory, School of Electrical and Computer Engineering, and Department of Nutrition Science, Purdue University, West Lafayette, IN 47907, USA.

**Tatiana Bracke** Faculty of Science and Technology, Department of Bio- and Food Sciences, University College Ghent-Campus Vesalius, Keramiekstraat 80, B-9000 Ghent, Belgium.

**Rita B. Buckley** Buckley/Swartz, 300 Lynn Shore Drive, #603, Lynn, MA 01902, USA.

**Tracy L. Burrows** Nutrition and Dietetics, School of Health Sciences, Faculty of Health and Medicine, and Priority Research Centre in Physical Activity and Nutrition, University of Newcastle, Newcastle 2300, Australia.

**Janet E. Cade** Nutritional Epidemiology Group, School of Food Science and Nutrition, University of Leeds, Leeds LS2 9JT, UK.

**Suzi A. Camey** Post-Graduate Program in Epidemiology and Department of Statistics—UFRGS, Porto Alegre 90000-000, Brazil.

**Margherita Caroli** Nutrition Unit, Department of Prevention, Azienda Sanitaria Locale Brindisi, Brindisi 72021, Italy.

**Michelle C. Carter** Nutritional Epidemiology Group, School of Food Science and Nutrition, University of Leeds, Leeds LS2 9JT, UK.

**Catherine B. Chan** Department of Physiology, and Department of Agricultural, Food and Nutritional Science, University of Alberta, Edmonton, AB T6G 2R3, Canada.

**Youn-OK Cho** Department of Food & Nutrition, Duksung Women's University, Seoul 132-714, Korea.

**Ji Young Choi** Department of Food & Nutrition, Duksung Women's University, Seoul 132-714, Korea.

**Morten R. Clausen** Department of Food Science, Aarhus University, Kirstinebjergvej 10, Aarslev DK-5792, Denmark.

**Clare E. Collins** Priority Research Centre for Physical Activity and Nutrition, School of Health Sciences, Faculty of Health and Medicine, University of Newcastle, Newcastle, NSW 2308, Australia.

**Sandra P. Crispim** Department of Nutrition, Federal University of Paraná (UFPR), Curitiba 80000-000, Brazil.

**Ross Crosby** Neuropsychiatric Research Institute, Fargo, ND 58103, USA; Department of Clinical Neurosciences, University of North Dakota, Grand Forks, ND 58202, USA.

**Scott Crow** Department of Psychiatry, University of Minnesota Medical School, Minneapolis, MN 55455, USA.

**Trine K. Dalsgaard** Department of Food Science, Aarhus University, Blichers Allé 20, Tjele DK-8830, Denmark.

**Alison Daly** School of Public Health, Curtin University, Kent Street, Perth 6845, Australia.

**Aline Martins de Carvalho** Department of Nutrition, School of Public Health, University of São Paulo, Av. Dr. Arnaldo 715, Consolação, São Paulo (SP) CEP 01246-904, Brazil.

**Stefaan De Henauw** Department of Public Health, Ghent University University Hospital 4K3, De Pintelaan, 185, B-9000 Ghent, Belgium; Faculty of Science and Technology, Department of Bio- and Food Sciences, University College Ghent-Campus Vesalius, Keramiekstraat 80, B-9000 Ghent, Belgium.

**Willem De Keyzer** Department of Public Health, Ghent University University Hospital 4K3, De Pintelaan, 185, B-9000 Ghent, Belgium; Faculty of Science and Technology, Department of Bio- and Food Sciences, University College Ghent-Campus Vesalius, Keramiekstraat 80, B-9000 Ghent, Belgium.

**Arnold L. M. Dekkers** Netherlands National Institute for Public Health and the Environment, Bilthoven 3720, The Netherlands.

**Edward J. Delp** School of Electrical and Computer Engineering Purdue University, Lafayette, IN 47907, USA; Video and Image Processing Laboratory, School of Electrical and Computer Engineering, Purdue University, West Lafayette, IN 47907-2035, USA.

**Satvinder S. Dhaliwal** School of Public Health, Curtin University, Perth, WA 6102, Australia.

**Kerith Duncanson** Nutrition and Dietetics, School of Health Sciences, and Priority Research Centre in Physical Activity and Nutrition, University of Newcastle, Newcastle 2300, Australia.

**Charlotte E. Evans** Nutritional Epidemiology Group, School of Food Science and Nutrition, University of Leeds, Leeds LS2 9JT, UK.

**Ariana Ferrari** Department of Pelvic Surgery, A.C. Camargo Cancer Center, Rua Professor Antônio Prudente, 211, Liberdade, São Paulo (SP) CEP 01509-010, Brazil.

**Gary S. Frost** Nutrition and Dietetic Research Group, Department of Investigative Medicine, Hammersmith Hospital, Imperial College London, London W12 0NN, UK.

**Victor L. Fulgoni III** Nutrition Impact, LLC, 9725D Drive North, Battle Creek, MI 49014, USA.

**Darren C. Greenwood** Division of Biostatistics, Leeds Institute of Genetics, Health and Therapeutics, University of Leeds, Leeds LS2 9JT, UK.

**Rachael T. Leon Guerrero** College of Natural and Applied Sciences University of Guam, Mangilao, GU 96923, USA.

**Maya Guest** Priority Research Centre in Physical Activity and Nutrition, and School of Health Sciences, Faculty of Health and Medicine, University of Newcastle, Newcastle 2300, Australia.

**Neil Hancock** Nutritional Epidemiology Group, School of Food Science and Nutrition, University of Leeds, Leeds LS2 9JT, UK.

**Vicki Harber** Faculty of Physical Education and Recreation , 3-100 University Hall, Van Vliet Complex, University of Alberta, Edmonton, AB T6G 2H9, Canada.

**Laura J. Hardie** Molecular Epidemiology Unit, Leeds Institute of Genetics, Health and Therapeutics, University of Leeds, Leeds LS2 9JT, UK.

**Amelia J. Harray** School of Public Health, Curtin University, GPO Box U1987, Perth 6845, Australia.

**Erin K. Howie** School of Physiotherapy and Exercise Science, Curtin University, GPO Box U1987, Perth 6845, Australia.

**Alexis J. Hure** School of Medicine and Public Health, University of Newcastle, New South Wales 2308, Australia; Hunter Medical Research Institute, New Lambton Heights, New South Wales 2305, Australia.

**Melinda J. Hutchesson** Nutrition and Dietetics, School of Health Sciences, Faculty of Health and Medicine, and Priority Research Centre in Physical Activity and Nutrition, University of Newcastle, Newcastle 2300, Australia.

**Inge Huybrechts** Department of Public Health, Ghent University University Hospital 4K3, De Pintelaan, 185, B-9000 Ghent, Belgium; International Agency for Research on Cancer (IARC), 150 Cours Albert Thomas, 69372 Lyon Cedex 08, France.

**Katsunari Ippoushi** National Food Research Institute, National Agriculture and Food Research Organization, Tsukuba, Ibaraki 305-8642, Japan.

**Lisa Jahns** USDA, ARS, Human Nutrition Research Center, Grand Forks, ND 58203, USA.

**LuAnn K. Johnson** USDA, ARS, Human Nutrition Research Center, Grand Forks, ND 58203, USA.

**Boris Kaganov** Nutrition and Health Clinic, Moscow 109012, Russia.

**Deborah A. Kerr** School of Public Health, Curtin University, Perth, WA 6102, Australia.

**Kay-Tee Khaw** Clinical Gerontology Unit, School of Clinical Medicine, University of Cambridge, Addenbrooke's Hospital, Cambridge CB2 2QQ, UK.

**Young-Nam Kim** Department of Food & Nutrition, Duksung Women's University, Seoul 132-714, Korea.

**Sharon Kirkpatrick** School of Public Health and Health Systems, University of Waterloo, Waterloo, ON N2L 3G1, Canada.

**Masuko Kobori** National Food Research Institute, National Agriculture and Food Research Organization, Tsukuba, Ibaraki 305-8642, Japan.

**Jun S. Lai** School of Medicine and Public Health, and Hunter Medical Research Institute, New Lambton Heights, New South Wales 2305, Australia.

**Rita Lau** Department of Agricultural, Food and Nutritional Science, University of Alberta, Edmonton, AB T6G 2R3, Canada.

**Greice H. C. Laureano** Post-Graduate Program in Epidemiology, Federal University of Rio Grande do Sul (UFRGS), Porto Alegre 90000-000, Brazil.

**Daniel Le Grange** Department of Psychiatry and Department of Pediatrics, University of California, San Francisco, San Francisco, CA 94143, USA.

**Haeng-Shin Lee** Nutrition Management Service and Policy Team, Korea Health Industry Development Institute, Chungbuk 363-700, Korea.

**Marleen A. H. Lentjes** Department of Public Health and Primary Care, Strangeways Research Laboratories, University of Cambridge, 2 Worts Causeway, Cambridge CB1 8RN, UK.

**Wanqing Li** School of Computing and Information Technology, University of Wollongong, Wollongong, NSW 2522, Australia.

**Robert N. Luben** Department of Public Health and Primary Care, Strangeways Research Laboratories, University of Cambridge, 2 Worts Causeway, Cambridge CB1 8RN, UK.

**Philippa Lyons-Wall** School of Exercise and Health Sciences, Edith Cowan University, Joondalup, Western Australia 6027, Australia.

**John Mamo** School of Public Health, Curtin University, Perth 6102, Australia.

**Dirce Maria Lobo Marchioni** Department of Nutrition, School of Public Health, University of São Paulo, Av. Dr. Arnaldo 715, Consolação, São Paulo (SP) CEP 01246-904, Brazil.

**Izumi Matsunaga** National Food Research Institute, National Agriculture and Food Research Organization, Tsukuba, Ibaraki 305-8642, Japan.

**Artur Mazur** Department of Pediatrics, University of Rzeszow, Rzeszow 35-350, Poland.

**Linda J. McCargar** Department of Agricultural, Food and Nutritional Science, 4-002 Li Ka Shing Centre for Health Research Innovation, University of Alberta, Edmonton, AB T6G 2E1, Canada.

**Mark McEvoy** School of Medicine and Public Health, University of Newcastle, New South Wales 2308, Australia; Hunter Medical Research Institute, New Lambton Heights, New South Wales 2305, Australia.

**Sarah A. McNaughton** Centre for Physical Activity and Nutrition Research, School of Exercise and Nutrition Sciences, Deakin University, 221 Burwood Highway, Melbourne, Victoria 3125, Australia.

**James E. Mitchell** Neuropsychiatric Research Institute, Fargo, ND 58103, USA; Department of Clinical Neurosciences, University of North Dakota, Grand Forks, ND 58202, USA.

**Michelle A. Morris** Nutritional Epidemiology Group, School of Food Science and Nutrition, and Centre for Spatial Analysis and Policy, School of Geography, University of Leeds, Leeds LS2 9JT, UK.

**Alanna J. Moshfegh** Beltsville Human Nutrition Research Center, Agricultural Research Service–USDA, 10300 Baltimore Ave., Beltsville MD 20705, USA.

**Syed Aqif Mukhtar** Centre for Population Health Research, Curtin University, GPO Box U1987, Perth 6845, Australia.

**Umme Z. Mulla** Global eHealth Unit, Department of Primary Care and Public Health, London School of Public Health, Imperial College London, London W6 8RP, UK.

**Angela A. Mulligan** Department of Public Health and Primary Care, Strangeways Research Laboratories, University of Cambridge, 2 Worts Causeway, Cambridge CB1 8RN, UK.

**Tadahiro Nagata** Department of Human Nutrition, Seitoku University, Matsudo, Chiba 271-8555, Japan.

**Shigehiro Naito** National Food Research Institute, National Agriculture and Food Research Organization, Tsukuba, Ibaraki 305-8642, Japan.

**Duc Thanh Nguyen** School of Computing and Information Technology, University of Wollongong, Wollongong, NSW 2522, Australia.

**Haruno Nishimuro** National Food Research Institute, National Agriculture and Food Research Organization, Tsukuba, Ibaraki 305-8642, Japan; Department of Human Nutrition, Seitoku University, Matsudo, Chiba 271-8555, Japan.

**Hirofumi Ohnishi** School of Medicine, Sapporo Medical University, Sapporo 060-8556, Japan.

**Mayumi Ohnishi-Kameyama** National Food Research Institute, National Agriculture and Food Research Organization, Tsukuba, Ibaraki 305-8642, Japan.

**Hideaki Oike** National Food Research Institute, National Agriculture and Food Research Organization, Tsukuba, Ibaraki 305-8642, Japan.

**Winsome Parnell** Division of Sciences, Department of Human Nutrition, University of Otago, PO Box 56, Dunedin 9054, New Zealand.

**Hélène Payette** Centre de Recherche sur le Vieillissement, CIUSSS de l\'Estrie-CHUS Sherbrooke, Sherbrooke J1J 3H5, QC, Canada; Sciences de la Santé Communautaire, Faculté de Médecine et des Sciences de la Santé, Université de Sherbrooke, Sherbrooke J1H 5N4, QC, Canada.

**Anna Peeters** Baker IDI Heart and Diabetes Institute, 75 Commercial Rd, Melbourne VIC 3004, Australia.

**Rosangela A. Pereira** Department of Social Nutrition, Instituto de Nutrição Josué de Castro, Federal University of Rio de Janeiro, Av. Carlos Chagas Filho 373, Cidade Universitária, Ilha do Fundão, Rio de Janeiro 21941-902, Brazil.

**Carol Peterson** Department of Psychiatry, University of Minnesota Medical School, Minneapolis, MN 55455, USA.

**Kristine Pezdirc** School of Health Sciences, Faculty of Health and Medicine, and Priority Research Centre in Physical Activity and Nutrition, University of Newcastle, Newcastle 2300, Australia.

**Michael Phillips** Harry Perkins Institute for Medical Research, University of Western Australia, 50 Murray Street, Perth 6000, Australia.

**Christina M. Pollard** School of Public Health, Curtin University, Kent Street, Perth 6845, Australia; Department of Health in Western Australia, 189 Royal Street, East Perth 6004, Australia.

**Yasmine Probst** School of Medicine, University of Wollongong, Wollongong, NSW 2522, Australia.

**Susan K. Raatz** USDA, ARS, Human Nutrition Research Center, Grand Forks, ND 58203, USA; Department of Food Science and Nutrition, University of Minnesota, Saint Paul, MN 55108, USA; Neuropsychiatric Research Institute, Fargo, ND 58103, USA.

**Stephanie M. Ramage** Department of Agricultural, Food and Nutritional Science, 4-002 Li Ka Shing Centre for Health Research Innovation, University of Alberta, Edmonton, AB T6G 2E1, Canada.

**Megan E. Rollo** Priority Research Centre in Physical Activity and Nutrition and School of Health Sciences, University of Newcastle, Callaghan, New South Wales 2308, Australia.

**Anthony W. Russell** Department of Diabetes and Endocrinology, Princess Alexandra Hospital, Woolloongabba, Queensland 4102, Australia.

**Maryam Sadegian** Department of Agricultural, Food and Nutritional Science, University of Alberta, Edmonton, AB T6G 2R3, Canada.

**Shigeyuki Saitoh** Sapporo Medical University School of Health Sciences, Sapporo, Hokkaido 060-8556, Japan.

**Midori Sato** Sobetsu-cho, Usugun, Hokkaido 052-0101 Japan.

**Jane Scott** School of Public Health, Curtin University, Perth 6102, Australia.

**Bryna Shatenstein** Centre de Recherche, Institut Universitaire de Gériatrie de Montréal, CIUSSS du Centre-est-de-l'Île-de-Montréal, Montréal H3W 1W5, QC, Canada.

**Jillian Sherriff** School of Public Health, Curtin University, Perth 6102, Australia.

**Kazuaki Shimamoto** Sapporo Medical University, Sapporo, Hokkaido 060-8556, Japan.

**Atul Singhal** Childhood Nutrition Research Centre, Institute of Child Health, London, WC1N 1EH, UK.

**Kyla L. Smith** School of Public Health, Curtin University, GPO Box U1987, Perth 6845, Australia.

**Diana C. Soria-Contreras** Department of Agricultural, Food and Nutritional Science, University of Alberta, Edmonton, AB T6G 2R3, Canada.

**Josiane Steluti** Department of Nutrition, School of Public Health, University of São Paulo, Av. Dr. Arnaldo 715, Consolação, São Paulo (SP) CEP 01246-904, Brazil.

**Leon M. Straker** School of Physiotherapy and Exercise Science, Curtin University, GPO Box U1987, Perth 6845, Australia.

**Natasha Tasevska** Nutrition Program, School of Nutrition and Health Promotion, Arizona State University, 500 North 3rd Street, Phoenix, AZ 85004, USA.

**the APrON Study Team** Department of Agricultural, Food and Nutritional Science, 4-002 Li Ka Shing Centre for Health Research Innovation, University of Alberta, Edmonton, AB T6G 2E1, Canada.

**Juliana Teixeira** Department of Nutrition, School of Public Health, University of São Paulo, Av. Dr. Arnaldo 715, Consolação, São Paulo (SP) CEP 01246-904, Brazil.

**Vanessa B. L. Torman** Post-Graduate Program in Epidemiology and Department of Statistics—UFRGS, Porto Alegre 90000-000, Brazil.

**Minh Khoi Tran** Faculty of Information Technology, University of Science Ho Chi Minh City 70000, Vietnam.

**Andrea Vania** Centre of Dietetics and Nutrition, Sapienza University, Rome 00161, Italy.

**Pieter van't Veer** Division of Human Nutrition, Wageningen University, Bomenweg 2, Wageningen 6703HD, The Netherlands.

**Nicholas J. Wareham** Medical Research Council, Epidemiology Unit, Institute of Metabolic Science, Addenbrooke's Hospital, Cambridge CB2 0QQ, UK.

**Petra A. Wark** Global eHealth Unit, Department of Primary Care and Public Health, London School of Public Health, Imperial College London, London W6 8RP, UK.

**Jane F. Watson** School of Health Sciences, Faculty of Health and Medicine, and Priority Research Centre in Physical Activity and Nutrition, University of Newcastle, Newcastle 2300, Australia.

**Ailsa A. Welch** Department of Population Health and Primary Care, Norwich Medical School, University of East Anglia, Norwich Research Park, Norwich NR4 7TJ, UK.

**Stephen A. Wonderlich** Neuropsychiatric Research Institute, Fargo, ND 58103, USA; Department of Clinical Neurosciences, University of North Dakota, Grand Forks, ND 58202, USA.

**Janine Wright** School of Public Health, Curtin University, Perth, WA 6102, Australia.

**Yunke Xu** Department of Agricultural, Food and Nutritional Science, University of Alberta, Edmonton, AB T6G 2R3, Canada.

**Hong Zheng** Department of Food Science, Aarhus University, Kirstinebjergvej 10, Aarslev DK-5792, Denmark.

# About the Guest Editors

**Clare Collins** is a National Health and Medical Research Council of Australia Senior Research Fellow in School of Health Sciences (Nutrition and Dietetics), at the University of Newcastle, Australia. Her research expertise is in the field of nutrition and dietetics, with a major focus on using technology to develop and evaluate nutrition interventions for prevention and treatment of diet and weight-related health conditions, at key life stages and in chronic disease. She has published over 250 journal articles, 320 conference papers and also authored a number of books. Currently, she is the Director of Research for the School of Health Sciences, in the Faculty of Health and Medicine, and Deputy Director of the Priority Research Centre for Physical Activity and Nutrition. Professor Collins is at the forefront of research to improve what people eat.

**Sharon Kirkpatrick**, PhD RD, is an assistant professor in the School of Public Health and Health Systems at the University of Waterloo, Canada. Dr. Kirkpatrick's research focuses on advancing methodologies for assessing diet and mitigating measurement error in dietary intake data. An area of emphasis is the use of technology to reduce researcher and respondent burden and allow the collection of high-quality comprehensive intake data in a range of contexts. Dr. Kirkpatrick works to enhance the capacity of researchers to collect robust dietary intake data through workshops and other training opportunities. Dr. Kirkpatrick also has interests in food security and food policy, as well as the environmental sustainability of current eating patterns.

# Preface to "Assessment of Nutrient Intakes"

Accurately measuring consumption of food, drinks and supplements is fundamental to nutrition and health research, including surveillance, epidemiology and intervention studies. However, assessing food intake is an area that is fraught with challenges (Thompson et al., 2015). What people eat is inherently complex given that it is a life-long and multifaceted behavior that changes over time and varies in relation to age, life stage, environment and many other factors. The challenges associated with assessing diet and nutrient intakes have led to the productive area of research that is the focus of this book, compiled from a Special Issue of the journal *Nutrients*.

Usual diet, or long-term average diet, is the phenomenon typically of interest in nutrition and health research. However, objective measures of usual diet are few and can be of limited use, while carrying high costs and substantial researcher and respondent burden (Thompson et al., 2010). As a result, researchers typically rely on self-report measures, such as 24-h recalls, food records, food frequency questionnaires, and brief instruments. The extent of error in dietary data collected using self-report instruments and tools has recently been debated (Archer et al., 2013; Mitka et al., 2013; Loannidis et al., 2013; Hébert et al., 2014; Subar et al., 2015), with some critics suggesting that such data be abandoned. However, the errors and their implications for interpreting the findings from nutrition research have long been recognized. Indeed, nutritionists, statisticians and epidemiologists in various parts of the world have made important advances over several years to better characterize and understand measurement error within self-reported dietary data and to identify ways to address it. These advances have included the use of recovery biomarkers, which provide objective measures of true intake for energy and a few specific nutrients, to ascertain the types and degree of error affecting data collected using different types of instruments (Freedman et al., 2014; Freedman et al., 2015). The findings of biomarker-based studies have informed recommendations for measuring diet in different types of studies (Thompson et al., 2015) and the development of statistical methods that allow for correction for error (Carriquiry et al., 2003; Dodd et al., 2006; Freedman et al., 2011; Mossavar-Rahmani et al., 2015). There has also been work to combine concentration biomarker and self-report data to mitigate measurement error (Freedman et al., 2011; Burrows et al., 2015). Further, the evolving understanding of limitations of existing tools, combined with technological advances, have enabled a new generation of dietary assessment instruments and strategies, including web-based tools, mobile apps, and image-based assessment, which are aimed at mitigating some of the challenges of traditional methods and modes of data collection (Thompson et al., 2010).

This book, compiled from a Special Issue of the journal *Nutrients*, provides examples of the diversity of research efforts underway internationally to advance the robust collection and use of dietary data. Included are 27 articles, with contributions from Australia, Brazil, Canada, Guam, Japan, Russia, South Korea, the United Kingdom, and the United States, as well as several countries in the European Union. The range of articles demonstrates efforts being made to improve the quality of dietary data collected from populations across the lifecycle and across contexts, with applications related to characterizing dietary intakes, as well as associations between diet and health. Articles within describe the development and/or evaluation of new tools, some of which take advantage of technology to address limitations in existing tools. Among these are mobile phone instruments, including a novel tool that incorporates not only health but also sustainability considerations related to diet, as well as a web-based 24-h recall developed in the UK. The use of biomarkers to assess intake and to evaluate self-report tools is also highlighted. For example, Tasevska examines evidence to support the use of urinary sugars as a biomarker for total sugar intake; Lai et al. examine the use of biomarkers to assess the validity of a food frequency questionnaire; and Zheng et al. explore the potential of metabolomics as markers of intake.

The articles included also highlight efforts to better understand the optimal use of existing tools. For example, Kerr et al. examine whether accuracy of recall among adolescents improves with a second administration of a 24-h dietary recall. Of interest in terms of understanding the comparability of data generated by surveillance systems in different countries, De Keyzer et al. provide a narrative review of methods used to assess diet in national food consumption surveys across continents. Such reviews and consideration of their findings are increasingly important as it is recognized that inconsistency in assessment methods complicates the interpretation of the larger evidence base, as well as posing a barrier to efforts to conduct pooled and cross-country analyses. Statistical methods for estimating usual intake of dietary components are also addressed, with a comparison of methods undertaken by Laureano et al.

Applied papers demonstrate the ways in which existing methods and resulting data contribute to our understanding of diet among populations, as well as the evaluation of interventions. Papers included also address dietary patterns and diet quality indices. These are growing areas within nutrition research, as the importance of embracing dietary patterns and capturing the complex interactions between all that we eat and drink is increasingly recognized.

This collection of papers demonstrates that dietary assessment research continues to be a lively area of inquiry. The advances in the use of technologic innovation and biomarkers to enhance measures of diet have the potential to contribute to the collection of higher quality data in future research. This compilation of articles also provides an opportunity to consider gaps in the evidence related to the assessment of diet and future research directions that could benefit from a more collaborative approach. Working together across institutions and countries can provide researchers with the opportunity to learn from one another, as well as to leverage scarce resources to advance the field internationally.

Clare Collins and Sharon Kirkpatrick
*Guest Editors*

# Section 1:
# Development and Evaluation of Measures to Collect Dietary Data from Populations across the Lifecycle and across Contexts

# The Reliability and Validity of the Perceived Dietary Adherence Questionnaire for People with Type 2 Diabetes

Ghada Asaad, Maryam Sadegian, Rita Lau, Yunke Xu, Diana C. Soria-Contreras, Rhonda C. Bell and Catherine B. Chan

**Abstract:** Nutrition therapy is essential for diabetes treatment, and assessment of dietary intake can be time consuming. The purpose of this study was to develop a reliable and valid instrument to measure diabetic patients' adherence to Canadian diabetes nutrition recommendations. Specific information derived from three, repeated 24-h dietary recalls of 64 type 2 diabetic patients, aged $59.2 \pm 9.7$ years, was correlated with a total score and individual items of the Perceived Dietary Adherence Questionnaire (PDAQ). Test-retest reliability was completed by 27 type 2 diabetic patients, aged $62.8 \pm 8.4$ years. The correlation coefficients for PDAQ items *versus* 24-h recalls ranged from 0.46 to 0.11. The intra-class correlation (0.78) was acceptable, indicating good reliability. The results suggest that PDAQ is a valid and reliable measure of diabetes nutrition recommendations. Because it is quick to administer and score, it may be useful as a screening tool in research and as a clinical tool to monitor dietary adherence.

Reprinted from *Nutrients*. Cite as: Asaad, G.; Sadegian, M.; Lau, R.; Xu, Y.; Soria-Contreras, D.C.; Bell, R.C.; Chan, C.B. The Reliability and Validity of the Perceived Dietary Adherence Questionnaire for People with Type 2 Diabetes. *Nutrients* **2015**, *7*, 5484–5496.

## 1. Introduction

There has been an increase in the incidence of diabetes worldwide. Over 347 million individuals have diabetes and it is estimated that by the year 2030, 552 million people will be living with diabetes [1]. In Canada, 2.4 million people had diabetes in 2009 and by 2019 the number is expected to reach 3.7 million [2]. The economic burden of diabetes in Canada is estimated to rise from $6.3 billion annually in 2000 and to $16.9 billion in 2020 [3]. Nutrition therapy is a crucial part of type 2 diabetes treatment and self-management. It has been well documented that improving dietary intake can reduce glycated hemoglobin (A1c) [4,5], improve clinical outcomes, and mediate weight loss [5,6]. The Canadian Diabetes Association (CDA) [7] recommends that diabetic patients to follow Eating Well with Canada's Food Guide (CFG) [8] in order to meet their nutrition requirements. Additional recommendations include limiting saturated fat and restricting added sucrose plus fructose to 10% of total energy while increasing consumption of low glycemic index foods, high-fiber foods, monounsaturated fats and foods rich in *n*-3 fatty acids [7].

While clinical outcomes such as A1c and blood pressure can easily be monitored by the medical team treating the diabetic patient, assessing dietary intake and creating a longitudinal record of dietary intake is not as practical [9]. However, being able to monitor a health outcome and provide timely feedback to the patient may help in long-term adherence to dietary goals [10]. Dietary intake is usually assessed by 24-h recalls, food frequency questionnaires (FFQ) and food records. These instruments require administration and analysis by a skilled health care professional [11]. Therefore, these instruments are not suitable for quick assessment by health care providers. They may also impose a significant patient burden [9–11]. Furthermore, these instruments are not specific for diabetes diet recommendations; therefore, the questionnaires may not be sensitive enough to assess how well a patient is adhering to a prescribed dietary pattern. For example, our previous study found no significant change in the Healthy Eating Index score calculated from 3-day food records after 12 weeks of following a menu plan for diabetes, despite significantly lower body mass index, waist circumference and A1c [12]. A shortcoming of the Healthy Eating Index is that it was not developed for people with diabetes; it incorporates general food guide serving recommendations but not specific diabetes recommendations. Few studies have developed a questionnaire to measure the adherence to disease-relevant guidelines [13,14] or specific diets [15,16] and there is no short questionnaire to measure a combination of the adherence to CFG [8] and CDA recommendations [7] in individuals with type 2 diabetes. Therefore, the Perceived Dietary Adherence Questionnaire (PDAQ) was developed to measure diabetic patients' perceptions of their dietary adherence. The present study aimed to measure the reliability of PDAQ and its validity relative to three repeated 24-h dietary recalls.

## 2. Experimental Section

### 2.1. Subjects

Data from the Physical Activity and Nutrition for Diabetes in Alberta (PANDA) intervention study (ClinicalTrials.gov registration NCT01625507) were used to test internal consistency and validity. Briefly, 73 participants were enrolled in the dietary intervention (Cohort I). Participants were recruited through a variety of avenues including posters, word-of-mouth, contact via a list of potential participants maintained by the Alberta Diabetes Institute and via an article about the project in a local newspaper. The inclusion criteria were: people diagnosed with type 2 diabetes and able to read and speak English. The exclusion criteria were: having severe gastrointestinal issues, type 1 diabetes or kidney disease. Anthropometric measures (height, weight, waist circumference), A1c, blood pressure, serum lipids, 24-h recall repeated on three successive days, and PDAQ were obtained at baseline and three months. Subsequently, additional type 2 diabetes patients ($n = 27$, Cohort II) were recruited through poster and database of the Alberta Diabetes Institute to measure the test and retest reliability of the PDAQ with a one-week interval. The inclusion and the exclusion criteria were the same as for the intervention study. The University of Alberta Human Research Ethics Board approved both studies. Written informed consent was obtained from all participants.

## 2.2. Perceived Dietary Adherence Questionnaire

The PDAQ was adapted from the Summary of Diabetes Self-care Activities measure [17]. The questionnaire was modified according to CFG [8] and the CDA Nutrition Therapy recommendations in place in the 2008 Clinical Practice guidelines [18]. To test item clarity, four experts were involved in reviewing the questionnaire items and the PDAQ was pre-tested on 10 non-diabetic volunteers. Questions raised by the pre-test cohort were addressed prior to using PDAQ in a research cohort.

The questionnaire consists of a total of nine questions structured to cover the CDA Nutrition Therapy guidelines [18] with reference to following CFG [8]: overall adherence to CFG, recommended fruits and vegetables servings, consumption of low glycemic index carbohydrate-containing foods, high sugar foods, high fiber foods, $n$-3 fatty acids, healthy (monounsaturated) oils, and high fat foods. One item addresses appropriate carbohydrate spacing. The response is based on a seven-point Likert scale to answer the question phrased as "On how many of the last 7 days did you . . . ?" (Table 1). Higher scores reflect higher adherence except for items 4 and 9, which reflect unhealthy choices (foods high in sugar or fat). For these items, higher scores reflect lower adherence, therefore, for computing a total PDAQ score, the scores for these items were inverted. Although based on a weekly timeframe, it was anticipated that the PDAQ would reflect usual dietary patterns based on knowledge that most people consume similar foods from week to week [19].

## 2.3. Assessment of Dietary Intake

Baseline dietary intake of Cohort I was measured by three 24-h dietary recalls (2 weekdays and 1 weekend day) using an internet-based questionnaire (WebSpan), which has been shown to reduce assessment error and bias [20]. Daily records were screened for duplicate entries for a single food item. Participants were excluded from the analysis if they did not completed three 24-h dietary recalls or implausible total energy values were reported (outside the range of 500–3500 kcal/day for women and 800–4000 kcal/day for men) [21]. The average daily total energy, macronutrient intake and intake from the four food groups described in CFG was obtained from WebSpan based on the 2001b Canadian Nutrient File database [22], and used for analysis. To calculate the Healthy Eating Index (HEI) [23] the food items reported by the participants and macronutrient analysis from WebSpan were used. Glycemic index (GI) score was calculated by following formula (daily GI = GL/net carbohydrate × 100). GI values were obtained from two databases [24,25]. Carbohydrate spacing was measured by calculating grams of carbohydrate consumed at each meal and snack [26], then giving a score from 1 to 6, where 1 represented poor spacing of carbohydrates (all in one meal) and six represented excellent spacing of carbohydrates (at least 15 g per meal and snack). PDAQ takes approximately 5 min for participants to complete and one minute to calculate the score, which was based on a maximum of 7 for each item (with the items for consumption of foods high in sugar and fat inversely scored), for a total maximum score of 63.

**Table 1.** Perceived Dietary Adherence Questionnaire (PDAQ).

| Item | Response * |
|---|---|
| 1. On how many of the last SEVEN DAYS have you followed a healthful eating plan such as Eating Well with Canada's Food Guide with appropriate serving sizes? | 0 1 2 3 4 5 6 7 |
| 2. On how many of the last SEVEN DAYS did you eat the number of fruit and vegetable servings you are supposed to eat based on Canada's Food Guide? | 0 1 2 3 4 5 6 7 |
| 3. On how many of the last SEVEN DAYS did you eat carbohydrate-containing foods with a low Glycemic Index? (Example: dried beans, lentils, barley, pasta, low fat dairy products) | 0 1 2 3 4 5 6 7 |
| 4. On how many of the last SEVEN DAYS did you eat foods high in sugar, such as cakes, cookies, desserts, candies, *etc.*? | 0 1 2 3 4 5 6 7 |
| 5. On how many of the last SEVEN DAYS did you eat foods high in fibre such as oatmeal, high fiber cereals, whole-grain breads? | 0 1 2 3 4 5 6 7 |
| 6. On how many of the last SEVEN DAYS did you space carbohydrates evenly throughout the day? | 0 1 2 3 4 5 6 7 |
| 7. On how many of the last SEVEN DAYS did you eat fish or other foods high in omega-3 fats? | 0 1 2 3 4 5 6 7 |
| 8. On how many of the last SEVEN DAYS did you eat foods that contained or was prepared with canola, walnut, olive, or flax oils? | 0 1 2 3 4 5 6 7 |
| 9. On how many of the last SEVEN DAYS did you eat foods high in fat (such as high fat dairy products, fatty meat, fried foods or deep fried foods)? | 0 1 2 3 4 5 6 7 |

\* Scoring: to obtain the total PDAQ score, the responses for items 4 and 9 were first inverted, e.g., a score of 7 becomes 0, then add all of the responses together. The maximum score was 63.

## 2.4. Statistical Methods

Statistical analyses were performed using SPSS version 22.0 (SPSS Inc., Chicago, IL, USA), Statistical significance was set at $p < 0.05$. Descriptive statistics were used to summarize demographic data. The mean $\pm$ SD was calculated for continuous variables, and percentage for categorical variables. Comparison of demographic characteristics between the first cohort (used to test validity) and the second cohort (used to do test-retest reliability) was assessed by Chi square and unpaired $t$-tests as appropriate. Spearman rank-order correlation coefficients were calculated between PDAQ questions to determine if the perceived adherence to CFG question score (Question (1)) correlated with the scores of Questions (2) through (9).

Validation: After screening the food intake data for implausible dietary intake or incomplete three 24-h dietary recalls, nine participants were removed ($n = 64$). Normality of nutrient intake distributions was checked statistically. If the normality assumption failed, data were log10-transformed. The questions of the PDAQ were individually correlated with specific information derived from the three 24-h dietary recalls (*i.e.*, mean servings of food groups, nutrient intakes, glycemic index). Specifically, the question related to CFG was correlated with the mean number of servings of the four food groups. The question related to vegetables and fruits consumption was correlated with the mean servings of vegetables and fruits. The question related to consumption of foods with low glycemic index was correlated with the mean glycemic index score. The question related to consumption of foods high in sugar was correlated with the average daily intake of added sugar. The question related to intake of foods high in fibre was correlated with the servings of whole grains. The question related to spacing carbohydrate throughout the day was correlated with the total carbohydrate spacing score. The question related to eating fish or foods high in $n$-3 fatty acids was correlated with the number of foods in the dietary recall that were high in $n$-3 fatty acids. The question related to using healthy oils was correlated with the intake of monounsaturated fatty acids. The question related to eating foods high in fat was correlated with the intake of total fat. The correlation coefficients were interpreted by using Dancey and Reidy's categorisation [27].

Reliability: the intra-class correlation coefficient (ICC) was calculated as an indication of test-retest reliability and internal consistency was measured by Cronbach's $\alpha$ coefficient [28].

## 3. Results

A total of 73 participants were enrolled in the PANDA study, which provided data for validity testing and internal consistency, and 27 participants were separately recruited for test-retest reliability testing. The characteristics of the participants are reported in Table 2. There were no significant differences between demographic characteristics of participants in the first *versus* second cohort except for employment status ($p = 0.008$).

The score for the PDAQ was normally distributed and ranged from 10 to 54. PDAQ scores were not statistically significant different between male ($32.5 \pm 10.6$, $n = 39$) and female ($32.9 \pm 12.2$, $n = 34$) participants. A significant positive correlation was found between PDAQ score and age with r = 0.46, 95% CI (0.19, 0.54), and inversely with weight with $r = -0.36$, 95% CI ($-0.52, -0.05$).

Total PDAQ scores were associated with nutrient intakes from the average of the three 24-h dietary recall and correlated moderately with HEI-score ($r = 0.41$, 95% CI (0.19, 0.54)), as well as with Vegetables and Fruits servings ($r = 0.25$, 95% CI (0.03, 0.50)). In contrast, total PDAQ scores were negatively correlated with added sugar intake ($r = -0.32$, 95% CI ($-0.51, -0.12$)) and saturated fat intake ($r = -0.25$, 95% CI ($-0.46, -0.05$)).

**Table 2.** Baseline characteristics of the first cohort ($n = 73$) and the second cohort ($n = 27$).

| Characteristics | Cohort I ($n = 73$) | Cohort II ($n = 27$) | $p$-Value |
|---|---|---|---|
| Age (years) | $59.2 \pm 9.7$ | $62.8 \pm 8.4$ | 0.096 |
| Duration of diabetes (years) | $9.1 \pm 8.3$ | $11.8 \pm 7.8$ | 0.127 |
| Gender, % | | | |
| Male | 53.4% | 59.3% | |
| Female | 46.6% | 40.7% | 0.603 |
| Ethnicity, % | | | |
| White | 87.7% | 70.3% | |
| Other | 12.3% | 29.7% | 0.223 |
| Education, % | | | |
| High school or less | 15% | 7.4% | |
| More than high school | 85% | 92.6% | 0.376 |
| Employment, % | | | |
| Wages and salaries | 56.2% | 18.5% | 0.008 |
| Household income, % | | | |
| ⩽$59,999 | 21.9% | 18.5% | 0.688 |
| ⩾$60,000 | 78.1% | 81.5% | |

To test the validity, we associated individual items of the PDAQ with nutrient intakes from the average of the three 24-h dietary recalls adjusted for total calories (Table 3). Following CFG more days per week was associated higher intake of servings from a variety of the four food groups ($p < 0.05$). Perceived eating of the recommended servings of Vegetables and Fruits more days per week was associated with higher intake of Vegetables and Fruits reported in 24-h recalls ($p < 0.05$). Reported consumption of foods with a low glycemic index more days per week predicted lower glycemic load ($p < 0.05$). Reporting eating of foods high in sugar (e.g., cookies) on more days was associated with higher added sugar intake ($p < 0.01$). Perceived eating of foods high in fiber (e.g., oatmeal) predicted higher intake of whole grains ($p < 0.001$). Reported consumption of foods high in fat (e.g., fried food) on more days predicted higher fat intake ($p < 0.01$). No significant association was found for spacing carbohydrate, foods high in $n$-3 fatty acids, and healthy oils *versus* the actual intake.

Table 3 presents the correlations between following CFG more days per week (Question (1) of PDAQ) with each subscale (Questions (2)–(9)). Higher perceived adherence to following CFG was moderately correlated with higher intake of Vegetables and Fruits ($r = 0.60$, 95% CI (0.42, 0.73)), higher intake of foods with low glycemic index ($r = 0.28$, 95% CI (0.04, 0.48)), higher intake of foods high in fiber ($r = 0.44$, 95% CI (0.22, 0.61)), more likely to space carbohydrate throughout the day ($r = 0.59$, 95% CI (0.40, 0.75)), and higher intake of fish high in $n$-3 fatty acids ($r = 0.27$, 95% CI (0.08, 0.45)). Conversely, there were negative correlations between perceived adherence of following CFG and intake of foods high in sugar ($r = -0.36$, 95% CI ($-0.55$, $-0.18$)) and foods high in fat ($r = -0.45$, 95% CI ($-0.63$, $-024$)).

**Table 3.** Validity of Perceived Dietary Adherence Questionnaire (PDAQ) *versus* three 24-h dietary recalls *.

| PDAQ Item | PDAQ Score (Mean $\pm$ SD) (Maximum 7) | 24 h Dietary Recall Item | Intake (Mean $\pm$ SD) | Linear Correlation Coefficient Between PDAQ Score and Intake |
|---|---|---|---|---|
| Following CFG | $3.0 \pm 2.5$ | Servings from the four food groups | $15.8 \pm 3.7$ | 0.33 * |
| F&V servings | $4.1 \pm 2.3$ | F&V servings | $4.9 \pm 1.9$ | 0.30 * |
| Low GI | $3.6 \pm 1.9$ | Glycemic load | $49.5 \pm 4.8$ | $-0.30$ * |
| High sugar foods | $2.7 \pm 2.2$ | Added sugar (g) | $47.4 \pm 37.1$ | 0.40 ** |
| High fiber foods | $5.0 \pm 1.9$ | Servings of whole grain foods | $5.6 \pm 2.2$ | 0.46 *** |
| Carb spacing | $3.5 \pm 2.6$ | At least 15 g carbohydrate per meal (maximum 6) | $4.3 \pm 0.8$ | 0.24 |
| $n$-3 FA | $1.7 \pm 1.6$ | $n$-3 PUFA (g) | $0.7 \pm 2.1$ | 0.11 |
| Healthy oils | $3.0 \pm 2.5$ | MUFA (g) | $28.7 \pm 11.2$ | 0.15 |
| High fat foods | $2.6 \pm 1.7$ | Total fat (g) | $83.9 \pm 30.7$ | 0.35 ** |

* $N = 64$ participants who completed three 24-h recalls. Abbreviations and explanation: CFG = Eating Well with Canada's Food Guide; F&V = Fruits and Vegetables; GI = glycemic index; Carb Spacing = Spacing carbohydrate throughout the day; FA = fatty acids; Healthy oils = consumption of foods like nuts, olive oil, canola oil; PUFA = polyunsaturated fatty acids; MUFA = monounsaturated fatty acids. Confidence intervals for significant correlations are reported in the text. * $p < 0.05$; ** $p < 0.001$; *** $p < 0.0001$.

Test and re-test reliability was assessed by the intra-class correlation. High correlations were obtained for five items on the PDAQ (Vegetables and Fruits, foods high in sugar, foods high in fiber, fish and other foods high in $n$-3 fatty acids, and healthy oils) as well as the total PDAQ score (Table 4). Cronbach's $\alpha$ was 0.78 with no significant change to the overall $\alpha$ with the deletion of any individual item.

Table 4. Spearman rank-order correlations between frequency of following Canada's Food Guide and other items in the Perceived Dietary Adherence Questionnaire (PDAQ).

| PDAQ Item | CFG |
|---|---|
| CFG | – |
| F&V servings | 0.604 ** |
| Low GI | 0.280 * |
| High sugar foods | −0.368 ** |
| High fiber foods | 0.414 ** |
| Carb spacing | 0.594 ** |
| $n$-3 FA | 0.272 * |
| Healthy oils | 0.19 |
| High fat foods | −0.453 ** |

Abbreviations and explanations: CFG = Eating Well with Canada's Food Guide; F&V = Fruits and Vegetables; GI = glycemic index; Carb Spacing = Spacing carbohydrate throughout the day; FA = fatty acids; Healthy oils = consumption of foods like nuts, olive oil, canola oil. * $p < 0.05$; ** $p < 0.001$; *** $p < 0.0001$.

## 4. Discussion

The aim of this study was to establish the validity and reliability of a dietary assessment tool for people with type 2 diabetes that would be simple to administer and score, as well as reflect current recommendations for a diabetes diet. Overall, the PDAQ appears to be a useful indicator of adherence to CFG and diet quality. Compared with a repeated 24-h recall, it also appears to be valid for assessing adherence to recommended servings of Vegetables and Fruit, and foods that have low glycemic index, are high in sugar, fiber or fat. The test-retest reliability was acceptable.

Other authors have developed short questionnaires to assess intake of various foods or nutrients in the general population whereas the PDAQ is targeted to specific nutrition recommendations for diabetes. The correlation obtained for Vegetables and Fruits intake between PDAQ and 24-h recall is comparable to previous studies that found moderate correlation ($r$ = 0.36–0.65) between Vegetables and Fruit and short food frequency questionnaires [29,30] or seven-day food records [31]. Likewise, other short questionnaires found similar moderate correlations with foods high in sugar, fat and fiber with food records or FFQs [30–32]. Poorer correlation was found for foods low in glycemic index in our study compared to other studies, which used short food frequency questionnaires [33,34]. The correlation between self-reported carbohydrate spacing and the carb spacing score derived from 24-h recalls was not significant, which may due to lack of knowledge among diabetic patients [35] as well as health care providers [36], who are thus unable to instruct patients in the technique. No significant relationship was observed between questions related to unsaturated fat and the actual intake of unsaturated fat, which is consistent with Francis and Stevenson´s questionnaire compared with a 4-day food diary [32]. Overall, the PDAQ performed similarly to other short questionnaires and has the advantage of being specific for a particular population, patients with diabetes living in Canada.

We determined that PDAQ had acceptable internal reliability since Cronbach's α was 0.78 (Cronbach's α scores for subscales were also acceptable and ranged from 0.74 to 0.79). The test-retest correlation coefficient for the entire questionnaire was acceptable ($r = 0.76$) suggesting that the PDAQ score is stable over time. Test-retest administration of PDAQ produced good correlations for questions related to Vegetables and Fruits, foods high in sugar and fibre, fish or foods high in $n$-3 fatty acids, and healthy oils; meanwhile, questions related to spacing carbohydrate and foods high in fat had moderate correlations ($r = 0.40$ and 0.53, respectively). The question related to CFG had poor test-retest correlation ($r = 0.21$). Low and moderate ICC values in some individual scores are due to the intra-individual variability [21], which is likely to be greater in foods that are consumed less often (like fish in the prairie provinces of Canada). Low test-retest reliability for high fat foods is interesting, suggesting either that there is true variation in intake or that fat may be "hidden" in some foods, such as processed foods [37].

The correlations produced in validity tests between following CFG more days per week and each subscale shows that the PDAQ ranked subjects quite well. We showed that reporting consistent following of CFG is more likely to be positively associated with the intake of low-caloric density foods, and negatively associated with high-caloric density foods. This finding indicates that the PDAQ is a good instrument to measure adherence to CFG recommendations. We were particularly interested in examining PDAQ's ability to assess intakes specifically mentioned in the CDA Nutrition Therapy Guidelines that may not be captured using scores like the Healthy Eating Index. PDAQ subscales for low GI foods, high sugar, fiber and fat foods were moderate predictors of intake substantiated by the 24-h recall data.

We also found correlations between PDAQ and demographic or biological variables. The positive relationship found between PDAQ and age is similar in direction to a previous study that examined the association between HEI and age [23]. The diet quality of Americans older adults measured using HEI was better than younger and middle-aged adults [38]. PDAQ scores were also significantly negatively correlated with weight, which is consistent with Pate and colleagues' finding that diet quality was inversely associated with weight status [39]. There was no significant relationship observed between PDAQ and gender.

Several other short questionnaires for dietary assessment have been developed. Calfas and colleagues [9] conducted a review to identify dietary measures that can be potentially used in a primary care setting. All of the instruments measured fat, and some of the instruments measured cholesterol, fruits, vegetables, and fiber. Pullen and Walker [13] used the Behavioral Risk Factor Surveillance Survey to assess adherence to the Dietary Guideline for Americans among midlife and older rural women. The Dutch Diet Index [14] and the Australian Recommended Food Score [40] were developed to measure the adherence to country-specific dietary guidelines. All the previous studies have assessed the reliability and validity of the instruments in the general population. Hemio and colleagues [31] developed a 16-Item Food Intake Questionnaire and used it in a type 2 diabetes prevention programme in Finland to estimate daily nutrient intake in a primary health care setting. To our knowledge, there are no other comparable questionnaires to assess adherence to diabetic recommendations in Canada. Therefore, PDAQ could be a useful tool for dietitians as well as practitioners who are not nutrition experts but who would like a snapshot of the dietary compliance of individuals with type 2 diabetes in Canada. It could also be easily adapted to other settings using the relevant disease and/or country-specific guidelines. In our ongoing research we are using PDAQ to assess longitudinal changes in dietary adherence in type 2 diabetes participants. Preliminary analyses suggest that PDAQ is useful for this purpose [41].

One strength of our study is that we used three internet-based, 24-h dietary recalls to estimate dietary intake, a method that has less bias than some others [20] and was also relatively simple for the participants to complete. The study developed a short, simple to administer and score questionnaire that covers the CDA Nutrition Therapy guidelines [18] with reference to following CFG [8]. Use of PDAQ could therefore reduce both client and practitioner burden but allow longitudinal monitoring of dietary adherence to recommendations. The study has some limitations that need to be recognised. This study has a relatively small sample size but some previous studies have validated dietary instruments with a similar number of participants [31,32,39]. However, the small sample size does limit our ability to conduct multivariate or subgroup analyses such as gender or age effects. All participants lived in an urban area, therefore, the result may not be generalizable to those living in rural areas. Another limitation is that participants in the intervention study were more educated and had higher income compared with the general population. Although this may not affect the validation study, our findings might be different if we apply it a population with lower education and income. Finally, although the CDA does not have a specific recommendation for sodium, our studies such as that reported in [41] consistently find sodium intake in excess of current Health Canada guidelines [42]. An item related to sodium intake could be a useful addition to the PDAQ.

## 5. Conclusions

Following the CDA nutrition therapy guidelines is important for improving health outcomes in people with type 2 diabetes, but there is a need to develop practical and quick tools that help clinicians and researchers to assess adherence to these guidelines. We suggest that the PDAQ may be useful to accomplish this objective and that it can be implemented in research. It may be worthwhile to test the PDAQ in a clinical setting.

**Acknowledgments:** The authors thank the participants for their dedication to the study. Research funding was from Alberta Diabetes Institute, University of Alberta. Ghada Asaad received personal funding from the Ministry for Higher Education, Kingdom of Saudi Arabia.

**Author Contributions:** Catherine B. Chan designed and wrote the grant that funded the cohort 1 study. Rhonda C. Bell and Catherine B. Chan designed the PDAQ. In cohort 1, Ghada Asaad and Diana C. Soria-Contreras carried out the participant recruitment and data collection. Diana C. Soria-Contreras conducted the intervention sessions. Ghada Asaad carried out the validity analysis. In cohort 2, Ghada Asaad, Maryam Sadegian, Rita Lau and Yunke Xu carried out the participant recruitment, data collection and reliability data analysis. Ghada Asaad wrote the manuscript. Catherine B. Chan provided critical feedback and edits on data analysis, data interpretation, and manuscript presentation. All authors reviewed the manuscript, provided their feedback and approval of its submission.

**Conflicts of Interest:** The authors declare no conflict of interest.

## References

1. International Diabetes Federation. Diabetes Atlas, 6th ed. Available online: http://www.idf.org/sites/default/files/EN_6E_Atlas_Full_0.pdf. (accessed on 7 April 2015).
2. Public Health Agency of Canada. Diabetes in Canada: Facts and Figures from a Public Health Perspective. Available online: http://www.phac-aspc.gc.ca/cd-mc/publications/diabetes-diabete/facts-figures-faits-chiffres-2011/index-eng.php (accessed on 7 April 2015).
3. Canadian Diabetes Association. An Economic Tsunami: The Cost of Diabetes in Canada. 2009. Available online: http://www.diabetes.ca/CDA/media/documents/publications-and-newsletters/advocacy-reports/economic-tsunami-cost-of-diabetes-in-canada-english.pdf (accessed on 7 April 2015).
4. Kulkarni, K.; Castle, G.; Gregory, R.; Holmes, A.; Leontos, C.; Powers, M.; Wylie-Rosett, J. Nutrition practice guidelines for type 1 diabetes mellitus positively affect dietitian practices and patient outcomes. *J. Am. Diet. Assoc.* **1998**, *1*, 62–70.
5. Pi-Sunyer, F.X.; Maggio, C.A.; McCarron, D.A.; Reusser, M.E.; Stern, J.S.; Haynes, R.B.; Oparil, S.; Kris-Etherton, P.; Resnick, L.M.; Chait, A. Multicenter randomized trial of a comprehensive prepared meal program in type 2 diabetes. *Diabetes Care* **1999**, *22*, 191–197.

6. Franz, M.J.; Monk, A.; Barry, B.; McClain, K.; Weaver, T.; Cooper, N.; Upham, P.; Bergenstal, R.; Mazze, R.S. Effectiveness of medical nutrition therapy provided by dietitians in the management of non-insulin-dependent diabetes mellitus: A randomized, controlled clinical trial. *J. Am. Diet. Assoc.* **1995**, *9*, 1009–1017.

7. Dworatzek, P.D.; Arcudi, K.; Gougeon, R.; Husein, N.; Sievenpiper, J.L.; Williams, S.L. Nutrition therapy. Canadian Diabetes Association 2013 clinical practice guidelines for the prevention and management of diabetes in Canada. *Can. J. Diabetes* **2013**, *37*, S54–S55.

8. Health Canada. Eating Well with Canada's Food Guide. 2011. Available online: http://www.hcsc.gc.ca/fn-an/food-guide-aliment/index-eng.php (accessed on 7 April 2015).

9. Calfas, K.; Zabinski, M.; Rupp, J. Practical nutrition assessment in primary care settings. *Am. J. Prev. Med.* **2000**, *18*, 289–299.

10. Jaacks, L.M.; Ma, Y.; Davis, N.; Delahanty, L.M.; Mayer-Davis, E.J.; Franks, P.W.; Brown-Friday, J.; Isonaga, M.; Kriska, A.M.; Venditti, E.M.; *et al.* Long-term changes in dietary and food intake behaviour in the diabetes prevention program outcomes study. *Diabet. Med.* **2014**, *12*, 1631–1642.

11. Rutishauser, I. Dietary intake measurement. *Public Health Nutr.* **2005**, *8*, 1100–1107.

12. Soria-Contreras, D.; Bell, R.; McCargar, L.; Chan, C. Feasibility and efficacy of menu planning combined with individual counselling to improve health outcomes and dietary adherence in people with type 2 diabetes: A pilot study. *Can. J. Diabetes* **2014**, *38*, 320–325.

13. Pullen, C.; Walker, S.N. Midlife and older rural women's adherence to U.S. dietary guidelines across stages of change in healthy eating. *Public Health Nurs.* **2002**, *19*, 170–178.

14. van Lee, L.; Geelen, A.; Hooft van Huysduynen, E.J.C.; de Vries, J.H.M.; van't Veer, P.; Feskens, E. The Dutch Healthy Diet index (DHD-index): An instrument to measure adherence to the Dutch Guidelines for a Healthy Diet. *Nutr. J.* **2012**, *11*, 49–57.

15. Mochari, H.; Mosca, L.; Gao, Q. Validation of the MEDFICTS Dietary Assessment Questionnaire in a Diverse Population. *J. Am. Diet. Assoc.* **2008**, *108*, 817–822.

16. Beliard, S.; Coudert, M.; Valéro, R.; Charbonnier, L.; Duchêne, E.; Allaert, F.A.; Bruckert, E. Validation of a short food frequency questionnaire to evaluate nutritional lifestyles in hypercholesterolemic patients. *Ann. Endocrinol.* **2012**, *73*, 523–529.

17. Toobert, D.; Hampson, S.; Glasgow, R. The summary of diabetes self-care activities measure: Results from 7 studies and a revised scale. *Diabetes Care* **2000**, *23*, 943–950.

18. Gougeon, R.; Aylward, N.; Nichol, H.; Quinn, K.; Whitham, D. Nutrition therapy. Canadian Diabetes Association 2008 clinical practice guidelines for the prevention and management of diabetes in Canada. *Can. J. Diabetes* **2008**, *32*, S40–S45.

19. Salvini, S.; Hunter, D.J.; Sampson, L.; Stampfer, M.J.; Colditz, G.A.; Rosner, B.; Willett, W.C. Food-based validation of a dietary questionnaire: The effect of week-to-week variation in food consumption. *Int. J. Epidemiol.* **1989**, *18*, 858–867.

20. Storey, K.; McCargar, L. Reliability and validity of Web-SPAN, a web-based method for assessing weight status, diet and physical activity in youth. *J. Hum. Nutr. Diet.* **2012**, *25*, 59–68.

21. Willet, W. *Nutritional Epidemiology*, 2nd ed.; Oxford University Press: New York, NY, USA, 1998.

22. Health Canada. Canadian Nutrient File (CNF). 2001. Available online: http://webprod3. hc-sc.gc.ca/cnf-fce/ (accessed on 7 April 2015).

23. Garriguet, D. Diet quality in Canada. *Health Rep.* **2009**, *20*, 41–52.

24. Foster-Powell, R.; Holt, S.H.; Brand-Miller, J.C. International table of glycemic index and glycemic load values: 2002. *Am. J. Clin. Nutr.* **2002**, *76*, 5–56.

25. The University of Sydney. Glycemic Index Database. Available online: http://www. glycemicindex.com (accessed on 7 April 2015).

26. Canadian Diabetes Association. Basic Carbohydrate Counting for Diabetes Management. Available online: http://www.diabetes.ca/CDA/media/documents/clinical-practice-and-education/professional-resources/carbohydrate-counting-resource-english.pdf (accessed on 7 April 2015).

27. Dancey, C.; Reidy, J. *Statistics without Maths for Psychology: Using SPSS for Windows*, 4th ed.; Pearson/Prentice Hall: Harlow, UK, 2007.

28. Weir, J.P. Quantifying test-retest reliability using the intraclass correlation coefficient and the SEM. *J. Strength Cond. Res.* **2005**, *19*, 231–240.

29. Andersen, L.; Johansson, L.; Solvoll, K. Usefulness of a short food frequency questionnaire for screening of low intake of fruit and vegetable and for intake of fat. *Eur. J. Public Health* **2002**, *12*, 208–213.

30. Osler, M.; Heitmann, B. The validity of a short food frequency questionnaire and its ability to measure changes in food intake: A longitudinal study. *Int. J. Epidemiol.* **1996**, *25*, 1023–1029.

31. Hemiö, K.; Pölönen, A.; Ahonen, K.; Kosola, M.; Viitasalo, K.; Lindström, J. A simple tool for diet evaluation in primary health care: Validation of a 16-item food intake questionnaire. *Int. J. Environ. Res. Public Health* **2014**, *11*, 2683–2697.

32. Francis, H.; Stevenson, R. Validity and test-retest reliability of a short dietary questionnaire to assess intake of saturated fat and free sugars: A preliminary study. *J. Hum. Nutr. Diet.* **2013**, *26*, 234–242.

33. Barclay, A.; Flood, V.; Brand-Miller, J.; Mitchell, P. Validity of carbohydrate, glycaemic index and glycaemic load data obtained using a semi-quantitative food-frequency questionnaire. *Public Health Nutr.* **2008**, *11*, 573–580.

34. Barrett, J.; Gibson, P. Development and validation of a comprehensive semi-quantitative food frequency questionnaire that includes FODMAP intake and glycemic index. *J. Am. Diet. Assoc.* **2010**, *110*, 1469–1476.

35. Watts, S.; Anselmo, J.; Kern, E. Validating the AdultCarbQuiz: A test of carbohydrate-counting knowledge for adults with diabetes. *Diabetes Spectr.* **2011**, *24*, 154–157.

36. Wynn, K.; Trudeau, J.; Taunton, K.; Gowans, M.; Scott, I. Nutrition in primary care: Current practices, attitudes, and barriers. *Can. Fam. Phys.* **2010**, *56*, 109–116.

37. Glanz, K.; Brug, J.; Assema, P. Are awareness of dietary fat intake and actual fat consumption associated?—A Dutch-American comparison. *Eur. J. Clin. Nutr.* **1997**, *51*, 542–547.

38. Hiza, H.; Casavale, K.; Guenther, P.; Davis, C. Diet quality of Americans differs by age, sex, race/ethnicity, income, and education level. *J. Acad. Nutr. Diet.* **2013**, *113*, 297–306.

39. Pate, R.; Ross, S.; Liese, A.; Dowda, M. Associations among physical activity, diet quality, and weight status in US adults. *Med. Sci. Sports Exerc.* **2015**, *47*, 743–750.

40. Collins, C.E.; Burrows, T.L.; Rollo, M.E.; Boggess, M.M.; Watson, J.F.; Guest, M.; Duncanson, K.; Pezdirc, K.; Hutchesson, M.J. The comparative validity and reproducibility of a diet quality index for adults: The Australian recommended food score. *Nutrients* **2015**, *7*, 785–798.

41. Soria-Contreras, D.; Chan, C. Monitoring adherence to the Canadian diabetes association nutrition therapy guidelines using the perceived dietary adherence questionnaire and a 3-day food record. *Can. J. Diabetes* **2012**, *36*, S66.

42. Health Canada. Sodium in Canada. Available online: http://www.hc-sc.gc.ca/fn-an/nutrition/sodium/index-eng.php (accessed on 7 April 2015).

# Evaluation of the Relative Validity of the Short Diet Questionnaire for Assessing Usual Consumption Frequencies of Selected Nutrients and Foods

Bryna Shatenstein and Hélène Payette

**Abstract:** A 36-item Short Diet Questionnaire (SDQ) was developed to assess usual consumption frequencies of foods providing fats, fibre, calcium, vitamin D, in addition to fruits and vegetables. It was pretested among 30 community-dwelling participants from the Québec Longitudinal Study on Nutrition and Successful Aging, "NuAge" ($n$ = 1793, 52.4% women), recruited in three age groups (70 ± 2 years; 75 ± 2 years; 80 ± 2 years). Following revision, the SDQ was administered to 527 NuAge participants (55% female), distributed among the three age groups, both sexes and languages (French, English) prior to the second of three non-consecutive 24 h diet recalls (24HR) and validated relative to the mean of three 24HR. Full data were available for 396 participants. Most SDQ nutrients and fruit and vegetable servings were lower than 24HR estimates ($p < 0.05$) except calcium, vitamin D, and saturated and *trans* fats. Spearman correlations between the SDQ and 24HR were modest and significant ($p < 0.01$), ranging from 0.19 (cholesterol) to 0.45 (fruits and vegetables). Cross-classification into quartiles showed 33% of items were jointly classified into identical quartiles of the distribution, 73% into identical and contiguous quartiles, and only 7% were frankly misclassified. The SDQ is a reasonably accurate, rapid approach for ranking usual frequencies of selected nutrients and foods. Further testing is needed in a broader age range.

Reprinted from *Nutrients*. Cite as: Shatenstein, B.; Payette, H. Evaluation of the Relative Validity of the Short Diet Questionnaire for Assessing Usual Consumption Frequencies of Selected Nutrients and Foods. *Nutrients* **2015**, *7*, 6362–6374.

## 1. Introduction

The Canadian Longitudinal Study on Aging (CLSA) is a national longitudinal study that will follow 50,000 men and women aged 45 to 85 years (y) at recruitment over a twenty-year period. The goal of the CLSA is to better understand the aging process and its determinants through the collection of information on biological, medical, psychological, social, lifestyle and economic aspects of people's lives, and their changes over time [1].

As an important lifestyle component, dietary data are being gathered at multiple time-points in the CLSA. Of interest were usual intakes of several key nutrients and

17

foods of current concern in health promotion and chronic disease prevention in both younger and older adults (OA), and which have been the focus of population-based nutritional health promotion campaigns. They include intakes of total fat, and fatty acid classes (saturated, polyunsaturated, monounsaturated, omega-3 and *trans* fatty acids), as well as dietary fibre, calcium, vitamin D, and consumption of fruits and vegetables. Because of interview time constraints and the challenging logistics related to administration of a full food frequency questionnaire (FFQ), a brief instrument was sought for assessment of usual frequency of consumption of these items. Existing dietary screeners that addressed the foods and nutrients of interest were initially considered, specifically, the Block Dietary Screener [2], which ranks individuals with regard to their usual intakes of fat, fibre, calcium and vitamin D. Also of interest was the six-item Fruit and Vegetable Food Frequency Questionnaire developed by the Centers for Disease Control and Prevention (CDC) for the US Behavioral Risk Factor Surveillance System Survey (BRFSS [3]). The BRFSS questionnaire collects intake frequency, as occasions per day, week or month, of six categories of vegetables and fruit [4]. It has been used at the state level in the United States since 1990 [5] and was incorporated into the Canadian Community Health Survey by Health Canada [6]. The fruit and vegetable module has been validated against three 24-hour recalls (24HR) in a young adult population by trained dietitian interviewers, and results indicate that it can be used as a proxy for quantified intake in population groups [7].

However, because of constraints set by developers on instrument modification (e.g., changing the food list), as well as handling and cost considerations related to their use, it was decided to adapt a previously validated Canadian FFQ [8] as it best fit the needs of the CLSA and was specific to the population [9]. This approach also allowed us to conserve the BRFSS in the new tool. Furthermore, it limited the additional work needed for instrument modification, database preparation and data entry and analysis software as we had already successfully used the full FFQ [8] at recruitment into an ongoing cohort study on nutrition and healthy aging. The present paper describes the development, pretest and evaluation of the relative validity of the Short Diet Questionnaire (SDQ), developed to estimate usual consumption frequencies of fat, fibre, calcium and vitamin D, and fruit and vegetables.

## 2. Methods

### 2.1. Study Context

At the time of SDQ development, the CLSA was not yet in the field. Consequently, the SDQ was developed, pretested and validated in the "Quebec Longitudinal Study on Nutrition and Successful Aging" ("NuAge"), a cohort study that we were conducting at the time, and which is described in detail elsewhere [10]. Briefly, NuAge is a five-year observational study of 1793 community-dwelling men and women recruited in three age groups (70 ± 2 years; 75 ± 2 years; 80 ± 2 years), from a random sample of the Québec Health Insurance database (RAMQ) in the areas of Montréal, Laval, and Sherbrooke in Québec, Canada. Participants were cognitively and functionally intact and in good general health at recruitment, that is, having common manageable conditions such as hypertension or diabetes, but no serious illness limiting their continued participation. The study was approved by the Institutional Review Board at the Institut universitaire de gériatrie de Sherbrooke and the Institut universitaire de gériatrie de Montréal.

## 2.2. SDQ Development

A validated Canadian self-administered 78-item semi-quantitative FFQ [8] was used as the template for the SDQ. Items were extracted from the full FFQ to address the goals of the SDQ (see Table A1 in Appendix). The food list underwent several iterations to address issues related to content, food order, syntax and nomenclature, and participant burden. The six fruit and vegetable questions from the BRFSS were incorporated into the SDQ food list, keeping the exact BRFSS wording to permit comparison with existing Canadian data on fruit and vegetable intakes from other studies having used this module. Two formulations of the frequency component were considered: (1) frequency categories, where the respondent is presented with a series of predetermined options for frequency of intakes which requires that he/she choose the appropriate frequency choice, and (2) precise frequencies, where the respondent provides a specific number indicating the number of times the food item is consumed in one of the provided time periods: per day, per week, per month, or never/rarely. Portion size was not questioned.

Several versions of the instrument were examined internally before arriving at the pre-test versions of the SDQ, one with frequency categories and the other with precise frequencies, in both French and English. The full food list of the SDQ contains 30 food items and six beverage items (see Table A2 in in Appendix), as well as four additional questions on dietary habits relevant to the SDQ objectives. It queries usual consumption frequency in the previous 12 months of food sources of fats, fibre, calcium, vitamin D, regular and low-fat food choices, whole grains, calcium-fortified foods and beverages, and of a series of fruits and vegetables. For consistency with other national Canadian studies, the tool was designed to be interviewer-administered.

## 2.3. Pretest

The pretest of the SDQ took place at the Montreal study site in the summer of 2006. Research agents identified 30 participants from their roster who had agreed on their consent form to be re-contacted for additional studies, targeting approximately one-third in each of the NuAge age groups (70 years, 75 years, 80 years), evenly distributed among men and women, with a representative number of English-speaking NuAge participants to permit assessment of both French and English versions of the SDQ. The pretest was designed as a cross-over study, where half of the participants completed the "frequency categories" version first, followed by the "precise frequencies" version while the other half was assigned to the reverse order. The pretest SDQ was self-administered and returned by mail. Respondents entered their start and finish times on the SDQ to verify whether it could be completed in the allotted 15-minute timeframe. Structured, telephone-based cognitive interviews [11] were then carried out to assess difficulties with the test version of both frequency types of the SDQ, in both languages. Participants' comments were used to clarify both language versions of the questionnaire following pretest. No quantitative analyses were carried out on the pretest questionnaires. A user's manual was prepared to train the NuAge research agents in standardized administration of the SDQ and to provide them with answers and solutions to potential problems encountered in the use of the SDQ.

## 2.4. Validation Study

Recruitment into the SDQ validation study took place in 2007. NuAge participants were invited sequentially over an 8-month period to take part in the validation study without imposing additional selection criteria, but targeting equivalent proportions in each of the three age groups, both sexes and representing both languages. A total of 527 NuAge subjects took part in this study; 154 were completing T3 (NuAge year three) interviews and 373 were in their T4 wave of data collection. Current diet was assessed using three non-consecutive 24-hour diet recalls (24HR) collected at each annual interview in face-to-face and telephone interviews by a research dietitian using the USDA 5-step multiple pass method [12], and the 24HR was designated as the reference instrument. The 24HR interviews were carried out by professional research dietitians who adhered to a strict protocol. Since the CLSA Tracking Cohort was to be assembled by Statistics Canada which carries out all assessments by interview (in-person or by telephone), the SDQ was administered in telephone interviews by trained NuAge research dietitians, prior to collecting the second of three 24HR.

## 2.5. Data Handling and Dietary Analysis: Validation Study

Because the purpose of this study was to determine the validity of the SDQ, daily consumption frequencies of each line item were not tabulated separately, but were data-entered from SDQ responses into WilliamTM customized data entry software (©Multispectra, 1997–2004) and output files were then imported directly into the

SDQ data entry and analysis utility based on a Microsoft AccessTM platform with a database and nutrient calculation algorithms adapted from the full FFQ [8]. Because portion size is not queried in the SDQ, it was imputed into the SDQ database as a standard (medium) portion in grams, from the NuAge study FFQ database to permit calculation of point estimates for comparison with the 24HR results. Nutrient analyses were thus done using the participants' reported frequencies of consumption of each line item, with the adapted SDQ database based on the 2007b Canadian Nutrient File (CNF) [13] and results were output as daily nutrient and food intake estimates. The 24HR were analyzed using CANDAT nutrient analysis software (version 10, ©Godin London Inc., London, ON, Canada), based on the then-current 2001b CNF [13]. The means of the three 24HR were used in validation analyses, and software developed by our group (CalculateurGAC©) was run on the 24HR food codes and Canada's Food Guide (CFG) subgroup codes to generate the four food groups of CFG in order to derive fruit and vegetable servings from the 24HR. Because the SDQ nutrient analysis targeted usual intakes of a limited set of nutrients and foods, the validation analyses were restricted to these target nutrients and foods from both the SDQ and the mean of the three non-consecutive 24HR.

*2.6. Statistical Analyses*

Estimated daily nutrient intakes for dietary fibre, calcium, vitamin D, total fat, cholesterol, saturated, monounsaturated, polyunsaturated, and *trans* fat, and servings of fruit and vegetables compiled from both instruments were examined using descriptive statistics to compute central tendencies. The test (SDQ) and reference (24HR) instruments were compared using paired t-tests for normally distributed data and Wilcoxon ranked non-parametric tests, and Spearman rank correlation analysis for data with skewed distributions. Joint classification of the targeted nutrient and food intake distributions from the SDQ and 24HR was assessed using cross-classification analyses, where participants were categorized into quartiles of consumption of nutrients and food group of interest, and the extent of exact and contiguous concordance, and frank misclassification was determined [14].

## 3. Results

Average completion time for both pretest versions of the SDQ was approximately 14 minutes (data not shown). The "precise frequencies" version of the pretest SDQ was retained in line with pretest participants' comments and to ensure consistency with diet modules based on the BRFSS previously used by Statistics Canada and to allow for easier comparison with other studies using this mode of questioning. The SDQ validation study was carried out among 396 NuAge participants (54.8% female) who had complete data in both the test and reference instruments (Table 1).

Most nutrient intakes and the number of servings of fruit and vegetables estimated from the SDQ were significantly lower than those estimated by the mean of three non-consecutive 24HR ($p < 0.05$), with the exception of calcium and vitamin D which were significantly higher compared to the 24HR, and saturated and trans fat (both NS) (Table 2). Spearman correlations between the SDQ and 24HR were low to moderate and statistically significant ($p < 0.01$), ranging from 0.19 (cholesterol: 27 mg/day lower than the 24HR) to 0.45 (fruits and vegetables: 1 portion/day lower than the 24HR) (Table 3). The arithmetic mean unadjusted Spearman correlation between the SDQ and the mean of three non-consecutive 24HR for the nine nutrients was 0.34, and it was 0.31 for the nine nutrients plus fruits and vegetables (data not shown). Finally, it can be seen in Table 4 that for all nutrients combined, 33.9% were jointly classified into identical quartiles of the distribution, 72.8% into identical and contiguous quartiles, and only 6.7% were frankly misclassified. Similar cross-classification results were observed in men and in women and there were no gender-related differences (data not shown).

**Table 1.** NuAge participants with complete data in both dietary data collection instruments, SDQ validation study ($n = 396$).

| Sex | Age Group (years) $n$ (%) | | | Total |
| --- | --- | --- | --- | --- |
| | 67–72 | 73–77 | 78–84 | |
| Male | 65 (46.1) | 46 (41.1) | 68 (47.6) | 179 (45.2) |
| Female | 76 (53.9) | 66 (58.9) | 75 (52.4) | 217 (54.8) |
| All | 141 (35.6) | 112 (28.3) | 143 (36.1) | 396 (100) |

**Table 2.** Estimated intakes of nutrients of interest from SDQ and mean of three non-consecutive 24HR, SDQ validation study ($n = 396$).

| Nutrient and Dietary Variables | Dietary Assessment Method | | | | $p$-Value [1] |
| --- | --- | --- | --- | --- | --- |
| | SDQ | | Mean of Three Non-Consecutive 24HR | | |
| | Mean | SD | Mean | SD | |
| Dietary fibre (g) | 15.4 | 6.2 | 19.6 | 7.7 | 0.0001 |
| Calcium (mg) | 946 | 465 | 768 | 334 | 0.0001 |
| Vitamin D (ug) | 5.70 | 2.91 | 5.06 | 3.87 | 0.003/0.0001 |
| Total fat (g) | 63.7 | 25.5 | 69.5 | 26.2 | 0.0001 |
| Cholesterol (mg) | 229 | 86 | 256 | 132 | 0.0001/0.006 |
| Saturated fat (g) | 22.4 | 9.2 | 23.3 | 10.9 | 0.163/0.423 |
| Monounsaturated fat (g) | 24.5 | 10.5 | 25.9 | 10.9 | 0.04/0.053 |
| Polyunsaturated fat (g) | 11.4 | 5.0 | 13.6 | 5.7 | 0.0001 |
| Trans fat (g) | 0.7 | 0.4 | 0.8 | 0.9 | 0.03/0.829 |
| Number of servings of fruit and vegetables [2] | 4.5 | 1.9 | 5.5 | 3.4 | 0.0001 |

[1] paired $t$-test/Wilcoxon signed rank test; [2] $n = 395$.

**Table 3.** Associations between nutrient estimates from SDQ and mean of three non-consecutive 24HR, SDQ validation study ($n = 396$).

| Nutrient and Dietary Variables | Spearman r [1,2] |
|---|---|
| Dietary fibre (g) | 0.34 |
| Calcium (mg) | 0.41 |
| Vitamin D (ug) | 0.33 |
| Total fat (g) | 0.26 |
| Cholesterol (mg) | 0.19 |
| Saturated fat (g) | 0.30 |
| Monounsaturated fat (g) | 0.28 |
| Polyunsaturated fat (g) | 0.22 |
| Trans fat (g) | 0.30 |
| Number of servings of fruit and vegetables | 0.45 |

[1] All correlations significant ($p$ ranged from <0.01 to <0.001); [2] Non-parametric correlations reported as variables did not follow a normal distribution.

**Table 4.** Cross-classification of nutrient estimates from SDQ and mean of three non-consecutive 24HR, SDQ validation study ($n = 396$).

| Nutrient and Dietary Variables | % in Identical Quartile | % in Identical and Contiguous Quartile | % in Opposite Quartile [1] |
|---|---|---|---|
| Dietary fibre (g) | 36.4 | 75.8 | 6.8 |
| Calcium (mg) | 41.7 | 77.1 | 5.3 |
| Vitamin D (ug) | 34.1 | 73.5 | 6.1 |
| Total fat (g) | 29.5 | 71.4 | 7.6 |
| Cholesterol (mg) | 30.8 | 68.7 | 9.8 |
| Saturated fat (g) | 32.1 | 73.5 | 8.6 |
| Monounsaturated fat (g) | 37.1 | 69.9 | 6.8 |
| Polyunsaturated fat (g) | 29.8 | 68.9 | 6.1 |
| Trans fat (g) | 36.1 | 73.7 | 6.6 |
| Number of servings of fruit and vegetables [2] | 32.2 | 77 | 3.5 |
| Mean % classification (10 nutrients plus fruit and vegetables) | 33.9 | 72.8 | 6.7 |

[1] Frank misclassification (Q1:Q4); [2] $n = 395$.

## 4. Discussion

Brief dietary measurement instruments have been developed to assess intakes of single nutrients or foods such as fat, fruits and vegetables and to examine relationships between certain dietary exposures and risk of chronic disease. Many have been compared to other dietary assessment measures with known validity [15]. The present study reports on the relative validity of a 36-item frequency-based Short Diet Questionnaire compared to the mean of three non-consecutive, quantitative 24HR, developed for use in the population-based Canadian Longitudinal Study on Aging, compared to the mean of three non-consecutive, quantitative 24HR. While many brief instruments have focussed mainly on fat intakes or on fruit and vegetables [15,16], the SDQ was developed to estimate older adults' usual consumption frequencies over a 12-month period of a set of key nutrients and foods that have been the focus of nutritional health promotion programmes targeting this segment of the population. Relative validation of the SDQ was carried out in a large sample ($n$ = 396) compared to other studies of this type, and the reference instrument was collected rigourously. To our knowledge, this is the first study of its type to be conducted among community-dwelling older adults. Consequently, while comparisons with other studies in this population group were not possible, because these older adults were cognitively intact there is no basis for expecting less accurate reporting of their intakes on either the test or reference instruments. Although the results showed some inconsistencies, where certain nutrients were underestimated while others were overestimated by the SDQ relative to the 24HR, others have observed that brief instruments tend to overestimate fat and underestimate fruits and vegetables [17]. However, almost three-quarters of participants were cross-classified into the same section of the distribution by both test and reference instruments, providing evidence of the SDQ's reasonable measurement properties.

While correlations between the key nutrients and foods estimated by the SDQ and the reference method (means of three non-consecutive 24HR) were quite modest, they were similar to those found in the literature for some of these variables. For example, a 43-item FFQ (Healthy Doc) administered by Spencer *et al.* [17] to 88 medical students estimated intakes of fruit and vegetables at 3.8 servings per day, only slightly lower than the 4.3 servings from the mean of five 24HR, with a Pearson correlation of 0.50. Using the 19-item NCI Fruit and Vegetable Screener (FVS) in an age and ethnically diverse sample of 590 adults, Greene *et al.* [18] obtained significant Pearson correlations ranging from 0.31 to 0.47 for men, and 0.43 to 0.63 for women between the FVS and multiple 24HR, depending on the sub-sample and version of their screener. Our results lined up closely to these findings, with 4.5 servings of fruits and vegetables per day estimated from the SDQ, compared to 5.5 servings daily from the three 24HR, and a significant, positive unadjusted Spearman rank correlation of 0.45.

Associations on fat from the SDQ and 24HR were also similar to those of Spencer *et al.* [17], with an unadjusted Spearman correlation of 0.26 between total fat estimated from the SDQ and the mean of the three 24HR, compared to the Spencer study which reported an adjusted, deattenuated Pearson correlation of 0.36 for fat between their brief FFQ and the mean of five 24HR.

Since the SDQ was not designed to assess the whole diet, we could not calculate energy intakes or estimate the percent of energy from fat. However, Thompson *et al.* [19] obtained a deattenuated Pearson correlation of 0.36 for percent energy from lipids from the 16-question NCI percentage of energy from fat short instrument (PFat) compared to multiple 24HR, suggesting that we can expect correlations between short diet questionnaires and quantitative, multiple 24HR to be in this modest range, similar to the present study.

It is difficult to contextualize results from this study with others, because of the heterogeneity of short dietary instruments and validation studies in the literature, including differing reference timeframes (for example the FVS asks for consumption frequencies over the last month), the use of implicit or explicit portion sizes in addition to frequency in some instruments [18], reporting on comparisons to "multiple" 24HR without specifying the number, and highly divergent samples and sample sizes. Although some studies have used a measurement error model to deattenuate correlations between the short dietary instrument and the reference measure, we have presented raw, unadjusted correlations from the SDQ and 24HR which fall into same range as adjusted correlations.

The study has limits. First, it must be acknowledged that all self-report dietary assessment methods are fraught with error. However, despite their age, the study participants were cognitively intact, which precludes expectation of poor results in this sample. Second, frequency-based dietary assessment instruments and quantitative tools such as 24HR call upon a different set of cognitive processes in order to respond to the food consumption questions. Consequently, respondents may have had difficulties with the notion of frequency on the SDQ, or could have forgotten to report some foods eaten on the 24HR assessment despite interviewer-prompts and cues on the 24HR, thus compounding errors and attenuating associations between the two instruments. Third, to permit calculation of point estimates for the validation analyses, SDQ portion sizes were imputed using medium portions from the parent NuAge FFQ nutrient database for all respondents, which may have induced a "regression to the mean" bias in comparing SDQ results to those from the 24HR, the "true" reference intakes. Fourth, the modest correlation coefficients could have been inflated due to the comparison of two potentially error-prone instruments, the SDQ and 24HR. Furthermore, this was a sub-study carried out within an ongoing cohort study, and certain participants reported confusion during the SDQ telephone interviews because the SDQ reminded them of the full FFQ that they had completed earlier in the study. In addition, based on comments noted by interviewers suggesting some uncertainty as to whether certain participants were aware that they had consumed fortified foods, the accuracy of their responses on consumption of omega-3 fatty acid or calcium-fortified foods may be questioned. Finally, because they had agreed to participate in the SDQ validation study, these respondents may have been particularly interested in diet, and thus not a representative sample.

# 5. Conclusions

The SDQ is a reasonably accurate, rapid, well-accepted approach for ranking usual consumption frequencies of selected nutrients and foods of interest. As such, it could serve in population health and chronic disease risk studies conducted among younger and older adults as a tool for rapid assessment of usual consumption frequencies of these foods and nutrients and to compare changes in patterns of consumption over time. Still, its limitations as a dietary assessment tool must be considered due to its focus only on selected nutrients and foods, as well as its qualitative nature which could result in underestimation of exposure to other dietary constituents. Consequently the SDQ would be inappropriate in studies where the objective is to obtain quantitative data on the whole diet. The first wave of administration of the SDQ to CLSA participants aged 45 to 85 years in the in-home interviews began in May 2012 and was completed in June 2015. Data entry is underway. Considering its intended use in the CLSA on multiple occasions over the 20-year follow-up, as well as the broader age range and more diverse population than the one that took part in the present relative validation study, further testing is necessary to determine its ability to accurately reflect consumption patterns of the target nutrients and foods considering different age groups, regional dietary variation and cognition in the older segment of the CLSA cohort. Additional testing of the SDQ against a full FFQ and a series of repeated 24HR would also permit further exploration of these issues, and allow for calibration of the SDQ to enhance its measurement properties.

**Acknowledgments:** The authors wish to thank the men and women of the NuAge cohort for their generous and enthusiastic participation in the study, and the study personnel for their highly professional and devoted work. We also wish to thank Katherine Gray-Donald, Véronique Boutier, Carole Coulombe, Catherine Huet, Mira Jabbour, and Marc-André Larochelle for their important contributions to the development and administration of the Short Diet Questionnaire. The NuAge study was supported by the Canadian Institutes for Health Research (CIHR), Grant number MOP-62842, and the Quebec Network for Research on Aging, a network funded by the Fonds de Recherche du Québec–Santé. CLSA is supported by the Canadian Institutes of Health Research (CIHR). The development, testing and validation of the Short Diet Questionnaire took place as part of the CLSA Phase II validation studies, CIHR 2006–2008. This work was previously presented as a poster at the 7th International Conference on Diet and Activity Methods (ICDAM), Washington, DC, 5–7 June 2009.

**Author Contributions:** Both authors conceived and designed the work; BS supervised data collection and analyses and drafted the manuscript. HP reviewed, commented on and approved the final manuscript.

**Conflicts of Interest:** The authors declare that they have no conflict of interest.

## Appendix A

**Table A1.** Sample food list modifications from the full FFQ to the SDQ.

| Full FFQ [1] | SDQ |
|---|---|
| High-fibre breakfast cereals (All Bran, 100% Bran, Bran Flakes, muesli...) | High-fibre breakfast cereals (All Bran, 100% Bran, Bran Flakes, muesli...) |
| 2 categories:<br>■ Bread: whole wheat, bran, multigrain, rye commercial sliced<br>■ Other whole-wheat bread (crusty bread, hamburger/hot dog buns, tortillas, bagels, pitas...) | Merged into 1 category:<br>■ Bread: whole wheat, bran, multigrain, rye (sliced, crusty, hamburger/hot dog buns, bagels, pita...) |
| 2 categories:<br>■ Beef (ground, hamburger, roast, steak, in cubes...)<br><br><br><br>■ Salmon, trout, sardines, herring, tuna | Merged into 1 category:<br>■ Beef, pork (ground, hamburger, roast, steak, in cubes...)<br>Other meats (veal, lamb, game...) (ground, hamburger, roast, steak, in cubes...)<br>Chicken, turkey<br>Addition of another species of fish:<br>■ Salmon, trout, sardines, herring, tuna, mackerel |
| 2 categories:<br>■ Sausages, hot dogs<br>■ Ham, cold cuts or smoked meats, bacon... | Merged into 1 category:<br>■ Sausages, hot dogs, ham, cold cuts or smoked meats, bacon... |

[1] Shatenstein *et al.* [8]

**Table A2.** Short Diet Questionnaire food and beverage list.

| Foods |
|---|
| High-fiber breakfast cereals (All Bran, 100% Bran, Bran Flakes, muesli...) |
| Whole-wheat breads, bran breads, multigrain breads, rye breads (sliced, crusty, hamburger bun, hot dog bun, bagel, pita, ...) |
| Beef, pork (ground, hamburgers, roast beef, steak, cubed...) |
| Other meats (veal, lamb, game...) (ground, hamburgers, roast, steak, cubed...) |
| Chicken, turkey |
| Salmon, trout, sardines, herring, tuna, mackerel (fresh, frozen or canned) |
| Sausages, hot dogs, ham, smoked meat, bacon... |
| Patés, cretons, terrines... |
| Sauces and gravies (brown, white, BBQ, ...) |
| **Omega-3** eggs |
| All egg dishes except omega 3 eggs (eggs, omelette, quiche...) |
| Legumes: beans, peas, lentils |
| Nuts, seeds and peanut butter |
| Fruit (fresh, frozen, canned) |
| Green salad (lettuce, with or without other ingredients) |
| Potatoes (boiled, mashed or baked) |

| Foods |
|---|
| French fries or pan-fried potatoes, poutine |
| Carrots (fresh, frozen, canned, eaten on their own or with other food, cooked or raw) |
| Other vegetables (except carrots, potatoes or salad) |
| All **low-fat** cheeses |
| All **regular** cheeses |
| Yogurt (**low-fat**) |
| Yogurt (**regular**) |
| **Calcium-fortified** foods (soy pudding, ...) |
| Ice cream, ice milk, frozen yogurt, milk-based desserts (puddings, ...) |
| Salty snacks (**regular** chips, crackers, ...) |
| Cakes, pies, doughnuts, pastries, cookies, muffins... |
| Chocolate bars |
| Butter or **regular** margarine on bread or on cooked vegetables **only** |
| **Regular** vinaigrettes, salad dressings, mayonnaise, homemade or commercial dips |

| Beverages |
|---|
| 100% pure fruit juices (orange, grapefruit or tomato, ...) |
| **Calcium-fortified** juices |
| Whole milk 3.25% milk fat for drinking |
| 2%, 1%, skim milk for drinking |
| **Calcium-fortified** milk (35% or more calcium) |
| Other **calcium-fortified** beverages (soy drink, ...) |

## References

1. Canadian Longitudinal Study on Aging. Available online: http://www.clsa-elcv.ca/scientific- executive-summary (accessed on 6 May 2015).
2. NutritionQuest. Available online: http://www.nutritionquest.com (accessed on 6 May 2015).
3. Centers for Disease Control and Prevention. Available online: http://www.cdc.gov/brfss/ (accessed on 6 May 2015).
4. Serdula, M.K.; Coates, R.J.; Byers, T.; Simoes, E.; Mokdad, A.H.; Subar, A.F. Fruit and vegetable intake among adults in 16 states: Results of a brief telephone survey. *Am. J. Public Health* **1995**, *85*, 236–239.
5. Li, R.; Serdula, M.; Bland, S.; Mokdad, A.; Bowman, B.; Nelson, D. Trends in fruit and vegetable consumption among adults in 16 us states: Behavioral risk factor surveillance system, 1990–1996. *Am. J. Public Health* **2000**, *90*, 777–781.
6. Perez, C.E. Fruit and vegetable consumption. *Health Rep.* **2002**, *13*, 23–31.
7. Traynor, M.M.; Holowaty, P.H.; Reid, D.J.; Gray-Donald, K. Vegetable and fruit food frequency questionnaire serves as a proxy for quantified intake. *Can. J. Public Health* **2006**, *97*, 286–290.
8. Shatenstein, B.; Nadon, S.; Godin, C.; Ferland, G. Development and relative validity of a food frequency questionnaire in Montreal. *Can. J. Diet. Pract. Res.* **2005**, *66*, 67–75.

9.  Willett, W. *Nutritional Epidemiology*; Oxford University Press: New York, NY, USA, 2012.

10. Gaudreau, P.; Morais, J.A.; Shatenstein, B.; Gray-Donald, K.; Khalil, A.; Dionne, I.; Ferland, G.; Fulop, T.; Jacques, D.; Kergoat, M.J.; *et al.* Nutrition as a determinant of successful aging: Description of the quebec longitudinal study nuage and results from cross-sectional pilot studies. *Rejuvenation Res.* **2007**, *10*, 377–386.

11. Subar, A.F.; Thompson, F.E.; Smith, A.F.; Jobe, J.B.; Ziegler, R.G.; Potischman, N.; Schatzkin, A.; Hartman, A.; Swanson, C.; Kruse, L.; *et al.* Improving food frequency questionnaires: A qualitative approach using cognitive interviewing. *J. Am. Diet. Assoc.* **1995**, *95*, 781–788.

12. Moshfegh, A.; Borrud, L.; Perloff, B.; LaComb, R. Improved method for the 24-hour dietary recall for use in national surveys. *FASEB J.* **1999**, *13*, A603.

13. Health Canada. *Canadian Nutrient File*; Health & Welfare Canada: Ottawa, ON, Canada, 1982.

14. Willett, W.C.; Sampson, L.; Stampfer, M.J.; Rosner, B.; Bain, C.; Witschi, J.; Hennekens, C.H.; Speizer, F.E. Reproducibility and validity of a semiquantitative food frequency questionnaire. *Am. J. Epidemiol.* **1985**, *122*, 51–65.

15. Thompson, F.E.; Subar, A.F. Dietary assessment methodology. In *Nutrition in the Prevention and Treatment of Disease*, 3rd ed.; Coulston, A.M., Boushey, C.J., Ferruzzi, M.G., Eds.; Elsevier: Oxford, UK, 2013.

16. Kim, D.J.; Holowaty, E.J. Brief, validated survey instruments for the measurement of fruit and vegetable intakes in adults: A review. *Prev. Med.* **2003**, *36*, 440–447.

17. Spencer, E.H.; Elon, L.K.; Hertzberg, V.S.; Stein, A.D.; Frank, E. Validation of a brief diet survey instrument among medical students. *J. Am. Diet. Assoc.* **2005**, *105*, 802–806.

18. Greene, G.W.; Resnicow, K.; Thompson, F.E.; Peterson, K.E.; Hurley, T.G.; Hebert, J.R.; Toobert, D.J.; Williams, G.C.; Elliot, D.L.; Goldman Sher, T.; *et al.* Correspondence of the nci fruit and vegetable screener to repeat 24-h recalls and serum carotenoids in behavioral intervention trials. *J. Nutr.* **2008**, *138*, 200S–204S.

19. Thompson, F.E.; Midthune, D.; Williams, G.C.; Yaroch, A.L.; Hurley, T.G.; Resnicow, K.; Hebert, J.R.; Toobert, D.J.; Greene, G.W.; Peterson, K.; *et al.* Evaluation of a short dietary assessment instrument for percentage energy from fat in an intervention study. *J. Nutr.* **2008**, *138*, 193S–199S.

# Validity of Two New Brief Instruments to Estimate Vegetable Intake in Adults

Janine Wright, Jillian Sherriff, John Mamo and Jane Scott

**Abstract:** Cost effective population-based monitoring tools are needed for nutritional surveillance and interventions. The aim was to evaluate the relative validity of two new brief instruments (three item: VEG3 and five item: VEG5) for estimating usual total vegetable intake in comparison to a 7-day dietary record (7DDR). Sixty-four Australian adult volunteers aged 30 to 69 years (30 males, mean age $\pm$ SD 56.3 $\pm$ 9.2 years and 34 female mean age $\pm$ SD 55.3 $\pm$ 10.0 years). Pearson correlations between 7DDR and VEG3 and VEG5 were modest, at 0.50 and 0.56, respectively. VEG3 significantly ($p < 0.001$) underestimated mean vegetable intake compared to 7DDR measures (2.9 $\pm$ 1.3 *vs.* 3.6 $\pm$ 1.6 serves/day, respectively), whereas mean vegetable intake assessed by VEG5 did not differ from 7DDR measures (3.3 $\pm$ 1.5 *vs.* 3.6 $\pm$ 1.6 serves/day). VEG5 was also able to correctly identify 95%, 88% and 75% of those subjects not consuming five, four and three serves/day of vegetables according to their 7DDR classification. VEG5, but not VEG3, can estimate usual total vegetable intake of population groups and had superior performance to VEG3 in identifying those not meeting different levels of vegetable intake. VEG5, a brief instrument, shows measurement characteristics useful for population-based monitoring and intervention targeting.

Reprinted from *Nutrients*. Cite as: Wright, J.; Sherriff, J.; Mamo, J.; Scott, J. Validity of Two New Brief Instruments to Estimate Vegetable Intake in Adults. *Nutrients* **2015**, 7, 6688–6699.

## 1. Introduction

A diet high in fruit and vegetable intake is known to decrease risk of chronic diseases including coronary heart disease CHD [1–3] and some cancers [4]. The World Health Organization recommends people eat at least 400 grams of fruit and vegetables daily (excluding potatoes) [1]. Increasing the intake of fruit and vegetables is a world-wide public health priority [5] with most countries having culturally-specific dietary recommendations to increase fruit and vegetables, which require monitoring [6,7]. There is a need for cost effective population-based monitoring tools for the purposes of nutritional surveillance and the targeting of nutrition interventions. Traditional dietary intake assessment methods such as 24 h recalls (24HR), diet records and long-form food frequency questionnaires (FFQ) are not suitable for many population monitoring and intervention settings as they are resource intensive, costly, and involve high respondent burden. Some short dietary questions [6] and abbreviated dietary intake assessment instruments have been developed [6,8] and are being increasingly used for both population-based monitoring [6] and assessing the impact of interventions [9].

Abbreviated instruments, used to estimate vegetable intake and assess other dietary behaviours, do not replace more detailed and comprehensive methods for measuring overall dietary intake such as diet records and 24HR but can provide valuable information on food group specific dietary behavior and level of consumption for population groups [6,10]. Brief instruments have advantages in situations where due to resource or time constraints it is not feasible to use more detailed measures of dietary intake [11]. However, the measurement characteristics of brief instruments should be considered and they should be used in appropriate contexts. Brief instruments with questions on self-reported fruit and vegetable consumption have been shown to be able to assess group mean/median intakes [6,8,10], a characteristic useful for monitoring and for identifying intervention target populations [10].

Brief dietary intake assessment instruments have a specific and limited focus [6]. This means that these instruments can be designed to specifically measure the population dietary behaviours of interest and relevance, an aspect particularly useful for targeting of behavioral-based interventions. For instance, a simple 1-item summary question on usual total vegetable intake in cups or serves has been routinely used in national and regional Australian studies [6,12] and has been widely used in the United States [12]. However, when evaluated this question was found to be valid only in discriminating between groups with significantly different intakes [6]. Furthermore, when used within a 2-item fruit and vegetable screener, this vegetable consumption question was found to underestimate median values for vegetables when compared to multiple 24HR [12]. Thus, in the area of vegetable intake estimation, there is a need to develop and assess the validity of alternative vegetable consumption questions or brief question sets [6,10,12].

The design of alternative questions for assessing vegetable consumption used in this study is informed by research evidence which indicates where improvements to questions could lead to useful and meaningful instruments with greater validity. The concept of what a serving size of vegetables is has been shown to be a factor adding to question difficulty in brief instruments [13] with Yarcoh *et al.* [12] recently reporting better performance of a 2-item fruit and vegetable screener that asked about intake in cups compared to intake in servings. Other difficulties in vegetable consumption questions relate to vegetable use in mixed dishes (e.g., vegetable soups) [8,10], the presence of multiple vegetable preparation forms (e.g., salads, cooked vegetables) [14], and the difficulty in interpreting questions which ask for the exclusion and inclusion of different types of potatoes [13]. Furthermore, it has been determined that it is desirable that vegetable consumption questions have less restrictive response categories [6], and in line with current dietary guidance [15] would also be able to assess consumption of vegetable sub-groups such as starchy vegetables and red and orange colored vegetables.

VEG3 and VEG5 are two new brief instruments for estimating usual total vegetable intake, consisting of three and five items respectively. The instruments were generated from six different questions on vegetable consumption, with five of these vegetable consumption questions having design aspects which address some of the identified challenges in estimating vegetable intake. This may lead to better measurement characteristics of these brief instruments. The aim of this paper is to assess the relative validity of VEG3 and VEG5 to estimate usual total vegetable intake for population monitoring and intervention targeting purposes through comparison to vegetable intake measured by a 7-day estimated dietary record (7DDR).

## 2. Methods

### 2.1. Participants

Sixty-four volunteers aged between 30 and 69 years were recruited. Recruitment was by newspaper and community announcements including a general practitioner (GP) surgery advertisement. Inclusion criteria were men and women aged between 30 and 69 years requiring primary or secondary prevention of cardio-vascular disease (CVD), that is, having one or more CVD risk factors. Exclusion criteria were: persons with non-insulin dependent diabetes; non-English speaking; unable to read or write; currently undertaking major dietary modification; major intercurrent illness. Eligibility was assessed by self-report via telephone interview. All participants provided written informed consent and the study was approved by the Curtin University of Technology Human Ethics Committee, approval reference number HR20/98.

### 2.2. Study Design

At baseline, subjects completed (1) a socio-demographic questionnaire; (2) a 63-item FFQ [16–18] containing the six vegetable consumption questions from which the 3-item (VEG3) and 5-item (VEG5) instruments are derived, and (3) were given instruction to commence the 7-day estimated diet record the following day. Four weeks later, subjects completed (1) a questionnaire on any dietary changes since baseline measures and (2) the second administration of the 63-item FFQ containing the vegetable consumption questions that make up VEG3 and VEG5. All materials were mailed to participants. Relative validity was determined through comparison of total vegetable intake estimates calculated from the first administration of VEG3 and VEG5 to total vegetable intake measured from the 7-day estimated dietary records.

Test-retest reliability was determined through comparison of total vegetable intake estimates between the two administrations of VEG3 and VEG5 (at baseline and four weeks later) in those not reporting dietary changes in the intervening period.

*2.3. Study Tools*

2.3.1. Seven-Day Estimated Dietary Records (7DDR)

The reference dietary assessment method was a 7-day estimated dietary record (7DDR) including food-photo serving size description aids, modified with permission from those used and validated by Raats and Geekie [19]. The booklet consisted of two pages of instructions, a sample day record, 12 blank pages for recording food and drinks and six pages of photographs depicting reference "medium" portion sizes of foods . The booklet also included two fold-out flaps with descriptions of "medium" portion sizes. Participants were asked to describe the "amount" eaten in terms of photographs and lists provided, in terms of household measures and weights taken from food packaging. Participants received telephone-based training on how to complete the 7DDR with phone call assistance available during the 7-day measuring period.

2.3.2. Brief Instrument (VEG3 and VEG5) Vegetable Consumption Questions

VEG3 and VEG5 were derived from six questions assessing vegetable consumption contained within a longer, validated 63-item combination FFQ [16–18]. The six questions were Ling and colleague's [14] 3-item set of questions (identified as C on Figure 1) on the consumption of vegetable soups, salads and cooked vegetables (excluding potato); a 1-item summary question (B on Figure 1) on usual total vegetable consumption (excluding potato); and two questions on non-fried potato intake (A on Figure 1) (the format and calculation of non-fried potato using these questions is further described in [18]). The time period of reference for all vegetable consumption questions was the previous month. Details of the questions and how they are combined to create the brief instruments are shown in Figure 1 with VEG3 = A + B and VEG5 = A + C.

*2.4. Data Analysis*

2.4.1. Dietary Analysis

Food groups were defined according to the specifications of the Australian Guide to Healthy Eating [20]. Food group data were determined through export of FoodWorks diet record food lists (FoodWorks Version 3.0 (Xyris software, Brisbane, QLD, utlilising the NUTTAB98 database ) into Microsoft Access (Microsoft Access

2007, Microsoft Enterprise Systems 2007) where all individual food and drink items were coded into food groups. This food group coding was then re-linked to each participant's dietary record to allow calculation of 7-day food group totals (total serves) and daily averages (servings/day). Food group outcome variables for vegetables were average daily serves of vegetables with and without non fried potato.

### 2.4.2. Brief Instrument (VEG3 and VEG5) Vegetable Intake Estimation

Total usual vegetable intake estimates were calculated using two different sets of questions as previously described and outlined in Figure 1. Both brief instruments were also used to calculate usual total vegetable intake excluding potato. For this the two questions related to non-fried potato intake were removed, in which case VEG3 had 1-item (B on Figure 1) and VEG5 had 3-items (the question set developed by Ling *et al.* [14] and shown as C on Figure 1).

### 2.5. Statistical Analysis

The relationship between the 7DDR measures with VEG3 and VEG5 estimates was assessed using Pearson's correlation coefficients. The ability of the brief instruments VEG3 and VEG5 to estimate group means for usual total vegetable intake (both including and excluding non-fried potatoes) in comparison to 7DDR measures was investigated using paired t-tests. The technique of Bland and Altman [21] was utilised to determine agreement between the 7DDR and brief instrument vegetable intake estimates, and to calculate mean bias and 95% limits of agreement (LOA). To examine how well the brief instruments could correctly classify subjects according to different intake levels the 7DDR, VEG3 and VEG5 measures were dichotomized for different serve intake levels (for example less than five servings/day or five or more servings/day), with data dichotomized four times in total (allowing examination of classification of intake from two to five serves/day). The predictive value of the VEG3 and VEG5 (both including and excluding non-fried potato) was examined using these dichotomized scores, with positive predictive value defined as those determined to be consuming less than the intake level serving/day cut-off by the brief instruments who also did not meet the same intake level serving/day cut-off according to the 7DDR measure. Test-retest reliability of the short instruments was assessed using Pearson's correlation coefficient. All data were analyzed using the Statistical Package for the Social Sciences (SPSS Version 17.0, Chicago, IL, USA). All data distributions (7DDR, VEG3 and VEG5) were checked for normality using a Shapiro-Wilk test. $p < 0.05$ was considered significant.

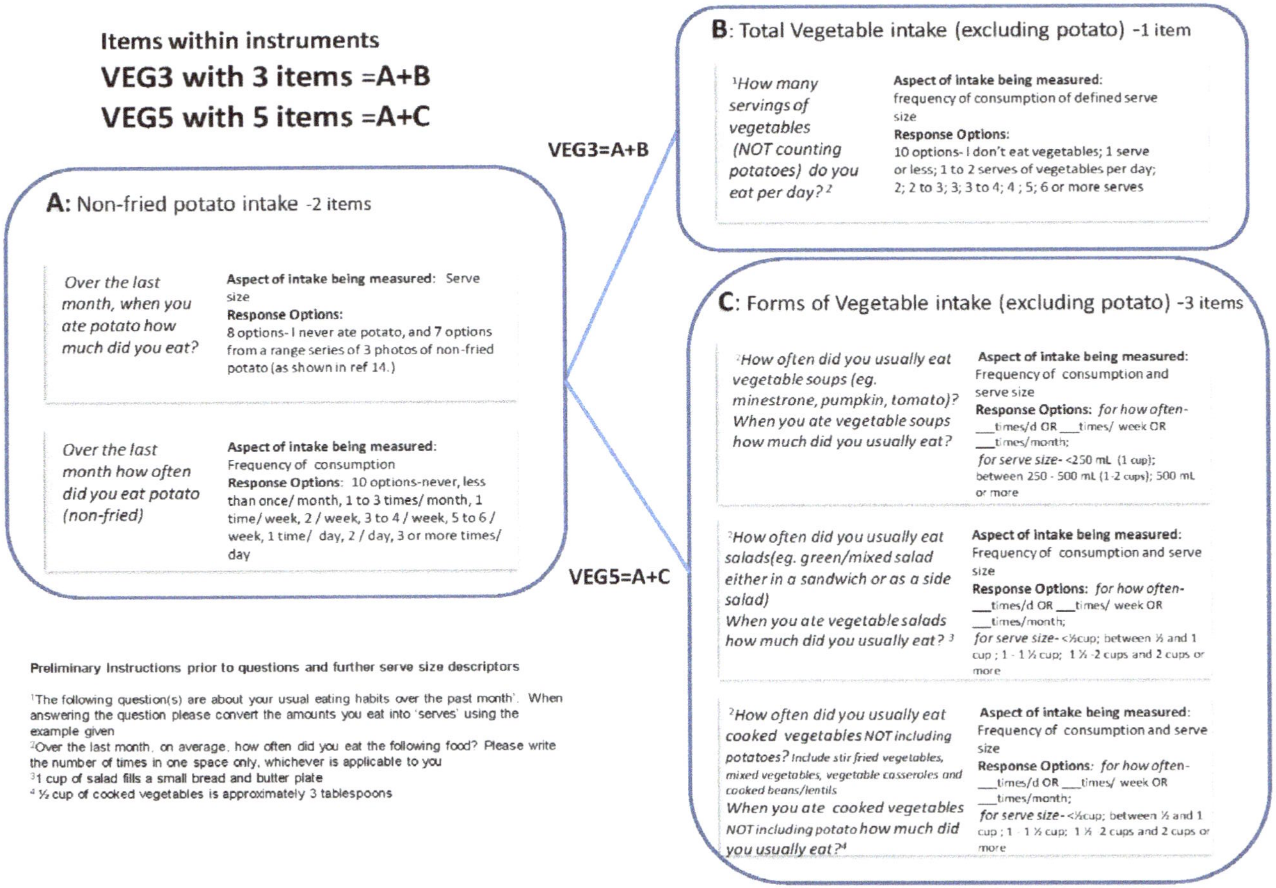

**Items within instruments**

**VEG3 with 3 items =A+B**

**VEG5 with 5 items =A+C**

---

**A: Non-fried potato intake - 2 items**

| | |
|---|---|
| *Over the last month, when you ate potato how much did you eat?* | **Aspect of intake being measured:** Serve size<br>**Response Options:**<br>8 options- I never ate potato, and 7 options from a range series of 3 photos of non-fried potato (as shown in ref 14.) |
| *Over the last month how often did you eat potato (non-fried)* | **Aspect of intake being measured:**<br>Frequency of consumption<br>**Response Options:** 10 options-never, less than once/ month, 1 to 3 times/month, 1 time/week, 2 / week, 3 to 4 / week, 5 to 6 / week, 1 time/ day, 2 / day, 3 or more times/ day |

**Preliminary Instructions prior to questions and further serve size descriptors**

[1]The following question(s) are about your usual eating habits over the past month. When answering the question please convert the amounts you eat into serves using the example given
[2]Over the last month, on average, how often did you eat the following food? Please write the number of times in one space only, whichever is applicable to you
[3]1 cup of salad fills a small bread and butter plate
[4]½ cup of cooked vegetables is approximately 3 tablespoons

---

**B**: Total Vegetable intake (excluding potato) -1 item

| | |
|---|---|
| [1]*How many servings of vegetables (NOT counting potatoes) do you eat per day?*[2] | **Aspect of intake being measured:**<br>frequency of consumption of defined serve size<br>**Response Options**<br>10 options- I don't eat vegetables; 1 serve or less; 1 to 2 serves of vegetables per day; 2; 2 to 3; 3; 3 to 4 ; 4 ; 5; 6 or more serves |

**VEG3=A+B**

---

**C**: Forms of Vegetable intake (excluding potato) -3 items

| | |
|---|---|
| [2]*How often did you usually eat vegetable soups (eg. minestrone, pumpkin, tomato)? When you ate vegetable soups how much did you usually eat?* | **Aspect of intake being measured:**<br>Frequency of consumption and serve size<br>**Response Options:** *for how often-*<br>___times/d OR ___ times/ week OR ___ times/month;<br>*for serve size-*<250 mL (1 cup); between 250 - 500 mL (1-2 cups); 500 mL or more |
| [2]*How often did you usually eat salads(eg. green/mixed salad either in a sandwich or as a side salad)*<br>*When you ate vegetable salads how much did you usually eat?*[3] | **Aspect of intake being measured:** *for how often-*<br>Frequency of consumption and serve size<br>**Response Options:** *for how often-*<br>___times/d OR ___ times/ week OR ___times/month;<br>*for serve size-*<½ cup; between ½ and 1 cup ; 1 - 1 ½ cup; 1 ½ - 2 cups and 2 cups or more |
| [2]*How often did you usually eat cooked vegetables NOT including potatoes? Include stir fried vegetables, mixed vegetables, vegetable casseroles and cooked beans/lentils*<br>*When you ate cooked vegetables NOT including potato how much did you usually eat?*[4] | **Aspect of intake being measured:**<br>Frequency of consumption and serve size<br>**Response Options:** *for how often-*<br>___times/d OR ___ times/ week OR ___times/month;<br>*for serve size-*<½ cup; between ½ and 1 cup ; 1 ½ cup; 1 ½ - 2 cups and 2 cups or more |

**VEG5=A+C**

**Figure 1.** Vegetable consumption question details for VEG3 and VEG5.

## 3. Results

### 3.1. Subject Characteristics

The mean age of the 64 adult volunteers was mean age $\pm$ SD 55.7 $\pm$ 9.6 years (30 males, mean age $\pm$ SD 56.3 $\pm$ 9.2 years and 34 female mean age $\pm$ SD 55.3 $\pm$ 10.0 years).

### 3.2. Test-Retest Reliability

Out of the 56 who completed the vegetable consumption questions making up VEG3 and VEG5 on two occasions four to six weeks apart , 19 reported making dietary changes in that period and thus a total of 37 persons (20 male mean $\pm$ SD age, 56.6 $\pm$ 9.1 years, 17 female mean age 56.5 $\pm$ 9.4) were included in an assessment of test-retest reliability. Total vegetable intake at baseline and at one month re-administration for VEG3 were mean $\pm$ SD 3.1 $\pm$ 1.4 and 3.1 $\pm$ 1.0 serves/day; and for VEG5 were 3.7 $\pm$ 1.3 and 3.1 $\pm$ 1.3 serves/day. The test-retest correlation coefficients between one-month re-administrations of VEG3 and VEG5 for total vegetable intake in serves/day were, for VEG3, $r$ = 0.64 95% CI (0.40,0.80) and for VEG5, $r$ = 0.58 95% CI (0.31,0.76), with both indicating reasonable to good test-retest reliability.

### 3.3. Relative Validity of Brief Instruments in Comparison to Dietary Record Measures

Pearson correlation coefficients between 7DDR measure of vegetable intake in serves/day and VEG3 and VEG5 estimates were modest at $r$ = 0.50 95% CI (0.29, 0.66) and $r$ = 0.56 95% CI (0.36, 0.71), respectively. For VEG3 the mean difference (7DDR-VEG3) or bias was 0.63 serves/day with 95% LOA of ($-2.20, 3.45$ serves/day). For VEG5 the mean difference (7DDR-VEG5) or bias was 0.24 serves/day with 95% LOA of ($-2.57, 3.04$ serves/day).

As shown in Table 1, VEG3 significantly ($p < 0.001$) underestimated mean vegetable intake compared to 7DDR measures (2.9 $\pm$ 1.3 *vs.* 3.6 $\pm$ 1.6 serves/day, respectively), whereas mean vegetable intake assessed by VEG5 did not differ from 7DDR measures (3.3 $\pm$ 1.5 *vs.* 3.6 $\pm$ 1.6 serves/day, respectively).

These differences between VEG3 and VEG5 were mirrored in prevalence estimates for intakes meeting different national food selection guide-specified serve intake levels (Table 1). VEG5 produced prevalence estimates of individuals meeting different intake levels (*i.e.*, from less than two serves to more than five serves) that were similar to 7DDR measures, with VEG3 produced prevalence estimates being somewhat different. VEG5 was able to correctly identify 91% of those not meeting the recommendation of five or more serves per day according to the 7DDR, and could correctly identify 71% and 72% of those not consuming at least four or three serves a day, respectively. When non-fried potato was excluded from VEG5, it identified 95%,

88% and 75% of those not consuming five, four, and three serves a day according to their 7DDR classification. VEG5 had superior positive predictive values to VEG3, the exception being for the less than five serves/day comparison point (95% *vs.* 97%).

## 4. Discussion

Wide 95% LOA for both VEG3 and VEG5 estimates of usual total vegetable intake in comparison to 7DDR measures indicates poor agreement between the brief instruments and the reference standard at the individual level. As such, neither VEG3 nor VEG5 can replace the comprehensive dietary measure of 7DDR in estimating vegetable intakes of individuals.

However, when assessing the brief instruments' estimation of vegetable intake at the group level, VEG5's estimation of mean vegetable intake did not differ from that measured by the 7DDR, whereas the VEG3's vegetable intake estimates at group level were significantly underestimated. Both of these results were found irrespective of whether non-fried potato was included or excluded in the estimation of vegetable intake. This result is consistent with the finding of the Kim and Holowaty review [10] in that the longer instrument had better relative validity than the shorter one.

These results indicate that VEG5, as an estimate of vegetable intake both including and excluding non-fried potato, is an instrument that could be used to assess mean vegetable intake in population groups. Although this study is smaller and has less generalizability than that of Yaroch and colleagues [12], their 16-item screener (with 12 vegetable consumption questions) was unable to estimate group mean vegetable intake.

VEG5 had superior positive predictive values to VEG3, the exception being for the less than five serves/day comparison point (95% *vs.* 97%). These high positive predictive values suggest that VEG5, in particular, is useful for confirming intake levels and will correctly classify sizeable and similar proportions of adults with vegetable intakes below, at or above three, four and five servings per day.

Overall, VEG5 shows measurement characteristics useful for population-level monitoring and for the targeting of interventions. VEG5 can identify those with intakes less than dietary recommendations, and was also able to identify and classify most people with consumption levels considerably lower than current recommendations. This maximizes potential uses of VEG5 in intervention targeting, as most consumers have intakes less than three serves a day [7,22] and represent the group that can make the greatest public health gains through increased consumption towards dietary recommendations [7].

**Table 1.** Estimation of usual total vegetable intake by VEG3 and VEG5 in comparison to 7-day estimated dietary records (7DDR) measures of mean vegetable intake, and predictive value of VEG3 and VEG5 for different vegetable intake levels.

| | Vegetable serves/day [a] | <5 serves/day Prevalence [b], % | <5 serves/day Positive Predictive Value | <4 serves/day Prevalence, % | <4 serves/day Positive Predictive Value | <3 serves/day Prevalence, % | <3 serves/day Positive Predictive Value | <2 serves/day Prevalence, % | <2 serves/day Positive Predictive Value |
|---|---|---|---|---|---|---|---|---|---|
| *Vegetable measures including potato (non-fried)* | | | | | | | | | |
| **All (n = 64)** | | | | | | | | | |
| 7DDR | 3.6 ± 1.6 (3.2,4.0) | 87.5 | … | 65.6 | … | 37.5 | … | 12.5 | … |
| VEG3 | 2.9 ± 1.3 * (2.6,3.3) | 92.2 | 0.90 | 81.2 | 0.68 | 53.1 | 0.59 | 26.6 | 0.29 |
| VEG5 | 3.3 ± 1.5 (3.0,3.7) | 87.5 | 0.91 | 60.9 | 0.71 | 39.1 | 0.72 | 17.2 | 0.45 |
| *Vegetable measures excluding potato* | | | | | | | | | |
| **All (n = 64)** | | | | | | | | | |
| 7DDR | 3.0 ± 1.5 (2.7,3.4) | 93.8 | … | 82.8 | … | 51.6 | … | 21.9 | … |
| VEG3-potato | 2.5 ± 1.1 * (2.2,2.7) | 93.8 | 0.97 | 92.2 | 0.85 | 64.1 | 0.63 | 31.3 | 0.35 |
| VEG5-potato | 2.8 ± 1.3 (2.5,3.2) | 96.9 | 0.95 | 79.7 | 0.88 | 50.0 | 0.75 | 23.2 | 0.40 |

[a] mean ± SD (95% CI); * $p \leqslant 0.05$ in comparison to 7DDR; [b] population prevalence estimates below each vegetable intake level using 7DDR, VEG3 or VEG5.

Furthermore, VEG5 has demonstrated characteristics useful for population-level monitoring independent of whether non-fried potato is included or excluded in the calculation of usual total vegetable intake. Thus VEG5 can be used in nations which differ in their treatment of non-fried potatoes in their vegetable intake recommendations; for example, Australia includes non-fried potatoes within their definition of total vegetable intake [7] whereas the US does not [15].

As a point of difference to many currently used short dietary questions and brief instruments, VEG5 includes open-ended response options for frequency estimates of consumption of soups, salad and cooked (non-potato) vegetables. VEG5 can therefore collect information on the full range of intakes including high vegetable consumers. VEG5 estimates may therefore remain relevant to monitoring contexts when and if the recommendations for vegetable intake increase from those currently used.

In this study, relative validity, rather than absolute validity, was assessed with only self-reported data compared. The use of the 7DDR as the reference standard is, however, a robust comparison method: the 7DDR is a comprehensive dietary intake measure which, importantly, has measurement errors most likely independent from the main systematic measurement errors common to brief instruments, which are the cognitive task of estimating usual intake over a period of time [11]. Also, the relative validity testing in this study did not test the vegetable consumption questions that are part of VEG3 and VEG5 as stand-alone items; rather the question items were administered as part of a longer 63-item FFQ. The impact of this is not known, but as potential applications of VEG5 include population monitoring, it is likely that in these settings, the brief instruments questions will also be used in combination with other dietary and health questions. The findings of this study were demonstrated with a relatively small volunteer sample size and further studies with larger and more diverse population groupings are needed to examine the generalisability of the findings.

## 5. Conclusions

When compared to the results from 7DDR, a 5-item set of questions (VEG5) better assessed vegetable intake of adult Australians at the group-level than a three item set of questions (VEG3). Both VEG3 and VEG5 were able to correctly classify high proportions of those subjects not consuming five, four and three serves/day of vegetables according to their 7DDR classification. Neither VEG3 nor VEG5 were accurate in assessing vegetable intake at an individual level and do not replace more thorough and comprehensive dietary intake measurement tools such as diet records for this purpose. VEG5 is a quick, inexpensive instrument that can assess mean intake of vegetables in population groups and can identify those not meeting public health-related vegetable consumption recommendations. Specifically, VEG5 has high predictive value in identifying those not consuming three serves to five serves of vegetables a day. These useful characteristics of VEG5 apply whether non-fried potato is included or excluded from its vegetable intake estimates. As a 5-item instrument to estimate usual total vegetable intake, VEG5 therefore appears useful for population-level monitoring and intervention targeting purposes.

**Acknowledgments:** We wish to thank the study participants and Deborah Kerr and Christina Pollard, who provided useful review comments on earlier versions of the manuscript.

**Author Contributions:** Janine Wright conceived and designed the study, collected, analysed and interpreted the data, and led the writing of the manuscript. Jill Sherriff, John Mamo and Jane Scott participated in the interpretation of data, and reviewed and edited the manuscript. All authors read and approved the final manuscript.

**Conflicts of Interest:** The authors declare no conflict of interest.

## References

1. Organization, W.H. Report of WHO/FAO Expert Consultation. In *Diet, Nutrition and the Prevention of Chronic Diseases*; Who Technical Report Series No. 916; World Health Organization/Food and Agriculture Organization: Geneva, Switzerland, 2003.
2. Dauchet, L.; Amouyel, P.; Hercberg, S.; Dallongeville, J. Fruit and vegetable consumption and risk of coronary heart disease: A meta-analysis of cohort studies. *J. Nutr.* **2006**, *136*, 2588–2593.
3. Pomerleau, J.; Lock, K.; McKee, M. The burden of cardiovascular disease and cancer attributable to low fruit and vegetable intake in the European union: Differences between old and new member states. *Public Health Nutr.* **2006**, *9*, 575–583.
4. World Cancer Research Fund/American Institute of Cancer Research. *Food, Nutrition, Physical Activity, and the Prevention of Cancer: A Global Perspective*; WRCR/AICR: Washington, DC, USA, 2007.
5. World Health Organization. *World Health Assembly Resolution Wha57.17-Global Strategy on Diet, Physical Activity and Health*; World Health Organisation: Geneva, Switzerland, 2003.
6. Coles-Rutishauser, I.; Webb, K.; Abraham, B.L.; Allsopp, R. *Evaluation of short dietary questions from the 1995 National Nutrition Survey*; Australian Food and Nutrition Monitoring Unit, The University of Queensland: Brisbane, Australia, 2001.
7. Pollard, C.M.; Miller, M.R.; Daly, A.M.; Crouchley, K.E.; O'Donoghue, K.J.; Lang, A.J.; Binns, C.W. Increasing fruit and vegetable consumption: Success of the Western Australian go for 2&5 campaign. *Public Health Nutr.* **2008**, *11*, 314–320.
8. Thompson, F.; Subar, A.; Smith, A.; Midthune, D.; Radimer, K.; Kahle, L.; Kipnis, V. Fruit and vegetable assessment: Performance of 2 new short instruments and a food frequency questionnaire. *J. Am. Diet. Assoc.* **2002**, *102*, 1764–1772.
9. Pollard, C.; Miller, M.; Woodman, R.J.; Meng, R.; Binns, C. Changes in knowledge, beliefs, and behaviors related to fruit and vegetable consumption among Western Australian adults from 1995 to 2004. *Am. J. Public Health* **2009**, *99*, 355–361.
10. Kim, D.J.; Holowaty, E.J. Brief, validated survey instruments for the measurement of fruit and vegetable intakes in adults: A review. *Prev. Med.* **2003**, *36*, 440–447.

11. Kirkpatrick, S.I.; Reedy, J.; Butler, E.N.; Dodd, K.W.; Subar, A.F.; Thompson, F.E.; McKinnon, R.A. Dietary assessment in food environment research: A systematic review. *Am. J. Prev. Med.* **2014**, *46*, 94–102.

12. Yaroch, A.L.; Tooze, J.; Thompson, F.E.; Blanck, H.M.; Thompson, O.M.; Colón-Ramos, U.; Shaikh, A.R.; McNutt, S.; Nebeling, L.C. Evaluation of three short dietary instruments to assess fruit and vegetable intake: The national cancer institute's food attitudes and behaviors survey. *J. Acad. Nutr. Diet.* **2012**, *112*, 1570–1577.

13. Wolfe, W.S.; Frongillo, E.A.; Cassano, P.A. Evaluating brief measures of fruit and vegetable consumption frequency and variety: Cognition, interpretation, and other measurement issues. *J. Am. Diet. Assoc.* **2001**, *101*, 311–318.

14. Ling, A.M.; Horwath, C.; Parnell, W. Validation of a short food frequency questionnaire to assess consumption of cereal foods, fruit and vegetables in Chinese Singaporeans. *Eur. J. Clin. Nutr.* **1998**, *52*, 557–564.

15. U.S. Department of Agriculture and U.S. Department of Health and Human Services. *Dietary Guidelines for Americans*, 7th ed.; Department of Health and Human Services: Washington, DC, USA, 2010.

16. Barkess, J.L.; Sherriff, J.L. *Relative Validity and Reliability of a Short Food Frequency Questionnaire to Assess Saturated Fat Intake Behaviours*; Dietitians Association of Australia: Cairns, Australia, 2003.

17. Barkess, J.L.; Sherriff, J.L. Relative validity of an Australian short food frequency questionnaire to assess intake of fruit, vegetables and cereal foods. In Proceedings of the XIV International Congress of Dietetics, Chicago, IL, USA, 28–31 May 2004.

18. Wright, J.; Sherriff, J.; Dhaliwal, S.; Mamo, J. Tailored, iterative, printed dietary feedback is as effective as group education in improving dietary behaviours: Results from a randomised control trial in middle-aged adults with cardiovascular risk factors. *Int. J. Behav. Nutr. Phys. Act.* **2011**, *8*, 43.

19. Raats, M.M.; Sparks, P.; Geekie, M.A.; Shepherd, R. The effects of providing personalized dietary feedback. A semi-computerized approach. *Patient Educ. Counsel.* **1999**, *37*, 177–189.

20. Smith, A.; Kellett, E.; Schmerlaib, Y. *Australian Guide to Healthy Eating*; Commonwealth Department of Health and Family Services: Canberra, Australia, 1998.

21. Martin Bland, J.; Altman, D.G. Statistical methods for assessing agreement between two methods of clinical measurement. *Lancet* **1986**, *327*, 307–310.

22. Australian Bureau of Statistics. 4364.0.55.003—Australian Health Survey: Updated Results, 2011–2012. Available online: http://www.abs.gov.au/ausstats/abs@.nsf/Lookup/C549D4433F6B74D7CA257B8200179569?opendocument (accessed on 4 December 2014).

# Fruit and Vegetable Intake Assessed by Food Frequency Questionnaire and Plasma Carotenoids: A Validation Study in Adults

Tracy L. Burrows, Melinda J. Hutchesson, Megan E. Rollo, May M. Boggess, Maya Guest and Clare E. Collins

**Abstract:** Dietary validation studies of self-reported fruit and vegetable intake should ideally include measurement of plasma biomarkers of intake. The aim was to conduct a validation study of self-reported fruit and vegetable intakes in adults, using the Australian Eating Survey (AES) food frequency questionnaire (FFQ), against a range of plasma carotenoids. Dietary intakes were assessed using the semi-quantitative 120 item AES FFQ. Fasting plasma carotenoids ($\alpha$- and $\beta$-carotene, lutein/zeaxanthin, lycopene and cryptoxanthin) were assessed using high performance liquid chromatography in a sample of 38 adult volunteers (66% female). Significant positive correlations were found between FFQ and plasma carotenoids for $\alpha$-carotene, $\beta$-carotene and lutein/zeaxanthin (52%, 47%, 26%, $p < 0.001, 0.003, 0.041$; respectively) and relationships between plasma carotenoids (except lycopene) and weight status metrics (BMI, waist circumference, fat mass) were negative and highly significant. The results of the current study demonstrate that carotenoid intakes as assessed by the AES FFQ are significantly related to plasma concentrations of $\alpha$-carotene, $\beta$-carotene and lutein/zeaxanthin, the carotenoids commonly found in fruit and vegetables. Lower levels of all plasma carotenoids, except lycopene, were found in individuals with higher BMI. We conclude that the AES can be used to measure fruit and vegetable intakes with confidence.

Reprinted from *Nutrients*. Cite as: Burrows, T.L.; Hutchesson, M.J.; Rollo, M.E.; Boggess, M.M.; Guest, M.; Collins, C.E. Fruit and Vegetable Intake Assessed by Food Frequency Questionnaire and Plasma Carotenoids: A Validation Study in Adults. *Nutrients* **2015**, *7*, 3240–3251.

## 1. Introduction

Regular consumption of fruit and vegetable intake in accordance with World Cancer Research Fund guidelines is associated with a reduced risk of some cancers and substantially lower risks of coronary heart disease [1,2], stroke [3,4] and possibly type 2 diabetes mellitus [5,6].

Plasma biomarkers can be used in studies validating dietary intake as independent proxy measures of intake [7] and to evaluate whether sources of random error are independent of errors associated with measurement by questionnaire and/or inaccuracies within nutrient databases [8]. Simultaneous measurement of plasma carotenoid concentrations have been reported in studies validating fruit and vegetable intakes [9,10] as carotenoids predominate in these foods [11]. It has been reported that a single carotenoid is not likely to be sufficient due to the diverse composition of plant foods [12]. Alpha-carotene, β-carotene, cryptoxanthin, lycopene and lutein are the carotenoids most commonly assessed in dietary validation studies [13].

Therefore, the aim of the current study was to compare fasting plasma carotenoid concentrations, as biomarkers of fruit and vegetables, with dietary carotenoids and intakes of fruit and vegetables, as assessed by the Australian Eating Survey (AES) food frequency questionnaire (FFQ) in a sample of adults.

## 2. Experimental Section

Data used in this analysis were obtained from a convenience sample of adults who had previously participated in a comparative validation study (The Family Diet Quality Study) [14] and who volunteered to give a blood sample for plasma carotenoid analysis. The methods have been published previously elsewhere [14]. Briefly, participants were recruited into the validation study through advertisements in newspapers, community notice boards and school newsletters in Newcastle, New South Wales, Australia. Eligibility included being an adult (>18 years), with no known medical conditions or taking medications that could influence body weight, (e.g., asthma, type 1 diabetes) and living full-time with at least one child aged 8–10 years, with data collected as part of a study of nutrition in families [14]. Demographic data including age, education, smoking status and self-rated health were measured. Anthropometric data, including height (cm), weight (kg) and body mass index (BMI) calculated as $kg/m^2$, waist circumference (cm) and fat mass (kg) were measured by trained assessors with full details reported elsewhere [15]. A trained research assistant explained and administered the AES FFQ, which consisted of 120 items, reporting intake over the previous six months. This instrument has previously been used compared in adults to weighed food records without use of independent biomarkers [14].

Fruit and vegetables were reported as servings per day. An individual response for each food or food type was recorded with seven frequency options ranging from "never" up to "4 or more times per day" and for some beverages up to "7 or more glasses per day". Nineteen FFQ items related directly to intake of vegetables. Vegetable types assessed were potatoes, pumpkin, sweet potato, cauliflower, green beans, spinach (*i.e.*, Swiss chard), cabbage/brussels sprouts, peas, broccoli, carrots, zucchini, eggplant, summer squash, capsicum (*i.e.*, red and green bell pepper), corn, mushrooms, tomatoes, lettuce, celery, cucumber, avocado, onion, spring onion, and leek. Eleven FFQ items related directly to the intake of fruit. Fruits assessed were: canned fruit, fruit salad, dried fruit, apple, pear, orange, mandarin, grapefruit, banana, peach, nectarine, plum or apricot, mango, paw-paw, pineapple, grapes, strawberries, blueberries and melon. The frequency categories for seasonal fruit for fruits such as peach and melon were calculated by adjusting for the number of months per year the fruit was available. Vitamin supplement use was assessed as "yes" or "no".

Standard adult portion sizes were used for each food item and derived from the most current Australian National Nutrition Survey using unpublished data purchased from the Australian Bureau of Statistics [16]. Daily carotenoid intakes of α-carotene, β-carotene, lycopene, cryptoxanthin and combined lutein-zeaxanthin were estimated from FFQ fruit and vegetable responses using the carotenoid database from the US Department of Agriculture National Cancer Institute [17].

## 2.1. Biochemical Assay

Phlebotomists collected blood samples in EDTA-coated tubes after an overnight fast and samples were analysed at an accredited pathology service (National Association of Testing Authorities, Australia). Serum was separated from red blood cells by centrifugation and remaining samples were frozen within 2 h to $-80\ °C$. Samples were thawed and high performance liquid chromatography (HPLC) methodology was used to determine β-carotene, lycopene, α-carotene, β-cryptoxanthin and lutein/zeaxanthin concentrations in serum. All extractions were carried out in a darkened laboratory under red light. In a 1:1 ratio, ethanol plus ethyl acetate containing internal standard (canthaxanthin) were added to the sample. The solution was vortexed, centrifuged (3000 g, 4 °C for 5 min) and the supernatant was collected. This process was repeated three times, adding ethyl acetate twice, then hexane to the pellet. Ultra-pure water was then added to pooled supernatant and the mixture was vortexed and centrifuged. The supernatant was decanted, the solvents evaporated with nitrogen and the sample reconstituted in dichloromethane:methanol (1:2 v/v). Chromatography was performed on a Hypersil ODS column (100 mm × 2.1 m × 5 µm) with a flow rate of 0.3 mL/min. Carotenoids were analysed using a mobile phase of acetonitrile: dichloromethane: methanol (containing 0.05% ammonium acetate) (85:10:5 v/v) and a diode array detector (470 nm) [18].

## 2.2. Ethics

The study protocol was approved by the University of Newcastle Human Research Ethics Committee (Approval No. H-2010-1170).

## 2.3. Statistical Methods

Median, minimum and maximum values were reported for reported FFQ fruit and vegetable intakes, FFQ carotenoids and plasma carotenoid concentrations. BMI was significantly associated with plasma carotenoids, as expected [19,20], and thus was used to stratify descriptive statistics. Participants were categorized as either healthy weight (BMI < 25 kg/m$^2$) or overweight (BMI $\geq$ 25 kg/m$^2$). Univariate effects (Tables 1 and 2) were assessed using Wilcoxon rank-sum tests. Comparisons of plasma carotenoids to FFQ carotenoids were made using Wilcoxon matched pairs signed-rank tests. Linear regression models were used to assess the relationship between plasma and FFQ carotenoid levels, whilst controlling for anthropometric variables (BMI, waist circumference and fat mass). Clustered, robust standard errors were used to account for the probable correlation of food intakes of participants in the same family [21]. The normality of the residuals from these models was assessed using the Shapiro-Wilk's test. Statistical significance is determined at the 5% level. All statistical analysis was performed using Stata MP version 12 [22].

**Table 1.** Anthropometric summary for $n$ = 38 participants from 26 families, by weight category.

| | All | | Healthy Weight (BMI < 25) | | Overweight (BMI $\geq$ 25) | | $p$ |
|---|---|---|---|---|---|---|---|
| | $n$ = 38 | | $n$ = 20 | | $n$ = 18 | | |
| Female | 25 (66%) | | 14 (70%) | | 11 (61%) | | 0.73 |
| Supplement use | 20 (53%) | | 10 (50%) | | 10 (56%) | | 0.76 |
| | Median | (Min–Max) | Median | (Min–Max) | Median | (Min–Max) | |
| Age (years) | 43.3 | (33.5–52.6) | 42.9 | (36.8–50.6) | 44.9 | (33.5–52.6) | 0.64 |
| Height (cm) | 169.3 | (151.4–188.0) | 169.8 | (161.6–184.5) | 168.3 | (151.4–188.0) | 0.24 |
| Weight (Kg) | 68.8 | (55.6–99.6) | 64.4 | (55.6–78.5) | 79.4 | (61.5–99.6) | <0.01 |
| BMI (kg/m$^2$) | 24.4 | (19.4–37.8) | 22.5 | (19.4–24.5) | 27.9 | (25.1–37.8) | <0.01 |
| Waist (cm) | 83.4 | (67.7–111.4) | 78.8 | (67.7–91.4) | 91.1 | (76.9–111.4) | <0.01 |
| Fat Mass (Kg) | 21.3 | (7.0–48.3) | 14.6 | (7.0–23.8) | 24.5 | (14.5–48.3) | <0.01 |
| Fat Mass (%) | 26.6 | (11.2–50.9) | 20.8 | (11.2–35.3) | 34.3 | (17.8–50.9) | <0.01 |
| Fat Free Mass (Kg) | 48.1 | (38.9–77.4) | 48.1 | (40.6–63.4) | 48.5 | (38.9–77.4) | 0.70 |
| Fat Free Mass (%) | 73.4 | (49.1–88.8) | 79.2 | (64.7–88.8) | 65.7 | (49.1–82.2) | <0.01 |

$p$ Value indicates differences between weight groups.

**Table 2.** Summary statistics (median, minimum and maximum) for plasma carotenoids, food frequency questionnaire (FFQ) carotenoids and fruit and vegetable intake, by weight category.

| | All | | Healthy Weight (BMI < 25) | | Overweight (BMI ≥ 25) | | p |
|---|---|---|---|---|---|---|---|
| | n = 38 | | n = 20 | | n = 18 | | |
| | Median | (Min–Max) | Median | (Min–Max) | Median | (Min–Max) | |
| Plasma Carotenoid (µg/dL) | | | | | | | |
| α-carotene | 6.40 | (0.80–29.30) | 7.35 | (1.90–29.30) | 3.85 | (0.80–28.40) | 0.05 |
| β-carotene | 40.65 | (3.50–176.80) | 46.4 | (7.30–162.40) | 25.4 | (3.50–176.80) | 0.01 |
| Lycopene | 40.85 | (7.20–114.30) | 38.7 | (7.20–114.30) | 43.3 | (13.40–94.60) | 0.64 |
| Lutein-zeaxanthin | 21.05 | (7.50–64.60) | 24.95 | (9.40–64.60) | 16.3 | (7.50–38.40) | 0.05 |
| Cryptoxanthin | 7.60 | (1.70–18.80) | 8.95 | (1.70–16.50) | 5.25 | (2.70–18.80) | 0.06 |
| | Median | (Min–Max) | Median | (Min–Max) | Median | (Min–Max) | |
| FFQ Carotenoid (µg/day) | | | | | | | |
| α-carotene | 12.78 | (3.67–74.16) | 12.8 | (3.67–74.16) | 12.15 | (4.30–26.89) | 0.88 |
| β-carotene | 57.72 | (11.98–191.3) | 57.65 | (11.98–191.33) | 59.84 | (26.09–98.53) | 0.98 |
| Lycopene | 95.27 | (34.09–194.3) | 89.15 | (34.09–194.28) | 96.11 | (39.27–176.69) | 0.54 |
| Lutein-zeaxanthin | 29.35 | (6.49–72.9) | 30.78 | (6.49–72.89) | 29.11 | (12.35–52.96) | 0.27 |
| Cryptoxanthin | 3.56 | (0.45–9.18) | 3.56 | (0.45–9.18) | 3.42 | (1.00–7.59) | 1 |
| FFQ Vegetables (serves/day) | | | | | | | |
| All | 4.26 | (1.07–9.07) | 4.43 | (1.57–9.07) | 3.94 | (1.07–6.71) | 0.24 |
| FFQ Fruit (serves/day) | | | | | | | |
| All | 2.57 | (0.20–4.71) | 2.57 | (0.20–4.01) | 2.55 | (0.30–4.71) | 0.77 |

p Value indicates differences between weight groups.

## 3. Results

### 3.1. Descriptive Statistics

A total of 38 participants (n = 25, 66% female) from 26 families completed the FFQ and provided a blood sample for plasma carotenoid measurement. Twenty participants (53%) were healthy weight and 18 (47%) were classified as overweight. Twenty nine participants reported having no health conditions; health conditions reported by 9 participants were back pain (n = 3), asthma (n = 3), depression (n = 2), arthritis (n = 2) and one each of anxiety, high blood pressure, low blood pressure, high cholesterol, heart murmur, stent due to cardio-vascular disease, and Crohn's disease. The majority had completed a high school or trade education (n = 34, 89%). Just over half (n = 20, 53%) reported using vitamin supplements. One participant was a current smoker and two were previous smokers. Table 1 reports anthropometric measures for the total sample and by BMI status category (over or under 25), with no significant differences between groups for age, sex, height and fat-free mass (kg).

Mean participant macronutrient intakes indicated that 18% of energy intake was derived from protein, 47% carbohydrate, 31% fat and 12% saturated fat and this did not differ by BMI status category. Mean fruit intake was 2.5 servings/day and 4.4 servings/day for vegetables with no difference by BMI status category.

Mean consumption of orange and yellow vegetables (carrot, pumpkin, sweet potato and corn) was 1.2 serves/day, red vegetables (tomato) 0.5 serves/day and green vegetables (spinach, cabbage and brussel sprouts) <0.5 serves/day with no difference by BMI status category.

Summary statistics for plasma and FFQ carotenoids and intakes of selected FFQ fruit and vegetables by BMI status category are reported in Table 2. While there were no significant differences in dietary carotenoid intakes by BMI status category (all $p$-values >0.2), there were significantly lower concentrations in plasma β-carotene carotenoids for overweight compared to healthy weight ($p = 0.01$), and marginally lower plasma concentrations for α-carotene, lutein-zeaxanthin and cryptoxanthin ($p = 0.05$, 0.05 and 0.06 respectively).

*3.2. Linear Regression Modelling*

Table 3 reports the correlations and partial correlations from multivariate regression models with plasma carotenoids as the response and anthropometrics, FFQ carotenoids and FFQ fruit and vegetable intakes as explanatory variables that were significant at the 5% level.

The correlation between plasma α-carotene concentration and FFQ dietary α-carotene intake was 0.52. FFQ dietary α-carotene was significantly ($p < 0.001$) related to plasma α-carotene concentration, whilst controlling for BMI ($p = 0.007$). For purposes of demonstration, Figure 1 shows estimated mean plasma α-carotene concentration, for an individual with BMI = 22.5 or 28, by α-carotene intake as reported in the FFQ. The strong positive slopes seen in Figure 1 demonstrate that plasma α-carotene increases in line with FFQ α-carotene intakes; more precisely for an increase in FFQ α-carotene intake of 1 mg/day there was a corresponding plasma α-carotene concentration increase of 0.310 mg/mL. The interaction term in the model was not significant, indicating that this relationship does not change with BMI. The model R-squared was 0.34, which was considerably higher than the univariate model containing BMI alone ($R$-squared = 0.11), or that with FFQ α-carotene alone ($R$-squared = 0.26), demonstrating that FFQ α-carotene dietary intake has substantial predictive power beyond that of BMI alone.

The correlation between plasma β-carotene concentration and FFQ dietary β-carotene intake was 0.47, and between plasma β-carotene concentration and FFQ dietary vegetable serves per day was 0.42. Plasma β-carotene was significantly related to FFQ β-carotene and BMI. The $p$-values from the model ($p = 0.001$, $p = 0.018$, respectively) indicated significant relationships between plasma β-carotene and FFQ β-carotene. The R-squared of this model was substantially greater ($R$-squared = 0.31) than for the model that included BMI alone ($R$-squared = 0.14). Figure 2 displays estimated mean plasma and FFQ β-carotene by BMI. More than any of the other plasma carotenoids, plasma β-carotene was significantly related to FFQ total vegetable intake, expressed as number of serves per day ($p = 0.013$), while controlling for fat mass, with $R$-squared equal to 0.25.

**Table 3.** Correlations between Food Frequency Questionnaire carotenoid intake and plasma carotenoid concentrations from multivariable linear regression modelling of plasma carotenoids, controlling for Body Mass Index and fat mass, significant at the 5% level.

| Anthropometric | $p$ | FFQ Intake | $p$ | Model R-squared | FFQ—Plasma Correlation | Correlation 95% CI |
|---|---|---|---|---|---|---|
| | | Plasma α-carotene | | | | |
| | | α-carotene | <0.001 | 0.26 | 0.52 | 0.35, 0.69 |
| BMI | 0.004 | α-carotene | <0.001 | 0.34 | 0.49 | 0.33, 0.64 |
| BMI | 0.001 | | | 0.11 | | |
| | | Plasma β-carotene | | | | |
| | | β-carotene | 0.003 | 0.21 | 0.47 | 0.18, 0.75 |
| | | Veg Serves | 0.007 | 0.17 | 0.42 | 0.12, 0.71 |
| BMI | 0.016 | β-carotene | 0.004 | 0.31 | 0.41 | 0.15, 0.68 |
| Fat mass | 0.013 | Veg Serves | 0.013 | 0.25 | 0.34 | 0.08, 0.61 |
| BMI | 0.004 | | | 0.14 | | |
| Fat mass | 0.003 | | | 0.14 | | |
| | | Plasma Lycopene | | | | |
| | | Lycopene | 0.756 | 0.00 | | |
| | | Plasma Lutein/zeaxanthin | | | | |
| | | Lutein/zeax | 0.041 | 0.09 | 0.26 | 0.01, 0.51 |
| BMI | <0.001 | Lutein/zeax | 0.095 | 0.20 | | |
| BMI | <0.001 | | | 0.14 | | |
| | | Plasma Cryptoxanthin | | | | |
| | | Cryptoxant | 0.236 | 0.08 | | |
| Fat mass | 0.005 | Supplements | 0.003 | 0.35 | | |
| Fat mass | <0.001 | | | 0.22 | | |

The correlation between plasma lutein-zeaxanthin concentration and FFQ dietary lutein-zeaxanthin intake was 0.29. Plasma lutein-zeaxanthin was significantly related to FFQ dietary lutein-zeaxanthin ($p = 0.041$), but the significance level was reduced when BMI was included in the model ($p = 0.095$).

In contrast to the other carotenoids, plasma concentrations of neither lycopene nor cryptoxanthin were significantly correlated with FFQ dietary intake ($p = 0.756, 0.236$, respectively). Lycopene was not significantly related to BMI, waist circumference or fat mass ($p = 0.55, 0.34, 0.16$, respectively).

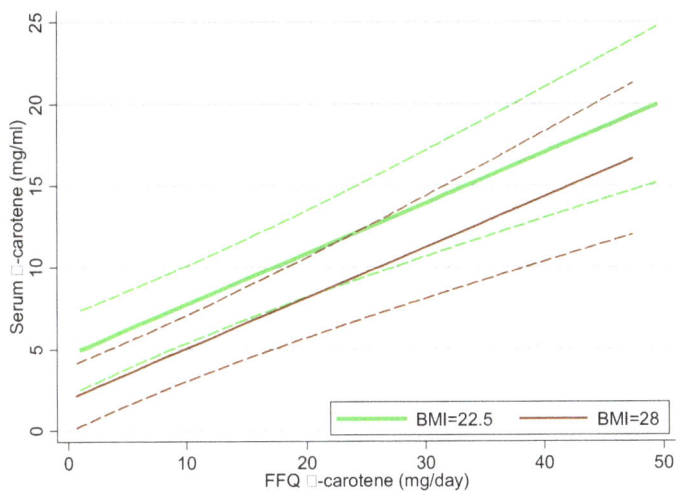

**Figure 1.** Estimated mean plasma α-carotene from multivariate linear regression model on FFQ α-carotene by BMI status, with 95% confidence interval. BMI = 22.5 and BMI = 28 were selected as these were the median BMI for the groups used in descriptive statistics shown Table 2.

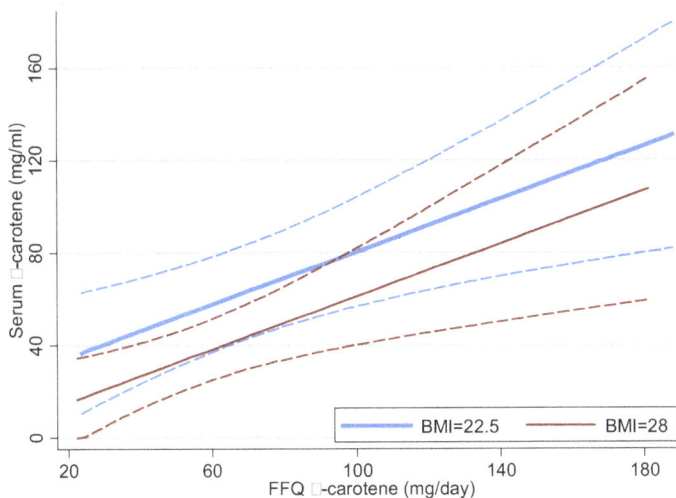

**Figure 2.** Estimate mean plasma β-carotene from multivariate linear regression model on FFQ β-carotene by BMI status, with 95% confidence interval.

Supplement use ($n$ = 20 out of 38 participants) was significantly associated with plasma cryptoxanthin ($p$ = 0.003), whilst controlling for fat mass ($p$ = 0.005), with an $R$-squared of 0.35. There was a negative relationship between plasma cryptoxanthin and fat mass, with plasma concentrations decreasing in line with increasing fat mass, and that supplement users have higher plasma cryptoxanthin. Supplement use was not significantly associated to plasma concentrations for $\alpha$-carotene, $\beta$-carotene, lycopene or lutein-zeaxanthin ($p$ = 0.37, 0.48, 0.20, 0.81, respectively).

Both fat mass and waist circumference were significantly related to plasma carotenoids, although the relationship with waist circumference was less significant, and thus it was not reported. Fat mass significance was reported in this study only if it was substantially greater than that of BMI. No significant relationships were found between any plasma carotenoid and age or sex.

## 4. Discussion

The aim of the current study was to compare plasma carotenoid concentrations, as biomarkers of fruit and vegetable intake, to examine the relative validity of fruit and vegetable intake self-reported using a semi-quantitative FFQ in a sample of adults. Highly significant correlations were found between dietary intake and plasma concentrations for two of the five measured carotenoids, $\alpha$- and $\beta$-carotene. These two are the most abundant carotenoids in the food supply and are primarily found in yellow and orange coloured fruits and vegetables. These foods were consumed commonly in this group, which is similar to another Australian report [19].

A dose-response relationship between food intake and appearance of carotenoids in plasma has been demonstrated by previous researchers in large prospective cohort studies in adults [23] providing support for their use as reliable biomarkers of intake. In the majority of previous studies, correlations between dietary carotenoid intake and plasma carotenoid concentrations have been variable, with correlations ranging from 0.2 to 0.7, and most studies showing statistical significance for at least one of the primary carotenoids measured [10,24,25]. The most commonly reported associations between diet and plasma carotenoids have been with the provitamin A compounds $\alpha$- and $\beta$-carotene and this has been confirmed in the current study. This may be attributed to both these carotenoids, having a higher bioavailability than other fruits and vegetables, as it is not part of a protein complex as in the case when found in green leafy vegetables [26]. A lack of correlation between plasma lycopene and dietary intake of lycopene [9] and fruit and vegetable intake [27] has been previously reported and suggests that not all food high in lycopene were captured by the FFQ or that other variable confound the relationship.

Weight status [19], supplementation [28] and smoking status [29] have been previously shown to influence plasma carotenoids concentrations in humans, and thus need to be accounted for when estimating the relationship between plasma carotenoids and food intake. In the current sample one person was a smoker and two were previous smokers so no effect of smoking could reliably be estimated. The impact of supplement use assessed in the current study was found to only significantly influence plasma levels for cryptoxanthin. This may be because dietary sources high in cryptoxanthin such as orange rind and papaya are not as frequently consumed, and are often in much smaller concentrations compared with other carotenoids including α and β-carotene. Previous studies have found supplements to have a general influence across a range of carotenoids rather than a specific one such as only cryptoxanthin as in the current study, although differences between supplement and non-supplement users have mixed [9,30].

The relationships between carotenoid concentrations and BMI found in this study concur with other studies in adults and children that suggest there may be a physiological mechanisms operating. For example, as BMI increases circulating carotenoids reduce secondary to increased utilization [31], or there may be differences in absorption and metabolism secondary to higher weight status [19,23,32].

A limitation of the current study was the small sample size and thus a possibly small variation in intakes. Also, the relatively small number of foods in the nutritional database used, although this is comparable with other dietary validation studies in adults [33]. Carotenoid databases available currently for use in estimating dietary intakes of carotenoids are not comprehensive and although the USDA database used in this study [17] was updated in 2006 there were still only 40 of the 120 items in the AES FFQ that have been evaluated for carotenoid content. However this was superior to the current Australian database which is even more limited, with approximately only 25 of the foods from the AES FFQ having values estimated. This limitation is likely to have reduced the likelihood of detecting relationships between dietary intakes and plasma carotenoid concentrations as significant. While the US carotenoid data values may not completely reflect current Australian food values, at the time of analysis it was the most comprehensive database of fruit and vegetable intake internationally.

A strength of the current study is that is demonstrates the approach to using a plasma biomarker as an independent assessment of dietary intake, in this case plasma carotenoids, dietary carotenoids and dietary fruit and vegetable intake. This approach can be used to guide researchers in the design of other such studies.

## 5. Conclusions

In conclusion, the results of the current study demonstrate that carotenoid intakes, as assessed by the AES FFQ are significantly related to plasma carotenoid concentrations of α-carotene, β-carotene and lutein/zeaxanthin, the carotenoids commonly found in fruit and vegetables. Lower levels of all plasma carotenoids, except lycopene, were found in individuals with higher BMI. We conclude that the AES can be used to measure fruit and vegetable intakes with confidence.

**Acknowledgments:** Hannah Lucas, Janne Beelen and Kristine Pezdirc for assistance with recruitment. Lisa Wood and Rebecca Williams for conducting the analysis of plasma carotenoids. The authors acknowledge the families who participated in the study as well as the research assistants involved in data collection and data entry. The current study was supported by funding from Meat and Livestock Australia (grant number G1000577).

**Author Contributions:** Clare E. Collins and Tracy L. Burrows designed the study. May M. Boggess and Maya Guest performed the statistical analysis. Tracy L. Burrows, Melinda J. Hutchesson, Megan E. Rollo and Clare E. Collins drafted the manuscript. All authors approve of the final manuscript.

**Conflicts of Interest:** The authors declare no conflict of interest.

## References

1. Dauchet, L.; Amouyel, P.; Hercberg, S.; Dallongeville, J. Fruit and vegetable consumption and risk of coronary heart disease: A meta-analysis of cohort studies. *J. Nutr.* **2006**, *136*, 2588–2593.

2. He, F.J.; Nowson, C.A.; Lucas, M.; MacGregor, G.A. Increased consumption of fruit and vegetables is related to a reduced risk of coronary heart disease: Meta-analysis of cohort studies. *J. Hum. Hypertens.* **2007**, *21*, 717–728.

3. Dauchet, L.; Amouyel, P.; Dallongeville, J. Fruit and vegetable consumption and risk of stroke: A meta-analysis of cohort studies. *Neurology* **2005**, *65*, 1193–1197.

4. He, F.J.; Nowson, C.A.; MacGregor, G.A. Fruit and vegetable consumption and stroke: Meta-analysis of cohort studies. *Lancet* **2006**, *367*, 320–326.

5. Villegas, R.; Shu, X.O.; Gao, Y.T.; Yang, G.; Elasy, T.; Li, H.; Zheng, W. Vegetable but not fruit consumption reduces the risk of type 2 diabetes in Chinese women. *J. Nutr.* **2008**, *138*, 574–580.

6. Hamer, M.; Chida, Y. Intake of fruit, vegetables, and antioxidants and risk of type 2 diabetes: Systematic review and meta-analysis. *J. Hypertens.* **2007**, *25*, 2361–2369.

7. Park, J.Y.; Vollset, S.E.; Melse-Boonstra, A.; Chajes, V.; Ueland, P.M.; Slimani, N. Dietary intake and biological measurement of folate: A qualitative review of validation studies. *Mol. Nutr. Food Res.* **2013**, *57*, 562–581.

8. Preis, S.R.; Spiegelman, D.; Zhao, B.B.; Moshfegh, A.; Baer, D.J.; Willett, W.C. Application of a repeat-measure biomarker measurement error model to 2 validation studies: Examination of the effect of within-person variation in biomarker measurements. *Am. J. Epidemiol.* **2011**, *173*, 683–694.

9. Andersen, L.F.; Veierød, M.B.; Johansson, L.; Sakhi, A.; Solvoll, K.; Drevon, C.A. Evaluation of three dietary assessment methods and serum biomarkers as measures of fruit and vegetable intake, using the method of triads. *Br. J. Nutr.* **2005**, *93*, 519–527.

10. McNaughton, S.; Marks, G.; Gaffney, P.; Williams, G.; Green, A. Validation of a food frequency questionnaire assessment of carotenoid and vitamin E intake using weighed food records and plasma biomarkers: The method of triads model. *Eur. J. Clin. Nutr.* **2005**, *59*, 211–218.

11. Block, G.; Norkus, E.; Hudes, M.; Mandel, S.; Helzlsouer, K. Which plasma antioxidants are most related to fruit and vegetable consumption? *Am. J. Epidemiol.* **2001**, *154*, 1113–1118.
12. Campbell, D.; Gross, M.; Martini, M.; Grandits, G.; Slavin, J.; Potter, J. Plasma carotenoids as biomarkers of vegetable and fruit intake. *Cancer Epidem. Biomar.* **1994**, *3*, 493–500.
13. Collins, C.; Burrows, T.; Truby, H.; Morgan, P.; Wright, I.; Davies, P.; Callister, R. Comparison of energy intake in toddlers assessed by food frequency questionnaire and total energy expenditure measured by the doubly labeled water method. *J. Acad. Nutr. Diet.* **2013**, *113*, 459–463.
14. Collins, C.; Watson, J.; Guest, M.; Boggess, M.; Duncanson, K.; Pezdirc, K.; Rollo, M.; Hutchesson, M.; Burrows, T. Reproducibility and comparative validity of a food frequency questionnaire for adults. *Clin. Nutr.* **2014**, *33*, 906–914.
15. Burrows, T.; Truby, H.; Morgan, P.; Callister, R.; Davies, P.; Collins, C. A comparison and validation of child *versus* parent reporting of children's energy intake using food frequency questionnaires *versus* food records: Who's an accurate reporter? *Clin. Nutr.* **2013**, *32*, 613–618.
16. Australian Bureau of Statistics. *National Nutrition Survey: Nutrient Intakes and Physical Measurements*; Australian Bureau of Statistics: Canberra, Australia, 1998.
17. Chug-Ahuja, J.; Holden, J.; Forman, M.; Reed Mangels, A.; Beecher, G.; Lanza, E. The development and application of a carotenoid database for fruits, vegetables and selected multi-component foods. *J. Am. Diet. Assoc.* **1993**, *93*, 318–323.
18. Barua, A.; Kostic, D.; Olsen, J. New simplified procedures for the extraction and simultaneous high-performance liquid chromatographic analysis of retinol, tocopherols, and carotenoids in human serum. *J. Chromatogr. B* **1993**, *617*, 257–264.
19. Burrows, T.; Warren, J.; Colyvas, K.; Garg, M.; Collins, C. Validation of overweight children's fruit and vegetable intake using plasma carotenoids. *Obesity* **2009**, *17*, 162–168.
20. Reitman, A.; Friedrich, I.; Ben-Amotz, A.; Levy, Y. Low plasma antioxidants and normal plasma B vitamins and homocysteine in patients with severe obesity. *Isr. Med. Assoc. J.* **2002**, *4*, 590–593.
21. Williams, R. A note on robust variance estimation for cluster-correlated data. *Biometrics* **2000**, *56*, 645–646.
22. StataCorp LP. *Stata MP*, version 12; Stata Statistical Software: College Station, TX, USA, 2012.
23. Al-Delaimy, W.; van Kappel, A.; Ferrari, P.; Slimani, N.; Steghens, J.; Bingham, S.; Johansson, I.; Wallstrom, P.; Overvad, K.; Tionneland, A.; *et al.* Plasma carotenoids as biomarkers of intake of fruits and vegetables: Ecological level correlations in the European Prospective Investigation into Caner and Nutrition (EPIC). *Eur. J. Clin. Nutr.* **2005**, *59*, 1397–1408.
24. Eliassen, A.; Hendrickson, S.; Brinton, L.; Buring, J.; Campos, H.; Dai, Q.; Dorgan, J.; Franke, A.; Gao, Y.; Goodman, M. Circulating carotenoids and risk of breast cancer: Pooled analysis of eight prospective studies. *J. Natl. Cancer Inst.* **2012**, *104*, 1905–1916.

25. Svilaas, A.; Sakhi, A.; Andersen, L.; Svilaas, T.; Ström, E.; Jacobs, D.; Ose, L.; Blomhoff, R. Intakes of antioxidants in coffee, wine, vegetables are correlated with plasma carotenoids in humans. *J. Nutr.* **2003**, *134*, 562–587.

26. Castenmiller, J.; West, C. Bioavailability and bioconversion of carotenoids. *Annu. Rev. Nutr.* **1998**, *18*, 19–38.

27. Coyne, T.; Ibiebele, T.I.; Baade, P.D.; Dobson, A.; McClintock, C.; Dunn, S.; Leonard, D.; Shaw, J. Diabetes mellitus and serum carotenoids: Findings of a population-based study in Queensland, Australia. *Am. J. Clin. Nutr.* **2005**, *82*, 685–693.

28. Satia, J.; Watters, J.; Galanko, J. Validation of an antioxidant nutrient questionnaire in whites and African Americans. *J. Am. Diet. Assoc.* **2009**, *109*, 502–508.

29. Coates, R.; Eley, J.; Block, G.; Gunter, E.; Sowell, A.; Grossman, C.; Greenberg, R. An evaluation of a Food Frequency Questionnaire for assessing dietary intake of specific carotenoids and vitamin E among low income black women. *Am. J. Epidemiol.* **1991**, *134*, 658–670.

30. Goodman, G.; Thornquist, M.; Kestin, M.; Methc, B.; Anderson, G.; Omenn, G. The association between participant characteristics and serum concentrations of beta-carotene, retinol, retinyl palmitate, and alpha-tocopherol among participants in the Carotene and Retinol Efficacy Trial (CARET) for prevention of lung cancer. *Cancer Epidem. Biomar.* **1996**, *5*, 815–821.

31. Molnar, D.; Decsi, T.; Koletzko, B. Reduced antioxidant status in obese children with multi-metabolic syndrome. *Int. J. Obesity* **2004**, *28*, 1197–1202.

32. Chung, H.-Y.; Ferreira, A.L.A.; Epstein, S.; Paiva, S.A.; Castaneda-Sceppa, C.; Johnson, E.J. Site-specific concentrations of carotenoids in adipose tissue: Relations with dietary and serum carotenoid concentrations in healthy adults. *Am. J. Clin. Nutr.* **2009**, *90*, 533–539.

33. Michaud, D.S.; Giovannucci, E.L.; Ascherio, A.; Rimm, E.B.; Forman, M.R.; Sampson, L.; Willett, W.C. Associations of plasma carotenoid concentrations and dietary intake of specific carotenoids in samples of two prospective cohort studies using a new carotenoid database. *Cancer Epidemiol. Biomarkers Prev.* **1998**, *7*, 283–290.

# Biochemical Validation of the Older Australian's Food Frequency Questionnaire Using Carotenoids and Vitamin E

**Jun S. Lai, John Attia, Mark McEvoy and Alexis J. Hure**

**Abstract:** Background: Validation of a food frequency questionnaire (FFQ) is important, as inaccurate and imprecise information may affect the association between dietary exposure and health outcomes. Objective: This study assessed the validity of the Older Australian's FFQ against plasma carotenoids and Vitamin E. Methods: A random subsample ($n = 150$) of 2420 participants in the Hunter Community Study, aged 55–85 years, were included. Correlations between crude and energy-adjusted FFQ estimates of carotenoids, Vitamin E, and fruit and vegetables with corresponding biomarkers were determined. Percentages of participants correctly classified in the same quartile, and in the same $\pm 1$ quartile, by the two methods were calculated. Results: Significant correlations ($P < 0.05$) were observed for $\alpha$-carotene ($r = 0.26$–$0.28$), $\beta$-carotene ($r = 0.21$–$0.25$), and $\beta$-cryptoxanthin ($r = 0.21$–$0.23$). Intakes of fruits and vegetables also showed similar correlations with these plasma carotenoids. Lycopene was only significantly correlated with fruit and vegetable intakes ($r = 0.19$–$0.23$). Weak correlations were observed for lutein + zeaxanthin ($r = 0.12$–$0.16$). For Vitamin E, significant correlation was observed for energy-adjusted FFQ estimate and biomarker ($r = 0.20$). More than 68% of individuals were correctly classified within the same or adjacent quartile, except for lutein + zeaxanthin. Conclusion: With the exception of lutein + zeaxanthin, the Older Australian's FFQ provides reasonable rankings for individuals according to their carotenoids, Vitamin E, fruit and vegetable intakes.

Reprinted from *Nutrients*. Cite as: Lai, J.S.; Attia, J.; McEvoy, M.; Hure, A.J. Biochemical Validation of the Older Australian's Food Frequency Questionnaire Using Carotenoids and Vitamin E. *Nutrients* **2014**, *6*, 4906–4917.

## 1. Introduction

A number of methods are used to measure dietary intake in epidemiological research including dietary recalls, food records, and food frequency questionnaires (FFQs) [1]. Of these, dietary recalls and food records are considered more precise, but they are limited in that they only measure short-term dietary intake. However, FFQs provide dietary data over a longer period of time [1], which in nutritional epidemiologic research is more important than intake on a few specific days. A number of FFQs have been developed to measure dietary intake among Australian adults [2–4]. Considering the fact that older people may differ in dietary habits and food patterns from younger adults [5], existing FFQs should be adapted to reflect these differences, and/or validated in older populations.

FFQs are often criticised for having a large number of measurement errors [1]. Consequently, much research has been concerned with the relative performance of FFQs in estimating dietary intake. Most studies have validated FFQs against food records or dietary recall [2,3], but self-reporting bias remains. Alternatively, biochemical indicators (or biomarkers) can act as objective measures in the validation of nutrient intake, as the errors recorded are assumed to be independent of self-report [1]. The body of literature on the performance of FFQs in older populations is relatively small, and validation against biochemical indicators is scarce. To date, we identified only one FFQ, developed by the Blue Mountains Eye Study (BMES), to measure dietary intake among older community-dwelling adults in Australia, which has been previously validated against 4-day food records [3]. In this study, we will further assess the validity of this FFQ against more objective biochemical indicators, using a sub-population of older Australian adults from the Hunter Community Study (HCS).

With increasing evidence that high intakes of fruits and vegetables are associated with better health outcomes [6,7], it is important that the FFQ used adequately captures these foods among the population of interest. The protective effects of fruit and vegetables may be due to their antioxidant properties. Nutrients such as carotenoids and Vitamin E have the ability to reduce inflammation and prevent free radical damage, all of which have been shown to play important functions in the biology of ageing [8,9]. Furthermore, concentrations of carotenoids and Vitamin E in blood are considered reliable markers of dietary intake [1] and have been previously used in a number of dietary validation studies [10–12]. Hence, this study aims to compare the dietary intakes of carotenoids and Vitamin E, estimated by Older Australian's FFQs, against plasma biomarkers, in a sample of 150 HCS participants.

## 2. Methods

### 2.1. Validation Quality

This study was developed based on the EURopean micronutrient RECommendations Aligned Network of Excellence (EURRECA) scoring system of a good quality validation study [13], scoring a total of 4 out of 7 points. The allocation of points was as follows: (1) 0.5 points for non-homogenous sample, and 0.5 points for a sample size of >50; (2) 1.5 points for reporting crude and energy-adjusted correlation coefficients, and including statistics to assess classification; and (3) 1.5 points for including supplements intake.

## 2.2. Subjects

The study subjects were drawn from the HCS. The HCS is a population based cohort study of adults aged 55–85 years residing in Newcastle, New South Wales state, randomly selected from the state's electoral roll [14]. Recruitment began in December 2004 and ended in December 2007. A total of 3253 individuals participated in the study. All participants were required to attend a clinical assessment, provide a blood sample and complete a series of self-administered questionnaires including Older Australian's FFQs [14]. Full methodological details have been published previously [14]. The HCS has received ethics approval from the University of Newcastle Research Ethics Committee (H-820-0504), and all participants provided written informed consent.

To be included in this study, participants needed to have completed the FFQ ($n$ = 3022) and provided a blood sample at baseline with enough volume for analysis ($n$ = 2534). Participants with more than 25 missing values or an entire blank page in their FFQ ($n$ = 132) were excluded from the final dataset. A subset of 150 subjects was selected from the remaining 2420 HCS participants. Stratified random sampling using computer-generated sequence was used to select 30 participants from each quintile of total energy intake, and ensuring an equal representation across gender and age groups (<65, 65+). A participant selection flow diagram is presented in Figure 1.

## 2.3. Food Frequency Questionnaire

Dietary intake was assessed by a self-administered, 145-item semi-quantitative FFQ [3], modified from the version developed by Willett [15], specifically for use with older Australians participating in the BMES [3]. The BMES previously validated this FFQ against 4-day weighed food records and demonstrated reasonable validity (*i.e.*, $r \geq 0.5$ for most nutrients including $r = 0.49$ for β-carotene; and $\geq 70\%$ correctly classified within same ± 1 quintile) [3]. Participants were required to indicate their usual frequency of foods consumed in the past year, with nine categorical frequency options, ranging from never to four or more times per day. Open-ended questions were included on the type of fruit juices, breakfast cereal, and other frequently consumed foods that were not included in the list. The FFQ also assessed dietary supplement usage. Participants completed the FFQ within three months of their blood collection. Dietary intake of carotenoids and Vitamin E was calculated using the US Department of Agriculture (USDA) data [16], and other nutrient intakes were derived from NUTTAB 2006, an Australian nutrient composition database [17]. Servings of fruits and vegetables were defined based on the Australian Dietary Guidelines (e.g., one serving of fruit = 150 g or 1 medium-sized fruit; one serving of vegetables = 75 g or $\frac{1}{2}$ cup cooked vegetables) [18]. Nutrient supplement information was obtained from manufacturers and added to the database. Approximately 2% of all FFQs were re-entered into the Food Works 2009, version 6 [19], by an Accredited Practicing Dietitian who was blinded to the original FFQ data entry to check for errors. Only minor discrepancies were observed and rectified prior to data analysis.

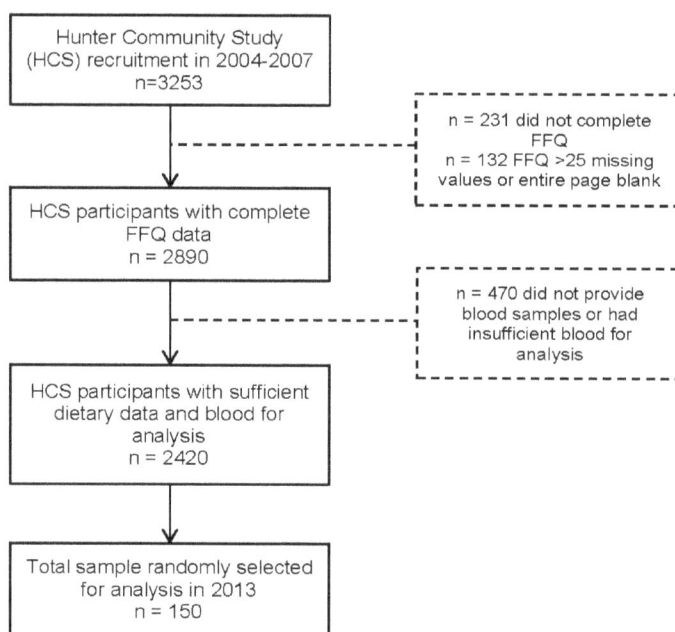

**Figure 1.** Participant flow diagram for a validation study of food frequency questionnaire (FFQ) estimated intakes against biomarkers.

## 2.4. Biomarkers Assays

The biomarkers included in this study were plasma concentrations of $\alpha$-carotene, $\beta$-carotene, $\beta$-cryptoxanthin, lycopene, lutein + zeaxanthin, and vitamin E ($\alpha$-tocopherol). The plasma and FFQ estimates of lutein and zeaxanthin are shown combined (lutein + zeaxanthin) because both the nutrient database and biochemical analysis combine lutein and zeaxanthin. Fasting venous blood was obtained using standard venepuncture techniques. All blood samples were centrifuged and stored in approximately 1 mL aliquots, cryopreserved in dimethyl sulfoxide (DMSO) at $-80^\circ$C immediately after collection [14]. These blood samples had been stored at $-80^\circ$C for approximately seven years at the time of assay, and were thawed immediately prior to analysis. Plasma carotenoids concentrations were determined using the high performance liquid chromatography method [20]. Measurements of red blood cell (RBC) folate concentration was carried out using the chemiluminescent immunoassay analyser (Access® Immunoassay Systems, Beckman Coulter, Inc., CA, USA) [21]. However, it was subsequently determined that DMSO had likely affected the integrity of RBC membrane, reducing the accuracy of the folate concentration. Therefore, subsequent results and discussion will focus on carotenoids and Vitamin E only.

*2.5. Statistical Analysis*

Dietary intakes were expressed as absolute amounts and as energy-adjusted intakes. Energy-adjusted intakes were computed for individual carotenoids, Vitamin E, servings of fruits and vegetables, using the residual method [22]. Adjusting for total energy intake accounts for between-person variation in total energy intake as a result of physiological differences such as body size and physical activity [22], thus reducing the potentially confounding effects of total energy intake. As the distribution of dietary intakes and biomarkers were skewed, Spearman rank correlation coefficients were used in all correlation analyses, unless otherwise specified. The significance level was set at $P < 0.05$. Aside from comparing individual dietary intakes of carotenoids and Vitamin E to their respective plasma biomarkers, fruit and vegetable intakes were also compared to each plasma carotenoid. Intakes of fruits and vegetables were restricted to those that contributed $\geq 5\%$ of daily mean intake for each carotenoid (e.g., carrot and pumpkin intakes to plasma $\alpha$-carotene). We did not compare intakes of fruits and vegetables to plasma Vitamin E, because Vitamin E comes from more diverse sources than each of the carotenoids.

Linear regression analyses were performed to identify potential confounders. Plasma carotenoids and Vitamin E were modelled as the dependent variables and the corresponding FFQ estimated intakes as the independent variables. This was performed using log-transformed values to comply with the assumptions for normality. The following variables were tested as potential confounders: age groups, gender, smoking status, body mass index (BMI) categories, medication use, supplement use and alcohol consumption. The significance level was set at $P < 0.05$.

Dietary intakes estimated by the FFQ and biomarkers were classified into quartiles to determine the ability of both methods to rank individuals. Percentages were calculated for participants correctly classified into the same quartile and within the adjacent quartile. All statistical analyses were performed using Stata, version 11 [23].

## 3. Results

Characteristics of the sampled subjects, along with their average daily nutrient intake values from the FFQ and measured biomarkers are presented in Table 1. The participants' ages ranged from 55–85 years. Stratified random sampling ensured a similar proportion of males and females. Mean BMI was 28.5 kg/m² indicating a high proportion of overweight and obesity, which is consistent with the broader Australian population of this age [24]. Only 6% of the sample currently smoked but many more were former smokers (41.3%). A large proportion of the sample

(78.6%) was taking at least one prescription medication, which is not surprising for an older population. Approximately 12% of the subjects reported taking supplements containing Vitamin A (including carotenoids) and/or Vitamin E. Approximately 63% of participants reported consuming alcoholic beverages at least once a week.

**Table 1.** Characteristics of Hunter Community Study participants ($n$ = 150) in a dietary validation study.

| Characteristics | |
|---|---|
| Age (years), mean ± SD | 66.2 ± 7.3 |
| Gender, $n$ (%) | |
| Male | 77 (51.3%) |
| Female | 73 (48.7%) |
| Body Mass Index, kg/m$^2$ | 28.5 ± 4.8 |
| Smoking status [a], $n$ (%) | |
| Non-smoker | 73 (48.7%) |
| Ex-smoker | 62 (41.3%) |
| Current smoker | 9 (6%) |
| Current use of medication, $n$ (%) | 118 (78.6%) |
| Supplement use, $n$ (%) | |
| Multivitamin [b] | 15 (10%) |
| Vitamin E only | 3 (2%) |
| Alcohol intake, $n$ (%) | |
| None | 55 (36.7%) |
| ≥1 drink/week | 95 (63.3%) |
| FFQ estimated nutrient intake, mean ± SD | |
| α-carotene, μg/day | 1810 ± 1499 |
| β-carotene, μg/day | 8449 ± 5005 |
| β-cryptoxanthin, μg/day | 590 ± 372 |
| Lycopene, μg/day | 6457 ± 6276 |
| Lutein + zeaxanthin, μg/day | 4026 ± 2538 |
| Vitamin E, mg/day | 5.8 ± 2.3 |
| FFQ estimated fruit + vegetable intakes, mean ± SD | |
| α-carotene sources, servings/day | 0.8 ± 0.6 |
| β-carotene sources, servings/day | 2.8 ± 1.4 |
| β-cryptoxanthin sources, servings/day | 2.2 ± 1.3 |
| Lycopene sources, servings/day | 0.8 ± 0.6 |
| Lutein + zeaxanthin sources, servings/day | 2.2 ± 0.9 |
| Plasma concentration, mean ± SD | |
| α-carotene, mg/L | 0.07 ± 0.06 |
| β-carotene, mg/L | 0.35 ± 0.40 |
| β-cryptoxanthin, mg/L | 0.14 ± 0.12 |
| Lycopene, mg/L | 0.29 ± 0.14 |
| Lutein + zeaxanthin, mg/L | 0.47 ± 0.27 |
| Vitamin E, mg/L | 13.61 ± 4.08 |

[a] $n$ = 6 did not report smoking status; [b] Multivitamin supplements containing carotenoids and Vitamin E.

Carrots and pumpkins were the main contributors to α-carotene intake. Sources of β-carotene included apricots or peaches, cantaloupe, broccoli, carrots, spinach or silverbeet, lettuce, peas, pumpkin, sweet potato. Intake of β-cryptoxanthin was from paw-paw, orange, pumpkin, apricots or peaches, carrots and corn. Lycopene was predominantly from tomato and tomato products, but also included watermelon and grapefruit. Lutein and zeaxanthin were mainly from dark green vegetables such as broccoli, brussel sprout, spinach or silverbeet, lettuce, and beans, peas, corn and pumpkin.

Results from linear regression showed that age, gender, smoking status, BMI, medication use, supplement use and alcohol consumption had little effect on correlation coefficients. As such, the correlation coefficients were only reported for crude intakes and energy-adjusted intakes.

Correlations between FFQ estimated intakes of individual carotenoids, Vitamin E, fruit and vegetables, and plasma concentrations are presented in Table 2. Both crude and adjusted correlations were significant for α-carotene ($r = 0.26$ and $0.28$), β-carotene ($r = 0.21$ and $0.25$) and β-cryptoxanthin ($r = 0.21$ and $0.23$). Energy-adjusted Vitamin E intake yielded a stronger correlation with plasma concentration ($r = 0.20$) compared to crude intake ($r = 0.08$). In contrast, weak correlations were observed for lycopene and lutein + zeaxanthin. Intakes of fruits and vegetables showed significant correlations with plasma α-carotene ($r = 0.23$ and $0.25$) and β-carotene ($r = 0.20$ and $0.25$), respectively. Interestingly, correlations between fruit and vegetable intakes, and plasma β-cryptoxanthin ($r = 0.31$ and $0.36$) and lycopene ($r = 0.19$ and $0.23$) were much higher than the corresponding nutrient intakes. Plasma lutein + zeaxanthin was weakly correlated with fruit and vegetable intakes ($r = 0.11$ and $0.14$).

**Table 2.** Correlations and 95% CI between FFQ estimated intakes and biomarkers.

| | Individual Nutrient Intakes | | | | Fruit and Vegetable Intakes | | | |
|---|---|---|---|---|---|---|---|---|
| | $r_{crude}$ [a] | 95% CI | $r_{adj}$ [b] | 95% CI | $r_{crude}$ [a] | 95% CI | $r_{adj}$ [b] | 95% CI |
| α-carotene | 0.26 [c] | 0.10, 0.38 | 0.28 [c] | 0.12, 0.42 | 0.23 [c] | 0.07, 0.38 | 0.25 [c] | 0.08, 0.39 |
| β-carotene | 0.21 [d] | 0.04, 0.35 | 0.25 [c] | 0.08, 0.39 | 0.20 [d] | 0.04, 0.36 | 0.25 [c] | 0.08, 0.38 |
| β-cryptoxanthin | 0.21 [d] | 0.04, 0.36 | 0.23 [c] | 0.07, 0.38 | 0.31 [c] | 0.16, 0.45 | 0.36 [c] | 0.21, 0.50 |
| Lycopene | 0.13 | −0.04, 0.27 | 0.17 | −0.01, 0.32 | 0.19 [d] | 0.02, 0.34 | 0.23 [c] | 0.07, 0.38 |
| Lutein + zeaxanthin | 0.12 | −0.05, 0.25 | 0.16 | −0.01, 0.31 | 0.11 | −0.01, 0.30 | 0.14 | −0.03, 0.27 |
| Vitamin E | 0.08 | −0.07, 0.24 | 0.20 [d] | 0.04, 0.36 | | | n/a [e] | |

[a] Spearman rank correlation using crude intakes and plasma biomarkers; [b] Spearman rank correlation using energy-adjusted intakes and plasma biomarkers; [c] $P<0.01$; [d] $P<0.05$; [e] No comparison made between plasma Vitamin E and fruit and vegetables because Vitamin E had more diverse sources.

Quartile agreements between individual nutrient intakes and their respective blood concentrations were in the range of 24%–31% for correctly classified within the same quartile and 62%–72% for correctly classified within the same or adjacent quartile (Table 3). Extremely low quartile agreements were observed for lutein + zeaxanthin. For fruit and vegetable intakes, quartile agreements were similar to those comparing individual carotenoid intakes. However, quartile agreements for fruit and vegetable intakes and β-cryptoxanthin were much higher (>34% within same quartile and >74% within the same/adjacent quartile).

**Table 3.** Agreement (%) between quartiles of FFQ estimated intakes and biomarkers.

| | Individual Nutrient Intakes | | | | Fruit and Vegetable Intakes | | | |
|---|---|---|---|---|---|---|---|---|
| | Crude [a] | | Energy-Adjusted [b] | | Crude [a] | | Energy-Adjusted [b] | |
| | Same | Adjacent | Same | Adjacent | Same | Adjacent | Same | Adjacent |
| α-carotene | 30 | 70 | 30 | 72 | 30 | 68 | 32 | 69 |
| β-carotene | 28 | 69 | 31 | 72 | 29 | 70 | 30 | 72 |
| β-crytoxanthin | 30 | 68 | 28 | 71 | 34 | 74 | 40 | 75 |
| Lycopene | 29 | 68 | 30 | 72 | 34 | 71 | 32 | 74 |
| Lutein + zeaxanthin | 24 | 62 | 24 | 65 | 22 | 62 | 21 | 62 |
| Vitamin E | 28 | 67 | 28 | 70 | | n/a[c] | | |

[a] Percentage correctly classified using crude intakes and plasma biomarkers; [b] Percentage correctly classified using energy-adjusted intakes and plasma biomarkers; [c] No comparison made between plasma Vitamin E and fruit and vegetables because Vitamin E had more diverse sources.

## 4. Discussion

This study determined the relative validity of the Older Australian's FFQs used in the BMES and HCS by comparing self-reported dietary carotenoid and Vitamin E intakes with more objective plasma biomarkers. Overall, we found that this FFQ performed reasonably well in assessing intakes of carotenoids, Vitamin E, and fruit and vegetables. Although all correlations presented were modest in magnitude ($\leq$0.36), they were comparable to those noted by other validation studies conducted in populations across Australia [10,11] and other countries [12,25–27]. More than 68% of individuals were correctly classified within the same or adjacent quartile, based on all nutrients assessed, with the exception of lutein + zeaxanthin.

We identified two other recent FFQ and biomarker validation studies conducted in Australia [10,11]. One of these studies was the validation study for the commercially available Dietary Questionnaire for Epidemiological Study used in a number of large epidemiological studies, including the Melbourne Collaborative Cohort Study, the Australian Prostate Cancer Family Study, and the Australian Longitudinal Study of Women's Health [28]. The correlations between dietary and plasma α-carotene and lycopene in our study were only slightly lower compared to these other two studies where correlations for α-carotene ranged between 0.35 and 0.47 and for lycopene ranged between0.19 and 0.28 [10,11]. Our correlations for β-carotene, β-cryptoxanthin and lutein + zeaxanthin were within the ranges reported in the two Australian studies (β-carotene: 0.22–0.28; β-cryptoxanthin: −0.002–0.46; lutein + zeaxanthin: 0.03–0.29).When we compared our results to four other FFQ-biomarker validation studies conducted in the United States of America, similar correlations were observed, althoughβ-cryptoxanthin showed a stronger correlation in the American studies [12,25–27]. These studies reported correlations as follows: α-carotene 0.18–0.35, β-carotene 0.25–0.36, β-cryptoxanthin 0.32–0.45, lycopene 0.002–0.37, lutein + zeaxanthin 0.10–0.47. A stronger correlation between energy-adjusted Vitamin E intake and plasma concentration was observed in our study ($r = 0.20$), compared to these other six studies which reported correlations of 0.05–0.07 for Vitamin E [10–12,25–27].

Plasma levels of carotenoids were significantly correlated with fruit and vegetable intakes except for lutein + zeaxanthin.   The observed correlation coefficients were also similar to other studies (α-carotene: 0.23–0.25; β-carotene: 0.13–0.29; β-cryptoxanthin: 0.17–0.35; lycopene: 0.06–0.21; lutein + zeaxanthin: 0.05–0.18) [12,29], indicating that fruit and vegetable intakes are reasonably well measured by the Older Australian's FFQs and comparable to other FFQs [12,29]. In fact, plasma β-cryptoxanthin and lycopene were more strongly correlated with fruit and vegetable intakes than with individual nutrients. A similar pattern was observed in another study that examined the correlation between plasma carotenoids and fruit and vegetable intakes [12]. Tucker et al. (1999) found that correlations were strongest for β-cryptoxanthin followed by lycopene, and the lowest correlation was observed for lutein + zeaxanthin [12].

Our study did not identify any important confounding variables. However, the study may have been under-powered for sub-group analyses and there could be other factors not accounted for, such as cholesterol levels in blood, which other studies have adjusted for [10–12]. Adjusting for these factors could potentially improve the correlations.

Quartile agreements between dietary intakes and plasma concentrations further demonstrated that the Older Australian's FFQs performed well in ranking individuals according to their carotenoid and Vitamin E intakes. As biomarkers are not a measure of absolute intake, the ability to rank individuals according to their consumption is more important [1]. Apart from lutein + zeaxanthin, the percentages of participants correctly classified within the same quartile, and within the same or adjacent quartile for carotenoids and Vitamin E were comparable to those observed in other studies (>25% within same quartile or >65% within same or adjacent quartile) [12,29]. A much lower quartile agreement was observed for lutein + zeaxanthin. Quartile agreement comparing fruit and vegetable intakes rather than individual carotenoid intakes showed similar results, indicating that simply measuring fruit and vegetable intakes provides a reasonable ranking. Subsequent studies examining the effects of nutrition on health outcomes can be confident that this FFQ not only has the ability to accurately capture individual carotenoid intakes but it is also a good measure of fruit and vegetable intakes.

The advantage of this validation method is that the error associated with biomarkers is unlikely to be associated with the error in self-report measures, thus offering an objective measure of nutrient intake [1]. Furthermore, our study methods comply with that of the EURRECCA scoring system, meeting the criteria of a good quality validation study [13]. The strength of this FFQ is that it is developed specifically for an older population and twice validated; firstly against weighed food records in the BMES [3] and now against nutritional biomarkers in the HCS. Validation against weighed food records demonstrated acceptable reproducibility and validity. The current study further demonstrates reasonable validityin reference to nutritional biomarkers, showing that this FFQ is useful in ranking individuals according to their consumption. However, due to the weaker correlation and low quartile agreements for lutein + zeaxanthin, we are less confident of the ability of this FFQ to measure intake of this nutrient.

## 5. Conclusions

In conclusion, results from the current study, together with findings from previous validation against weighed food records, indicate that the Older Australian's FFQs can reasonably rank individuals according to their consumption of carotenoids (with the exception of lutein + zeaxanthin), Vitamin E, fruit and vegetables. Future studies can use this FFQ to collect dietary data from the older population knowing that it has acceptable validity.

**Acknowledgments:** We thank Paul Mitchell and Victoria Flood of the Blue Mountains Eye Study for permission to use their food frequency questionnaire. Grateful acknowledgements to Narelle Eddington and Lynn Clark at the Hunter Area Pathology Service, and Lisa Wood and Michelle Wong-Brown at the University of Newcastle, for their assistance with the biomarker assays. Thanks are also extended to Stephen Hancock for his assistance in the development of the nutrient-analysis program and sampling of study subjects. The present study was supported by a research grant from the John Hunter Hospital Charitable Trust Fund (No. G1200266).

**Author Contributions:** All authors were involved in the overall conception and design of the validation study, and the interpretation of data. JSL conducted the research including reviewing data coding errors, performed statistical data analyses, and wrote the paper. All authors contributed to the editing and proof-reading of the final manuscript.

**Conflicts of Interest:** The authors declare no conflict of interest. The founding sponsors had no role in the design of the study; in the collection, analyses, or interpretation of data; in the writing of the manuscript, and in the decision to publish the results.

## References

1. Willett, W. *Nutritional Epidemiology*; Oxford University Press: New York, NY, USA, 2012; Volume 40.

2. Collins, C.E.; Boggess, M.M.; Watson, J.F.; Guest, M.; Duncanson, K.; Pezdirc, K.; Rollo, M.; Hutchesson, M.J.; Burrows, T.L. Reproducibility and comparative validity of a food frequency questionnaire for australian adults. *Clin. Nutr.* 2013.

3. Smith, W.; Mitchell, P.; Reay, E.M.; Webb, K.; Harvey, P.W.J. Validity and reproducibility of a self-administered food frequency questionnaire in older people. *Aust. N. Z. J. Public Health* **1998**, *22*, 456–463.

4. Marks, G.C.; Hughes, M.C.; van der Pols, J.C. Relative validity of food intake estimates using a food frequency questionnaire is associated with sex, age, and other personal characteristics. *J. Nutr.* **2006**, *136*, 459–465.

5. Van Staveren, W.A.; de Groot, L.C.; Blauw, Y.H.; van der Wielen, R.P. Assessing diets of elderly people: Problems and approaches. *Am. J. Clin. Nutr.* **1994**, *59*, 221S–223S.

6. Lai, J.S.; Hiles, S.; Bisquera, A.; Hure, A.J.; McEvoy, M.; Attia, J. A systematic review and meta-analysis of dietary patterns and depression in community-dwelling adults. *Am. J. Clin. Nutr.* **2014**.

7. Brennan, S.F.; Cantwell, M.M.; Cardwell, C.R.; Velentzis, L.S.; Woodside, J.V. Dietary patterns and breast cancer risk: A systematic review and meta-analysis. *Am. J. Clin. Nutr.* **2010**, *91*, 1294–1302.

8. Stanner, S.; Denny, A. Healthy ageing: The role of nutrition and lifestyle—A new british nutrition foundation task force report. *Nutr. Bull.* **2009**, *34*, 58–63.

9. Young, S. The use of diet and dietary components in the study of factors controlling affect in humans: A review. *J. Psychiatry Neurosci.* **1993**, *18*, 235–244.

10. Hodge, A.M.; Simpson, J.A.; Fridman, M.; Rowley, K.; English, D.R.; Giles, G.G.; Su, Q.; O'Dea, K. Evaluation of an ffq for assessment of antioxidant intake using plasma biomarkers in an ethnically diverse population. *Public Health Nutr.* **2009**, *12*, 2438–2447.

11. McNaughton, S.A.; Marks, G.C.; Gaffney, P.; Williams, G.; Green, A. Validation of a food-frequency questionnaire assessment of carotenoid and vitamin e intake using weighed food records and plasma biomarkers: The method of triads model. *Eur. J. Clin. Nutr.* **2005**, *59*, 211–218.

12. Tucker, K.L.; Chen, H.; Vogel, S.; Wilson, P.W.F.; Schaefer, E.J.; Lammi-Keefe, C.J. Carotenoid intakes, assessed by dietary questionnaire, are associated with plasma carotenoid concentrations in an elderly population. *J. Nutr.* **1999**, *129*, 438–445.

13. Serra-Majem, L.; Andersen, L.F.; Henríque-Sánchez, P.; Doreste-Alonso, J.; Sánchez-Villegas, A.; Ortiz-Andrelluci, A.; Negri, E.; la Vecchia, C. Evaluating the quality of dietary intake validation studies. *Br. J. Nutr.* **2009**, *102*, S3–S9.

14. McEvoy, M.; Smith, W.; D'Este, C.; Duke, J.; Peel, R.; Schofield, P.; Scott, R.; Byles, J.; Henry, D.; Ewald, B.; *et al.* Cohort profile: The hunter community study. *Int. J. Epidemiol.* **2010**, *39*, 1452–1463.

15. Willett, W.C.; Sampson, L.; Browne, M.L.; Stampfer, M.J.; Rosner, B.; Hennekens, C.H.; Speizer, F.E. The use of a self-administered questionnaire to assess diet four years in the past. *Am. J. Epidemiol.* **1988**, *127*, 188–199.

16. U.S. Department of Agriculture, Agricultural Research Service. USDA National Nutrient Database for Standard Reference, Release 18. Available online: http://www.ars.usda. gov/ba/bhnrc/ndl (accessed on 10 July 2014).

17. Food Standards Australia New Zealand (FSANZ). *Nuttab 2006: Australian Food Composition Tables*; FSANZ: Canberra, Australia, 2007.

18. National Health and Medical Research Council. *Australian Dietary Guidelines*; NHMRC: Canberra, Australia, 2013.

19. Xyris Software. *Foodworks Premium 2009, Version 6*, Xyris: Queensland, Australia, 2012.

20. Barua, A.B.; Kostic, D.; Olson, J.A. New simplified procedures for the extraction and simultaneous high-performance liquid chromatographic analysis of retinol, tocopherols and carotenoids in human serum. *J. Chromatogr. B Biomed. Sci. Appl.* **1993**, *617*, 257–264.

21. Beckman Coulter Inc. *Access Immunoassay Systems: Folate rbc*; Beckman Coulter: Sydney, Australia, 2011.

22. Willett, W.; Stampfer, M.J. Total energy intake: Implications for epidemiologic analyses. *Am. J. Epidemiol.* **1986**, *124*, 17–27.

23. Stata Corp LP. *Stata, Version 11*; StataCorp LP: Texas, TX, USA, 2009.

24. Australian Institute of Health and Welfare. *Older Australia at a Glance*, 4th ed.Cat. No. Age 52; AIHW: Canberra, Australia, 2007.

25. Signorello, L.B.; Buchowski, M.S.; Cai, Q.; Munro, H.M.; Hargreaves, M.K.; Blot, W.J. Biochemical validation of food frequency questionnaire-estimated carotenoid, α-tocopherol, and folate intakes among african americans and non-hispanic whites in the southern community cohort study. *Am. J. Epidemiol.* **2010**, *171*, 488–497.

26. Arab, L.; Cambou, M.C.; Craft, N.; Wesseling-Perry, K.; Jardack, P.; Ang, A. Racial differences in correlations between reported dietary intakes of carotenoids and their concentration biomarkers. *Am. J. Clin. Nutr.* **2011**, *93*, 1102–1108.

27. Talegawkar, S.A.; Johnson, E.J.; Carithers, T.C.; Taylor, H.A.; Bogle, M.L.; Tucker, K.L. Carotenoid intakes, assessed by food-frequency questionnaires (ffqs), are associated with serum carotenoid concentrations in the jackson heart study: Validation of the jackson heart study delta niri adult ffqs. *Public Health Nutr.* **2008**, *11*, 989–997.

28. Giles, G.G.; Ireland, P. *Dietary Questionnaire for Epidemiological Studies (Version 2)*; The Cancer Council Victoria: Melbourne, Australia, 1996.

29. Sauvageot, N.; Alkerwi, A.A.; Albert, A.; Guillaume, M. Use of food frequency questionnaire to assess relationships between dietary habits and cardiovascular risk factors in nescav study: Validation with biomarkers. *Nutr. J.* **2013**, *12*, 143.

# Feasibility and Use of the Mobile Food Record for Capturing Eating Occasions among Children Ages 3–10 Years in Guam

Tanisha F. Aflague, Carol J. Boushey, Rachael T. Leon Guerrero, Ziad Ahmad, Deborah A. Kerr and Edward J. Delp

**Abstract:** Children's readiness to use technology supports the idea of children using mobile applications for dietary assessment. Our goal was to determine if children 3–10 years could successfully use the mobile food record (mFR) to capture a usable image pair or pairs. Children in Sample 1 were tasked to use the mFR to capture an image pair of one eating occasion while attending summer camp. For Sample 2, children were tasked to record all eating occasions for two consecutive days at two time periods that were two to four weeks apart. Trained analysts evaluated images. In Sample 1, 90% (57/63) captured one usable image pair. All children (63/63) returned the mFR undamaged. Sixty-two children reported: The mFR was easy to use (89%); willingness to use the mFR again (87%); and the fiducial marker easy to manage (94%). Children in Sample 2 used the mFR at least one day at Time 1 (59/63, 94%); Time 2 (49/63, 78%); and at both times (47/63, 75%). This latter group captured 6.21 ± 4.65 and 5.65 ± 3.26 mean (±SD) image pairs for Time 1 and Time 2, respectively. Results support the potential for children to independently record dietary intakes using the mFR.

Reprinted from *Nutrients*. Cite as: Aflague, T.F.; Boushey, C.J.; Leon Guerrero, R.T.; Ahmad, Z.; Kerr, D.A.; Delp, E.J. Feasibility and Use of the Mobile Food Record for Capturing Eating Occasions among Children Ages 3–10 Years in Guam. *Nutrients* **2015**, 7, 4403–4415.

## 1. Introduction

Traditional dietary assessment methods for children are challenging related to literacy levels, limited cognitive abilities, and difficulties estimating portion size at different developmental stages [1]. The day-to-day composition of young children's diets varies reflecting changing and developing taste and flavor perceptions [2]. Measuring dietary intake in children provides insight into food choices and eating habits, like fruit and vegetable consumption, which is lowest in children compared to adults in the United States (US) [3,4]. A systematic review of dietary assessment methods in children found the most accurate method for reporting energy intake among 4 to 11 year olds was the multiple pass 24 h dietary recall as reported by the parent [5]. For children aged 0.5 to 4 years, the authors concluded that the weighed food record provided the best estimate for energy intake [5]. However, due to the burden associated with keeping weighed food records, they are less useful in community dwelling populations [6]. Additionally, many young children have multiple eating occasions in different settings outside of home, such as childcare centers, or schools where parents are not the primary informants in all settings [7]. Therefore, proxy dietary assessments reported by parents may not be as accurate as desired.

New self-reported methods shown to be useful for adolescents, 11–18 years old, are image-based dietary assessments using mobile devices, such as the mobile food record (mFR) [8,9]. The mFR is a dietary record application that uses the embedded camera in a mobile device (e.g., mobile telephone, iPod) to record dietary intake. Images can enhance self-reported data and, in this case, provide the primary record of dietary intake to obtain valid estimates of energy intake. Briefly, methods of automated image analysis or a trained analyst can be used to identify the food in the image and estimate volume of food consumed [8,10,11]. In addition to real-time data collection, this method eliminates reliance on the respondent's memory, proxy reports, and ability to write and/or estimate portions [8]. Thus, the usability of the mFR with young children is worthwhile to examine.

The current generation of children, born into the digital age, lends to a high level of technology readiness. Use of technologies, such as web- and mobile-based applications may address many of the barriers to gathering accurate dietary data from children. Research involving children will contribute to research to advance mFR technology by addressing age-specific developments. This will allow the mFR to serve as a more accurate and feasible method of dietary assessment for children.

The overall goal of the analyses described in this paper was to determine if children 3 to 10 years could successfully use the mFR, previously tested with 11 to 18 year olds [8,9]. The first sample of children was evaluated using the mFR on three defined skill sets: (1) capturing a usable image pair; (2) demonstrating responsibility for the mobile device; and (3) reporting the feasibility and usability of using the mFR. A usable image pair is an image taken before an eating occasion that includes foods and/or beverages and the fiducial marker, as well as an image taken after the same eating occasion including an appropriate scene (e.g., an empty plate or food wrapper) and the fiducial marker. The second sample of children was assessed for cooperation using the mFR to capture usable image pairs of eating occasions over two days during two time periods as a method to collect fruit and vegetable intake among community-dwelling children (3 to 10 years).

## 2. Methods

Data were collected from two samples of boys and girls registered in preexisting summer day camps in Guam [10]. For the analyses reported here, only those children between 3 and 10 years old were included. These ages represent ages for which no previous studies have examined use of the mFR. All summer programs were open to children of all race/ethnic groups. Recruitment materials for the studies were made available in the registration areas or the camp registration packets. Children were recruited during drop-off or pick-up times. Informed consent was obtained from the parents and assent from their children. The Human Studies Program of the University of Hawaii and the University of Guam Committee on Human Subjects Research approved the study methods described here.

For the first sample (Sample 1) children were recruited from two summer day camps in 2013: A cultural immersion camp for 3 to 12 year olds and a recreational sports camp for children 5 to 15 years old [10]. Participants from these camps were tasked to use the mFR to take an image pair of, at least, one eating occasion on one day while at camp. Children were in possession of the mFR from the time after instruction and during, at least, one eating occasion, plus the time in between, and variable amounts of time after. Upon returning the mFR to researchers, participants were asked to complete a brief questionnaire on feasibility and usability of the mFR and fiducial marker (FM).

During 2014, the second sample of children was recruited from the same cultural immersion camp described in Sample 1 and a university-based day camp for children 6 to 12 years. Participants were tasked to capture image pairs of all eating occasions over two-days during two time periods for a total of 4 days. The data collected from the mFR was used to assess whole fruit and vegetable intake before ($\pm$2 weeks) and after ($\pm$1 week) the summer day camp (*i.e.*, Time 1 and Time 2). Data from both time periods were included in this analysis. Figure 1 shows the data collection flow for the two samples.

## 2.1. Description of the mFR

The mFR is an application based on one of the technology assisted dietary assessment (TADA) protocols [9,11,12]. Ideally, users are tasked to take an image pair at each eating occasion. Methods of image analysis [13] are used to assess foods and beverages captured in the images. A critical method for image analysis is the inclusion of the FM in the captured image [9,14,15]. The FM is an object of known dimensions and markings, in particular a color checkerboard (noted in Figure 2), that is used for spatial and color calibration of the camera and aids in identification of the foods and beverages and estimation of portion sizes [15].

Assess for eligibility and inclusion in analyses
*Data from studies among young children attending summer camps in Guam*

**Sample 1**
*Summer 2013*
$n = 65$

**Sample 2**
*Summer 2014*
$n = 72$

Excluded ($n = 2$):
Not meeting inclusion criteria, age > 10 y ($n = 2$)

Excluded ($n = 9$):
Not meeting inclusion criteria, age > 10 y ($n = 9$)

Children provided the mFR ($n = 63$)

Children provided the mFR at Time 1 ($n = 63$)

Missing image pairs ($n = 6$):
Images lost ($n = 2$)
Before or after image only ($n = 4$)

Missing 2-d mFR ($n = 4$):
Before or after image only ($n = 4$)

Number of children with, at least, one image pair ($n = 57$)

Children who captured eating occasions over 1st set of 2-days ($n = 51$)

Children who returned the mFR undamaged ($n = 63$)

Children who returned the mFR undamaged ($n = 63$)

Loss to follow-up ($n = 1$):
Unable to contact ($n = 1$)

Children provided the mFR at Time 2 ($n = 63$)

Children who provided mFR feedback ($n = 62$)

Missing 2-d mFR ($n = 19$):
Before or after image only ($n = 14$)
1-d mFR ($n = 5$)

Children who captured eating occasions over 2nd set of 2-days ($n = 44$)

1st Distribution of mFR Eligibility

2nd Distribution of mFR

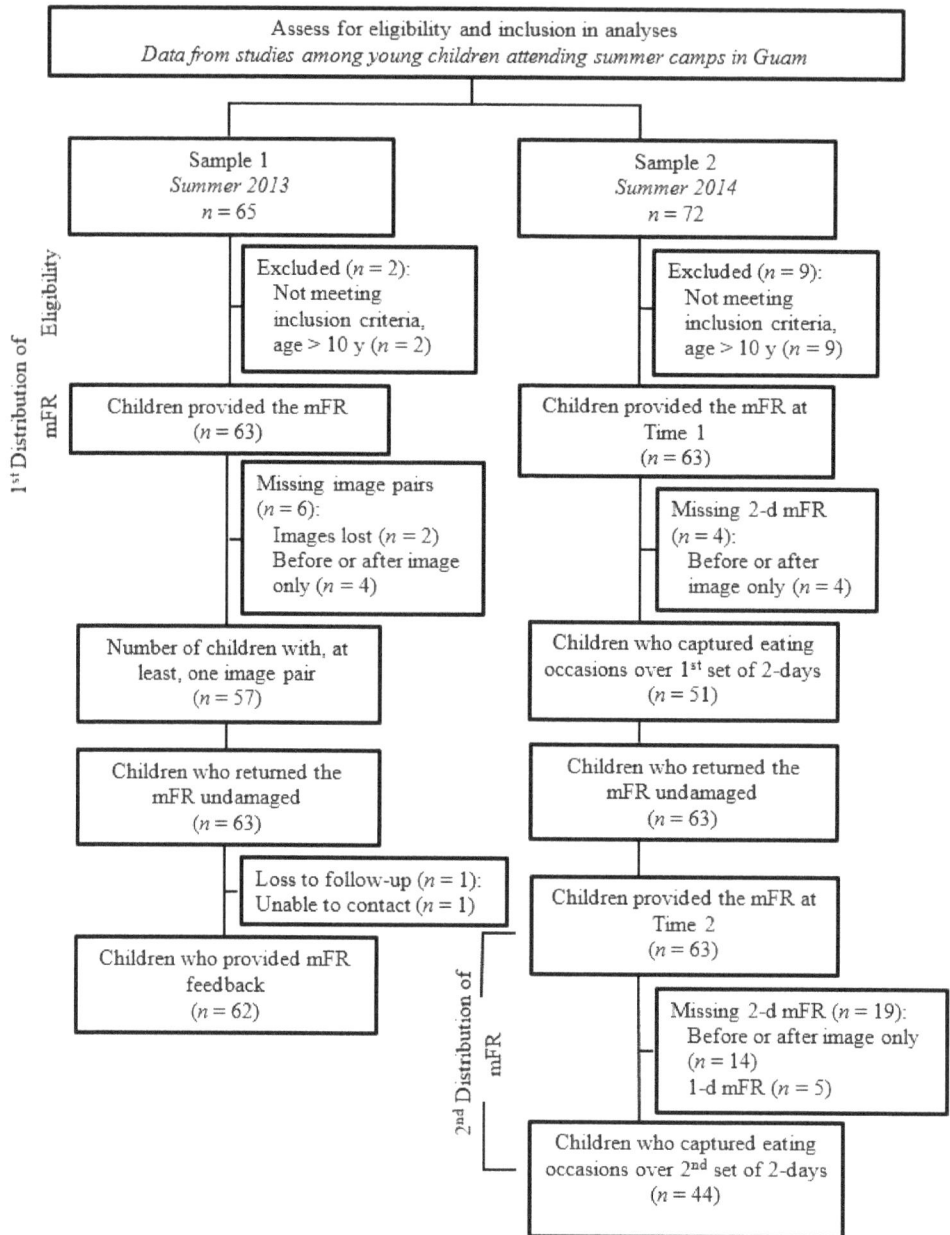

**Figure 1.** Assessment of eligibility for inclusion in analyses among children attending summer day-camps in Guam during summer 2013 (Sample 1) and during summer 2014 (Sample 2).

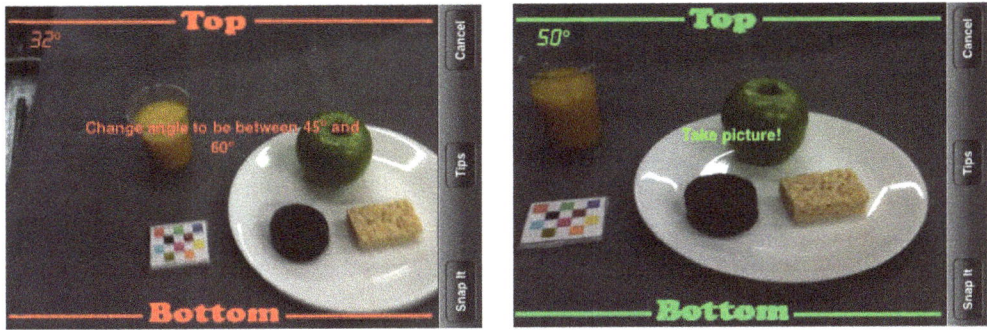

**Figure 2.** Field of view colored borders that appear when in camera settings of the TADA app to aid with proper angle. A red border (image on left) indicates the camera is not at the correct angle. Children from Samples 1 and 2 were to capture the image when the border was green (image on right). Note the fiducial marker (FM) is the color checkerboard seen of the left of the plate.

The TADA app includes parameters to guide users on when to take the image using the embedded information within the mobile device. This is defined by an interchangeable color border (*i.e.*, red or green) shown in Figure 2. Users are tasked to capture the image when the mobile device is held at an angle maintaining a green border by pressing a button labeled, 'snap-it'. After the image is captured, users are able to view the image and select 'use' if the image is acceptable or 'retake' (the image) if unacceptable. All captured images are automatically uploaded to a secure TADA website, when a wireless connection is available. Researchers can login to the website to view images among other features. In addition to the system features described here, the devices were preloaded with child appropriate games.

### 2.2. mFR Instructions Provided to Children

Participants were given instruction on how to use the mFR application available on either an Apple iPhone 3Gs running iOS6 (for Sample 1) or an Apple iPod Touch 5th generation (with a rear facing camera) running on iOS7 (for Sample 2). The instruction included a demonstration of launching the application, using the application to capture images (e.g., following the red and green lines in the camera's view screen, Figure 2), and managing the mFR and FM.

After the introduction instruction, children were given a FM and a colorful silicone wristband to place on the left wrist. The silicone wristband was given to children to guide placement of the FM to the left of the food and/or beverage. Children were asked to wear the wristband for the duration of the time they possessed the mFR. For Sample 2, children were provided four wristbands in the event of misplacing one. Children were asked to demonstrate taking a usable image pair using plastic food replicas, if time permitted or it did not interrupt camp activities. All instructions were provided in an out-of-the-way area within view of camp staff.

During eating occasions at the campsite, researchers and/or camp staff reminded children, ad libitum, to take images of before and after eating, observed the use of the mFR, and assisted children with the mFR as needed. For Sample 1, the mFR, FM, and silicone wristband were collected at the end of the day. The next camp day all were redistributed to a new group of participants until each participant had the opportunity to take, at least, one image of an eating occasion. Children in Sample 2 were assigned two-days to use the mFR before camp started (±2 weeks) and after camp ended (±1 week). When distribution, collection, and redistribution of the mFR and accessories occurred outside of camp, a pre-arranged setting, such as the child's home or public space (e.g., a mall), was used. Scheduling participants to use the mFR for two-days was dictated by study registration date and availability of the mFR.

*2.3. Description of the Methods for the Three Defined Skill Sets (Sample 1)*

2.3.1. Skill Set 1: Capturing a Usable Image Pair

While in possession of the mFR, all participants were asked to take images of one eating occasion. The camp situation was unique in that the eating occasions were limited to morning snack, lunch, and afternoon snack. Therefore, depending upon the time of the mFR distribution, children had four opportunities to take images during instructions and/or at three eating occasions. To assess the first skill set, a trained human analyst examined before and after images uploaded to the TADA website.

2.3.2. Skill Set 2: Responsibility for the Device

Children were responsible for storing the mFR and FM between and during eating occasions. Camp staff members were trained a priori on how to use the mFR and were informed that children had been asked to independently retrieve the mFR and FM from stored locations during eating occasions.

2.3.3. Skill Set 3: Usability and Acceptability of Using the mFR and FM

Children completed a questionnaire that was interview-administered in an out-of-the-way area within view of camp staff. The questionnaire was comprised of three (3) 'Yes' or 'No' choice questions. Examples of questions asked were "Was the iPhone (mFR) easy to use for taking pictures of your food and drinks?" and "Would it be easy to carry the checkerboard square (the fiducial marker) around with you?" Copies of the questionnaire can be requested from the corresponding author. If a child answered 'No', they were probed to elaborate, e.g., "What did you think was not easy about using the mFR?", and comments were noted. Similarly, when responses other than 'Yes' or 'No', were used and the responses better aligned with personal willingness the response was considered 'Yes'. For example, the phrase, "Maybe if my mom or teacher says it's 'okay'", was considered 'Yes'.

For participation and cooperation, participants received a $5 gift card upon return of the mFR and completion of the mFR Feedback Questionnaire.

### 2.4. Description of the Methods for the Community Dwelling Sample (Sample 2)

Participants were asked to use the mFR to collect images of all eating occasions over two days at two time points. Each participant was loaned the mFR. Children were instructed to capture image pairs of all eating occasions using an mFR as previously described. Intentionally parents were not given the instructions, unless they asked. The days a child used the mFR varied in that some used it on a weekend day, camp day, or non-camp summer weekday. Observations from Sample 1 informed mFR management methods for Sample 2 and children were given a waterproof carrying case to manage the mFR, FMs, and a charging cord. When the children returned the mFR, researchers asked the children to assist with identifying food items that were indistinguishable, e.g., opaque containers, occluded foods, and to recall foods at eating occasions that were not captured as an image. A trained human analyst examined all images using the TADA server to enumerate and evaluate image pairs. Collectively, these methods were used to assess whole fruit and vegetable intake as part of another study.

For participation and cooperation, participants received $5 and $10 gift cards before and after camp, respectively.

### 2.5. Data Analysis

For this study a trained human analyst examined all images on the TADA server and data were entered into Microsoft Access files specifically designed for each study and then imported into IBM SPSS statistics version 21 for data analysis (IBM Corporation, Armonk, NY, USA). Participant's responses to the mFR questionnaire provided by Sample 1 were entered and analyzed using the same programs.

For Sample 1, information about each image was entered including date and time stamps, before image or after image, all foods and beverages and/or FM present, and other objects captured in the image. Number of image pairs were examined and assessed as meeting skill set 1 (*i.e.*, FM, all food and beverage, or both present). Statistical examination to compare girls and boys and age group included frequencies, chi-square test, Fisher's exact test, and independent sample *t*-test. Statistical significance was set at $p < 0.05$ (two-sided).

Data entered for Sample 2 included date and time stamps, image number and order, and amount of whole fruits and vegetables consumed. For whole fruit and vegetables intake, fruit and/or vegetable (100%) juices were excluded [16]. Fruit and vegetable servings/day were calculated by dividing the total fruit and vegetable servings consumed by the total number of days that eating occasions were captured using the mFR. The number of days a child used the mFR was determined by the total number of days the child captured at least one image pair of their food and/or beverage using the mFR. Descriptive statistics were used to describe image pairs. The same statistical tests described under Sample 1 were used for Sample 2. In addition, examination of the number of images within child, between collection periods were assessed using paired $t$-tests.

## 3. Results

A total of 126 children, 3–10 years old, used the mFR. Forty-two were boys and 84 were girls of diverse ethnic backgrounds. The majority of the children were Chamorro (55% Chamorro or 36% Chamorro Mix). The descriptive characteristics of both samples are shown in Table 1. Participants in Sample 1 ($n = 63$) were loaned the mFR over 3–8 h in one day. The second sample of children ($n = 63$) were tasked to use the mFR for two days at two time points.

Skill set 1 was evaluated in Sample 1. For the task of taking, at least, one image pair of an eating occasion, or the practice image, two image pairs were lost because of technical errors and four image pairs were excluded as four children took only a before or an after image. Therefore, 95% (57/63) were able to demonstrate taking one image pair as shown in Table 2. Of these children, at least 70% (40/57) had the FM present, 95% (54/57) had the food and beverages present, and 70% (40/57) had both in the before and after images (Figure 3). With regard to capturing one image pair, boys were less likely to take an image pair ($x^2 = 5.755$, $p = 0.026$) than girls. Although children were tasked to take only one image pair, some children captured more than one image pair when they possessed the mFR longer (Table 2). Thirty percent (17/57) took two image pairs and 37% (21/57) took three to four image pairs. Of those that took two or more image pairs ($n = 38$), 68% (26/38) were girls and 32% (12/38) were boys. There were no significant differences found between younger (3–6 years) and older (7–10 years) age groups for capturing one image pair and this was also true accounting for more than one image pair. However, boys were more likely to miss including the FM ($x^2 = 5.216$, df $= 1$, $p = 0.022$), food and/or beverages ($x^2 = 5.292$, df $= 1$, Fisher's exact 0.045), or both ($x^2 = 5.216$, df $= 1$, $p = 0.022$). This significant difference in usable image pairs was primarily due to no after image captured.

**Table 1.** Characteristics of children, 3 to 10 years old, attending summer camp in Guam who used the mobile food record and/or provided feedback in 2013 or 2014.

| Characteristics | Sample 1 n = 63 | | Sample 2 n = 63 | |
|---|---|---|---|---|
| | n | % | n | % |
| Sex | | | | |
| Boys | 24 | 38 | 18 | 29 |
| Girls | 39 | 62 | 45 | 71 |
| Age groups (years) | | | | |
| 3–6 | 27 | 43 | 18 | 29 |
| 7–10 | 36 | 57 | 45 | 71 |
| Ethnic group | | | | |
| Chamorro, only | 32 | 51 | 37 | 59 |
| Chamorro, mixed | 24 | 38 | 21 | 33 |
| Other | 7 | 11 | 5 | 8 |

**Table 2.** Descriptive data of usable image pairs by number of image pairs captured using the mobile food record among children, 3–10 years old, in Sample 1 (n = 57 children) attending summer camps in Guam during 2013.

| Image Pair(s) [a] | Total Image Pairs [a] | FM Present | | Food Present | | FM and Food Present | |
|---|---|---|---|---|---|---|---|
| | | Before | After | Before | After | Before | After |
| | 57 | 56 | 57 | 50 | 53 | 47 | 51 |
| | ← | | | n (Percent, %) | | | → |
| 1 | 19 (33) | 18 (32) | 19 (33) | 19 (38) | 18 (34) | 18 (38) | 18 (35) |
| 2 | 17 (30) | 17 (30) | 17 (30) | 15 (30) | 16 (30) | 15 (32) | 16 (32) |
| 3+ [b] | 21 (37) | 21 (38) | 21 (37) | 16 (32) | 19 (36) | 14 (30) | 17 (33) |
| Total | 57 (100) | 56 (100) | 57 (100) | 50 (100) | 53 (100) | 47 (100) | 51 (100) |

FM is fiducial marker; [a]: An image pair is the before and after image for an eating occasion; [b]: Includes 3 and 4 image pairs.

All children in Sample 1 were able to demonstrate responsibility for the mFR, *i.e.*, skill set 2, as 100% (63/63) returned the mFR undamaged. For the third skill set, all but one child (n = 62) completed the questionnaire about usability and feasibility of the mFR and FM. Questionnaire responses by sex are shown in Table 3. Eighty-nine percent (55/62) of participants found the mFR easy to use; 87% (54/62) of children would use the mFR again; and 94% (58/62) reported the FM was easy to carry around. Children volunteered the comment that the FM is "small enough to fit in my pocket". No differences between boys and girls were found. Among those participants that said the mFR was not easy, when asked why, examples of responses were "it was hard to make it green" (establishing the green border in the mFR camera settings to obtain the correct camera angle), "it was hard to get the board in the image" (fitting the FM in the field of view), and "taking the after eating image". When asked if they would borrow the mFR again and carry the FM, children who reported, 'no', stated "I might lose it". With regard to carrying the FM a couple of children shared that they would carry it "if it sticks to the iPhone".

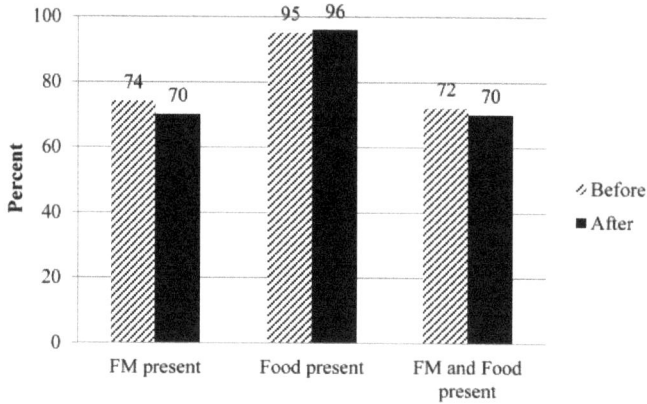

**Figure 3.** Representation of children's demonstration of skill set 1 for capturing, at least, one usable image pair ($n = 57$) among Sample 1 in Guam during summer 2013.

**Table 3.** Responses to mobile food record (mFR) questionnaire among children, 3–10 years old, in Sample 1 after using the mFR ($n = 62$) while at summer camp during 2013.

| Statement, As Presented: | Boys ($n = 23$) | | Girls ($n = 39$) | |
| --- | --- | --- | --- | --- |
| | 'Yes' | | 'Yes' | |
| | $n$ | % | $n$ | % |
| The mFR was easy to use | 21 | 91 | 34 | 87 |
| I would borrow and use the mFR again | 19 | 83 | 35 | 90 |
| Carry the fiducial marker around | 21 | 91 | 37 | 95 |

The community dwelling participants in Sample 2 ($n = 63$) captured 0 to 21 image pairs at Time 1 and Time 2 which were approximately four weeks apart. When the images were reviewed with the children at Time 1 ($n = 55$) and at Time 2 ($n = 56$), five participants reported missing images due to unknown reasons. Technical difficulties aside, 4 of the 63 children (6%) did not take any images at Time 1 compared to 14 of 63 (22%) at Time 2. Two of the children that did not take images at either time point reported only playing the games available on the mFR device. Among those children that took images, the mean number of days were 2.4 (SD ± 1.2) and 2.8 (SD ± 1.1) for Time 1 and Time 2, respectively. The majority of children captured their food and/or beverages using the mFR over, at least, one day at Time 1 (59/63, 94%) and at Time 2 (49/63, 78%). Older participants were more likely to use the mFR longer than younger children as shown in Table 4. However, no statistically significant differences by age and sex were detected with regard to the number of image pairs or the number of days the mFR was used. Seventy-five percent (47/63) of children took images at both time points. Of these children, the mean (±SD) numbers of images captured were 6.21 ± 4.65 for Time 1 and 5.65 ±3.26 for Time 2. There were no significant differences between Time 1 and Time 2 for total number of images and days that the 47 children with repeat measures used the mFR. Estimated servings of whole fruit and vegetables among those children who had images were 0.83 and 0.44 cups per day of fruit and vegetables for Time 1 and Time 2, respectively.

**Table 4.** Descriptive data of images captured using the mobile food record (mFR) among children, 3–10 years old, in Sample 2 ($n$ = 63) attending summer camps in Guam during 2014.

| Length of Time mFR Used [a] | Number of Children | Age | Number of Image Pairs [b] Per Day | |
|---|---|---|---|---|
| (Days) | $n$ (Percent, %) | Mean (Years) | Mean ± SD | Median (Min-Max) |
| | | Time 1 | | |
| 0 | 4 (6) | 5.5 | 0 | 0 |
| 1 | 8 (13) | 7.7 | 1.50 ± 1.07 | 1.00 (1.00–4.00) |
| 2 | 20 (32) | 8.2 | 2.28 ± 0.83 | 2.00 (1.00–4.00) |
| 3 | 20 (32) | 8.2 | 2.73 ± 1.16 | 2.42 (1.33–6.00) |
| 4+ [c] | 11 (17) | 9.8 | 2.80 ± 0.87 | 2.67 (1.33–4.25) |
| | | Time 2 | | |
| 0 | 14 (22) | 7.8 | 0 | 0 |
| 1 | 5 (8) | 7.8 | 1.20 ± 0.45 | 1.00 (1.00–2.00) |
| 2 | 16 (25) | 8.3 | 2.34 ± 1.29 | 2.00 (1.00–5.00) |
| 3 | 18 (29) | 8.3 | 2.07 ± 0.80 | 1.83 (1.00–3.33) |
| 4+ [c] | 10 (16) | 8.0 | 1.94 ± 0.81 | 1.75 (1.20–3.75) |

SD is standard deviation; [a]: Number of days at least 1 image pair was captured using the mFR; [b]: An image pair is the before and after image for an eating occasion; [c]: Includes image pairs captured over 4 and 5 days.

## 4. Discussion

This is the first study to: (1) evaluate the use of the mFR among young children; and (2) capture self-reported dietary intake among children this age. Results of this study demonstrated that the mFR is potentially a feasible method of dietary assessment in 3 to 10 year olds. Given instructions with demonstration and practice, children 3 to 10 years old were able to use the mFR to record their dietary intakes. Children in both samples were provided unique tasks to capture image pairs, such as at one eating occasion for Sample 1 and any and all eating occasions for a two-day food record over two time periods for Sample 2. The majority of the children exceeded the assigned task in both scenarios. Although responsibility for the mFR was not an objective for Sample 2, it is noteworthy that all participants returned the mFR undamaged as well. Additionally, three-fourths (75%) of children in Sample 2 used the mFR to capture eating occasions at two time points. These results are indicative of their willingness to cooperate and participate. Children in both samples were given the freedom to manage and store the mobile devices where they pleased, such as the carrying cases provided or their lunch boxes. Moreover, every mobile device was returned undamaged which demonstrates that even very young children can be responsible for these devices.

For capturing a two-day food record in a community dwelling situation, children may require reminders and prompts for taking an image pair at all eating occasions. Many children in Sample 2 had used the mFR while at camp where the camp staff were aware of the purpose and knowledgeable on how to use it. When examined by skill set, differences were found only between boys and girls. Children were provided instructions for how to take an image pair for different after eating occasions (e.g., some food leftover or all food eaten). In Sample 1, boys were less likely than girls to take the after eating image, which may suggest the need for an operation incorporated into the mFR to remind children to take after images. One reason this may have occurred is that boys usually ate all of their food. In a previous study [8], adolescents recommended a selection for "ate all food and beverages" in the after image camera setting. This suggestion may address the issue of the missing after images. For the young children included in this study, especially the three to five year olds, attentiveness can be another challenge to remembering to take the after eating image or any image for that matter. Therefore, further research is necessary to determine the age that children can use the mFR independently, as well as the age where a parent or caregiver is needed to prompt and/or assist the child with managing the mFR for taking images.

Age appropriate games were preloaded onto the mFR devices for children to use while they possessed the mFR, which was observed to motivate children to agree to use the mFR and likely maintained engagement for capturing images. Of the children in Sample 2 that did not take any image pairs at either time point, these two children voluntarily disclosed that they used the mFR device for playing games only. These observations corroborate the premise proposed by Lu and colleagues [17] that children's self-report of diet can be enhanced with animated, customizable agents (e.g., games). The TADA system has the potential to be modified along these lines. On the other hand, some of the age appropriate games were described by the children as being 'hard to figure out'. Therefore, enhancements to any technology assisted dietary assessment should be designed to be age appropriate in that cognitive abilities, such as literacy level needs to be addressed for children in early childhood (*i.e.*, three to five year olds). For example, the mFR used for studies described in this paper has an automated operation to remind users to include the FM when missing that is a pop-up statement, "fiducial marker is missing [12]". This enhancement was developed with the input of adolescents [8]. This type of enhancement and any future enhancements for younger children would be better addressed through replacing text with images.

Based on the voluntary comments provided by participants in Sample 1, this study is not without limitations. The challenges that the children reported with regard to using the mFR may be attributed to the small stature of the children and size of their hands. Short-statured children were often observed standing, tip-toeing, or kneeling on a chair to capture the best image. This was also reported by adolescents when they used the mFR [8]. In response to the first reports of issues in achieving the green border, researchers for this study taught children the 'cup' and 'alligator' holds to improve management and control of the mFR in camera settings given their small hand sizes. These were simple hand positions that symbolized assigned names. With regard to carrying the FM, one child suggested that the FM be fastened to the backside of the mobile device when not in use, but detachable during capturing images at eating occasions. Despite these comments, children still perceived that capturing images with the mFR was easy. In the studies described here, the parents were minimally involved. A large proportion of the community dwelling children were active participants, especially during the first time period. However, a quarter of the children did not complete the second assessment period. Therefore, the right balance between child and parent involvement needs to be examined, as well as methods to generate continuous motivation in the children.

## 5. Conclusions

An image-based dietary assessment method using a mobile device may eliminate the bias of surrogate reporting (e.g., parent or caregiver) of children's food and beverage intake throughout the day. The children's high level of technology readiness suggests that dietary methods using technology, like the mFR, may alleviate the burden associated with current dietary assessment methods for children. The significance of this study is that it is the first to evaluate the use of the mFR among young children and moreover, the first study to capture self-reported dietary intake among children this age.

**Acknowledgments:** The authors thank the summer camps and the families and children who participated in the study; Research Assistant, Rosae Calvo, for her contributions to the study. Sources of financial support include NIH, NCI, 1U01CA130784-01; Agriculture and Food Research Initiative Grant no 2011-68001-30335 from the USDA NIFA.

**Author Contributions:** Authors T.A., C.B. and R.T. designed the study and took part in data analysis and collection. D.A.K. advised on analysis and interpretation. E.D. and Z.A. led the mFR and image data base technology development. All authors read and contributed to the final manuscript.

**Conflicts of Interest:** The authors declare no conflict of interest.

## References

1. Livingstone, M.B.E.; Robson, P.J.; Wallace, M.W. Issues in dietary intake assessment of children and adolescents. *Br. J. Nutr.* **2004**, *92*, S213–S222.

2. Ventura, A.K.; Worobey, J. Early influences on the development of food preferences. *Curr. Biol. CB* **2013**, *23*, R401–R408.

3. Guenther, P.M.; Dodd, K.W.; Krebs-Smith, S.M. Most Americans eat much less than recommended amounts of fruits and vegetables. *J. Am. Diet. Assoc.* **2006**, *106*, 1371–1379.

4. Centers for Disease Control and Prevention. State Indicator Report on Fruits and Vegetables, 2013. Centers for Disease Control and Prevention, U.S. Department of Health and Human Services: Atlanta, GA, USA, 2013.

5. Burrows, T.L.; Martin, R.J.; Collins, C.E. A systematic review of the validity of dietary assessment methods in children when compared with the method of doubly labeled water. *J. Am. Diet. Assoc.* **2010**, *110*, 1501–1510.

6. Willet, W. *Nutritional Epidemiology*, 3rd ed.; Oxford University Press: New York, NY, USA, 2013.

7. Institute of Medicine (IOM). *Preventing Childhood Obesity: Health In The Balance*; National Academies Press: Washington, DC, USA, 2005.

8. Daugherty, B.L.; Schap, T.E.; Ettienne-Gittens, R.; Zhu, F.M.; Bosch, M.; Delp, E.J.; Ebert, D.S.; Kerr, D.A.; Boushey, C.J. Novel Technologies for Assessing Dietary Intake: Evaluating the Usability of a Mobile Telephone Food Record Among Adults and Adolescents. *J. Med. Interent Res.* **2012**, *14*, e58.

9. Six, B.L.; Schap, T.E.; Zhu, F.M.; Mariappan, A.; Bosch, M.; Delp, E.J.; Ebert, D.S.; Kerr, D.A.; Boushey, C.J. Evidence-based development of a mobile telephone food record. *J. Am. Diet. Assoc.* **2010**, *110*, 74–79.

10. Aflague, T.F.; Leon Guerrero, R.T.; Boushey, C.J. Adaptation and evaluation of the WillTry tool to assess willingness to try fruits and vegetables among children 3-11y in Guam. *Prev. Chronic Dis.* **2014**, *11*, 140032.

11. Zhu, F.M.; Bosch, M.; Khanna, N.; Boushey, C.J.; Delp, E.J. Multiple hypotheses image segmentation and classification with application to dietary assessment. *IEEE J. Biomed. Health Inform.* **2015**, *19*, 377–388.

12. Ahmad, Z.; Khanna, N.; Kerr, D.A.; Boushey, C.J.; Delp, E.J. A mobile phone user interface for image-based dietary assessment. In Proceedings of the IS & T/SPIE Conference on Mobile Devices and Multimedia: Enabling Technologies, Algorithms, and Applications, San Francisco, CA, USA, 2 February 2014.

13. Schap, T.E.; Zhu, F.M.; Delp, E.J.; Boushey, C.J. Merging dietary assessment with the adolescent lifestyle. *J. Hum. Nutr. Diet.* **2014**, *27*, 82–88.
14. Zhu, F.M.; Bosch, M.; Woo, I.; Kim, S.; Boushey, C.J.; Ebert, D.S.; Delp, E.J. The use of mobile devices in aiding dietary assessment and evaluation. *IEEE J. Sel. Top. Signal Proc.* **2010**, *4*, 756–766.
15. Xu, C.; Zhu, F.M.; Khanna, N.; Boushey, C.J.; Delp, E.J. Image enhancement and quality measures for dietary assessment using mobile devices. In Proceedings of the IS&T/SPIE Conference on Computational Imaging X, Burlingame, CA, USA, 22 January 2012; Volume 8296.
16. Chiuve, S.E.; Fung, T.T.; Rimm, E.B.; Hu, F.B.; McCullough, M.L.; Wang, M.; Stampfer, M.J.; Willett, W.C. Alternative dietary indices both strongly predict risk of chronic disease. *J. Nutr.* **2012**, *142*, 1009–1018.
17. Lu, A.S.; Baranowski, J.; Islam, N.; Baranowski, T. How to engage children in self-administered dietary assessment programmes. *J. Hum. Nutr. Diet.* **2014**, *27*, 5–9.

# Evaluation of a Mobile Phone Image-Based Dietary Assessment Method in Adults with Type 2 Diabetes

Megan E. Rollo, Susan Ash, Philippa Lyons-Wall and Anthony W. Russell

**Abstract:** Image-based dietary records have limited evidence evaluating their performance and use among adults with a chronic disease. This study evaluated the performance of a 3-day mobile phone image-based dietary record, the Nutricam Dietary Assessment Method (NuDAM), in adults with type 2 diabetes mellitus (T2DM). Criterion validity was determined by comparing energy intake (EI) with total energy expenditure (TEE) measured by the doubly-labelled water technique. Relative validity was established by comparison to a weighed food record (WFR). Inter-rater reliability was assessed by comparing estimates of intake from three dietitians. Ten adults (6 males, age: $61.2 \pm 6.9$ years old, BMI: $31.0 \pm 4.5$ kg/m$^2$) participated. Compared to TEE, mean EI (MJ/day) was significantly under-reported using both methods, with a mean ratio of EI:TEE $0.76 \pm 0.20$ for the NuDAM and $0.76 \pm 0.17$ for the WFR. Correlations between the NuDAM and WFR were mostly moderate for energy ($r = 0.57$), carbohydrate (g/day) ($r = 0.63$, $p < 0.05$), protein (g/day) ($r = 0.78$, $p < 0.01$) and alcohol (g/day) ($r_s = 0.85$, $p < 0.01$), with a weaker relationship for fat (g/day) ($r = 0.24$). Agreement between dietitians for nutrient intake for the 3-day NuDAM (Intra-class Correlation Coefficient (ICC) = 0.77–0.99) was lower when compared with the 3-day WFR (ICC = 0.82–0.99). These findings demonstrate the performance and feasibility of the NuDAM to assess energy and macronutrient intake in a small sample. Some modifications to the NuDAM could improve efficiency and an evaluation in a larger group of adults with T2DM is required.

Reprinted from *Nutrients*. Cite as: Rollo, M.E.; Ash, S.; Lyons-Wall, P.; Russell, A.W. Evaluation of a Mobile Phone Image-Based Dietary Assessment Method in Adults with Type 2 Diabetes. *Nutrients* **2015**, *7*, 4897–4910.

## 1. Introduction

Nutrition therapy provided by a dietitian and self-management education and support are important strategies for the effective long-term management of type 2 diabetes mellitus (T2DM) [1]. The measurement of dietary intake is necessary to inform, support and evaluate these interventions. Traditional prospective methods of recording intake, such as weighed or estimated food records, are ideal as they allow for the natural day-to-day variation in intake to be captured [2], however these methods are often associated with high burden and changes to usual intake [3–5].

Image-based dietary records continue to show promise in alleviating the issues associated with subject burden relating to the collection of dietary intake information among adults [6,7], including those with T2DM [8]. Evaluation of the performance of image-based dietary records as an independent prospective method to estimate nutrient intake in adults has predominantly been limited to relative validity [9–13] and inter-rater reliability [11,13,14]. However, evaluation with an objective reference method is essential to determine the true accuracy or criterion validity (defined as the comparison to a criterion value to determine the extent to which the test method captures a true representation of the dietary variable it intends to measure [15]). The doubly labelled water (DLW) technique is a method used to assess total energy expenditure (TEE) and is considered the "gold standard" method to validate self-reported dietary energy intake (EI) [16,17]. Only one study [7] has determined criterion validity of self-reported energy intake (EI) derived from image-based dietary records.

Therefore, this study aimed to establish the preliminary validity (both relative and criterion) and inter-rater reliability of the Nutricam Dietary Assessment Method (NuDAM) in adults with T2DM. The usability and acceptability of the NuDAM in this group was also assessed.

## 2. Experimental Section

### 2.1. Subjects and Study Design

In this pilot study, a pre-determined sample size of 10 adults with T2DM was used with subjects recruited through a research study database and internal university staff email list serves. To be eligible to participate in the study, subjects needed to meet the following criteria: be aged 18–70 years; have a diagnosis of T2DM of >3 months; not currently receiving treatment for cancer or have a previous diagnosis of liver, kidney or thyroid diseases; not currently trying to lose weight; and have a stable body weight (assessed as not having lost or gained more than 4 kg in the past 6 months). The study was approved by the Queensland University of Technology Human Research Ethics Committee and each subject provided written informed consent.

For the evaluation of new dietary assessment methods it is recommended that test and reference methods are used separately, with the test method used first [18]. Therefore, dietary intake was assessed using the NuDAM (test method) in week 1 and the weighed food record (WFR) (reference method) in week 2. Intake was assessed over a three day period (two week days and one weekend day; non-consecutive) for both methods. Demographic information was collected on Day 0, in addition to height to the nearest 0.1 cm using a stadiometer (Model PE087, Mentone Educational, Moorabbin, Australia) and body weight to the nearest 0.1 kg using calibrated electronic scales (Model HD319, Tanita Corporation, Tokyo, Japan). Weight was also measured on Days 8 and 15. To account for factors which may explain mis-reporting of intake [17], dietary restraint was also measured on Day 0 using a 10-item scale [19]. At the end of each dietary recording period, subjects were asked to complete a brief questionnaire on the experience of using the NuDAM and the WFR. Response options to questions included Likert and categorical scales in addition to open-ended text.

## 2.2. Total Energy Expenditure (TEE)

TEE was measured over a two week period using the DLW technique and coincided with the collection of dietary intake using the NuDAM and WFR. Administration of the DLW occurred on Day 0, with subjects in a fasted state. Subjects were orally dosed with 1.25 g 10% $^{18}O$ + 0.1g 99% $^{2}H$/kg and a post-dose urine sample was collected 6 hours after drinking the DLW. During Days 1–14 subjects were required to collect one urine sample each day. The level of enrichment of $^{18}O$ and $^{2}H$ isotopes contained in the urine samples were measured in triplicate by isotope ratio mass spectrometry (Hydra 20/20 CF-IRMS, Sercon, Cheshire, UK). Isotope dilution spaces were derived [20] and used to calculate carbon dioxide production [21]. Indirect calorimetry principles were applied and TEE derived via using the modified Weir [22] equation, with a standard respiratory quotient of 0.85 used for all subjects.

## 2.3. Nutricam Dietary Assessment Method (NuDAM)

The NuDAM consisted of a prospective mobile phone Nutricam image-based dietary record and brief phone call to the subject the following day (Figure 1). Details of the development and early testing of Nutricam have been described previously [8]. Building on this earlier work, the NuDAM method was modified to incorporate a follow-up phone call component to clarify items in the Nutricam record and probe for commonly forgotten foods. In addition, the current study used a standardized analysis protocol including an aid (called the Dietary Estimation and Assessment Tool) to assist in the quantification of food portions contained in the images.

The Nutricam dietary record was recorded using a Sony Ericsson K800i mobile phone (Sony Ericsson Mobile Communications AB, Lund, Sweden) installed with the software application Nutricam (Alive Technologies, Pty. Ltd., Arundel, Australia). When recording the image, subjects were instructed to place the reference object (a 9 cm × 5 cm card which also acted as a prompt for recording an entry) next to the food items, hold the phone at an angle of approximately 45° and ensure all items were clearly visible. After capturing the image, subjects were automatically prompted to make a voice recording describing the location, meal occasion, and the foods (name, type, brand/product name, and preparation/cooking method) contained in the image. Information documenting any food leftover at the end of the eating occasion was also collected in a similar manner. All subjects were trained in the use of the Nutricam mobile phone prior to the collection of the 3-day dietary record and were provided with written instructions for reference during the recording period. The Nutricam record was automatically sent to a secure website accessed only by the researchers. Additional intake information consisting of the clarification of foods within the Nutricam record and probing for forgotten foods was collected from subjects during a brief structured phone call by a Dietitian (D1) on the morning following each recording day.

## 2.4. Weighed Food Record (WFR)

In the second week, dietary information was collected using a 3-day WFR. Subjects were provided with a set of digital food scales (Model HR 2385, Koninklijke Philips Electronics N.V., Amsterdam, The Netherlands) (accurate to 1 g) and were required to weigh all food items prior to consumption and record all information (including recipes) into the paper-based diary supplied. Any food which was served and recorded in the diary but then not eaten was also required to be weighed and documented. At the completion of the recording period, the WFR was reviewed by a dietitian (D1) in the presence of the subject to ensure that the information was complete.

## 2.5. Nutrient Analysis from the NuDAM and WFR

The two sets of dietary records were analysed independently by three dietitians (D1 and two additional dietitians, D2 and D3) using the *AUSNUT 1999* food composition databases [23] in the nutrient analysis software program FoodWorks® Professional 2009 (Xyris Software, Brisbane, Australia). The Nutricam dietary records were analysed first. Using both the image and accompanying voice recording for each eating occasion, each dietitian identified and quantified food items contained in the Nutricam records and entered this information directly into the nutrient analysis program. To assist with the quantification of foods in the images, each dietitian used a portion size estimation aid, called the Dietary Estimation and Assessment Tool (DEAT), previously developed by the research team (Figure 1). The tool consisted of various reference images of foods, serving vessels, amorphous mounds and generic shapes and was based on aids developed for other dietary assessment methods [24,25]. The reference object (9 cm × 5cm card) also appeared in the DEAT and provided perspective to the dietitian during the analysis. Dietitians were then provided with a recording of the phone calls to each subject following each Nutricam recording day and used this information to make any adjustments to the NuDAM analysis. For the WFRs, information on the types and amounts of foods consumed contained within the diaries was entered directly into the FoodWorks® program.

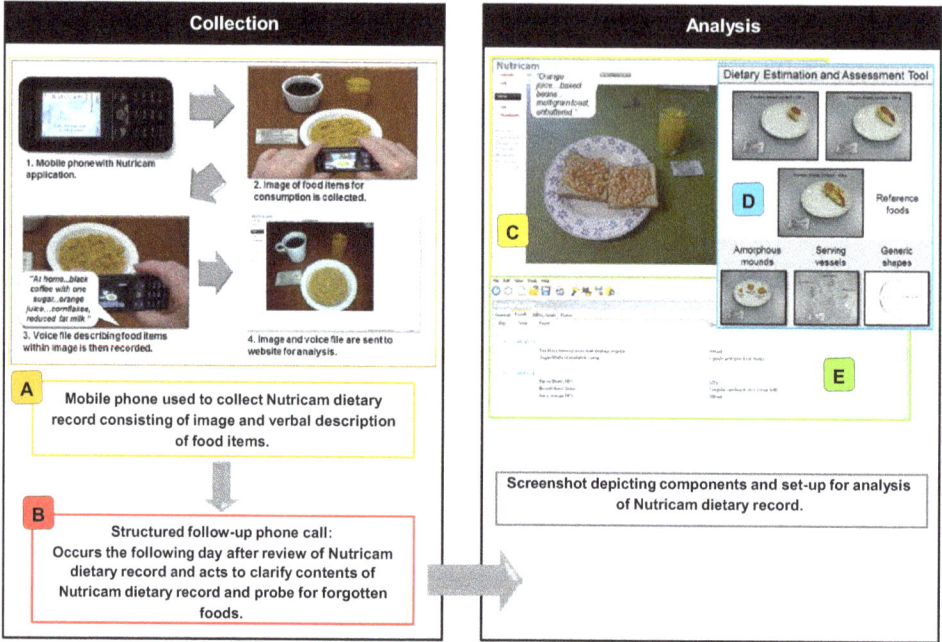

**Figure 1.** Overview of the Nutricam Dietary Assessment Method (NuDAM). For the collection of dietary intake data, a mobile phone is used to capture the Nutricam image-based dietary record (**A**) and is combined with information collected via a phone call (using a standardized interview protocol) (**B**) Analysis consisted of the dietitian identifying and quantifying food items contained in each Nutricam dietary record entry (**C**) A standardized protocol and the Dietary Estimation and Assessment Tool (DEAT) (a two-dimensional portion size estimation aid (**D**)) was used to assist in the task of quantifying the food items. Dietary data was entered directly into the nutrient analysis software program, FoodWorks® (**E**) to obtain an estimate of nutrient intake. Data from the follow-up phone call (**B**) is used to supplement the Nutricam dietary record, with adjustments made by the dietitian to the analysis (**E**) as required.

## 2.6. Statistical Analysis

Data analysis was performed using SPSS for Windows (version 17.0, 2008, SPSS Inc., Chicago, IL, USA). For both dietary assessment methods, the estimates of energy and macronutrient intake were averaged for the three days for each subject and then separately for each of the three dietitians. Intra-class correlation coefficients (ICC) evaluated agreement between dietitians' estimates of energy and macronutrient intake for each method. Repeated-measures ANOVA or Friedman's ANOVA were used to assess differences between dietitians' estimates (Bonferroni correction post hoc analysis applied). Paired $t$-tests or Wilcoxon signed-rank test assessed differences in the overall nutrient intake (average of the three dietitians' estimates) between methods and for EI and TEE. Correlation coefficients were used to determine the relationship between estimates of nutrient intake derived from the NuDAM and WFR. Validation of self-reported EI was based on the principle of EI = TEE ± body stores, where in the absence of non-significant weight change at the group level, the expected ratio of EI:TEE is 1.00 [17]. At the individual level with the 95% confidence limits (CL) calculated to determine mis-reporting [26]. The calculated 95% CL for the NuDAM were 0.72 and 1.28; and for the WFR were 0.76 and 1.24.

## 3. Results

Six men and four women with T2DM ranging in age between 48–69 years participated, with all 10 subjects completing the study. Five were classified as obese (body mass index (BMI) $\geq$30.0 kg/m$^2$), four as overweight (BMI 25.0–29.9 kg/m$^2$), and one was within the normal BMI range (18.5–24.9 kg/m$^2$). The group showed a low level of dietary restraint, with individual scores ranging between 1.3 to 3.2 (out of 5). At the group level, there were no significant changes in mean body weight during Week 1 (baseline to Day 8), $-0.7 \pm 1.2$ kg, Week 2 (Day 8 to Day 15), $0.4 \pm 0.9$ kg and overall (baseline to Day 15) $-0.3 \pm 1.2$ kg.

### 3.1. Criterion and Relative Validity

The overall mean EI was $8.8 \pm 2.0$ MJ/day from the NuDAM and $8.8 \pm 1.8$ MJ/day from the WFR; both were significantly lower than mean TEE of $11.8 \pm 2.3$MJ/day ($p < 0.01$). The mean EI:TEE ratio was $0.76 \pm 0.20$ and $0.76 \pm 0.17$ for the NuDAM and WFR, respectively. At the individual level, three males and four males were classified as under-reporters for the NuDAM and WFR, respectively. NuDAM under-reporters were also found to be under-reporting EI with the WFR. When using the NuDAM, all three under-reporters of EI lost weight in the first recording week ($-2.8$ kg each for two subjects and $-0.3$ kg for one subject). In comparison among the under-reporters identified using the WFR, two subjects had no change in weight while the other two subjects gained weight ($+0.6$ kg and $+2.4$ kg) in the second week. No individuals were found to be over-reporting EI. Overall, the mean nutrient intakes were not significantly different between the two dietary assessment methods (Table 1). Associations between intakes were stronger for protein and alcohol, moderate for energy and carbohydrate, and weaker for fat.

## 3.2. Inter-Rater Reliability

The inter-rater reliability and comparison of the dietitians' estimated energy and nutrient intakes from the NuDAM and WFR are shown in Table 1 Bonferonni post-hoc analysis between dietitians showed estimates by D1 to be significantly different for energy compared to both D2 and D3, protein compared to D3, and fat and carbohydrate compared to D2.

**Table 1.** Comparison of energy and nutrient intake obtained from NuDAM and WFR between dietitians and between methods ($n$ = 10 subjects).

| | | Mean ($\pm$ SD) Intake as Assessed by Each Dietitian [†] | | | ICC (95% CI) between Dietitians | Overall [‡] | |
| --- | --- | --- | --- | --- | --- | --- | --- |
| | | D1 | D2 | D3 | | Mean ($\pm$ SD) Intake [§] | Correlation ^ between Methods |
| Energy | NuDAM | 8.2 $\pm$ 1.7 | 9.0 $\pm$ 2.3 * | 9.1 $\pm$ 2.0 * | 0.88 (0.58–0.98) *** | 8.8 $\pm$ 2.0 | 0.57 |
| (MJ/day) | WFR | 8.5 $\pm$ 1.6 | 8.9 $\pm$ 2.0 | 8.9 $\pm$ 1.8 | 0.92 (0.80–0.98) *** | 8.8 $\pm$ 1.8 | |
| Protein | NuDAM | 89.3 $\pm$ 20.2 | 99.0 $\pm$ 31.4 | 98.1 $\pm$ 23.1 * | 0.79 (0.53–0.94) *** | 95.5 $\pm$ 23.7 | 0.78 ** |
| (g/day) | WFR | 89.1 $\pm$ 26.8 | 91.9 $\pm$ 28.2 | 91.5 $\pm$ 24.9 | 0.97 (0.92–0.99) *** | 90.8 $\pm$ 26.4 | |
| Fat (g/day) | NuDAM | 75.6 $\pm$ 18.3 | 87.0 $\pm$ 25.4 * | 86.6 $\pm$ 20.1 | 0.77 (0.45–0.93) *** | 83.1 $\pm$ 20.3 | 0.24 |
| | WFR | 79.5 $\pm$ 16.8 | 85.4 $\pm$ 27.4 | 80.9 $\pm$ 24.2 | 0.82 (0.59–0.95) *** | 81.9 $\pm$ 21.8 | |
| CHO | NuDAM | 194.9 $\pm$ 52.8 | 212.0 $\pm$ 52.7 * | 215.3 $\pm$ 60.8 | 0.91 (0.71–0.98) *** | 207.4 $\pm$ 54.4 | 0.63 * |
| (g/day) | WFR | 206.3 $\pm$ 53.8 | 207.2 $\pm$ 54.9 | 211.9 $\pm$ 57.8 | 0.92 (0.79–0.98) *** | 208.5 $\pm$ 53.9 | |
| Alcohol | NuDAM | 15.0 $\pm$ 29.4 | 13.6 $\pm$ 28.0 | 14.4 $\pm$ 29.5 | 0.99 (0.98–0.99) *** | 14.3 $\pm$ 28.9 | 0.85 ** |
| (g/day) [#,¶] | WFR | 16.1 $\pm$ 23.4 | 17.4 $\pm$ 30.2 | 16.5 $\pm$ 28.4 | 0.99 (0.98–0.99) *** | 16.7 $\pm$ 28.3 | |

Abbreviations: D1: dietitian No.1; D2: dietitian No.2; D3: dietitian No.3; CHO: carbohydrate; NuDAM: Nutricam dietary assessment method; WFR: weighed food record; [†] Repeated-measures ANOVA (GLM) between dietitians for each dietary method, except for alcohol ([#]) which was Friedman's ANOVA: * $p < 0.05$, compared to D1, all others not significant; ICC: Intra-class Correlation Coefficient significant: *** $p < 0.001$; Difference within each dietitian's mean estimates of nutrient intake, NuDAM *vs.* WFR (paired $t$-test or [#] Wilcoxon Signed Ranked test): not significant; [‡] Overall mean ($\pm$ SD) intake = mean (D1, D2, and D3 intake per day); [§] difference between overall mean ($\pm$ SD) estimate of nutrient intake, NuDAM *vs.* WFR: not significant for energy or macronutrient intakes; ^ Correlations are Pearson's correlation coefficient ($r$); except for alcohol ([¶]) which is Spearman's rank correlation coefficient ($r_s$): * $p < 0.05$, ** $p < 0.01$.

## 3.3. Usability, Acceptability and Changes to Eating Behaviours

All subjects preferred to use the NuDAM to record intake compared to the WFR, with "convenience", "ease of use", and "portability" used to explain preferences. All subjects would be willing to use both recording methods again. For the Nutricam mobile phone, the majority ($n$ = 9) would be willing to use again to record their intake for periods of up 7 days or longer, whereas up to 3 days was the maximum recording period most commonly reported ($n$ = 5) for the WFR. Subject responses to additional questions relating to the experience of the NuDAM and WFR are summarized in Table 2.

88

**Table 2.** Evaluation of Nutricam dietary assessment method and weighed food record ($n = 10$ subjects).

| Questions (as Presented): | Count | | | |
|---|---|---|---|---|
| Usability and Acceptability ^ | Strongly Agree | Agree | Neutral | Disagree |
| Overall, I found the Nutricam mobile phone easy to use: | 7 | 2 | 1 | 0 |
| Overall, I found weighing my foods and drinks easy: | 0 | 3 | 4 | 3 |
| NuDAM only: | | | | |
| I found taking photographs of food and drink items easy *: | 5 | 5 | 0 | 0 |
| I found recording the voice file easy *: | 5 | 5 | 0 | 0 |
| I found that the Prompt Card was useful for remembering how to use Nutricam: | 5 | 1 | 4 | 0 |
| When prompted during the call: I found it easy to clarify the details of the food and/or drink items that I had eaten during the previous day: | 8 | 1 | 1 | 0 |
| I found it easy to remember if there were any food and/or drink items I had not recorded using the Nutricam mobile phone the previous day: | 7 | 3 | 0 | 0 |
| I found it easy to remember the description of the food and/or drink items I had not recorded using the Nutricam mobile phone the previous day: | 6 | 4 | 0 | 0 |
| I found it easy to remember the quantities of the food and/or drink items I had not recorded using the Nutricam mobile phone the previous day: | 6 | 3 | 1 | 0 |
| Overall, I found that the length of the calls I received were appropriate: | 5 | 4 | 1 | 0 |
| Change to eating behaviours | No | | Yes | |
| Was there any difference in how you used the Nutricam mobile phone to record your diet when you were alone compared to when you were with other people or in public? | 4 | | 6 | |
| Was there any difference in how you recorded your diet using the weighed record method when you were alone, compared to when you were with other people or in public? | 2 | | 8 | |
| Did you record all food and drink items that you consumed during the test period using the Nutricam mobile phone? | 5 | | 5 | |
| Did you record all food and drink items that you consumed during the test period using the weighed record method? | 4 | | 6 | |
| Where there any foods and/or drinks that you usually eat, but did not eat during the Nutricam test period? | 9 | | 1 | |
| Where there any foods and/or drinks that you usually eat, but did not eat during the weighed record method test period? | 6 | | 4 | |

Abbreviations: ^ These questions were answered on a 5-point Likert Scale (Strongly agree/Agree/Neutral/Disagree /Strongly disagree); however no responses for the "strongly disagree" category were recorded; * Questions refer to using the Nutricam mobile phone to collect the image-based dietary record.

Changes in eating behaviours were reported for both methods (Table 2). More than half of the subjects reported a difference in how the methods were used when in the presence of others as opposed to when they were alone. The most common reason for this response was feeling more self-conscious and/or requiring to explain why they were recording their intake when in public compared to at home. Regardless of the method used, forgetting to record prior to eating was the main reason for not recording all food items consumed. Making changes to the types of foods typically consumed was more common for the WFR, with simplifying intake in order to facilitate recording often reported for this method.

## 4. Discussion

This study assessed the criterion and relative validity and the inter-rater reliability of the NuDAM for the estimation nutrient intake, with the findings demonstrating the performance and feasibility of this method in a small sample of adults with T2DM. Compared to TEE, similar levels of under-reporting of EI were found for the NuDAM ($-23.7\%$) and WFR ($-23.9\%$). The level of under-reporting for the NuDAM is comparable to using 3-day food records where the difference between EI and TEE may be up to $-24\%$ in older adults [27–29]; and more favourable to using a 3-day food recall in obese adults with T2DM where a difference of up $-60\%$ was reported [30]. Martin *et al.* [7] used DLW to validate EI collected over 6 days using a mobile phone image-based dietary record among free-living overweight and obese adults. When used with generic meal time reminders sent to the phone mean participant error between EI and TEE was $-34.3\%$, compared to when the reminders were tailored to the specific meal times of the individual under-reporting decreased to $-3.7\%$ [7]. The combination of a longer recording period and customised meal-time prompts may have contributed to the greater reporting accuracy and will be considered for future use of the NuDAM.

The associations between the NuDAM and WFR for estimated intakes of energy, protein, and carbohydrate were similar to some studies [9,10], although others have found stronger correlations [11,12]. Compared to these studies, estimates of fat intake between the NuDAM and WFR showed a weaker relationship ($r = 0.24$). However in these studies intake was recorded concurrently and therefore differs from our study where records were collected one week apart and higher within-subject variation is expected. Alcohol intake was highly correlated between methods ($r_s = 0.85$) and displayed the strongest agreement between dietitians. The use of standardized serving vessels and detailed descriptions (e.g., "pint" glass) may have contributed to the strength of the relationship observed for alcohol. It is important to note, the observed correlations for estimates of energy and nutrient intake between the two dietary assessment methods are based on the assumption that the errors between the methods are independent [18]. Therefore the validity of the NuDAM should be interpreted in the context of the other measures of agreement.

Inter-rater reliability for the nutrients assessed ranged from moderate to high for the NuDAM. Although discrepancies existed between dietitians' nutrient estimates for the NuDAM, these did not translate to significant differences between methods in the overall mean intakes of the group. Similar studies have also found acceptable agreement between dietitians for estimates of nutrient intake derived from image-based records [13,14]. While these studies were conducted in controlled settings of single meal occasions or using pre-prepared food items, the NuDAM was used in a free-living situation over multiple days with opportunity for greater food variety.

Nine subjects were classified as either overweight or obese in our study and this may in part explain the level of reporting accuracy observed. Increasing BMI is generally associated with an increase in the likelihood of under-reporting, however some variation does occur at the individual level [17]. The dietary restraint scale used measured both actual restriction of intake and intention to restrict [31], with scores of ≤3 categorised as "low-restraint" [32]. In the current group, overall dietary restraint was low, even among those subjects identified as under-reporting intake who all had restraint scores ≤3 Therefore, the level of dietary restraint did not appear to influence the accuracy of self-reported EI in the current study.

Forgetting to record intake prior to consumption was commonly reported as reasons for not collecting all intake information for both the NuDAM and WFR and remains a challenge with prospective dietary records. Although, the phone call component of the NuDAM was designed to capture food items consumed but not recorded, it is possible that selective mis-reporting may have been present. Snacks and foods eaten at times other than main meals are most commonly mis-reported [33] and could also explain the difference between TEE and EI observed in our study.

Change in behaviours were reported for both methods, although there appeared to be a slightly greater change in eating behaviours during the period recording with the WFR compared to the NuDAM. At the individual level, those identified as under-reporters of EI using the NuDAM all lost weight and may suggest under-eating [34]. In contrast with the WFR, two of the four under-reporters had no change in weight which may be indicative of under-recording of intake [34]. However, replication in a larger sample would be necessary to confirm these conclusions regarding changes in intake and/or recording using the NuDAM and WFR. An increased awareness and changes to intake behaviours are common when diet is recorded [3–5], including when wearable devices are used to automatically collect image-based records [35]. Further exploration into the effect of using wearable devices and mobile/smartphone to collect image-based records has on eating behaviours and dietary intake is needed.

Similar to other studies which have found a preference for image-based methods over traditional dietary assessment methods [8–11], the NuDAM was also well received among this group of older adults with T2DM. Subjects were willing to use the NuDAM again and for longer recording periods. However, some refinement to the method could be incorporated to improve efficiency in the collection of the dietary data, such as replacing the follow-up phone call with an in-built feature in the Nutricam application to collect missed eating occasions. As use of the method in its current form may not be feasible in large groups, further modifications to the NuDAM are required to minimize the effect on analysis time that occurred with shifting some of the subject burden to the dietitian. New techniques which automate all or some of the quantification of foods within the image-based dietary record hold promise for improving efficiency in the analysis [36,37].

Strengths of this study are the use of a "gold standard" DLW technique to validate EI and the use of standardized analysis protocol, including aids to estimate portion size of foods in the Nutricam records. Limitations include the small sample which restricts generalisability of these results to the greater population of adults with T2DM. However, when using DLW, small samples have been used initially to validate measures of EI [17] and justify evaluation in larger numbers. It is possible that the use of the NuDAM first may have introduced a training effect for the WFR. The administration sequence of the two dietary assessment methods was standardised for all subjects and based on recommendations [18], however randomisation of the administration order will be considered for future NuDAM validation studies. The use of the same dietitian (D1) (MER) to review and clarify the dietary data and then to code the records is another potential limitation. Although, a standardized protocol was followed for all dietitians, increased familiarity with the subject intakes in the NuDAM and WRF could have contributed to the difference in nutrient intake estimates.

## 5. Conclusions

This pilot study assessed the validity (criterion and relative) and inter-rater reliability of a novel image-based dietary assessment method, the NuDAM, in 10 adults with T2DM. The results demonstrated that in comparison to an objective measure of TEE the NuDAM performed equally well to the WFR, however EI was significantly under-estimated by both methods. Relative validity was comparable to other image-based prospective food records for all nutrients, except for fat. Agreement between dietitians for estimates of nutrient intake was slightly lower for the NuDAM compared to WFR. All subjects preferred using the NuDAM and were willing to use it again for longer recording periods. These findings demonstrate the performance and feasibility of the NuDAM to assess energy and macronutrient intake in a small group of adults with T2DM. However, some modifications to the method are necessary to improve efficiency, particularly for use with a greater number of individuals. Evaluation in a larger group is needed to be able to generalise the results to the broader population of adults with T2DM.

**Acknowledgments:** Megan E. Rollo was supported by a Queensland University of Technology (QUT) Post-graduate Research Award Scholarship and an Australian Post-graduate Award Scholarship during her candidature. This study was also partially supported by funding from a Novo Nordisk®Regional Diabetes Support Scheme Grant. The authors would like to acknowledge Jamie Sheard and Chloe McKenna, Connie Wishart, Rachel Wood, Ainsley Groves and Nuala Byrne for their assistance with the study.

**Author Contributions:** Megan E. Rollo was involved in the study conception and design; data collection; statistical analysis and interpretation; drafting and critical revision of the manuscript. Susan Ash was involved in the study conception and design; critical revision of the manuscript; statistical analysis and interpretation; and supervision. Philippa Lyons-Wall was involved in the study conception and design; critical revision of the manuscript; statistical analysis and interpretation; and supervision. Anthony Russell was involved in the study conception and design; critical revision of the manuscript; and supervision. All authors have reviewed and approved the final manuscript.

**Conflicts of Interest:** The authors declare no conflict of interest.

# References

1. American Diabetes Association. Standards of medical care in diabetes—2014. *Diabetes Care* **2014**, *37*, S14–S80.

2. Nelson, M.; Bingham, S.A. Assessment of food consumption and nutrient intake. In *Design Concepts in Nutrional Epidemiology*; Margetts, B., Nelson, M., Eds.; Oxford University Press: New York, NY, USA, 1997.

3. Mela, D.J.; Aaron, J.I. Honest but invalid: What subjects say about recording their food intake. *J. Am. Diet. Assoc.* **1997**, *97*, 791–793.

4. Rebro, S.M.; Patterson, R.E.; Kristal, A.R.; Cheney, C.L. The effect of keeping food records on eating patterns. *J. Am. Diet. Assoc.* **1998**, *98*, 1163–1165.

5. Vuckovic, N.; Ritenbaugh, C.; Taren, D.L.; Tobar, M. A qualitative study of participants' experiences with dietary assessment. *J. Am. Diet. Assoc.* **2000**, *100*, 1023–1028.

6. Daugherty, L.B.; Schap, E.T.; Ettienne-Gittens, R.; Zhu, M.F.; Bosch, M.; Delp, J.E.; Ebert, S.D.; Kerr, A.D.; Boushey, J.C. Novel technologies for assessing dietary intake: Evaluating the usability of a mobile telephone food record among adults and adolescents. *J. Med. Internet Res.* **2012**, *14*, e58.

7. Martin, C.K.; Correa, J.B.; Han, H.; Allen, H.R.; Rood, J.C.; Champagne, C.M.; Gunturk, B.K.; Bray, G.A. Validity of the remote food photography method (RFPM) for estimating energy and nutrient intake in near real-time. *Obesity* **2012**, *20*, 891–899.

8. Rollo, M.E.; Ash, S.; Lyons-Wall, P.; Russell, A. Trial of a mobile phone method for recording dietary intake in adults with type 2 diabetes: Evaluation and implications for future applications. *J. Telemed. Telecare* **2011**, *17*, 318–323.

9. Kikunaga, S.; Tin, T.; Ishibashi, G.; Wang, D.H.; Kira, S. The application of a handheld personal digital assistant with camera and mobile phone card (Wellnavi) to the general population in a dietary survey. *J. Nutr. Sci. Vitaminol. (Tokyo)* **2007**, *53*, 109–116.

10. Wang, D.H.; Kogashiwa, M.; Kira, S. Development of a new instrument for evaluating individuals' dietary intakes. *J. Am. Diet. Assoc.* **2006**, *106*, 1588–1593.

11. Wang, D.H.; Kogashiwa, M.; Ohta, S.; Kira, S. Validity and reliability of a dietary assessment method: The application of a digital camera with a mobile phone card attachment. *J. Nutr. Sci. Vitaminol. (Tokyo)* **2002**, *48*, 498–504.

12. Bird, G.; Elwood, P.C. The dietary intakes of subjects estimated from photographs compared with a weighed record. *Hum. Nutr. Appl. Nutr.* **1983**, *37*, 470–473.

13. Lassen, A.D.; Poulsen, S.; Ernst, L.; Andersen, K.K.; Biltoft-Jensen, A.; Tetens, I. Evaluation of a digital method to assess evening meal intake in a free-living adult population. *Food Nutr. Res* **2010**, *54*.

14. Martin, C.K.; Han, H.M.; Coulon, S.M.; Allen, H.R.; Champagne, C.M.; Anton, S.D. A novel method to remotely measure food intake of free-living individuals in real time: The remote food photography method. *Br. J. Nutr.* **2009**, *101*, 446–456.

15. Gleason, P.M.; Harris, J.; Sheean, P.M.; Boushey, C.J.; Bruemmer, B. Publishing nutrition research: Validity, reliability, and diagnostic test assessment in nutrition-related research. *J. Am. Diet. Assoc.* **2010**, *110*, 409–419.

16. Black, A.E.; Prentice, A.M.; Goldberg, G.R.; Jebb, S.A.; Bingham, S.A.; Livingstone, M.B.; Coward, W.A. Measurements of total energy expenditure provide insights into the validity of dietary measurements of energy intake. *J. Am. Diet. Assoc.* **1993**, *93*, 572–579.

17. Livingstone, M.B.E.; Black, A.E. Markers of the validity of reported energy intake. *J. Nutr.* **2003**, *133*, 895S–920S.

18. Nelson, M. The validation of dietary assessment. In *Design Concepts in Nutritional Epidemiology*, 2nd ed.; Margetts, B.M., Nelson, M., Eds.; Oxford University Press: New York, NY, USA, 1997.

19. Van Strien, T.; Frijters, J.E.R.; Bergers, G.P.A.; Defares, P.B. The dutch eating behavior questionnaire (DEBQ) for assessment of restrained, emotional, and external eating behaviours. *Int. J. Eat. Disord.* **1986**, *5*, 295–315.

20. Schoeller, D.A. Hydrometry. In *Human Body Composition*; Roche, A.F., Ed.; Human Kinetics: Champaign, IL, USA, 1996.

21. Racette, S.B.; Schoeller, D.A.; Luke, A.H.; Shay, K.; Hnilicka, J.; Kushner, R.F. Relative dilution spaces of 2h- and $^{18}$O-labeled water in humans. *Am. J. Physiol.* **1994**, *267*, E585–E590.

22. Weir, J.B. New methods for calculating metabolic rate with special reference to protein metabolism. *J. Physiol.* **1949**, *109*, 1–9.

23. Australia New Zealand Food Authority. *AUSNUT 1999—Australian Food and Nutrient Database 1999*; Australia New Zealand Food Authority: Canberra, Australia, 1999.

24. McBride, J. Was it a slice, a slab or a sliver? *Agric. Res.* **2001**, *3*, 4–7.

25. Nelson, M.; Atkinson, M.; Darbyshire, S. Food photography II: Use of food photographs for estimating portion size and the nutrient content of meals. *Br. J. Nutr.* **1996**, *76*, 31–49.

26. Black, A.E.; Cole, T.J. Biased over- or under-reporting is characteristic of individuals whether over time or by different assessment methods. *J. Am. Diet. Assoc.* **2001**, *101*, 70–80.

27. Goran, M.I.; Poehlman, E.T. Total energy expenditure and energy requirements in healthy elderly persons. *Metabolism* **1992**, *41*, 744–753.

28. Johnson, R.K.; Goran, M.I.; Poehlman, E.T. Correlates of over-and underreporting of energy intake in healthy older men and women. *Am. J. Clin. Nutr.* **1994**, *59*, 1286–1290.

29. Tomoyasu, N.J.; Toth, M.J.; Poehlman, E.T. Misreporting of total energy intake in older men and women. *J. Am. Geriatr. Soc.* **1999**, *47*, 710–715.

30. Sallé, A.; Ryan, M.; Ritz, P. Underreporting of food intake in obese diabetic and nondiabetic patients. *Diabetes Care* **2006**, *29*, 2726–2727.

31. Van Strien, T. Success and failure in the measurement of restraint: Notes and data. *Int. J. Eat. Disord.* **1999**, *25*, 441–449.

32. Rennie, K.L.; Siervo, M.; Jebb, S.A. Can self-reported dieting and dietary restraint identify underreporters of energy intake in dietary surveys? *J. Am. Diet. Assoc.* **2006**, *106*, 1667–1672.

33. Poppitt, S.D.; Swann, D.; Black, A.E.; Prentice, A.M. Assessment of selective under-reporting of food intake by both obese and non-obese women in a metabolic facility. *Int. J. Obes. Relat. Metab. Disord.* **1998**, *22*, 303–311.

34. Goris, A.H.; Westerterp-Plantenga, M.S.; Westerterp, K.R. Undereating and underrecording of habitual food intake in obese men: Selective underreporting of fat intake. *Am. J. Clin. Nutr.* **2000**, *71*, 130–134.

35. Gemming, L.; Doherty, A.; Kelly, P.; Utter, J.; Ni Mhurchu, C. Feasibility of a sensecam-assisted 24-h recall to reduce under-reporting of energy intake. *Eur. J. Clin. Nutr.* **2013**, *67*, 1095–1099.

36. Jia, W.; Chen, H.C.; Yue, Y.; Li, Z.; Fernstrom, J.; Bai, Y.; Li, C.; Sun, M. Accuracy of food portion size estimation from digital pictures acquired by a chest-worn camera. *Public Health Nutr.* **2014**, *17*, 1671–1681.

37. Lee, C.D.; Chae, J.; Schap, T.E.; Kerr, D.A.; Delp, E.J.; Ebert, D.S.; Boushey, C.J. Comparison of known food weights with image-based portion-size automated estimation and adolescents' self-reported portion size. *J. Diabetes Sci. Technol.* **2012**, *6*, 428–434.

# A Novel Dietary Assessment Method to Measure a Healthy and Sustainable Diet Using the Mobile Food Record: Protocol and Methodology

Amelia J. Harray, Carol J. Boushey, Christina M. Pollard, Edward J. Delp, Ziad Ahmad, Satvinder S. Dhaliwal, Syed Aqif Mukhtar and Deborah A. Kerr

**Abstract:** The world-wide rise in obesity parallels growing concerns of global warming and depleting natural resources. These issues are often considered separately but there may be considerable benefit to raising awareness of the impact of dietary behaviours and practices on the food supply. Australians have diets inconsistent with recommendations, typically low in fruit and vegetables and high in energy-dense nutrient-poor foods and beverages (EDNP). These EDNP foods are often highly processed and packaged, negatively influencing both health and the environment. This paper describes a proposed dietary assessment method to measure healthy and sustainable dietary behaviours using 4-days of food and beverage images from the mobile food record (mFR) application. The mFR images will be assessed for serves of fruit and vegetables (including seasonality), dairy, eggs and red meat, poultry and fish, ultra-processed EDNP foods, individually packaged foods, and plate waste. A prediction model for a *Healthy and Sustainable Diet Index* will be developed and tested for validity and reliability. The use of the mFR to assess adherence to a healthy and sustainable diet is a novel and innovative approach to dietary assessment and will have application in population monitoring, guiding intervention development, educating consumers, health professionals and policy makers, and influencing dietary recommendations.

Reprinted from *Nutrients*. Cite as: Harray, A.J.; Boushey, C.J.; Pollard, C.M.; Delp, E.J.; Ahmad, Z.; Dhaliwal, S.S.; Mukhtar, S.A.; Kerr, D.A. A Novel Dietary Assessment Method to Measure a Healthy and Sustainable Diet Using the Mobile Food Record: Protocol and Methodology. *Nutrients* **2015**, *7*, 5375–5395.

## 1. Introduction

Recent evidence would suggest that eating a diet that increases environmental sustainability has the potential to also benefit health [1–4]. Worldwide overweight and obesity rates are rising, posing significant costs at an individual and societal level [5]. In Australia, the direct cost spent annually on overweight and obesity is estimated to be at least $21 billion [6]. The overconsumption of kilojoules above an individual's energy requirements (resulting in weight gain) is environmentally unsustainable and places burden on the future food supply [7]. Hence, there may be considerable health and environmental benefits in assessing the impact of dietary behaviours and practices on the food supply [8,9]. Research on the effects of diet on the environment is rapidly emerging, particularly the area of life cycle assessment- a method for measuring the carbon footprint (amount of greenhouse gas emissions) of food products throughout production [10,11]. However, identifying a healthy and sustainable diet that meets the nutrient requirements of all populations groups and cultures is complex and challenging [1,8,12,13]. Researchers have identified the need to identify dietary patterns that provide adequate nutrition at a low environmental cost [14], but methods to do so have focused on the assessment of typical diets and food choices at a population level [2,13] rather than individual dietary behaviours. Therefore, there is limited evidence on whether current individual dietary patterns align with a sustainable diet.

The Australian Dietary Guidelines, which provide the evidence-base for dietary recommendations and directions for nutrition policy in Australia, have highlighted the issue of food, nutrition and environmental sustainability over the last decade. The 2013 review of the Guidelines sought to assess the evidence to make dietary recommendations that were protective of health as well as the environment. However, no specific guidelines to address a sustainable diet were made as a result of inadequate evidence in the area, rather an appendix containing key messages regarding food, nutrition and environmental sustainability. These recommendations include advice to: try to eat seasonal produce; reduce food and packaging waste; and avoid overconsuming kilojoules [7]. Several of the Australian Dietary Guidelines form indirect synergies between eating a diet for good health and a sustainable diet to reduce burden on the environment (represented graphically in Figure 1). For example, the overconsumption of kilojoules is associated with overweight and obesity, but is also creating an avoidable environmental burden due to the resources used in the production, storage and preparation of food [7,15,16]. While attempts to create awareness of the impact of dietary choices on the environment exist, the absence of set guidelines relating to sustainable diets in Australia is the probable result of limited evidence in this area of nutrition and no dietary assessment method to accurately measure an individual's healthy and sustainable dietary behaviours.

There is no agreed definition for what constitutes a "healthy and sustainable diet". Separately, healthy diets conform to the Australian Dietary Guidelines [7], while sustainable diets have been defined by the Food and Agriculture Organization of the United Nations as "those diets with low environmental impacts which contribute to food and nutrition security and to healthy life for present and future generations. Sustainable diets are protective and respectful of biodiversity and ecosystems, culturally acceptable, accessible, economically fair and affordable; nutritionally adequate, safe and healthy; while optimizing natural and human resources." [4]. Several European countries have developed guidelines for a healthy and sustainable diet [17,18] and research examining associations between other dietary recommendations and dietary patterns and their associations with environmental sustainability is becoming available [3,13]. Even with strengthening evidence on the health benefits of diets with lower environmental impact, the revised Australian Dietary Guidelines failed to include specific sustainable eating dietary recommendations [3,19].

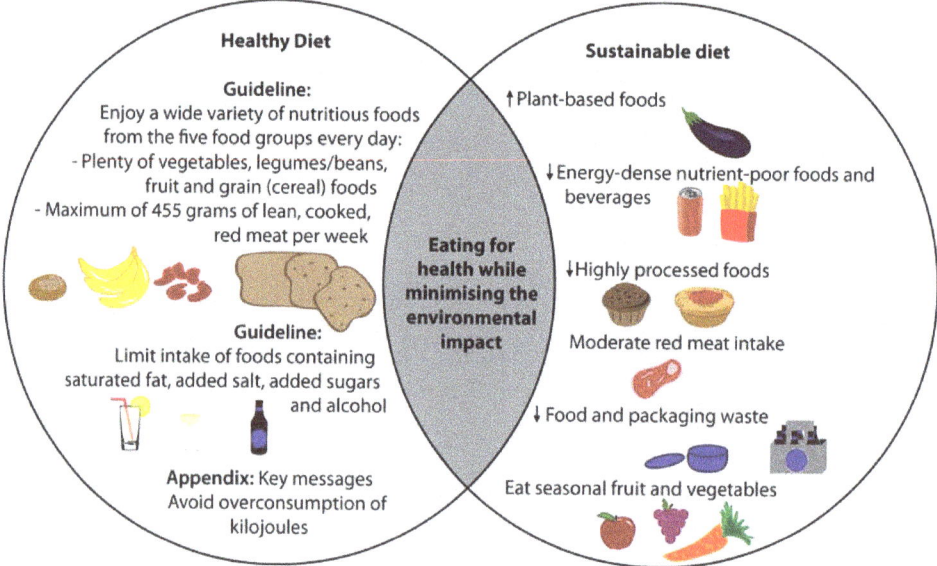

**Figure 1.** Graphic representation of the direct synergies between the 2013 Australian Dietary Guidelines and sustainable dietary behaviours outlined in the Australian Dietary Guidelines [7].

There is a plethora of evidence suggesting climate change and poor health are two major public health concerns, both of which would benefit from government policy promoting more sustainable dietary behaviours [2,9,20,21]. However, dietary recommendations and policies cannot be developed without an evidence base. In order to collect evidence on how current dietary patterns adhere to a sustainable diet, surveillance and monitoring of individual dietary behaviours using a comprehensive dietary assessment method is required.

To the authors' knowledge there is no feasible dietary assessment method to accurately measure an individual's healthy and sustainable dietary behaviours and the need for such a method has been highlighted in a recent review by Johnston et al. [22]. To date methods of dietary assessment have focused mostly on nutrients and food groups and not considered the assessment of sustainable dietary practices, such as reducing food packaging and waste. Brief assessment instruments, commonly used in population surveillance, have been used to reliably estimate the quality of diets in Australia [23]. These methods typically use a short questionnaire or several questions to assess knowledge and specific diet and nutrition behaviours [24,25]. Other frequently used dietary assessment methods, such as written food records, provide more objective data on what individuals are eating and in some cases individuals may be asked to record food waste. However, a limitation of written food records is there is no way to verify the recording and researchers must rely on good literacy levels, the ability of people to accurately estimate portion sizes and remember to write down all meals, snacks and beverages, creating burden on participants. The use of technology in dietary assessment, and more specifically image-based food records, is a new and rapidly emerging area that will reduce the burden for participants through the elimination of detailed writing and portion size estimation. Image-based dietary assessment methods, including the mobile food record (mFR) application, enable people to capture their intake by taking a momentary image and do not allow users to review, edit or alter earlier images [26–30]. This feature may reduce the chances of people reflecting on their prior consumption and consequently underreporting further intake. In addition, before and after eating images taken using the mFR application allow for the assessment of plate waste and packaging use, as well as the estimation of serving and portion sizes. For such reasons the existing mFR application shows great potential as a feasible method for individual and population-wide nutrition monitoring of sustainable dietary behaviours. Food image data previously collected from a population-based sample of adults using the mFR will enable the validation of a *Healthy and Sustainable Diet Index*.

Diet quality indices assist in translating intake data collected using dietary assessment methods to values or scores that are more easily interpretable and allow for consistent comparisons between groups of interest. Such indices are developed to measure dietary patterns, behaviours and adherence to particular eating recommendations in populations [31]. Diet quality indices consider multiple components of a diet and apply weighting factors to each component to calculate a final diet quality score [32]. Developing and validating indices for use in dietary assessment can assist in guiding nutrition interventions, population monitoring, informing policy makers, monitoring the effectiveness of programs and research [33]. Examples of validated diet quality indices include the Healthy Eating Index [33], Mediterranean Diet Score [34], Diet Quality Index [35], Dietary Guideline Index [31], Dietary Quality Score [36], Australian Recommended Food Score [23] and Dietary Approaches to Stop Hypertension (DASH) Diet Score [37].

Traditionally, dietary indices have been developed to monitor specific or general nutrient intake and predict the effect of dietary behaviours on health outcomes.

But, there is increasing need to measure impacts of dietary behaviours on external factors due to the potential negative impact on the future of the food supply (e.g., the environment) [22]. A recent review by Johnston and colleagues highlighted the urgent need to develop innovative approaches to measuring and promoting sustainable diets so consumers and policymakers can become aware of the benefits on individual and population health and the environment [22]. In doing so, the authors emphasised the need for culturally acceptable and locally appropriate indices to accurately assess sustainable diets, suggesting the development of such indices would enable the measurement of a suite of indicators relating to the impact of dietary behaviours on health and the food system to inform policy makers [22]. This paper addresses the gap in the literature by proposing a feasible method to assess multiple elements of a healthy and sustainable diet.

This paper describes the protocol and methodology for a proposed novel dietary assessment method to measure indicators of an individual's healthy and sustainable diet not typically measured in traditional methods. Due to a lack of consensus of what constitutes a healthy and sustainable diet, the five dietary behaviours selected for assessment were chosen based on the evidence documented in the Australian Dietary Guidelines, and Appendix G on Environmental Sustainability [7]. The five characteristics of a healthy and sustainable diet selected relate to nutritional status and/or future food supplies to maintain good health. As the proposed dietary assessment method uses images to assess healthy and sustainable dietary behaviours, the selection has been confined to those that can be objectively assessed from food and beverage images using a mFR. The five indicators to be assessed using the mFR application include the intake of ultra-processed EDNP foods and beverages, individually packaged foods and beverages, fruit and vegetables (including seasonality), dairy, eggs and meat, and plate waste.

Food intake data, collected using the image-based mFR during the Connecting Health and Technology study, will provide evidence to assist the development of this method and a *Healthy and Sustainable Diet Index*, which will provide evidence for policy makers, health professionals, and others interested in promoting environmental sustainability through dietary recommendations (e.g., the agricultural sector). A validated index to accurately assess healthy and sustainable dietary behaviours, and ultimately gather evidence on individual eating behaviours, is timely and urgent. It is yet to be determined but the mFR may have the potential to be a cost effective method to gather valuable data on healthy and sustainable dietary behaviours, an area of nutrition in need of evidence. The dietary assessment method described in this paper when implemented will provide evidence on current adherence to a healthy and sustainable diet, addressing a gap in the literature both in Australia and globally. This protocol paper outlines the methods used to assess healthy and sustainable dietary behaviours using an mFR, providing detail to assist with further advancements in this field of dietary assessment and allowing for future reproducibility. Importantly, the methods proposed in this paper may address the lack of dietary assessment methods to assess sustainable dietary behaviours, as highlighted in the review by Johnston *et al.* [22].

## 2. Experimental Section

### 2.1. Study Participants

The study sample to be used for developing the proposed methods will consist of 247 adults aged from 18 to 30 years, comprising of 162 (66%) women and 85 (34%) men previously recruited for another study, the Connecting Healthy and Technology study, referred to as CHAT [26]. Recruitment involved sending letters of invitation to 15,000 residents from 57 suburbs (using the Socio-Economic Indexes for Areas) in the Perth Metropolitan Area from the Federal Electoral Roll, a compulsory enrolment system for Australians aged over 18 years. Participants were screened either online, using a survey website, or on the telephone to ensure the inclusion criteria were satisfied (aged between 18 and 30 years and owned a mobile phone). For the original study, potential participants were excluded if they were: (a) unable to attend on four occasions to complete the 6-month randomised controlled trial; (b) studied nutrition; (c) took part in extreme forms of exercise; (d) followed a restrictive diet; or (e) pregnant or breastfeeding. The CHAT study was conducted between July 2012 and June 2013.

The Connecting Health and Technology study was registered on the Australian and New Zealand Clinical Trials Registry (ACTRN12612000250831) and approved by the Curtin University Human Resources Ethics Committee (HR181/2011) and the Western Australian Department of Human Research Ethics Committee (#2011/90).

### 2.2. Study Design

During the Connecting Health and Technology study, participants completed four day mFRs using the CHAT application at baseline and at the end of the 6-month randomised controlled trial. During both visits height and weight data were collected. Participants were asked to capture before and after images of all eating occasions using a mobile device (iPod Touch) provided by the research team. On the initial visit participants were taught how to use the specifically designed dietary assessment method, the CHAT application, uploaded onto the iPod Touch (iOS6). Participants were asked to place a small fiducial marker in the bottom left hand corner of every image to assist in portion size and colour estimation [38]. Details of the mFR CHAT application have been previously described by Kerr *et al.* [39].

Participants were asked to take images over four consecutive days, from Wednesday to Saturday. On completion of the food record, participant's clarified the contents of images with an Accredited Practising Dietitian, and verified plate waste or if the leftover food or beverage was consumed at a later stage. Each image obtained during the CHAT study contains metadata on the time, date and location it was taken, allowing for the assessment of whether fresh produce were in season at time of consumption. The food images collected during the CHAT study will be used to validate and test the *Healthy and Sustainable Diet Index.*

For the development of the proposed methodology, participants completed an mFR at baseline ($n$ = 247) and repeated this six months later ($n$ = 220). A secondary analysis by the Accredited Practising Dietitian who was involved in the original analysis of all food images collected during the CHAT study will take place. A purpose built Microsoft Access database will be developed to assess the contents of images, and the review of each image pair (including a before and after eating image). A minimum of one image pair per day will be required to be considered a valid day. Five indicators of a healthy and sustainable diet will be assessed using the images captured using the mFR. An objective of this study is to determine whether the five selected dietary behaviours can be assessed from image-based food records without interaction with participants. This is therefore a "proof of concept" approach to developing the Index before replication in possible future interventions. A flowchart outlining the design of the proposed study can be seen in Figure 2.

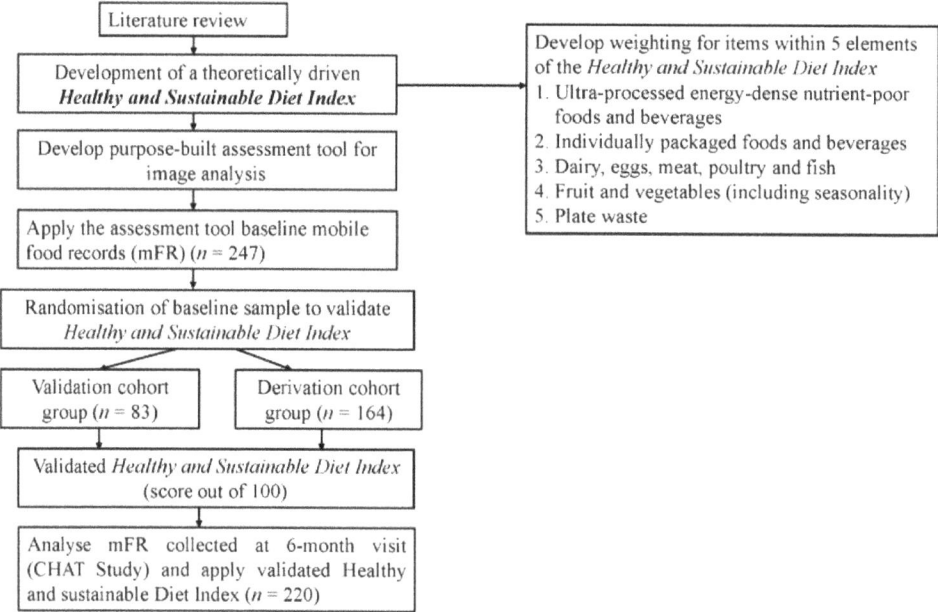

**Figure 2.** Flow chart of study design.

## 2.3. Assessment of Healthy and Sustainable Dietary Behaviours

For the development of a *Healthy and Sustainable Diet Index*, dietary behaviours were identified from evidence of their supportive or unsupportive role within a healthy and/or a sustainable diet and the inclusion of details that can be assessed using images. Descriptions of each component's role within the context of a healthy and sustainable diet are outlined below. The five indicators to be assessed using the mFR application include: the intake of ultra-processed EDNP foods and beverages, individually packaged foods and beverages, fruit and vegetables (including seasonality), dairy, eggs and meat portions, and plate waste. These dietary behaviours will be assessed using the following proposed methodologies.

### 2.3.1. Ultra-Processed EDNP Foods and Beverages

Processed foods form a large component of modern diets and have been linked to the growing rates of overweight and obesity [7,40–42]. A definition of food processing is "all methods and techniques used by industry to turn whole fresh foods into food products" [43]. Food processing is important to ensure an adequate and safe food supply [44], however, high levels of food processing often increases the energy density of food due to "ultra-processing" with the addition of added fat and sugar. In general, foods that have been highly or ultra-processed are more likely to contain high levels of saturated fats, added sugars and/or sodium and minimal levels of micronutrients therefore are often categorised as "energy-dense nutrient-poor" choices [41,45]. Energy-dense nutrient-poor foods and beverages are associated with poor diet quality, overweight, obesity and chronic disease [45,46], as well as being some of the most emissions-intensive food products due to the processing, packaging and landfill necessary to produce these foods in certain locations [9]. Although all EDNP foods may not negatively affect the environment more than other food items, these foods are generally low in nutrients [7]. In addition, the excessive intake of kilojoules above an individual's energy requirements, from these EDNP foods and beverages, is a dietary behaviour unsupportive of health whilst creating unnecessarily burden on natural resources [7,15]. Highly processed takeaway foods and poor diet quality are associated with abdominal obesity in young adults [40,47] and compared to older age groups, young adults are more likely to consume EDNP that are convenient, highly processed and packaged, such as meat pies, fried potatoes, pizzas, crisps, confectionary, savoury pastries, chocolate and sugar-sweetened beverages [40,48]. Hence, processed food is not the issue in a healthy and sustainable diet, the issue is EDNP ultra-processed foods.

Ultra-processed foods are defined as those that require minimal, if not any, culinary preparation [41]. Previous studies have relied on household expenditure surveys and semi-quantitative food frequency questionnaires to assess the intake of ultra-processed foods [41–43], yet no studies have investigated the consumption of ultra-processed foods in Australia. A unique aspect of the methods to be used is that EDNP ultra-processed foods will be assessed using image-based mFRs. For inclusion in this component only ultra-processed foods and beverages categorised as energy-dense and nutrient-poor, such as cakes, crisps, commercial burgers and sugar-sweetened beverages will be used [7]. Ultra-processed EDNP foods and beverages will be assessed according to the Australian Dietary Guidelines serve sizes-one serve of EDNP food or beverage being equivalent to 600 kJ (143 kcal) [7]. Nutrient dense foods that are highly processed, such as bread, will be excluded due to associated health benefits.

An example image of ultra-processed EDNP foods collected using the mFR application can be seen in Figure 3. Using the proposed assessment protocol, this eating occasion would be recorded as 14 serves of ultra-processed EDNP foods. The two pieces of fried chicken appearing in the after eating image would not be counted as ultra-processed EDNP serves but rather non-compostable food waste.

We can appreciate all EDNP foods may not necessarily be worse for the environment than other food items, however, in regard to health consequences, these food items offer minimal, if any, nutritional benefit. In addition, the excessive intake of kilojoules above an individual's energy requirements, from these EDNP foods and beverages, is a dietary behaviour unsupportive of health whilst creating unnecessarily burden on natural resources.

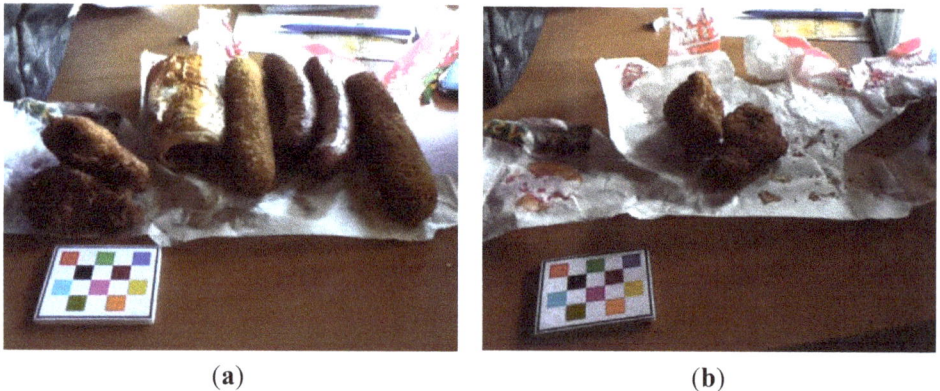

(a)  (b)

Figure 3. Example of using an mobile food record (mFR) to assess ultra-processed energy-dense nutrient-poor foods. (a) Before eating image; (b) After eating image shows the food waste. The number of energy-dense nutrient-poor food and beverage (EDNP) serves consumed were: 1 sausage roll (commercial, 175 g) = 2100 kJ, fried sausage (large) 1300 kJ × 2 = 2600 kJ, crumbed fried sausage (large) 1800 kJ × 2 = 3600 kJ → Total: 8300 kJ/600 kJ = 14 serves of EDNP foods.

### 2.3.2. Individually Packaged Foods and Beverages

Food packaging plays a crucial role in maintaining a safe food supply and has the ability to reduce waste by retaining the effect of food processing to extend shelf life [49]. However, food packaging negatively impacts the environment at a number of stages including during production, transport and land fill [15]. Individually packaged foods are convenient and are becoming more common in Australian supermarkets. An Australian study assessed attitudes towards environmentally friendly eating behaviours and found people believe food packaging has a greater impact on the environment compared to the consumption of meat [50].

Key messages in Appendix G of the Australian Dietary Guidelines encourage people to select foods with appropriate packaging and recycle due to the impact on natural resources [7]. Food packaging is not assessed by traditional dietary assessment methods. Images from mFRs show great potential for the accurate assessment of the intake of individually packaged products as they are easily identifiable from the before eating images. Due to the negative impact of packaging on the environment, all individually packaged items will be recorded regardless of the nutrient composition of the food it originally contained. However, individually packaged foods, classified as either EDNP or healthy, will be counted separately to allow for further assessment of adherence to a healthy and sustainable diet. Foods and beverages served from larger packages (so not individually packaged) such as a glass of milk poured from a two litre bottle will not be recorded due to the unavoidable use of larger packages to ensure a safe food supply. A limitation of this method is that some food or beverages may be removed from individual packaging prior to the before eating image being taken. This challenge could be avoided by requesting participants do not remove individual packaging prior to taking images using the mFR.

An example of an image containing individually packaged items collected using the mFR application can be seen in Figure 4. Using the proposed protocol, this eating occasion would likely be assessed as containing two individually packaged EDNP food items and one individually packaged EDNP beverage item.

### 2.3.3. Fruit and Vegetables

A diet consistent with the Australian Dietary Guidelines can help maintain a healthy weight and assist in the prevention of chronic diseases, such as cardiovascular disease, type 2 diabetes and some cancers [7,8,20,51]. Previous studies have found Australian adults eat less than the recommended daily serves of fruit and vegetables [52], supported by the most recent Australian Health Survey which found only three per cent of young adults meet the recommended two 150 gram serves of fruit and five 75 gram serves of vegetables per day, compared to 9.6% of older adults [53]. The reasons why people are not eating enough fruit and vegetables are complex but household income and the expense of fruit and vegetables have been shown to be significant factors [54,55]. In recent years, changes in climate have influenced the availability and affordability of some fresh fruits and vegetables in Australia [22,56]. The cost of fresh fruit and vegetables in Australia appears to be increasing at a higher rate than other food categories, evidenced by an 18.8% increase in the cost of fresh fruit and 10.7% increase in fresh vegetables in Western Australia since 2010 [57].

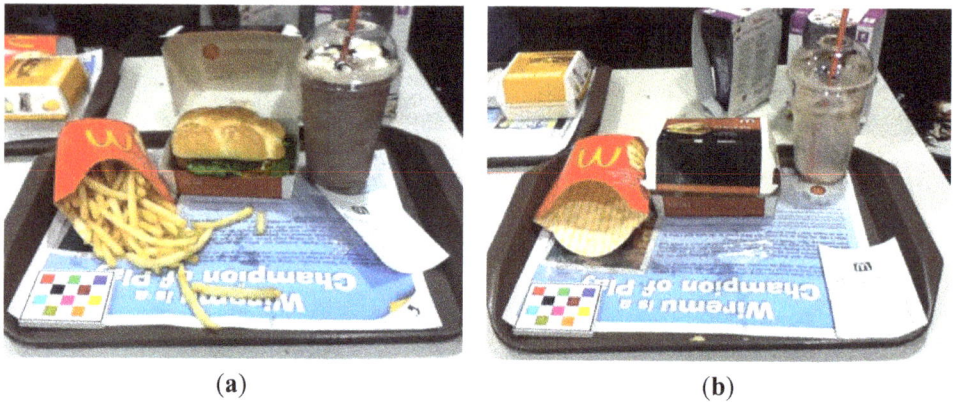

**(a)**           **(b)**

**Figure 4.** Example of using the mobile food record (mFR) to assess individually packaged foods. (**a**) Before eating image; (**b**) After eating image.

Diets high in fruit and vegetables have a lesser impact on the environment than those high in processed foods or animal-based foods [3,15]. Although the consumption of a diet that consists of mostly fresh fruits and vegetables is encouraged [7], it has been suggested that additional considerations need to be included, for example, produce grown locally and in season. This is because fruits and vegetables grown locally or in season are less likely to require a climate controlled environment and typically undergo less processing, packaging, transportation and storage [58,59]. However, other studies have suggested the benefits of consuming locally grown seasonal produce is not the determining factor of environmental impact because food production has more impact on the environment than transportation [12,60,61]. A recent study by Drewnowski *et al.* [11] assessed the relationship between nutrient and energy density and carbon footprint, and found that processed and frozen fruit and vegetables had a low carbon footprint when considered as per 100 grams in comparison to meat and dairy products. But when looking at energy density per 100 kcal, the carbon footprint of frozen and processed fruit and vegetables increased dramatically [11]. This study pointed out that carbon footprint is only one of many metrics to assess the environmental impact of food. Overall, it is widely accepted that some fruits and vegetables are more emissions-intensive than others depending on several factors, including country of origin, the need for protected conditions, storage and cooking.

Choosing seasonal local fruits and vegetables requires specific knowledge of where food was grown. This information is not always evident or available to consumers [7] particularly when meals are prepared by others (e.g., meals eaten at a restaurant). Studies have shown people are prepared to buy local produce, although factors such as convenience, price, accessibility and perceived quality also determine purchasing habits [50,62].

Using the protocol outlined in this paper, the intake of fruit and vegetables will be analysed from each eating image pair and classified according to the Australian Dietary Guidelines serve sizes (1 serve of vegetables = 75 grams, $\frac{1}{2}$ cup cooked vegetables or 1 cup of salad vegetables, and 1 serve of fruit = 150 grams, 1 medium piece or 2 small pieces of fruit). A Microsoft Access database tool will be created to record the estimated serve size and type of fruit and vegetable consumed separately. This feature will allow for further assessment of the environmental impact of different varieties. As the time and date stamp is available from images collected with the mFR, the date fruits and vegetables were consumed can be recorded and merged within the database containing information on when each fruit and vegetable is in season. For example, in Western Australia bananas are in season in summer and autumn, meaning if someone consumed a banana between 1st December and the 30th May then the banana will be recorded as "eaten in season". For this study, seasonal fruits and vegetables will be classified according to the Western Australia (WA) Seasonal Fruit and Vegetable Calendar [63].

Dietary assessment of seasonal and local fruit and vegetable intake poses significant challenges including: the additional burden of recording "place of origin" at time of purchase; prepared food not carrying this information (e.g., buying a salad at a café): and the sale of fruits and vegetables all year around, regardless of seasonality. A limitation of assessing the intake of seasonal fruit and vegetable intake is that there is no way of determining the origin of fresh produce, for example a banana from Queensland could be eaten in Western Australia, 4341 kilometres away by road (the main transportation method used). However, consuming seasonally available produce, regardless of origin, is likely to reflect an aspect of a healthy and sustainable diet. There is currently limited data on the intake of seasonal fruits and vegetables by adults in Australia. As less than 7% of Australians consume the recommended daily serves of vegetables and less than half consume the recommended two serves of fruit [64], increasing intake alone, regardless of seasonality, would result in health benefits.

An example of fruit to be consumed can be seen in the mFR image (as it appears using the web application hosted on a secure server) in Figure 5. Using this example containing the date of the image, one serve of fruit (e.g., one medium banana) would be entered in the database and because this eating occasion took place in September in Western Australia, this piece of fruit would be considered eaten "out of season".

**Before Image:**

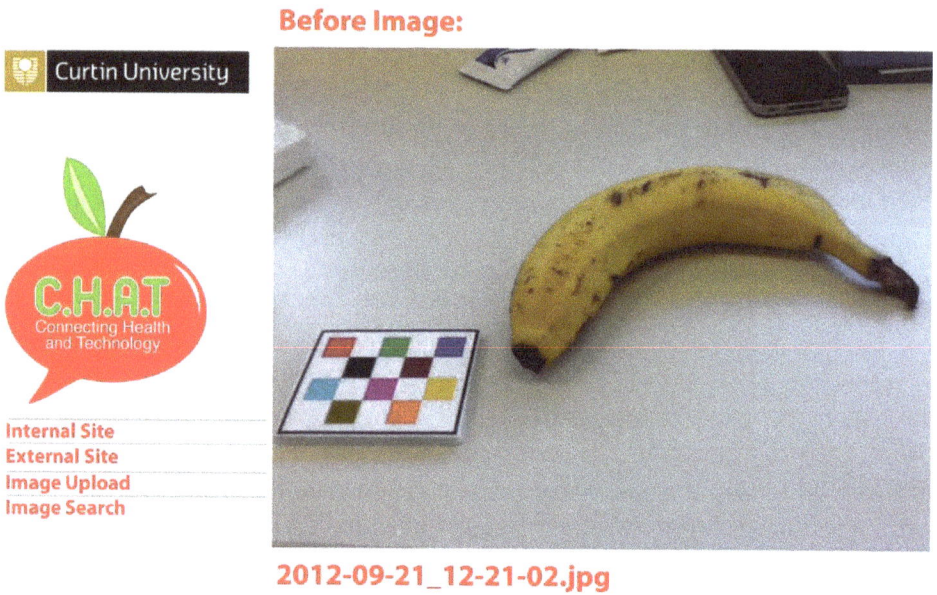

2012-09-21_12-21-02.jpg

**Figure 5.** Example of using the mobile food record to assess seasonal fruit and vegetable intake.

## 2.3.4. Dairy, Eggs and Meat Products

There is substantial evidence supporting the additional environmental impact of meat and dairy foods, compared to plant-based foods [2,14,65]. Along with a growing population and urbanisation, there is a global transition from largely plant-based diets to diets higher in EDNP foods and animal-based foods [45], increasing burden on the food system. While the consumption of dairy foods in Australia is generally below dietary recommended levels, Australians traditionally consume large volumes of meat, with the consumption of beef constituting the highest amount [15]. Meat and dairy products from ruminant cattle and sheep are some of the greatest greenhouse gas contributors in modern diets [8,9].

Previous research in the area of sustainable diets has highlighted a healthy and sustainable diet can be followed without the complete exclusion of dairy and meat [1,2,8,65], however, excessive red meat and processed meat consumption has been linked to an increased risk of colorectal cancer [7,66]. To accommodate this, the latest review of the Australian Dietary Guidelines reduced the standard serving size of lean red meat to a set 65 grams from the previous range of 65 to 100 grams of cooked meat, with a maximum of seven serves, or 455 grams, of red meat per week [7].

In Australia, only 2.1% of people avoid red meat [53]. Therefore, comparing meat intake between small, moderate and large meat consumers is relevant in assessing a healthy and sustainable diet when only a small percentage of the population are vegetarians [67].

When applying the proposed method to this component, food images will be used to estimate average daily intake of milk, cheese and yoghurt, eggs and meat products (including red meat, poultry and fish). The volume of specific types of dairy, eggs and meat products (e.g., beef mince) will be recorded as an approximate gram or millilitre weight and compared to the Australian Dietary Guidelines recommendations [7]. Meat consumed in other food products assessed using this method, such as a beef patty in a commercial burger, will be counted as ultra-processed EDNP food serves and also meat serves.

### 2.3.5. Food Waste

Australians throw away $5.3 billion Australian dollars (AUD) worth of food each year. This includes fresh food (AUD $2.9 billion), frozen food (AUD $241 million), take-away food (AUD $630 million), unfinished drinks (AUD $596 million) and leftover food (AUD $876 million) [68]. Young adults waste more food than older adults with 38% of 18–24 year olds wasting more than AUD $30 on fresh produce per fortnight, compared to only seven percent of older adults [68]. Reducing food waste from production to consumption will decrease burden on the food system, in turn benefiting the environment [69]. Discrepancies were detected in an Australian study comparing reported household fresh food waste (AUD $4.6 million) and actual fresh food waste (AUD $8 billion), collected during a household garbage bin audit [68]. The methods proposed here will accurately capture an important element of food waste, consumer plate waste, through the use of before and after eating food images, to support an area of research with a lack of sufficient data [69].

Image pairs allow for the accurate assessment of plate waste due to the presence of before eating and after eating images. Plate waste will be estimated as a percentage of food or beverage not consumed in the after eating image. Food waste in each image will also be classified as compostable (e.g., fruit, vegetables, egg shells), not compostable (e.g., meat and dairy) or unable to determine.

An example of red meat intake and food waste can be seen in Figure 6. Using the described protocol, this eating occasion will be assessed as four serves of roast beef, and having 30% edible plate waste. Note, one serve of cooked beef is 65 grams [7].

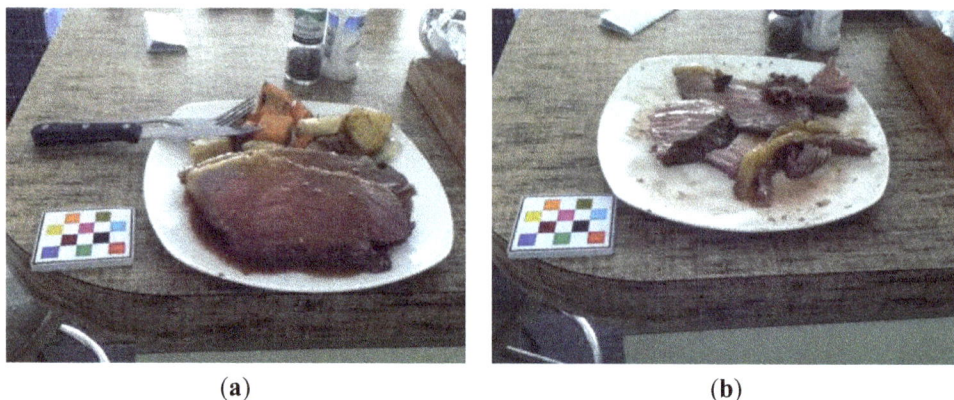

**Figure 6.** Example of using the mobile food record (mFR) to assess food waste and meat intake. (**a**) Before eating image; (**b**) After eating image.

### 2.4. Outcome Variables

The outcome variables measured using the proposed dietary assessment method include:

- number of serves and types of fruit and vegetables and whether they were in season at the time and location of consumption,
- intake of ultra-processed energy-dense nutrient-poor foods and beverages, separated by type and number of serves,
- intake of foods and beverages that are individually packaged, separated into "healthy" or "EDNP" foods or beverages,
- portion sizes and total amount of dairy, eggs and meat products
- percentage of plate waste and whether the food wasted was compostable.

### 2.5. Development of Healthy and Sustainable Diet Index

Existing diet quality indices will be reviewed to investigate the processes undertaken in development, validation, and evaluation and will guide the development of the *Healthy and Sustainable Diet Index*. This will be a theoretically driven Index, which will be internally validated using food image data collected during the CHAT study. Each indicator incorporated in the Index will be categorised into one or more of the following elements; impact on human health and/or impact on the environment. For example, ultra-processed EDNP foods and beverages impact health (contributing excess kilojoules and contributing to chronic disease risk) and the environment (use of water, electricity, transport and packaging). Another example is food waste, which has a direct negative impact on the environment (landfill) and a potential influence on health as fresh fruit and vegetables are perishable and often thrown away, creating a barrier for purchase and consumption.

The influence of dietary behaviours on human health will be given the highest weighting, followed by impact on the environment, for example plate waste. Weighting of different food items will involve a thorough assessment of available evidence, including evidence on the life cycle assessment of particular foods (which takes into account green-house gas emissions), and additional effects on ecosystems and biodiversity. The final Index may need to be modified when applied in other countries to take into account differences in the environmental impact of foods produced in various areas and climates, including climate conditions, farming, agricultural and production methods. For example the environmental impact of fruit that requires a climate controlled environment, *versus* seasonal fruit grown outside. A maximum number of total points will be allocated to each component of the *Healthy and Sustainable Diet Index*. A high weighting will not be given to components of the Index that cannot be measured accurately using image-based food records, for example whether fruits and vegetables consumed were locally grown and in season, due to the amount of error.

Each component incorporated into the *Healthy and Sustainable Diet Index*, will be given a weighting used to calculate a final score measuring adherence to a healthy and sustainable diet. For example, typically indices have a maximum score of 100, with a higher score indicating greater adherence to the preferred dietary pattern [23]. Individual components will be given a weighting to reflect consistency with the recommended dietary and sustainable eating outcomes, for example, fruit and vegetable intake may be given a higher weighting as it contributes to both healthy and sustainable eating.

The theoretically driven *Healthy and Sustainable Diet Index* will be internally validated for reliability, content validity and construct validity using 4-days image-based food records collected during a 6-month randomised controlled trial. The baseline data collected during the CHAT study ($n = 247$) will be randomised into thirds using age- and sex-stratified random sample techniques. Two-thirds of the sample will be randomly selected as the derivation cohort and the image-based mFRs of those selected will be used to develop the *Healthy and Sustainable Diet Index* using regression techniques. The remaining one-third of the sample will be used as the validation cohort for the *Healthy and Sustainable Diet Index*. This Index will also be used in the assessment of food images from the 6-month follow up ($n = 220$), and the results compared with baseline.

To assess content validity, components of the *Healthy and Sustainable Diet Index* will be assessed against the Australian Dietary Guidelines [7]. Construct validity will quantitatively assess how well the Index measures conformance to a healthy and sustainable diet.

111

To determine a total score using the *Healthy and Sustainable Diet Index*, density scores for each component will be calculated. Internal consistency, one form of reliability, will be assessed using Cronbach's coefficient $\alpha$. This test has previously been used in the evaluation of the Healthy Eating Index [70] to examine the degree of association between components, to determine if a diet only has one dimension. The relationship between the components of the *Healthy and Sustainable Diet Index* will be assessed using Pearson correlations coefficient. Principle component analysis will be used to assess if there are independent components of the Index. This will measure if there are any significant independent predictors of an overall score.

## 3. Discussion

The proposed methodologies described in this paper aim to determine if the mobile food record can be used to accurately measure five key indicators of a healthy and sustainable diet. The availability of dietary intake data collected from 4-day mFRs during the CHAT study enables the refinement of the assessment tool and internal validation of a theoretically driven *Healthy and Sustainable Diet Index*. This Index will be tested on a duplicate sample and a longitudinal sample of adults' 4-day image-based food records to measure content validity, construct validity and reliability.

The *Healthy and Sustainable Diet Index* will be unique in two ways; firstly it will combine the assessment of eating behaviours that influence health outcomes (e.g., EDNP foods and beverages) and dietary behaviours that significantly burden the environment (e.g., ultra-processed foods, food waste). Secondly, it will require the use of image-based food records, which will enable the accurate assessment of dietary behaviours not assessed in traditional forms of dietary assessment (e.g., individually packaged foods).

Using an mFR application to assess the five healthy and sustainable dietary behaviours described in this paper has the potential for further enhancement of the mFR applications capability as a new dietary assessment method. For example, a current fiducial marker probe exists to alert users when the fiducial marker is not located in the image, as described by Ahmad *et al.* [29]. A similar mechanism to ask the user whether food waste detected in the after image was thrown in the rubbish bin, composted, saved for consumption at a later time or other could be incorporated into the mFR application.

Currently there is limited evidence on whether Australian adults have dietary habits consistent with a sustainable diet. Without adequate evidence in this area, appropriate changes to dietary recommendations and nutrition policy are challenging. Results from the Australian Health Survey indicate most Australian's have eating habits inconsistent with the Dietary Guidelines, contributing to the burden of diet-related diseases in this country [63]. However, to the authors' knowledge, there is currently no dietary assessment tool or indexing system to assess and monitor whether individuals have dietary behaviours inconsistent with a sustainable diet, such as the use of individual food packaging and plate waste.

Similar to other dietary assessment methods, using the mobile food record to assess dietary behaviours does not come without limitations. The primary limitation being if a participant forgets to take an image of an eating occasion. This can be minimized by the ability to set alerts on the mobile device to remind participants to take images of all foods and beverages consumed.

Although this method of dietary assessment was tested on a population-based sample of young adults during the CHAT study, the mFR has also been tested in other ages groups [71]. A unique aspect of this proposed work is that images collected using the mFR application have not previously been used to measure these important and topical dietary behaviours, and hold potential for accurate dietary assessment. In addition to the development and validation of a novel dietary assessment method, findings from the work proposed will provide evidence on the current healthy and sustainable dietary habits of young Australian adults.

## 4. Conclusions

The strengths of the protocol and methodology proposed include the development of a dietary assessment method to accurately assess key indicators of a healthy and sustainable diet that are not measured during traditional dietary assessment methods. This innovative method will enable the development of a *Healthy and Sustainable Diet Index* to assess an individual's adherence to these dietary behaviours. The use of the mFR to assess adherence to a healthy and sustainable diet is a novel and innovative approach to dietary assessment. The steps outlined in this paper only capitalise on the images captured with the mFR, however other features in mobile devices, such as activity measures, could also be considered. Future applications of this method may strengthen this area of research, influence behaviour and raise the awareness of the potential benefits on individual and population health and the environment.

**Acknowledgments:** This Connecting Healthy and Technology study was funded by a three-year Heathway Project Grant with funding from the Department of Health, Western Australia. The authors are grateful to the Purdue University TADA project team, Marc Bosch, Ziad Ahmad, Maggie Zhu, and Brendon Wade and Andrew Buttsworth, Curtin University IT Services, for their ongoing technical support for the mobile food record application. We wish to thank the study participants.

**Author Contributions:** Amelia J. Harray, Deborah A. Kerr, Carol J. Boushey and Christina M. Pollard designed the protocol. Amelia J. Harray and Deborah A. Kerr took part in data collection and image analysis. Edward J. Delp, Carol J. Boushey and Deborah A. Kerr developed the mobile CHAT Application and backend server. Deborah A. Kerr, Carol J. Boushey, Christina M. Pollard, Edward J. Delp and Ziad Ahmad designed the CHAT study. Amelia J. Harray, Deborah A. Kerr, Carol J. Boushey drafted the manuscript. Satvinder S. Dhaliwal and Syed Aqif Mukhtar advised on statistical analysis and database development. All authors read and contributed to the final manuscript.

**Conflicts of Interest:** The authors declare no conflict of interest.

## References

1. Macdiarmid, J.I. Is a healthy diet an environmentally sustainable diet? *Proc. Nutr. Soc.* **2013**, *72*, 13–20.

2. Macdiarmid, J.I.; Kyle, J.; Horgan, G.W.; Loe, J.; Fyfe, C.; Johnstone, A.; McNeill, G. Sustainable diets for the future: Can we contribute to reducing greenhouse gas emissions by eating a healthy diet? *Am. J. Clin. Nutr.* **2012**, *96*, 632–639.

3. Reynolds, C.J.; Buckley, J.D.; Weinstein, P.; Boland, J. Are the dietary guidelines for meat, fat, fruit and vegetable consumption appropriate for environmental sustainability? A review of the literature. *Nutrients* **2014**, *6*, 2251–2265.

4. Burlingame, B.; Dernini, S. *Sustainable Diets and Biodiversity: Directions and Solutions for Policy, Research and Action*; Food and Agriculture Organization: Rome, Italy, 2012.

5. Swinburn, B.A.; Sacks, G.; Hall, K.D.; McPherson, K.; Finegood, D.T.; Moodie, M.L.; Gortmaker, S.L. The global obesity pandemic: Shaped by global drivers and local environments. *Lancet* **2011**, *378*, 804–814.

6. Colagiuri, S.; Lee, C.M.; Colagiuri, R.; Magliano, D.; Shaw, J.E.; Zimmet, P.Z.; Caterson, I.D. The cost of overweight and obesity in Australia. *Med. J. Aust.* **2010**, *192*, 260–264.

7. National Health and Medical Research Council. *Eat for Health: The Australian Dietary Guidelines*; National Health and Medical Research Council: Canberra, Australia, 2013.

8. Riley, H.; Buttriss, J.L. A UK public health perspective: What is a healthy sustainable diet? *Nutr. Bull.* **2011**, *36*, 426–431.

9. Lowe, M. Obesity and climate change mitigation in Australia: Overview and analysis of policies with co-benefits. *Aust. N. Zeal. J. Public Health* **2014**, *38*, 19–24.

10. Roy, P.; Nei, D.; Orikasa, T.; Xu, Q.; Okadome, H.; Nakamura, N.; Shiina, T. A review of life cycle assessment (LCA) on some food products. *J. Food Eng.* **2009**, *90*, 1–10.

11. Drewnowski, A.; Rehm, C.D.; Martin, A.; Verger, E.O.; Voinnesson, M.; Imbert, P. Energy and nutrient density of foods in relation to their carbon footprint. *Am. J. Clin. Nutr.* **2015**, *101*, 184–191.

12. Garnett, T. *What is a Sustainable Healthy Diet? A Discussion Paper*; Food Climate Research Network: Oxford, UK, 2014.

13. Tilman, D.; Clark, M. Global diets link environmental sustainability and human health. *Nature* **2014**, *515*, 518–522.

14. Drewnowski, A. Healthy diets for a healthy planet. *Am. J. Clin. Nutr.* **2014**, *99*, 1284–1285.

15. Bradbear, C.; Friel, S. *Food Systems and Environmental Sustainability: A Review of the Australian Evidence*; National Centre for Epidemiology and Population Health: Canberra, Australia, 2011.

16. Friel, S.; Barosh, L.J.; Lawrence, M. Towards healthy and sustainable food consumption: An Australian case study. *Public Health Nutr.* **2014**, *17*, 1156–1166.

17. Dixon, J.; Isaacs, B. Why sustainable and "nutritionally correct" food is not on the agenda: Western Sydney, the moral arts of everyday life and public policy. *Food Policy* **2013**, *43*, 67–76.

18. Clonan, A.; Holdsworth, M. The challenges of eating a healthy and sustainable diet. *Am. J. Clin. Nutr.* **2012**, *96*, 459–460.

19. Selvey, L.A.; Carey, M.G. Australia's dietary guidelines and the environmental impact of food "from paddock to plate". *Med. J. Aust.* **2013**, *198*, 18–19.

20. Morgan, E. *Fruit and Vegetable Consumption and Waste in Australia*; Victorian Health Promotion Foundation, State Government of Victoria: Melbourne, Australia, 2009.

21. Bradbear, C.; Friel, S. Integrating climate change, food prices and population health. *Food Policy* **2013**, *43*, 56–66.

22. Johnston, J.L.; Fanzo, J.C.; Cogill, B. Understanding sustainable diets: A descriptive analysis of the determinants and processes that influence diets and their impact on health, food security, and environmental sustainability. *Adv. Nutr.* **2014**, *5*, 418–429.

23. Collins, C.E.; Burrows, T.L.; Rollo, M.E.; Boggess, M.M.; Watson, J.F.; Guest, M.; Duncanson, K.; Pezdirc, K.; Hutchesson, M.J. The comparative validity and reproducibility of a diet quality index for adults: The Australian recommended food score. *Nutrients* **2015**, *7*, 785–798.

24. Thompson, F.E.; Subar, A.F. Assessment methods for research and practice. In *Nutrition in the Prevention and Treatment of Disease*, 3rd ed.; Ferruzzi, M., Coulston, A.M., Boushey, C.J., Eds.; Academic Press: London, UK, 2013; pp. 5–46.

25. Kirkpatrick, S.I.; Reedy, J.; Butler, E.N.; Dodd, K.W.; Subar, A.F.; Thompson, F.E.; McKinnon, R.A. Dietary assessment in food environment research: A systematic review. *Am. J. Prev. Med.* **2014**, *46*, 94–102.

26. Zhu, F.; Bosch, M.; Woo, I.; Kim, S.; Boushey, C.J.; Ebert, D.S.; Delp, E.J. The use of mobile devices in aiding dietary assessment and evaluation. *IEEE J. Sel. Top. Signal Proc.* **2010**, *4*, 756–766.

27. Daugherty, B.L.; Schap, T.E.; Ettienne-Gittens, R.; Zhu, F.M.; Bosch, M.; Delp, E.J.; Ebert, D.S.; Kerr, D.A.; Boushey, C.J. Novel technologies for assessing dietary intake: Evaluating the usability of a mobile telephone food record among adults and adolescents. *J. Med. Intern. Res.* **2012**, *14*, e58.

28. Zhu, F.; Bosch, M.; Khanna, N.; Boushey, C.J.; Delp, E.J. Multiple hypotheses image segmentation and classification with application to dietary assessment. *IEEE J. Biomed. Health Inform.* **2015**, *19*, 377–388.

29. Ahmad, Z.; Khanna, N.; Kerr, D.A.; Boushey, C.J.; Delp, E.J. A Mobile Phone User Interface for Image-Based Dietary Assessment. In Proceedings of the IS&T/SPIE Conference on Mobile Devices and Multimedia: Enabling Technologies, Algorithms, and Applications, San Francisco, CA, USA, 2–6 February 2014.

30. Xu, C.; He, Y.; Khanna, N.; Boushey, C.; Delp, E. Model-Based Food Volume Estimation Using 3D Pose. In Proceedings of IEEE International Conference on Image Processing, Melbourne, Australia, 15–18 September 2013; pp. 2534–2538.

31. McNaughton, S.A.; Ball, K.; Crawford, D.; Mishra, G.D. An index of diet and eating patterns is a valid measure of diet quality in an australian population. *J. Nutr.* **2008**, *138*, 86–93.

32. Sofi, F.; Macchi, C.; Abbate, R.; Gensini, G.F.; Casini, A. Mediterranean diet and health status: An updated meta-analysis and a proposal for a literature-based adherence score. *Public Health Nutr.* **2014**, *17*, 2769–2782.

33. Guenther, P.M.; Reedy, J.; Krebs-Smith, S.M. Development of the healthy eating index-2005. *J. Am. Diet. Assoc.* **2008**, *108*, 1896–1901.

34. Trichopoulou, A.; Costacou, T.; Bamia, C.; Trichopoulos, D. Adherence to a mediterranean diet and survival in a Greek population. *N. Engl. J. Med.* **2003**, *348*, 2599–2608.

35. Patterson, R.E.; Haines, P.S.; Popkin, B.M. Diet quality index: Capturing a multidimensional behavior. *J. Am. Diet. Assoc.* **1994**, *94*, 57–64.

36. Toft, U.; Kristoffersen, L.H.; Lau, C.; Borch-Johnsen, K.; Jorgensen, T. The dietary quality score: Validation and association with cardiovascular risk factors: The inter99 study. *Eur. J. Clin. Nutr.* **2007**, *61*, 270–278.

37. Harrington, J.M.; Fitzgerald, A.P.; Kearney, P.M.; McCarthy, V.J.; Madden, J.; Browne, G.; Dolan, E.; Perry, I.J. Dash diet score and distribution of blood pressure in middle-aged men and women. *Am. J. Hypertens.* **2013**, *26*, 1311–1320.

38. Xu, C.; Zhu, F.; Khanna, N.; Boushey, C.J.; Delp, E.J. Image Enhancement and Quality Measures for Dietary Assessment Using Mobile Devices. In Proceedings of SPIE-The International Society for Optical Engineering, Burlingame, CA, USA, 9 February 2012; p. 82960.

39. Kerr, D.A.; Pollard, C.M.; Howat, P.; Delp, E.J.; Pickering, M.; Kerr, K.R.; Dhaliwal, S.S.; Pratt, I.S.; Wright, J.; Boushey, C.J. Connecting health and technology (CHAT): Protocol of a randomized controlled trial to improve nutrition behaviours using mobile devices and tailored text messaging in young adults. *BMC Public Health* **2012**, *12*, 477.

40. Rangan, A.M.; Schindeler, S.; Hector, D.J.; Gill, T.P.; Webb, K.L. Consumption of "extra" foods by Australian adults: Types, quantities and contribution to energy and nutrient intakes. *Eur. J. Clin. Nutr.* **2009**, *63*, 865–871.

41. Monteiro, C.; Levy, R.B.; Claro, R.M.; Ribeiro de Castro, I.R.; Cannon, G. A new classification of foods based on the extent and purpose of their processing. *Cadernos de Saude Publica* **2010**, *26*, 2039–2049.

42. Tavares, L.F.; Fonseca, S.C.; Garcia R., M.L.; Yokoo, E.M. Relationship between ultra-processed foods and metabolic syndrome in adolescents from a Brazilian family doctor program. *Public Health Nutr.* **2012**, *15*, 82–87.

43. Moubarac, J.-C.; Martins, A.P.B.; Claro, R.M.; Levy, R.B.; Cannon, G.; Monteiro, C.A. Consumption of ultra-processed foods and likely impact on human health. Evidence from Canada. *Public Health Nutr.* **2013**, *16*, 2240–2248.

44. Monteiro, C. World nutrition. *J. World Public Health Nutr. Assoc.* **2010**, *1*, 237–269.

45. World Health Organization. *Diet, Nutrition and the Prevention of Chronic Disease: Report of a Joint Who/Fao Expert Consultation*; World Health Organization: Geneva, Switzerland, 2003.

46. Smith, K.J.; Blizzard, L.; McNaughton, S.A.; Gall, S.L.; Dwyer, T.; Venn, A.J. Daily eating frequency and cardiometabolic risk factors in young australian adults: Cross-sectional analyses. *Br. J. Nutr.* **2012**, *108*, 1086–1094.

47. Smith, K.J.; McNaughton, S.A.; Gall, S.L.; Blizzard, L.; Dwyer, T.; Venn, A.J. Takeaway food consumption and its associations with diet quality and abdominal obesity: A cross-sectional study of young adults. *Int. J. Behav. Nutr. Phys. Act.* **2009**, *6*, 29.

48. Drewnowski, A.; Specter, S.E. Poverty and obesity: The role of energy density and energy costs. *Am. J. Clin. Nutr.* **2004**, *79*, 6–16.

49. Marsh, K.; Bugusu, B. Food packaging-roles, materials, and environmental issues. *J. Food Sci.* **2007**, *72*, R39–R55.

50. Lea, E.; Worsley, A. Australian consumers' food-related environmental beliefs and behaviours. *Appetite* **2008**, *50*, 207–214.

51. Martínez-González, M.Á.; de la Fuente-Arrillaga, C.; López-del-Burgo, C.; Vázquez-Ruiz, Z.; Benito, S.; Ruiz-Canela, M. Low consumption of fruit and vegetables and risk of chronic disease: A review of the epidemiological evidence and temporal trends among Spanish graduates. *Public Health Nutr.* **2011**, *14*, 2309–2315.

52. Pollard, C.M.; Miller, M.R.; Daly, A.M.; Crouchley, K.E.; O'Donoghue, K.J.; Lang, A.J.; Binns, C.W. Increasing fruit and vegetable consumption: Success of the Western Australian Go for 2&5 campaign. *Public Health Nutr.* **2008**, *11*, 314–320.

53. Australian Bureau of Statistics. *Australian Health Survey: Nutrition First Results-Foods and Nutrients; 2011–2012 No. 4364.0.55.007*; Australian Bureau of Statistics: Canberra, Australia, 2014.

54. Kamphuis, C.B.; Giskes, K.; de Bruijn, G.J.; Wendel-Vos, W.; Brug, J.; van Lenthe, F.J. Environmental determinants of fruit and vegetable consumption among adults: A systematic review. *Br. J. Nutr.* **2006**, *96*, 620–635.

55. Pollard, C.; Miller, M.; Woodman, R.J.; Meng, R.; Binns, C. Changes in knowledge, beliefs, and behaviors related to fruit and vegetable consumption among western Australian adults from 1995 to 2004. *Am. J. Public Health* **2009**, *99*, 355–361.

56. Barosh, L.J.; Friel, S.; Engelhardt, K.; Chan, L. The cost of a healthy and sustainable diet-who can afford it? *Aust. N. Zeal. J. Public Health* **2014**, *38*, 7–12.

57. Australian Bureau of Statistics. *Consumer Price Index, Australia; No. 6401.0*; Australian Bureau of Statistics: Canberra, Australia, 2013.

58. Larsen, K.; Ryan, C.; Abraham, A.B. *Sustainable and Secure Food Systems for Victoria: What do We Know? What do We Need to Know?*; Victorian Eco-Innovation Lab: Melbourne, Australia, 2008.

59. Lake, I.R.; Hooper, L.; Abdelhamid, A.; Bentham, G.; Boxall, A.B.; Draper, A.; Fairweather-Tait, S.; Hulme, M.; Hunter, P.R.; Nichols, G.; *et al.* Climate change and food security: Health impacts in developed countries. *Environ. Health Perspect.* **2012**, *120*, 1520–1526.

60. Avetisyan, M.; Hertel, T.; Sampson, G. Is local food more environmentally friendly? The GHG emissions impacts of consuming imported *vs.* domestically produced food. *Environ. Resour. Econ.* **2014**, *58*, 415–462.

61. Macdiarmid, J.I. Seasonality and dietary requirements: Will eating seasonal food contribute to health and environmental sustainability? *Proc. Nutr. Soc.* **2014**, *73*, 368–375.

62. Vermeir, I.; Verbeke, W. Sustainable food consumption among young adults in Belgium: Theory of planned behaviour and the role of confidence and values. *Ecol. Econ.* **2008**, *64*, 542–553.

63. Department of Agriculture and Food. *Western Australian Seasonal Calendar for Fruit and Vegetables*; Department of Agriculture and Food: Waroona, Australia, 2013.

64. Australian Bureau of Statistics. *Australian Health Survey: First Results, 2011–2012*; No. 4364.0.55.001; Australian Bureau of Statistics: Canberra, Australia, 2012.

65. Masset, G.; Soler, L.; Vieux, F.; Darmon, N. Identifying sustainable foods: The relationship between environmental impact, nutritional quality, and prices of foods representative of the French diet. *J. Acad. Nutr. Diet.* **2014**, *114*, 862–869.

66. World Cancer Research Fund. *Food, Nutrition, Physical Activity, and the Prevention of Cancer: A Global Perspective*; American Institute for Cancer Research: Washington, DC, USA, 2007.

67. De Boer, J.; Hoogland, C.T.; Boersema, J.J. Towards more sustainable food choices: Value priorities and motivational orientations. *Food Q. Prefer.* **2007**, *18*, 985–996.

68. Hamilton, C.; Denniss, R.; Baker, D. *Wasteful Consumption in Australia*; The Australia Institute: Manuka, Australia, 2005.

69. Mason, L.; Boyle, T.; Fyfe, J.; Smith, T.; Cordell, D. *National Food Waste Assessment: Final Report*; Institute for Sustainable Futures, Univeristy of Technology: Sydney, Australia, 2011.

70. Guenther, P.M.; Reedy, J.; Krebs-Smith, S.M.; Reeve, B.B. Evaluation of the healthy eating index-2005. *J. Am. Diet. Assoc.* **2008**, *108*, 1854–1864.

71. Six, B.L.; Schap, T.E.; Zhu, F.M.; Mariappan, A.; Bosch, M.; Delp, E.J.; Ebert, D.S.; Kerr, D.A.; Boushey, C.J. Evidence-based development of a mobile telephone food record. *J. Am. Diet. Assoc.* **2010**, *110*, 74–79.

# Dietary Assessment on a Mobile Phone Using Image Processing and Pattern Recognition Techniques: Algorithm Design and System Prototyping

Yasmine Probst, Duc Thanh Nguyen, Minh Khoi Tran and Wanqing Li

**Abstract:** Dietary assessment, while traditionally based on pen-and-paper, is rapidly moving towards automatic approaches. This study describes an Australian automatic food record method and its prototype for dietary assessment via the use of a mobile phone and techniques of image processing and pattern recognition. Common visual features including scale invariant feature transformation (SIFT), local binary patterns (LBP), and colour are used for describing food images. The popular bag-of-words (BoW) model is employed for recognizing the images taken by a mobile phone for dietary assessment. Technical details are provided together with discussions on the issues and future work.

Reprinted from *Nutrients*. Cite as: Probst, Y.; Nguyen, D.T.; Tran, M.K.; Li, W. Dietary Assessment on a Mobile Phone Using Image Processing and Pattern Recognition Techniques: Algorithm Design and System Prototyping. *Nutrients* **2015**, *7*, 6128–6138.

## 1. Introduction

Assessment of dietary intake is a process vital to dietetic care across different disciplines and specialties of practice. As a fundamental skill taught during early dietetic training, the manual process of conducting a dietary assessment with a participant is inherently flawed due to various forms of bias depending on the method of assessment being applied [1] in addition to the format of the assessment. Traditionally, assessments were completed using a paper-and-pen format to record *usual* intake through diet history interview, repeated 24-h recall and food frequency questionnaire and are often impacted by memory and cognition of the person recalling their intake. In addition, the time burden of the process and the literacy of the target group for which dietary intake data is required are also factors that affect the data being recorded. This is particularly evident in assessing the intakes of children where the age of the child plays an important role on the method employed. Whether the recall is obtained from the child who consumed the food or whether the recall is provided by the child's carer or parents, may have impact on the accuracy of what has been consumed [2]. With the combination of these challenges and technological advances, many dietary assessment methods have been partially or fully automated in an attempt to reduce bias, ease the burden for the participants and also streamline the steps applied within each method [1].

Automation of dietary assessment appears to have begun during the 1960s with early movements towards computerized processing of intake data [3]. Along with the move to the computerized analysis of the nutrients, there has been an expansion to the automation of the intake assessment process itself. This initially began with the use of software on a standalone desktop computer and later advanced to interactive processes through the Internet [1]. Today, web-based dietary recalls are not uncommon in large cohort studies due to their efficiency and ability to streamline processes within one study time point [3]. The automated version of the 24-hour recall for example minimizes the need for an interviewer by employing the use of on-screen avatars [4] and probing questions to guide the participants through the recall. This change has also resulted in reduced resource requirements overall allowing it to be implemented with a very large number of participants.

Contrary to this, the most common method of dietary assessment used within the randomized controlled trials remains as that of the food record or food diary [5], a record of *actual* food intake. This method places increased burden on the person completing the assessment and may involve a process of estimating or measuring the food portion size after recording the name of the food item that has been consumed. The method is retrospective in nature and due to the participant burden, modifications made to the intake during the recording period often occur with a longer recording periods resulting in greater bias or underestimation of intake [6]. Automation of the food record method aims to address this issue. More recently, the food record method has shifted to portable devices such as Tablets and Smartphones [1]. This shift should not simply be thought of as the creation of data collection forms on a phone but rather be considered as essential changes to the method within which data collection occurs. During the past decade research in this area has been expanding rapidly. Although there are many applications (apps) available for download to a Smartphone, the credibility of these apps remains questionable. Key groups in the United States have developed credible, evidence-based applications used within the research setting [1]. The Technology Assisted Dietary Assessment (TADA) project, for example, has employed a process of image segmentation to accurately detect food items, with an initial prototype trialed on iPhones/iPods. This group reported challenges of detecting colour and texture [7] and employed the use of a fiducial marker to assist with the accuracy of the detection process. Illumination and the angle of the photos being taken have been further noted as concerns [8]. The Bag-of-Words model, used as the basis for the prototype described in this paper, was also used by the TADA team. Also using image recognition, the Food Intake Visual and voice Recognizer (FIVR) project similarly used a fiducial marker to assist with the image recognition. Contrasting to the TADA project, which initially used text to assist with image tagging, FIVR used voice for this process, and in addition, it relied on the user's descriptions (text or voice) to identify the food in the photograph [9]. While the above tools aim to automate the assessment, notable progress has also been made with the Remote Food Photography Method (RFPM), which uses a semi-automated food photograph classification approach. The RFPM is focused on portion size of the food items and uses bilateral filtering to reduce the noise in the images taken [10]. User training is required in order to ensure that photographs are captured correctly [11].

This paper describes the development of a baseline prototype of an automated food record by using image processing and pattern recognition algorithms. To the knowledge of the authors, the automated food record described in this paper is the first Australian developed prototype of this nature. The described prototype supports automation of the food recording and recognition. The prototype facilitates an extension to determine the portion size of the food and finally all data can be easily matched to food composition databases. Determination of food portion is crucial for nutrient calculations and automation of this process can reduce the need for manual calculations from the recognized foods. The focus of this paper is to provide a comprehensive overview of a baseline prototype with the function of image recognition and addresses the challenges that are potentially faced when moving an algorithm from a laboratory-based test environment [12] to a user-based application.

The baseline prototype also adopts the Bag-of-Words model for recognition due to computational efficiency and promising results obtained recently [11,16]. Many challenging issues mentioned above are dealt by the careful selection of features. However, the work differs from the previous studies [11,16] in the following dimensions. Firstly, the system does not require any fiducial markers or addition user annotation such as text or voice. Secondly, the system aims to recognize multiple foods in a single image, *i.e.*, more than one food type can be present in an input image. Our system is thus more realistic in practice. Thirdly, we are also simultaneously deploying the food image recognition on mobile phones. This enables us to investigate the practical factors of the proposed dietary assessment prototype including the discriminative power of each feature type, the combination of features to particular food categories and the computational speed of various interest point detectors.

## 2. Experimental Section: Image Classification Using Bag-of-Words (BoW) Model

The BoW model was originally devised for text classification [13]. In the model, a text document is encoded by a histogram representing the frequency of the occurrence of codewords. The codewords are predefined in a discrete vocabulary referred to as a codebook. The codeword histograms obtained from training samples (small collections of text documents) are used to train a discriminative classifier, e.g., Support Vector Machine (SVM) [14]. The trained classifier is then used to classify test documents (larger collections of text).

To automate the food record, the BoW model was applied for classification of food images captured using a person's mobile phone. In this task, the features of an image are used as codewords. The images employed in this study, are the photographs of foods recorded as part of the food record method. Rather than recording the text-based name of the food risking poor quality detail about the food due to long food selection lists, incorrect spelling or typographical errors, a photograph can provide additional details about the foods. Using photographs also provides the potential to minimize the burden on the person completing the dietary assessment. The food image classification method in this study was implemented in C++ programming language. The training phase and evaluation of the food image recognition were conducted on a desktop computer using Microsoft Windows 7.0. The prototype was deployed on a Smartphone using the Android mobile operating system.

Image classification using the BoW model requires feature selection, codebook creation, discriminative training. In the following sections, each of these components is described in further detail.

## 2.1. Feature Selection

For the purpose of image recognition, the features are used to describe the visual properties of the foods in the photographs. In this study, we investigated three common types of features including Scale Invariant Feature Transformation (SIFT) [15], Local Binary Pattern (LBP) [16], and Colour [17]. *SIFT* [15] is used to describe the local *shape* of visual objects. It is constructed by a histogram of the orientations of edges in the food photographs. *LBP* [16] is used to capture the *texture* information of the foods. The LBP is known for its simplicity in implementation, low computational complexity and robustness under varying illumination conditions. *Colour* [17] plays an important role in food image classification, e.g., the red colour of a tomato is useful to distinguish it from an apple sharing a similar shape. In our experiments, we quantise each colour channel (Red, Green, and Blue) of an image pixel into four bins (intervals). The colour features of an image then can be constructed as the histogram of the colour of all pixels in that image.

## 2.2. Codebook Creation

Suppose that there are $N$ food categories $C_1, C_2, \ldots, C_N$ (e.g., carrots, muscle meat, *etc.*) and $A$ is the set of training images. The SIFT interest point detector of Lowe [15] was invoked to detect interest points on the training images of $A$. SIFT [14] and LBP [15] features were then extracted at interest points. Let $v_p$ be the $D$-dimensional features extracted at interest points $p$. These features were then clustered into $K$ groups using a K-means algorithm. Idendennn clustering, the dissimilarity (based on distance) between two features was computed using a metric, e.g., $\chi^2$ distance (as in our implementation). Equation (1) outlines the dissimilarity between features as follows,

$$(v_p, v_q) = \frac{1}{2} \sum_{i=1}^{D} \frac{[v_p(i) - v_q(i)]^2}{v_p(i) + v_q(i)} \tag{1}$$

where $v_p(i)$ is the $i$-th element of $v_p$.

Completion of this step resulted in a codebook $G = \{w_1, w_2, \ldots, w_K\}$ in which codewords $w_i$ were considered to be the centres of the $i$'th clusters.

### 2.3. Discriminative Training

To classify $N$ food categories, $N$ binary classifiers $f_1, f_2, \ldots, f_N$ were used. Each classifier $f_i$ classified a given test sample (food image in this context) into two classes: $C_i$ or non-$C_i$. Given a food image and codebook $G$, the SIFT interest point detector was used to detect a set of interest points from the food image. Let $p$ and $v_p$ be an interest point and the feature extracted at $p$. The best matching codeword $w(p) \in G$ was determined as outlined in Equation (2),

$$\mathbf{w}(p) = \operatorname*{argmin}_{w_i \in G} d(v_p, w_i) \tag{2}$$

where $d(v_p, w_i)$ is defined in Equation (1).

Figure 1 provides an example of describing a food image by codewords. In this figure, the red points are SIFT interest points, where $w_1, w_2, w_3$ are the best matching codewords of the features extracted at each of these interest points. The food image was then encoded by a histogram of occurrence of the codewords. Such histograms were collected from all training images of the food category $i$'th and from the training images of other categories to train the classifier $f_i$. In our implementation, SVMs were used as classifiers for $f_i$.

### 2.4. Testing

Given a test image, $I$, similar to the training phase, the histogram of the occurrence of the codewords obtained on $I$ was computed and denoted as $h(I)$. Let $f_i(h(I))$ be the classification score of the trained classifier $f_i$ applied on $h(I)$. If the image $I$ contains only one food category, this food category was determined as shown in Equation (3)

$$C_i \text{ if } f_i = \max_{j \in \{1, \ldots, N\}} f_j(h(I)) \tag{3}$$

If $I$ contains more than one food category (such as for a meal on a plate), the food category $C_i$ was considered to be present in $I$ if $f_i\left(h\left(I\right)\right) > \epsilon$, where $\epsilon$ is a user-defined threshold, referred to as recognition sensitivity.

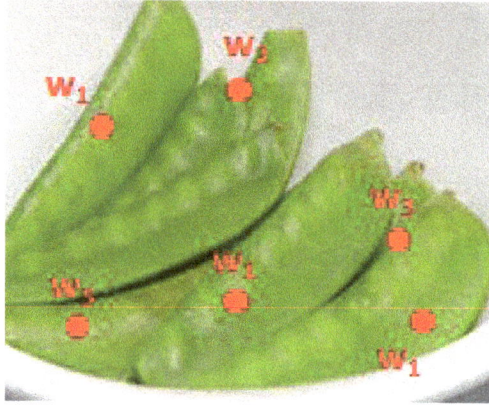

**Figure 1.** An image of snowpeas showing interest points shown as red points and the corresponding best matching codewords labelled $w_1$, $w_2$, $w_3$.

## 3. Results

The SIFT interest point detector took on average approximately 74 seconds for an image captured by a smartphone's camera. To speed-up the interest point detector, input images were resized by a factor of two if either the width or height of the input image was over 2000 pixels. Through the experiments it was found that by reducing the image's size, the speed of the interest point detector could be improved and also the number of interest points overall could be reduced. In the experiments, the detection of interest points on the resized images took approximately 20 s. Note that the time also depends on the computing resource available in the Smartphone. Different implementations of the SIFT interest point detector outlined by Lowe [15] were also trialed. Table 1 shows the times taken by those interest point detectors.

**Table 1.** Processing time of interest point detectors.

| Interest Point Detector | Processing Time (s/image) [†] |
|---|---|
| Original interest point detector [9] | 74 |
| ezSift | 14 |
| openCV | 60–65 |
| zerofog | 15–20 |

[†] Obtained without resizing the input image.

The ezSift interest point detector was found to be the fastest detector with less than 15 s. The number of interest points generated by this detector was less than that generated by other detectors, likely due to a lower number of scales used in the ezSift detector. However, the number of detected interest points was usually sufficient for recognition as this has been found empirically. The study also found that the zerofog had been optimized using openmp to run on parallel processors.

To describe the appearance of food images, three codebooks corresponding to three different feature types were created for each food category. The codebook size (*i.e.*, the number of codewords) for the SIFT, LBP, and colour feature was 100, 40, and 50, respectively. To combine the three features, for each food image, three histograms of codewords corresponding to the three codebooks were concatenated to form a longer histogram. Linear SVMs [18] were employed as classifiers.

The food image classification method was evaluated on a newly created dataset [19–21]. Table 2 summarises the dataset used in the evaluation. Note that in this dataset, one food image may contain more than one food category (see Figure 2). The dataset was organised so that the training sets (used during codebook creation) and test sets were separated.

**Table 2.** Summary of the dataset used for training and testing of the food image recognition method. Positive images of a food category indicate the number of images contained in each food category.

| Food Category | Positive Training Images, $n$ | Test Images, $n$ |
|---|---|---|
| Beans | 4 | 18 |
| Carrots | 7 | 47 |
| Cheese | 4 | 53 |
| Custards | 5 | 64 |
| Milk | 4 | 44 |
| Muscle meat | 7 | 34 |
| Oranges | 8 | 61 |
| Peas | 5 | 13 |
| Tomato | 6 | 24 |
| Yoghurt | 6 | 52 |

Since more than one food category could be contained in a food image, as would be consumed in real life, a food category $C_i$ was considered to be contained in the food image $I$ if $f_i(h(I)) > \epsilon$. Thus, the classification (recognition) performance was investigated by varying the threshold $\epsilon$. Let $M$ be a set of test images, $M_i$ be a subset of $M$ and contain the food category $C_i$. For a given $\epsilon$, let $M_i^R(\epsilon)$ $M$ be the set of images whose classification score is greater than $\epsilon$, i.e., $M_i^R(\epsilon)$ is the set of images recognised as containing instances of $C_i$. The recognition performance associated with $\epsilon$ of the food category $C_i$ was represented by $r_i(\epsilon)$ and defined in Equation (4) as follows,

$$r_i(\epsilon) = \frac{\left| M_i^R(\epsilon) \cap M_i \right|}{\left| M_i^R(\epsilon) \cup M_i \right|} \tag{4}$$

where $\cap$ and $\cup$ is the intersection and union operator, respectively, and $|M|$ is the cardinality of the set $M$.

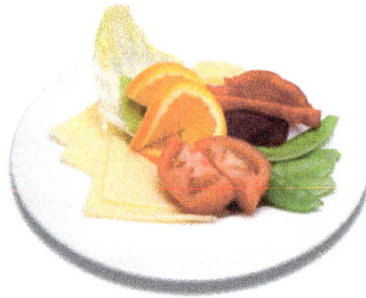

**Figure 2.** An example of a food image containing five food categories: cheese, tomato, oranges, beans, and carrots.

As shown in Equation (4), the higher $r(\epsilon)$ is, the better the recognition performance is. In this study, $\mathbf{r}_i = \max_{\epsilon} r_i(\epsilon)$; was used as the recognition accuracy of the food image recognition method on the food category $C_i$. Table 3 represents the accuracy of the method with the various feature types. The accuracy was computed for each food category and for the overall food categories.

**Table 3.** Recognition accuracy of the food image recognition method with various feature types. SIFT, scale invariant feature transformation; LBP, local binary patterns.

|  | SIFT | LBP | Colour | SIFT + LBP + Colour |
|---|---|---|---|---|
| Beans | 0.33 | **0.53** | 0.19 | 0.43 |
| Carrots | 0.37 | 0.44 | 0.46 | **0.51** |
| Cheese | **0.16** | **0.16** | **0.16** | **0.16** |
| Custards | 0.60 | 0.22 | 0.24 | **0.62** |
| Milk | 0.13 | **0.78** | 0.3 | 0.13 |
| Muscle meat | 0.40 | 0.32 | 0.5 | **0.55** |
| Oranges | 0.23 | 0.44 | 0.5 | **0.57** |
| Peas | 0.65 | 0.85 | **1.0** | 0.93 |
| Tomato | **0.35** | 0.29 | 0.29 | 0.33 |
| Yoghurt | **0.54** | 0.2 | 0.2 | 0.42 |
| *Overall* | *0.37* | *0.42* | *0.38* | ***0.47*** |

SIFT: scale invariant feature transformation, LBP: local binary patterns

## 4. Discussion

A prototype of an automated dietary assessment on mobile devices has been described in this paper. Various challenges have been identified through this progressive step with future work continuing to address these challenges. Challenges faced were similar to existing studies [7] in this field with colour and multiple food items being of particular focus. As shown in Table 3, on average, the LBP outperformed both the SIFT and colour histogram and the SIFT gave the poorest performance overall. The combination of all features (SIFT, LBP and Colour) gave a better performance overall as anticipated due to the various advantages and disadvantages of each feature. One particular note was for the "Cheese" category, where the accuracy was low. This was likely due to the presence of other food types in the same image with cheese. The accuracy could be improved if the "Cheese" items could be captured at a closer distance, *i.e.*, outliers and other food items other than cheese are not present in the image.

In the current implementation, linear SVMs were used. More sophisticated SVMs such as radial basis function (RBF) and polynomial kernel SVMs often gain better performance. Thus, those kernel types will be implemented, tested, and compared with the linear kernel in future studies. In addition, some advanced machine learning techniques, e.g., deep learning [22], extreme learning [23], will also be considered to improve the recognition accuracy. These techniques are recent developments in the area of pattern recognition.

Since multiple food types can co-occur on the same image, extracting individual food items would help to improve the recognition accuracy. Therefore, the aim is to simultaneously detect and recognise food as for future work. The accuracy of the food image recognition may also be improved if the classifiers were trained on large and diverse datasets including various illumination conditions, complex background, food images captured at various viewpoints. More challenging datasets with more food categories have been collected and will be released in our future work.

## 5. Conclusions

Applying image processing and pattern recognition techniques on a mobile device has allowed for the development of an automated food record via the use of a Smartphone. Continuing the prototype developed in this study to the subsequent stages of the food record, namely portion identification and translation to nutrient data, will complete the process and allow for a practical user-friendly approach to dietary data collection within the Australian context. It is vital that the mapping of food images to their corresponding food items within a food composition database is performed carefully to allow for the most accurate output data to be provided. Development of applications for the use in dietetic practice needs to encompass the inherent bias of the underpinning method of dietary assessment.

127

They should also consider the advancements in technology to potentially reduce some of these biases. This will provide impetus for more robust dietary assessment processes that are streamlined in their methods but also less resource intensive in their nature. Considering these two concepts together will mean that nutrition researchers or clinicians in practice can spend additional time with the clients working on behaviour changes for better health rather than data entry and nutrient analysis as was previously the case. Embracing credible and suitably selected technologies to work within the existing nutrition care processes should be considered to the advantage of both the clients and clinicians. The work of this study is one of the first of this nature in the Australian context.

**Acknowledgments:** The authors would like to thank the University of Wollongong Science Medicine and Health Advancement funding for supporting the prototype development work of this project. The authors would also like to acknowledge the contribution to the image dataset provided by Dr Megan Rollo during the earlier phases of this project.

**Author Contributions:** YP conceived the initial project idea, sourced funding support and contributed the initial test images and main proportion of training images to the dataset. DT and WL performed the experiments to refine the image recognition algorithm from the original Bag-of-Words model and MT assisted with transferring the developed algorithm to Android, testing and intensive experimentation on Android. DT, WL contributed to the analysis of the data and all authors contributed to the writing and editing of the manuscript.

**Conflicts of Interest:** The authors declare no conflict of interest.

## References

1.  Probst, Y.; Nguyen, D.T.; Rollo, M.; Li, W. mHealth diet and nutrition guidance. In *mHealth Multidisciplinary Verticals*; CRC Press—Taylor & Francis Group: Boca Raton, FL, USA, 2014.
2.  Bell, L.; Golley, R.; Magarey, A. Short tools to assess young children's dietary intake: A systematic review focusing on application to dietary index research. *J. Obes.* **2013**, *2013*.
3.  Probst, Y.C.; Tapsell, L.C. Overview of computerized dietary assessment programs for research and practice in nutrition education. *J. Nutr. Educ. Behav.* **2005**, *37*, 20–26.
4.  Subar, A.F.; Kirkpatrick, S.I.; Mittl, B.; Zimmerman, T.P.; Thompson, F.E.; Bingley, C.; Willis, G.; Islam, N.G.; Baranowski, T.; McNutt, S.; *et al.* The automated self-administered 24-hour dietary recall (ASA-24): A resource for researchers, clinicians, and educators from the national cancer institute. *J. Acad. Nutr. Diet.* **2012**, *112*, 1134–1137.
5.  Probst, Y.; Zammit, G. Predictors for reporting of dietary assessment methods in food-based randomized controlled trials over a ten year period. *Crit. Rev. Food Sci. Nutr.* **2015**, in press.
6.  Black, A.E.; Paul, A.A.; Hall, C. Footnotes to food tables. 2. The underestimations of intakes of lesser b vitamins by pregnant and lactating women as calculated using the fourth edition of mccance and widdowson's "the composition of foods". *Hum. Nutr. Appl. Nutr.* **1985**, *39*, 19–22.

7.  Zhu, F.; Bosch, M.; Boushey, C.J.; Delp, E.J. An image analysis system for dietary assessment and evaluation. *Proc. Intl. Conf. Image Proc.* **2010**, 1853–1856.

8.  Bosch, M.; Zhu, F.; Khanna, N.; Boushey, C.J.; Delp, E.J. Combining global and local features for food identification in dietary assessment. *IEEE Trans. Image Process.* **2011**, 1789–1792.

9.  Weiss, R.; Stumbo, P.J.; Divakaran, A. Automatic food documentation and volume computation using digital imaging and electronic transmission. *J. Am. Diet. Assoc.* **2010**, *110*, 42.

10. Ming, Z.; Gunturk, B.K. Multiresolution bilateral filtering for image denoising. *IEEE Trans. Image Process.* **2008**, *17*, 2324–2333.

11. Martin, C.K.; Han, H.; Coulon, S.M.; Allen, H.R.; Champagne, C.M.; Anton, S.D. A novel method to remotely measure food intake of free-living people in real-time: The remote food photography method (RFPM). *Br. J. Nutr.* **2009**, *101*, 446–456.

12. Nguyen, D.T.; Zong, Z.; Ogunbona, P.O.; Probst, Y.; Li, W. Food image classification using local appearance and global structural information. *Neurocomputing* **2014**, *140*, 242–251.

13. Nigam, K.; Lafferty, J.; McCallum, A. Using maximum entropy for text classification. In Proceedings of the International Joint Conference on Artificial Intelligence Workshop on Machine Learning for Information Filtering, Stockholm, Sweden, 31 July–6 August 1999; pp. 61–67.

14. Burges, C.C. A tutorial on support vector machines for pattern recognition. *Data Min. Knowl. Discov.* **1998**, *2*, 121–167.

15. Lowe, D. Distinctive image features from scale-invariant keypoints. *Int. J. Comput. Vis.* **2004**, *60*, 91–110.

16. Zong, Z.; Nguyen, D.; Ogunbona, P.; Li, W. On the combination of local texture and global structure of food classification. In Proceedings of the IEEE International Symposium on Multimedia, Taichung, Taiwan, 13–15 December 2010; pp. 204–211.

17. Chen, M.; Dhingra, K.; Wu, W.; Yang, L.; Sukthankar, R.; Yang, J. PFID: Pittsburgh fast-food image dataset. In Proceedings of the 16th IEEE International Conference on Image Processing; IEEE: Piscataway, NJ, USA, 2009; pp. 289–292.

18. Chang, C.; Lin, C. Libsvm: A library for support vector machines. *ACM Trans. Intell. Syst. Technol.* **2011**, *2*, 1–27.

19. Probst, Y.; Jones, H.; Sampson, G.; Smith, K. Development of australian portion size photographs to enhance self-administered online dietary assessments for adults. *Nutr. Diet.* **2010**, *67*, 275–280.

20. Rollo, M.; Ash, S.; Lyons-Wall, P.; Russell, A. Trial of a mobile phone method for recording dietary intake in adults with type 2 diabetes: Evaluation and implications for future applications. *J. Telemed. Telecare* **2011**, *17*, 318–323.

21. Walton, K.; Mcmahon, A.; Brewer, C.; Baker, J.; Fish, J.; Manning, F.; Grafenauer, S.; Kennedy, M.; Probst, Y.C. Novel digital food photos resource enhances knowledge of nutrition and dietetics students. In Proceedings of the Higher Education Research and Development Society of Australasia Conference, Hobart, TAS Australia, 2–5 July 2012.

22. He, K.; Zhang, X.; Ren, S.; Sun, J. *Delving Deep into Rectifiers: Surpassing Human-Level Performance on Imagenet Classification*; Microsoft Research: Redmond, WA, USA, 2015.
23. Zhang, S.; He, B.; Nian, R.; Wang, J.; Han, B.; Lendasse, A.; Yuan, G. Fast image recognition based on independent component analysis and extreme learning machine. *Cogn. Comput.* **2014**, *6*, 405–422.

# Development of a UK Online 24-h Dietary Assessment Tool: myfood24

Michelle C. Carter, Salwa A. Albar, Michelle A. Morris, Umme Z. Mulla,
Neil Hancock, Charlotte E. Evans, Nisreen A. Alwan, Darren C. Greenwood,
Laura J. Hardie, Gary S. Frost, Petra A. Wark and Janet E. Cade

**Abstract:** Assessment of diet in large epidemiological studies can be costly and time consuming. An automated dietary assessment system could potentially reduce researcher burden by automatically coding food records. myfood24 (Measure Your Food on One Day) an online 24-h dietary assessment tool (with the flexibility to be used for multiple 24 h-dietary recalls or as a food diary), has been developed for use in the UK population. Development of myfood24 was a multi-stage process. Focus groups conducted with three age groups, adolescents (11–18 years) ($n = 28$), adults (19–64 years) ($n = 24$) and older adults ($\geq 65$ years) ($n = 5$) informed the development of the tool, and usability testing was conducted with beta (adolescents $n = 14$, adults $n = 8$, older adults $n = 1$) and live (adolescents $n = 70$, adults $n = 20$, older adults $n = 4$) versions. Median system usability scale (SUS) scores (measured on a scale of 0–100) in adolescents and adults were marginal for the beta version (adolescents median SUS = 66, interquartile range (IQR) = 20; adults median SUS = 68, IQR = 40) and good for the live version (adolescents median SUS = 73, IQR = 22; adults median SUS = 80, IQR = 25). Myfood24 is the first online 24-h dietary recall tool for use with different age groups in the UK. Usability testing indicates that myfood24 is suitable for use in UK adolescents and adults.

Reprinted from *Nutrients*. Cite as: Carter, M.C.; Albar, S.A.; Morris, M.A.; Mulla, U.Z.; Hancock, N.; Evans, C.E.; Alwan, N.A.; Greenwood, D.C.; Hardie, L.J.; Frost, G.S.; Wark, P.A.; Cade, J.E. Development of a UK Online 24-h Dietary Assessment Tool: myfood24. *Nutrients* **2015**, *7*, 4016–4032.

## 1. Introduction

Reliable assessments of the associations between diet and health require estimation of usual diet. Traditional methods of dietary assessment such as multiple 24-h dietary recall interviews and food diaries can be impractical for large cohort studies often requiring costly and time-consuming manual nutrition coding. Food frequency questionnaires (FFQs) have been used in epidemiological studies due to their relative ease of administration and low participant burden. However, FFQs are subject to measurement error due to imprecision with respect to portion sizes, limited food lists, lack of detail regarding food preparation and the potential for misclassification of participants according to intake [1,2]. Multiple 24-h dietary recalls effectively represent habitual dietary intake and have shown less bias in reporting of energy and protein intakes when compared with FFQs using biomarker measures [3]. Along with convenience and scalability, incorporation of an online 24h dietary recall into large prospective cohort studies may advance our understanding of the nutritional determinants of disease [1] through possibly improved assessment of diet. Ultimately, this would allow for more reliable evidence-based formulations of health policies.

A number of online dietary assessment systems have already been developed [4–9]. In the United States, Subar *et al.* (2010) [10] have developed ASA24 (Automated Self-Administered 24 h Recall), which is currently being used in many studies. ASA24 is based on the USDA's "Automated Multiple Pass Method" (AMPM) [11], which involves recording intake in a series of defined "passes" to elicit a detailed recall. The AMPM has been validated against doubly-labeled water and shown to accurately estimate mean total energy intake in "normal"-weight individuals [12].

While an online 24-h dietary checklist for the UK exists (the Oxford WebQ [9]), there is currently no automated 24-h recall dietary assessment tool appropriate for the UK population. To address this gap, a fully automated online 24-h dietary assessment system, myfood24 (Measure Your Food on One Day) was developed with the flexibility to be self- or interviewer-administered as required and to be used as either a 24-h dietary recall or a food diary. This paper aims to describe the myfood24 development process and provide an overview of its features and functionality relating to self-administered use.

## 2. Experimental Section

Development of myfood24 was a multi-stage process, as summarized in Figure 1. Features of myfood24 are described in Table 1. Methods and results are presented together by stage of the project. Results comprise both qualitative and quantitative data. Ethical approval for this work was provided by the University of Leeds Research Ethics Committee (reference number MEEC 11-146).

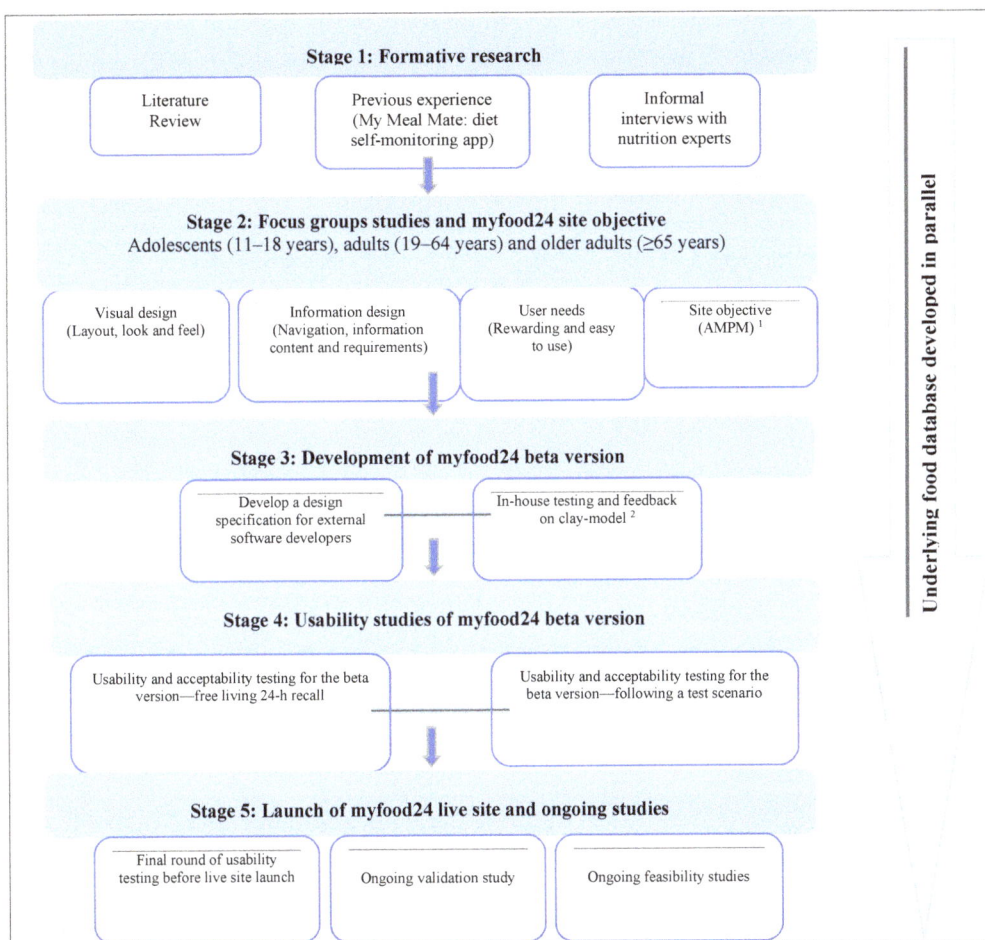

**Stage 1: Formative research**

Literature Review

Previous experience (My Meal Mate: diet self-monitoring app)

Informal interviews with nutrition experts

**Stage 2: Focus groups studies and myfood24 site objective**
Adolescents (11–18 years), adults (19–64 years) and older adults (≥65 years)

Visual design (Layout, look and feel)

Information design (Navigation, information content and requirements)

User needs (Rewarding and easy to use)

Site objective (AMPM) [1]

**Stage 3: Development of myfood24 beta version**

Develop a design specification for external software developers

In-house testing and feedback on clay-model [2]

**Stage 4: Usability studies of myfood24 beta version**

Usability and acceptability testing for the beta version—free living 24-h recall

Usability and acceptability testing for the beta version—following a test scenario

**Stage 5: Launch of myfood24 live site and ongoing studies**

Final round of usability testing before live site launch

Ongoing validation study

Ongoing feasibility studies

Underlying food database developed in parallel

**Figure 1.** Flow chart illustrating the development process of myfood24. [1] AMPM = Automated Multiple-Pass Method; [2] "Clay model" = static clickable wire-frame without database functionality.

## 3. Results

### 3.1. Stage 1: Formative Research

In preparation for the development of myfood24, substantial formative research was conducted by reviewing the literature on existing computerized dietary assessment tools and discussion with experts in the field of dietary assessment. Consideration was also given to factors which enhance usability and engagement with websites in general (Figure 2). The findings were used to inform the focus groups among all ages in Stage 2 and in particular to focus on the design of the "food search" and "portion size estimation" components of the system. Several existing dietary assessment tools from other countries were inspected and presented to focus group participants in order to aid discussion; these included: ASA24 (Automated Self-Administered 24-hour Recall) [5], DietDay [4] and NutriNet-Santé [6].

**Table 1.** Features of myfood24.

| Participant Area | Researcher Area |
| --- | --- |
| • "Getting started" instructions displayed on first screen<br>• Search function (with options to filter by category or brand)<br>• "Make a List" searching (an optional small area to list everything consumed with free text. Once completed, the search function works its way through this list. The participant is then able to add individual items remembered afterwards)<br>• Portion size selection area (including photos; standard pack sizes; enter own amount)<br>• Recipe Builder (user is able to search and log ingredient combinations as individual recipes in a separate section)<br>• Recently used items to allow quick entry of repeated foods/drinks<br>• Food lists by meal (with time of meal optional for researcher)<br>• Drag-and-drop between meals<br>• Prompt for commonly missed accompaniments for a number of items (e.g., milk with cereal, spread on bread)<br>• Final review screen encouraging user to check before submission. Includes list of commonly forgotten food items.<br>• Supplementary questions (e.g., did you take any vitamins, minerals or other supplements during your day? Was the food consumed representative of a typical day?—Optional to researcher)<br>• Login area where the participant can select which recall day to complete<br>• Help—(including a specific area of the site with detailed help text, mouseovers/hover text over specific parts of the website and help videos)<br>• Nutrient feedback (energy, protein, fat, carbohydrate, fiber, and salt—Optional to researcher). | • Customization<br>• Add project specific text and logo<br>• Tailored additional help text (in addition to default help text)<br>• Tailored invitation and reminder emails to participants (how many and how frequently)<br>• Tailored optional "thank you" email to go out at the end of the study<br>• Select recall or diary option<br>• Select whether to record time of meals or not<br>• Option to display nutrient summary details to participant or not<br>• Supplementary questions (optional).<br>• Study participant management—upload email addresses; send automatic reminders at specified dates<br>• "Take control" function for interviewer mode (The researcher is able to use this button to access the tool and complete and submit the recall/diary on the participants behalf)<br>• Export of summary macronutrient and micronutrient analysis output (from potential 120 nutrients) to a CSV file<br>• Export of detailed food and nutrient analysis (120 nutrients) output to a CSV file |

Several methods for finding foods have been employed in existing online dietary assessment tools. The food list in ASA24 [5] is hierarchically organized into food categories, with a free-search option. Young Adolescents' Nutrition Assessment on Computer (YANA-C) [13] uses a "tree" structure (if there are no matches, the closest food must be selected), and others like DietDay [4] have a "fast track" option, which allows the respondent to save commonly-consumed foods. Standard food portion sizes have been used in several tools, such as Synchronised Nutrition and Activity Program™ (SNAP™) [14], Oxford WebQ [9], and Reality [15], while others like ASA24 [5] and NutriNet-Santé [6] have used portion size images to guide selection of appropriate portion sizes.

Experience was drawn upon from the previous development of a smartphone app supporting self-monitoring of diet for weight loss, "My Meal Mate" (MMM) [16]. In the pilot trial of MMM, the food composition database was found to be a limiting factor in engaging with the app, and participants struggled to find the correct food and drink items. With this in mind, we created an extensive new UK food composition database for incorporation into the tool. The database currently includes ~45,000 UK branded and generic foods with their associated pack and portion sizes (by comparison, the existing British food composition tables contain ~3500 generic food items) [17].

In the new database, 5669 food items contain portion images [18]. Portion images were added for the 100 most commonly consumed food types, and for all other foods for which they were relevant. For example, the image for sliced chicken breast was also applied to other white sliced meats, such as turkey and pork. Each food type with associated portion images has the option for the user to select from seven portion sizes images. The foods with portion size images are the top 100 foods in terms of frequency of consumption, weight of consumption and contribution to energy intake, identified from data collected during the National Diet and Nutrition Survey conducted with young people (4–18 years) [19]. All the food items in the database have been mapped via their back-of-pack nutrient information to the McCance and Widdowson composition of food codes [17]. Details of the development of the food database are reported elsewhere [20].

### 3.2. Stage 2: Focus Groups

The findings of Stage 1 were used to inform the focus group questions among all ages in Stage 2, in particular, to focus on the design of the "food search" and "portion size estimation" components of the system. Focus groups were conducted with adolescents, adults and older adults to understand what features people might prefer in an online dietary assessment tool and whether or not they might use such a tool. These discussions were <60 min in duration, facilitated by a moderator and assistant moderator, audiotaped and transcribed *verbatim* alongside field notes taken by a research assistant. Group discussions were allowed to flow naturally but were divided into semi-structured sections with prompts on the following topics: preference for how to search a food composition database; preferences for estimating portion size; lay-out; usability features; potential incentives for use; and the maximum amount of time that individuals would be willing to spend using the system.

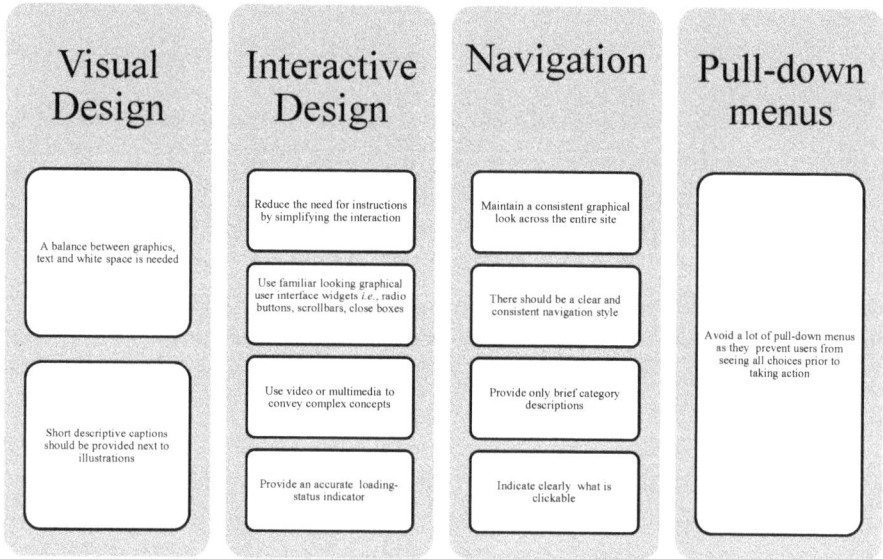

**Figure 2.** Key requirements to be considered in website design identified from the literature [21–26].

Adolescent participants were recruited by email and posters from two secondary schools in Leeds. Adults were recruited by email and posters advertising the study to staff at the University of Leeds and older people were recruited by contacting the Leeds branch of the University of the Third Age (an international educational organization aimed at retired people).

Data were analyzed using a basic thematic analysis. Findings were organized according to predefined topics (linked to the website design and key functions) and not data-derived themes, as the data were used to inform the website specification. Results are summarized in Table 2. All age groups preferred images to aid portion size estimation and a clean design with no "pop-ups". Whereas adults and older adults were prepared to spend a bit longer completing the tool, adolescents were unwilling to spend more than 15 min. All expressed a desire for feedback on their nutritional intake.

**Table 2.** Summary of feedback from focus groups on preferred options for an online dietary assessment tool, by age and discussion topic on which views were sought.

| | Adolescents (11–18 Years) (*n* = 28) | Adults (19–64 Years) (*n* = 24) | Older Adults (≥65 Years) (*n* = 5) |
|---|---|---|---|
| **Summary characteristics** | | | |
| **Mean age years (SD)** | 14 (2) | 36 (13) | 67 (3) |
| **Male, %** | 61 | 37 | 40 |
| **Topics on which views were sought during focus groups** | | | |
| | *Focus group feedback on topics discussed* | | |
| Database searching | Keyword or category preferred Predictive text useful | Keyword preferred Speed important Concerns expressed about long lists | Keyword preferred Speed important Concerns expressed about long lists |
| Portion size estimation | Images desired Variety of options (e.g., plate, packet) preferred | Images desired Manual input from packaging useful | Images desired Portion size plate image suggested |
| Layout | Balance between text and images important No pop-ups No "childish" design or colors | Uncluttered look desired Health neutral in terms of color and design No pop-ups | Uncluttered look desired No pop-ups |
| Usability features/support | 10–15 min for completion, maximum 15 min | 10–20 min acceptable for completion but depends on required frequency of use Recipe function "Frequently used" function Typical day indicator | 20–30 min acceptable completion time, up to 60 min if infrequent |
| Help option | Trial and error preferred; short video or avatar helpful (only young adolescents) | Hover features; FAQs; no avatar or video | Paper based written wanted. Help by telephone support desirable |
| Incentives | Feedback on intake and guidance on improving diet preferred Cash desired | General report on intake desired | General report on intake desired Incentive enough to benefit the overall study |

137

## 3.3. Stage 3: Development of myfood24 Beta-Version

### 3.3.1. Develop a Design Specification

Using results of the initial focus groups, the design specification was developed in collaboration with software developers and the myfood24 project consortium. The myfood24 consortium combines researchers from the University of Leeds and Imperial College London. Members of the consortium bring a wide range of expertise, including nutritional epidemiology, dietetics, dietary assessment, public health, biostatistics and molecular epidemiology. The two major sections for development were the participant area and the researcher area of the website. The researcher area was required so that projects could be set up and data extracted with ease. A typical example of workflow using myfood24 is displayed in Figure 3.

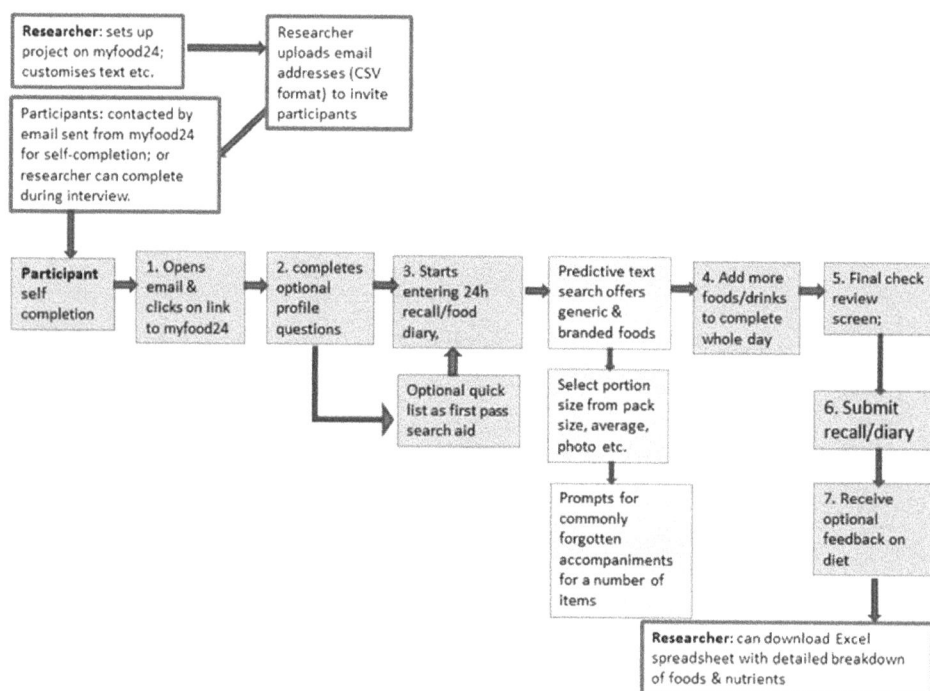

**Figure 3.** Typical myfood24 workflow for researcher and participant (shaded boxes represent participant actions; unshaded boxes represent researcher actions).

### 3.3.2. In House Testing/Feedback on "Clay Model"

The first prototype of myfood24 was a static "clay model" without database searching functionality (individual wireframes with the ability to click-through the screens to understand the navigation) (Figure S1a, b in supplementary materials).

It was subjected to in-house testing rather than external user testing, as it was not yet deemed to be at the required standard for external users. The clay model feedback informed the development process of the beta model. An iterative development approach was adopted throughout the project, the project team as well as a small number of employees and students of the University of Leeds were involved in user testing and feedback to the software developers at regular intervals.

### 3.4. Stage 4: Usability Testing of the Beta Version

User testing took place using the beta version of the software. This involved using myfood24 to self-complete a 24-h recall. The beta version of myfood24 only contained a sample of items from the food composition database. Fourteen adolescents, eight adults and one older person were involved in testing the beta version of myfood24. There is debate about the sample size needed to identify usability problems, but it has been reported that 80% of usability problems are uncovered with the inclusion of around five participants [27,28]. These studies also show diminishing returns in uncovering problems as sample size increases [27,28]. Questionnaires were administered to gather data on user demographic characteristics, usability (using the Systems Usability Scale (SUS)) and confidence in using technology. The SUS is a 10-item scale with users asked to rate their level of agreement with 10 usability statements (1 = strongly disagree; 5 = strongly agree), which gives an overall usability score from 0 to 100 [29]. In general, a product with an SUS of 70 is considered to be good and products with less than a score of 70 would be judged as marginal. Products with a score of less than 50 are considered to be a cause for concern [30]. Participants were also asked to self-rate their confidence in using technology on a Likert scale of 1 to 10. The key issues identified with the beta version of myfood24 during usability testing are presented in Table 3, and all reported issues were fed back to the software developers to inform the final phase of development. The sample characteristics, SUS score and self-rated technology confidence score of those who conducted usability testing of the beta and live version of myfood24 can be found in Table 4.

**Table 3.** Key issues identified with the beta version of myfood24 during usability testing.

| Problem Identified | Improvements Made to myfood24 |
|---|---|
| • List of foods presented after database search appeared to confuse users. This was because brand and generic items were mixed | • Generic items were displayed first in the search list |
| • Users could not find foods if they misspelt them (e.g., zucchini, avocado and baguette) | • A large database of misspellings and synonyms was created to improve searching the underlying food composition database |
| • Problems in finding two-word food items were identified (e.g., cheese sandwich, chocolate biscuit) | • Search was improved to match on more than one search term |
| • Portion-size options for generic foods were challenging for users as only one option could be selected (e.g., for generic orange juice only a 200ml glass could be selected) | • Significant work was done on providing a range of appropriate portion-size options for generic food items |
| • "Bug" in final nutrient summary output which lead to miscalculation of total macronutrients displayed | • "Bug" fixed and nutrient summary output, which was checked against a sample of manually coded diaries |
| • Recipe builder was not intuitive and difficult to use | • Text in the recipe builder was reworded to make the flow easier to follow |
| • People disliked having to add in meal slot details each time for each individual food item | • Meal slots were defaulted to previously selected so only needs to be clicked when moving to a different meal slot rather than each individual food. Drag-and-drop between meal slots enabled. Ability to select meal slot on left side of diary in advance and then add foods was added |
| • Long food descriptors were not displayed in full | • Text was wrapped so that entire food description displayed |
| • It was not clear on final screen that the food diary has been completed | • Text was added to confirm that diary is complete and safe to close browser |

**Table 4.** Sample characteristics by age group and system usability scale (SUS) scores for participants completing usability testing of the beta and live versions of myfood24.

| Age group | Adolescents (11–18 Years) | | Adults (19–64 Years) | | Older Adults ($\geq$65 Years) | |
|---|---|---|---|---|---|---|
| Sample characteristic | Beta | Live | Beta | Live | Beta | Live |
| N | 14 | 70 | 8 | 20 | 1 | 4 |
| Female (%) | 57 | 50 | 75 | 74 | 100 | 75 |
| System Usability Scale score (Median (IQR)) | 66 (20) | 73 (22) | 68 (40) | 80 (25) | 38 | 29 (63) |
| Technology confidence [a] (Median, (IQR)) | 9 (1) | 9 (2) | 8 (1) | 8 (2) | 8 | 3 (2) |

[a] Self-rated based on a 10-point Likert scale (1 = not confident at all; 10 = extremely confident).

## 3.5. Stage 5: Launch of Live Site

Figure 4a,b are examples of the myfood24 participant interface. To assess usability before the tool was launched as live for the validation study, a further round of usability testing took place.

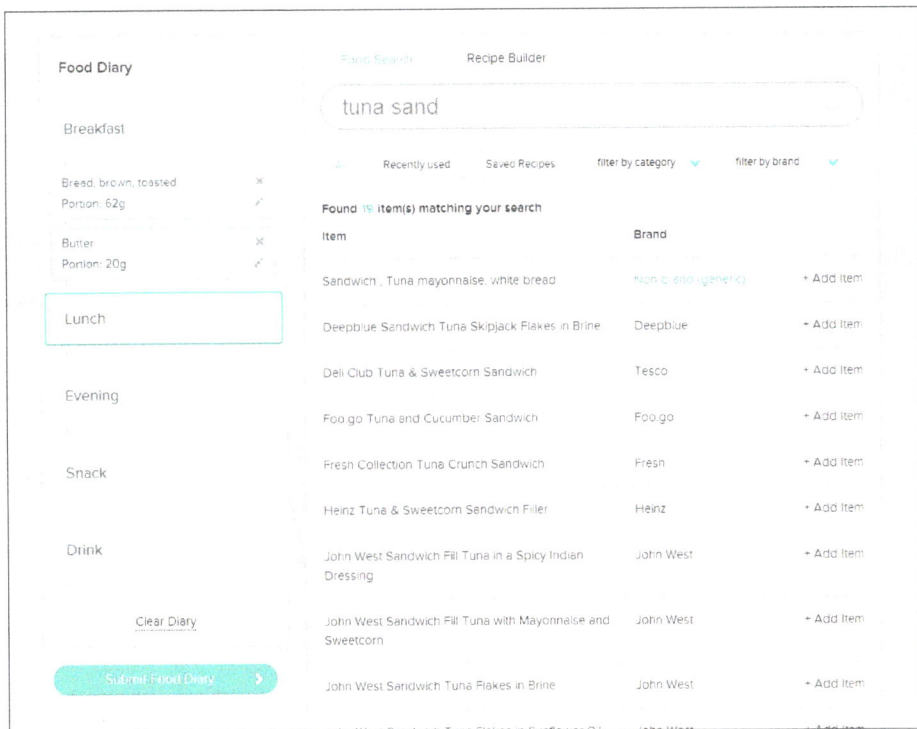

(a)

**Figure 4.** *Cont.*

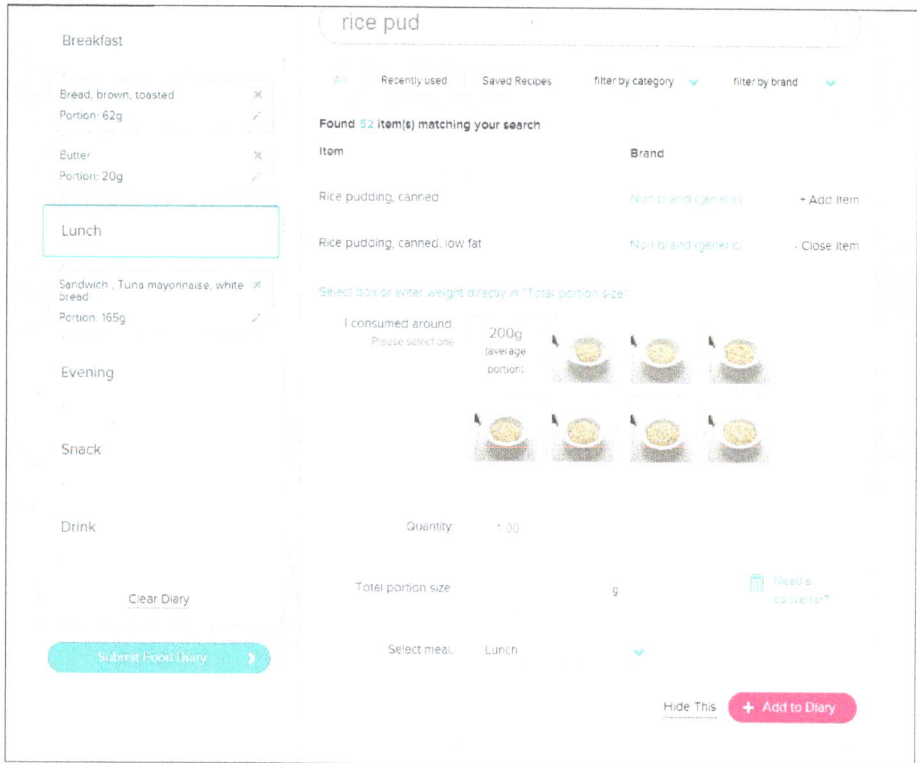

**(b)**

**Figure 4.** (a) Screenshot to show searching and logging items consumed using myfood24. (b) Screenshot to show estimating portion sizes using myfood24.

The adolescent participants were recruited from two high schools in different areas of Leeds. The adult participants were recruited from a convenience sample in London and Leeds. Older people were recruited from a convenience sample in Leeds. Anyone who had used myfood24 before, or had been involved with the development in any way, was not eligible to take part. The participants were required to report their food intake over the previous 24-h using myfood24. Basic demographic data were collected and the SUS was administered. Participants gave feedback relating to specific features of myfood24.

The live version of myfood24 was tested by 70 adolescents, 20 adults and four older adults. Attempts were made to contact 10 older adults but only four responded. The sample characteristics, SUS score and self-rated technology confidence score of those who conducted usability testing of the beta and live version of myfood24 can be found in Table 4. Qualitative results relating to testing of the live version of myfood24 with adults can be found in Table 5. A noteworthy result from this stage of testing is the length of time it took adult participants to complete their 24-h dietary recalls. In the sample of 24 adults using the live site, the mean completion time was 19 (SD: 7) minutes.

Median SUS in adolescents and adults were moderate for the beta version of myfood24 (adolescents median SUS = 66, (interquartile range) IQR = 20; adults median SUS = 68, IQR = 40) and good for the live version (adolescents median SUS = 73, IQR = 22; adults median SUS = 80, IQR = 25). Among older adults the median SUS score was poor for both the beta (median SUS = 38) and live version (median SUS = 29, IQR = 63).

**Table 5.** A summary of qualitative findings relating to specific areas of the live version of myfood24 with a sample of adult users.

| Features of myfood24 | Answer % (*n/n*) | Notes |
|---|---|---|
| MY PROFILE-Are you able to load the webpage and enter your details successfully? | Yes—100 (20/20) | All able to enter details |
| GETTING STARTED-Have you read the instructions and is the language appropriate and easy to understand? | Yes—95 (18/19) | Mostly straightforward; 1 person was not sure how to complete the diary page |
| MAKE A LIST-Did you use the "Make a list" function. If so, did you find it easy to use? | Used—40 (8/20) Easy—75 (3/4) | Some did not notice feature |
| SEARCH-Was the search function easy to use? Could you find items easily? | Easy—89 (17/19) Find items—29 (4/14) | Some brands not listed and some lists too long |
| PROMPTS-Did you find any prompts that came after you entered certain foods to be helpful? Did you respond to the prompts? | Helpful—94 (17/18) Respond—67 (8/12)) | Useful overall |
| PORTION SIZE ENTRY-Did you find it easy to understand how to enter portion size? Did you find it confusing to have both pictures *and* grams displayed on the screen? | Easy—89 (16/18) Confusing—21 (3/14)) | Pictures found to be helpful |
| RECENTLY USED ITEMS-Could you find and use the "Recently used items" list? | Used—29 (5/17) | Not widely used but no negative comments |
| RECIPE BUILDER-Was the recipe builder easy to use? | Yes—88 (7/8) | Convenient; some found it confusing and time investment required |
| SUBMITTING FOOD DIARY-Could you submit your food diary? | Yes—85 (17/20) | Some had error messages on submission |
| TIME TAKEN TO COMPLETE-How long did it take you to complete your intake and submit your diary? | Mean (SD) 19 (7) minutes | |
| HELP-Did you use the help text or the help video? If so, did you find it useful? | Used—5 (1/20) Useful—100 (1/1) | |

## Availability of myfood24

In order that myfood24 remains up-to-date with respect to new products or reformulations of existing foods, the tool will be hosted and maintained by the University of Leeds. The tool has been developed such that it can be made available to researchers worldwide through a unique login. For enquiries relating to use of myfood24 in research please contact myfood24@leeds.ac.uk. myfood24 has a demonstration feature so it is possible to try the front-end (participant side) of the tool by visiting: www.myfood24.org and using the "demo" button.

## 4. Discussion

myfood24 is the first online 24-h dietary recall tool targeted for use with the UK population. The findings from the focus groups were used to inform the specifications of myfood24. After development of a beta version, usability testing was conducted to further refine the tool. The focus groups highlighted that an overriding requirement from potential system users was a system that is quick and easy to use. During the development, we balanced the needs of the researchers to collect detailed and accurate dietary assessments with the users' desires to spend minimal time using the tool. To reduce the time taken to complete the food intake, we therefore chose not to pursue the detailed AMPM method. Within myfood24, users are asked to move through as few screens as possible to complete food recalls and "pop-ups" and prompts are limited. However, the myfood24 tool has retained some aspects of the AMPM, with an optional quick-list as the first pass, detailed food search, forgotten-item prompts for commonly-forgotten foods, and final review before submission. Although checks and final checks are built into the system most pages within myfood24 can be reached within a few clicks. This design approach was adopted based on the desires of focus group participants and experience with the MMM app (see Section 3.1). Thus, although myfood24 does not fully embrace the AMPM method, the strengths of this method have still been applied.

To ensure the system is intuitive and easy to use, a new food composition database was developed for the tool, and consideration has gone in to refining the database search function [20]. Whilst the existing British food composition tables contain ~3500 generic food items [17], the food database developed for myfood24 contains ~45,000 UK branded and generic foods with their associated pack and portion sizes. The median adult SUS score of the myfood24 live version at 80/100 is in the "good" range for websites and compares favorably with other behavior-assessment websites, such as a smoking cessation website rated at 67 [31] and a physical activity website rated at 73 [32].

### 4.1. Strengths and Challenges

A major strength of myfood24 is that it is the first UK online 24-h dietary assessment tool aimed at the UK adult population and incorporates a novel and extensive food composition database to generate instant nutrient values without the need for coding. The system has been informed by the views of three different age groups (adolescents, adults and older adults) to be user-friendly among a wide range of people. The flexible researcher website permits a range of study types and personalization of information presented to participants. A strength of the myfood24 development process has been the iterative approach which has facilitated the creation of a user friendly tool. The usability testing discussed in this study has shown myfood24 to be highly rated in adolescents and adults.

A limitation of the development process was the small number of older adults who were involved in focus groups and undertook testing of the beta and live versions of the system. Ten older adults were contacted at both testing points (beta and live), however at the beta stage only one was able to complete the tool and only four (with low computer literacy) were able to complete the final version. The SUS for those older adults who did complete the tool was very low in comparison to the other two age groups, which were considerably higher. There are a number of factors such as general lack of technical knowledge, fine motor control issues and hearing and vision loss which can affect an older adult's ability to use the Internet [33]. These factors may have affected their ability to use myfood24. It is also worth noting that self-rated confidence in using technology was much lower for the older adults (median = 3, IQR = 2 for the live site) than the other two age groups (adolescents median = 9, IQR = 2; adults median = 8, IQR = 2), which may have influenced engagement with myfood24. The low SUS score is in line with the observation that SUS scores generally decrease with age of the user [34]. Further research is planned to investigate what changes could be made to myfood24 to improve its usability with older adults. There is a facility for a researcher to "take control" of the recall so that it can be administered over the phone or face-to-face by an interviewer. This might be a more suitable option for using the tool with older people.

Given the complexity and detailed requirements of the tool, barriers encountered during working with an external software company included separate geographical location, communication and effective project management. This was overcome in the later stages with additional face-to-face meetings and introduction of financial milestones. This has been identified as a common difficulty when nutrition researchers work with external software companies [35]. Maintaining an up-to-date food composition database will be an ongoing challenge given that food and beverage manufacturers regularly reformulate products or introduce new products to the market. Ongoing funding will therefore be necessary to host and maintain the website.

### 4.2. Planned Future Work

myfood24 is being validated in a sample of adults against reference measures of 3 researcher-administered 24-h dietary recalls over 3 months and 3 blood and urine collection biomarker assessments. The tool will be piloted in (1) a sample of the UK Women's Cohort Study, which includes 35,000 women [36]; (2) in a clinical sample of women with gestational diabetes mellitus; and (3) within the Airwaves Health

Monitoring Study cohort at Imperial College London [37]. Furthermore, a relative validity study has been conducted among adolescents (11–18 years old) to compare myfood24 *vs.* interviewer-administered 24-h dietary recall.

A new feature will be added to incorporate a range of different food composition tables from different nationalities. This will allow the researcher to determine which food composition databases will be displayed in the myfood24 food search so that databases for different countries can be made available with relative ease. Furthermore, regular maintenance will be performed to the system to ensure that the food composition database remains up to date.

## 5. Conclusions

Myfood24 is the first online multiple-pass 24-h dietary assessment tool for the UK population. Foods are selected from a new comprehensive food composition database, which has been specifically designed for and built into the tool. Focus groups undertaken with three age groups have informed the development of the tool, and usability testing has been conducted with beta and live versions of myfood24 to facilitate an iterative development process. Usability testing indicated that myfood24 is suitable for use in UK adolescents and adults. For enquiries relating to use of myfood24 please contact myfood24@leeds.ac.uk.

**Acknowledgments:** This study was Medical Research Council (MRC) funded (ref: G1100235/1). The authors would like to acknowledge the software company Rippleffect for their contribution to the design and development of myfood24. The authors would like to acknowledge additional past and present members of the myfood24 consortium not listed as authors on this paper: Heather Ford, Claire Mcloughlin, Kay White, Helen Brown and Aikaterina Petropoulou. We would also like to thank Alexandra Hatherly, Catherine E Rycroft and Emilie Steen who were involved in the nutrient mapping for the myfood24 database. Also, thank you to Amy Subar for sharing her experience and expert advice during the project.

**Author Contributions:** The Principle Investigator on this project is JEC. In terms of individual contributions, JEC, DCG, PAW, LJH, GSF, CEE, NAA were involved in the grant application and conception of the myfood24 project. JEC, MCC and SAA were involved in the study design, data collection, analysis and interpretation of the focus group data and usability testing of the beta version of myfood24. JEC, MAM, and UZM were involved in the design, data collection, analysis and interpretation of the usability testing of the live version of myfood24 in adults. MCC wrote the initial draft of the manuscript. All authors have been involved in the overall development of myfood24. All authors have contributed to writing this paper.

**Conflicts of Interest:** The authors declare no conflict of interest

## References

1. Schatzkin, A.; Subar, A.F.; Moore, S.; Park, Y.; Potischman, N.; Thompson, F.E.; Leitzmann, M.; Hollenbeck, A.; Morrissey, K.G.; Kipnis, V. Observational Epidemiologic Studies of Nutrition and Cancer: The Next Generation (with Better Observation). *Cancer Epidemiol. Biomark. Prev.* **2009**, *18*, 1026–1032.

2. Bingham, S.A.; Luben, R.; Welch, A.; Wareham, N.; Khaw, K.T.; Day, N. Are imprecise methods obscuring a relation between fat and breast cancer? *Lancet* **2003**, *362*, 212–214.

3. Subar, A.F.; Kipnis, V.; Troiano, R.P.; Midthune, D.; Schoeller, D.A.; Bingham, S.; Sharbaugh, C.O.; Trabulsi, J.; Runswick, S.; Ballard-Barbash, R.; *et al.* Using intake biomarkers to evaluate the extent of dietary misreporting in a large sample of adults: The OPEN study. *Am. J. Epidemiol.* **2003**, *158*, 1–13.

4. Arab, L.; Tseng, C.H.; Ang, A.; Jardack, P. Validity of a multipass, web-based, 24-h self-administered recall for assessment of total energy intake in blacks and whites. *Am. J. Epidemiol.* **2011**, *174*, 1256–1265.

5. Subar, A.F.; Kirkpatrick, S.I.; Mittl, B.; Zimmerman, T.P.; Thompson, F.E.; Bingley, C.; Willis, G.; Islam, N.G.; Baranowski, T.; McNutt, S.; *et al.* The Automated Self-Administered 24-h dietary recall (ASA24): A resource for researchers, clinicians, and educators from the National Cancer Institute. *J. Acad. Nutr. Diet* **2012**, *112*, 1134–1137.

6. Touvier, M.; Kesse-Guyot, E.; Mejean, C.; Pollet, C.; Malon, A.; Castetbon, K.; Hercberg, S. Comparison between an interactive web-based self-administered 24 h dietary record and an interview by a dietitian for large-scale epidemiological studies. *Br. J. Nutr.* **2011**, *105*, 1055–1064.

7. Foster, E.; Hawkins, A.; Delve, J.; Adamson, A.J. Reducing the cost of dietary assessment: Self-completed recall and analysis of nutrition for use with children (SCRAN24). *J. Hum. Nutr. Diet* **2014**, *27* (Suppl. 1), 26–35.

8. UK Biobank. 24-hour Dietary Recall Questionnaire. Available online: http://biobank. ctsu.ox.ac.uk/crystal/docs/DietWebQ.pdf (accessed on 18 December 2014).

9. Liu, B.; Young, H.; Crowe, F.L.; Benson, V.S.; Spencer, E.A.; Key, T.J.; Appleby, P.N.; Beral, V. Development and evaluation of the Oxford WebQ, a low-cost, web-based method for assessment of previous 24 h dietary intakes in large-scale prospective studies. *Public Health Nutr.* **2011**, *14*, 1998–2005.

10. Subar, A.F.; Crafts, J.; Zimmerman, T.P.; Wilson, M.; Mittl, B.; Islam, N.G.; McNutt, S.; Potischman, N.; Buday, R.; Hull, S.G.; *et al.* Assessment of the accuracy of portion size reports using computer-based food photographs aids in the development of an automated self-administered 24-h recall. *J. Am. Diet Assoc.* **2010**, *110*, 55–64.

11. Conway, J.M.; Ingwersen, L.A.; Vinyard, B.T.; Moshfegh, A.J. Effectiveness of the US Department of Agriculture 5-step multiple-pass method in assessing food intake in obese and nonobese women. *Am. J. Clin. Nutr.* **2003**, *77*, 1171–1178.

12. Moshfegh, A.J.; Rhodes, D.G.; Baer, D.J.; Murayi, T.; Clemens, J.C.; Rumpler, W.V.; Paul, D.R.; Sebastian, R.S.; Kuczynski, K.J.; Ingwersen, L.A.; *et al.* The US Department of Agriculture Automated Multiple-Pass Method reduces bias in the collection of energy intakes. *Am. J. Clin. Nutr.* **2008**, *88*, 324–332.

13. Vereecken, C.A.; Covents, M.; Matthys, C.; Maes, L. Young adolescents' nutrition assessment on computer (YANA-C). *Eur. J. Clin. Nutr.* **2005**, *59*, 658–667.

14. Moore, H.J.; Hillier, F.C.; Batterham, A.M.; Ells, L.J.; Summerbell, C.D. Technology-based dietary assessment: Development of the Synchronised Nutrition and Activity Program (SNAP). *J. Hum. Nutr. Diet* **2014**, *27* (Suppl. 1), 36–42.

15. Jackson, D.; Craig, L.; Creaton, M. Evaluation and relative validation of a web based 24-h dietary recall in children aged 9–11 years. In Proceedings of the 8th International Conference on Diet and Activity Methods, Rome, Italy, 14–17 May 2012.

16. Carter, M.C.; Burley, V.J.; Nykjaer, C.; Cade, J.E. "My Meal Mate" (MMM): Validation of the diet measures captured on a smartphone application to facilitate weight loss. *Br. J. Nutr.* **2013**, *109*, 539–546.

17. McCance, R.A.; Widdowson, E.M. *McCance and Widdowson's The Composition of Foods*, 6th ed.; Royal Society of Chemistry: Cambridge, UK, 2002.

18. Foster, E.; Hawkins, A.; Adamson, A. *Young Person's Food Altas-Secondary*; Food Standards Agency Publications: London, UK, 2010.

19. Gregory, J.; Lowe, S.; Bates, C.J.; Prentice, A.; Jackson, L.V.; Smithers, G.; Wenlock, R.; Farron, M. *National Diet and Nutrition Survey: Young People Aged 4 to 18 Years*; TSO: London, UK, 2000.

20. Cade, J.; Hancock, N.; Carter, M.; McLoughlin, C.; Wark, P.; Hatherley, A.; Steen, E.; Ryecroft, C.; Alwan, N.; Morris, M. PP38 Development of a new UK food composition database. *J. Epidemiol. Community Health* **2014**, *68*, A62–A63.

21. Yan, Z. What influences children's and adolescents' understanding of the complexity of the Internet? *Dev. Psychol.* **2006**, *42*, 418–428.

22. Nielsen, J. Usability of Websites for Teenagers. Available online: http://www.nngroup.com/articles/usability-of-websites-for-teenagers/ (accessed on 18 December 2014).

23. Nielsen, J. Ten Usability Heuristics for User Interface Design. Available online: http://www.nngroup.com/articles/ten-usability-heuristics/ (accessed on 18 December 2014),.

24. Norman, D. Emotion & design: Attractive things work better. *Interactions* **2002**, *9*, 36–42.

25. Courage, C.; Baxter, K. *Understanding Your Users: A Practical Guide to User Requirements Methods, Tools, and Techniques*; Morgan Kaufmann Publishers Inc.: San Fransisco, CA, USA, 2005.

26. Holzwarth, M.; Janiszewski, C.; Neumann, M. The Influence of Avatars on Online Consumer Shopping Behavior. *J. Mark.* **2006**, *70*, 19–36.

27. Virzi, R.A. Streamlining the Design Process: Running Fewer Subjects. *Proceed. Hum. Factors Ergon. Soc. Ann. Meet.* **1990**, *34*, 291–294.

28. Nielsen, J.; Landauer, T.K. A mathematical model of the finding of usability problems. In Proceedings of the INTERACT '93 and CHI '93 Conference on Human Factors in Computing Systems, Amsterdam, The Netherlands, 24–29 April 1993; pp. 206–213.

29. Brooke, J. SUS-A quick and dirty usability scale. *Usability Eval. Ind.* **1996**, *189*, 194.

30. Bangor, A.; Kortum, P.T.; Miller, J.T. An Empirical Evaluation of the System Usability Scale. *Int. J. Hum.-Comput. Interact.* **2008**, *24*, 574–594.

31. Krebs, P.; Burkhalter, J.E.; Snow, B.; Fiske, J.; Ostroff, J.S. Development and Alpha Testing of QuitIT: An Interactive Video Game to Enhance Skills for Coping With Smoking Urges. *JMIR Res. Protoc.* **2013**, *2*, e35.

32. Bossen, D.; Veenhof, C.; Dekker, J.; de Bakker, D. The usability and preliminary effectiveness of a web-based physical activity intervention in patients with knee and/or hip osteoarthritis. *BMC Med. Inform. Decis. Mak.* **2013**, *13*.

33. Lynch, K.R.; Schwerha, D.J.; Johanson, G.A. Development of a Weighted Heuristic for Website Evaluation for Older Adults. *Int. J. Hum.-Comput. Interact.* **2012**, *29*, 404–418.

34. Bangor, A.; Kortum, P.; Miller, J. Determining what individual SUS scores mean: Adding an adjective rating scale. *J. Usability Stud.* **2009**, *4*, 114–123.

35. Buday, R.; Tapia, R.; Maze, G.R. Technology-driven dietary assessment: A software developer's perspective. *J. Hum. Nutr. Diet* **2014**, *27* (Suppl. 1), 10–17.

36. Cade, J.E.; Burley, V.J.; Greenwood, D.C. The UK Women's Cohort Study: Comparison of vegetarians, fish-eaters and meat-eaters. *Public Health Nutr.* **2004**, *7*, 871–878.

37. Elliott, P.; Vergnaud, A.C.; Singh, D.; Neasham, D.; Spear, J.; Heard, A. The Airwave Health Monitoring Study of police officers and staff in Great Britain: Rationale, design and methods. *Environ. Res.* **2014**, *134*.

# Does an Adolescent's Accuracy of Recall Improve with a Second 24-h Dietary Recall?

Deborah A. Kerr, Janine L. Wright, Satvinder S. Dhaliwal and Carol J. Boushey

**Abstract:** The multiple-pass 24-h dietary recall is used in most national dietary surveys. Our purpose was to assess if adolescents' accuracy of recall improved when a 5-step multiple-pass 24-h recall was repeated. Participants ($n = 24$), were Chinese-American youths aged between 11 and 15 years and lived in a supervised environment as part of a metabolic feeding study. The 24-h recalls were conducted on two occasions during the first five days of the study. The four steps (quick list; forgotten foods; time and eating occasion; detailed description of the food/beverage) of the 24-h recall were assessed for matches by category. Differences were observed in the matching for the time and occasion step ($p < 0.01$), detailed description ($p < 0.05$) and portion size matching ($p < 0.05$). Omission rates were higher for the second recall ($p < 0.05$ quick list; $p < 0.01$ forgotten foods). The adolescents over-estimated energy intake on the first (11.3% $\pm$ 22.5%; $p < 0.05$) and second recall (10.1% $\pm$ 20.8%) compared with the known food and beverage items. These results suggest that the adolescents' accuracy to recall food items declined with a second 24-h recall when repeated over two non-consecutive days.

Reprinted from *Nutrients*. Cite as: Kerr, D.A.; Wright, J.L.; Dhaliwal, S.S.; Boushey, C.J. Does an Adolescent's Accuracy of Recall Improve with a Second 24-h Dietary Recall?. *Nutrients* **2015**, *7*, 3557–3568.

## 1. Introduction

The evidence linking the adolescent diet with risk for chronic diseases later in life, including obesity and some cancers continues to increase [1,2]. This makes adolescents an important target group however, assessing diet in this age group is challenging. The methods most commonly used to evaluate diet in adolescents are dietary records, the 24-h dietary recall and food frequency questionnaires. However, acceptability of these methods by adolescents is not ideal [3]. Early adolescents, ages 11 to 14 years, in particular, are in that period of time when the novelty and curiosity of self-reporting food intakes starts to wane and the assistance from parents is seen as an intrusion [4].

The 24-h dietary recall is the method used in most national dietary surveys and has been recommended for use in European children aged 7 to 14 years [5]. The Food Surveys Research Group (FSRG) of the United States Department of Agriculture (USDA) has devoted considerable effort to improving the accuracy of the 24-h recall through development and refinement of the multiple-pass method. The 5-step multiple-pass method provides a structured interview format with specific probes and involves five structured sets of probing [6]. As the 24-h recall is conducted by interview, this may be less burdensome to participants, compared to other methods such as dietary records [7].

In children under 11 years comparisons of the 24-h recall with energy expenditure, as measured by doubly labelled water (DLW) show mixed results. One study showed a 14% greater energy intake than DLW estimated energy expenditure [8] and another showed only group estimates of energy intake as being valid [9]. An automated self-administered web version has been developed and is still undergoing evaluation in comparison to interviewer-administered 24-h recall [10].

The most common method of evaluating the accuracy of the multiple-pass 24-h recall with children is through observation of school meals comparing foods recalled with foods either observed as eaten or foods actually weighed [11,12]. These recalls have demonstrated both under-reporting and over-reporting, and incorrect identification of foods and rely on the dietitian being able to accurately assess the food type and quantity. A controlled feeding study offers a unique opportunity to assess the accuracy of dietary assessment. In a controlled feeding study, as the food and nutrient intake is known, it does not require the participants to be observed to confirm food and beverages consumed. There are occasions when adolescents are exposed to foods unfamiliar to them (e.g., new school lunch menus) and the controlled feeding study can duplicate this type of environment. The purpose of the study was to assess if adolescents' accuracy of recall improved when a 5-step multiple-pass method for 24-h recall was repeated. Our hypothesis was that adolescents' accuracy would improve when the 24-h recall was repeated. In addition, we determined the rates of intrusions and omissions and if these differed between the repeated recalls.

## 2. Methods

### 2.1. Participants and Study Design

Thirty-one Chinese-American boys and girls (11–15 years) were recruited to participate in a 7-week metabolic study where they lived in a campus residence hall facility converted into a metabolic unit for two 3-week balances in the summer separated by a 1-week washout when they returned to their homes [3,13]. During the balance, participants were scheduled for a variety of educational and recreational activities coordinated as a summer-camp environment. The participants were required to eat all meals, snacks and beverages provided. A camp supervisor sat at the table with a group of four to five participants for all meals and snacks and ensured that all food and beverages were consumed. On days two and five of the first week, 24 participants participated in the 24-h recall for both days and six participants participated in the 24-h recall for at least one of the two days. Only the

24 participants (11 boys and 13 girls) who completed two 24-h recall were included in the final analysis. Some participants were unavailable to complete the second recall due to other research commitments. The menu was a 4-day cycle and items were selected to reflect foods commonly eaten by Chinese-American youth. Participants did not know in advance what was to be served (Table 1). All food and beverages served were weighed and participants were required to consume all foods and beverages served. The study was approved by the Purdue University Institutional Review Board.

**Table 1.** Number and percentage of participants ($n = 24$) who reported omissions for each menu item in the first and second 24-h dietary recalls.

| Eating Occasion | 1st Recalled Day Menu | $n$ (%) Omissions [a] | 2nd Recalled Day Menu | $n$ (%) Omissions |
|---|---|---|---|---|
| Breakfast | Pillsbury biscuit | 0 | Frosted flakes cereal | 1 (4%) |
| | Jam (in packet) | 2 (8%) | Milk | 0 |
| | Margarine (in packet) | 2 (8%) | Sliced pears | 5 (21%) |
| | Fruit cup | 10 (42%) | | |
| | Milk | 4 (17%) | | |
| Lunch | Turkey sandwich | 1 (4%) | Hot dog (with bun) | 2 (8%) |
| | Shrimp chips | 2 (8%) | Steak fries | 7 (29%) |
| | Sliced apples | 2 (8%) | Ketchup (in packet) | 2 (8%) |
| | Orange juice | 0 | Grapes | 9 (38%) |
| | | | Orange juice | 2 (8%) |
| Snack | Oatmeal cookies | 4 (17%) | Gummi savers confectionary | 7 (29%) |
| Dinner | Chicken thigh | 0 | Pasta | 1 (4%) |
| | Orange marmalade sauce | 2 (8%) | Pork & vegetable stir fry | 5 (21%) |
| | Sliced carrots | 3 (13%) | Pineapple pieces | 10 (42%) |
| | Margarine (in packet) | 13 (54%) | Milk | 18 (75%) |
| | Rice | 1 (4%) | Orange juice | 1 (4%) |
| | Orange juice | 3 (13%) | | |
| Snack | Juice bar | 0 | Flavor pop | 1 (4%) |
| | Orange juice | 10 (42%) | Orange juice | 5 (21%) |

[a]: refers to the number of participants reporting omission for each food item.

## 2.2. 24-h Dietary Recall

Dietitians completed training in the 5-pass 24-h recall method prior to commencement of the study. Seven dietitians conducted the 24-h recalls, with each individual dietitian conducting between two and three 24-h recalls on each occasion. The allocation of dietitian to participant was based on availability. The dietitians were not familiar with the menu and were not present at any meals or snacks prior to the data collection. By ensuring that the dietitians did not view any of the meals consumed reduced the likelihood of bias or prompting due to knowing the menu when interviewing. A standard interview protocol was followed with each dietitian having a standard set of aids for portion size estimation. The target period for the interview was a recall of the previous day's intake. Each recall covered a different menu day. To standardize the time of recall, the interviews took place following lunch and before dinner (commencing at 12:30 and finishing at 6:00 pm). The time taken for each participant to complete the 24-h recall on two separate occasions was recorded.

The procedure for the 5-step multiple-pass method was as previously described [14]. In the first step, participants were asked to provide a 'quick list' where they listed all foods and beverages consumed without interruption. In the second step, they were asked about "forgotten foods" where the interviewer followed a standard set of probes. The third step detailed "time and eating occasion" for each food item identified. In the fourth step, known as the "detail cycle," standard probes were followed to obtain detailed information on the food and drinks consumed as well as how much they ate or drank. The fifth step was a "final review probe" for any forgotten food or beverage items.

## 2.3. Analyses

Key errors in the 5-step multiple-pass method were assessed with a separate score (number of correct matches divided by the number of known food and beverages) for the first four steps (quick list; forgotten foods; time and eating occasion; detailed description of the food/beverage) of the 24-h recall. A higher percent value was a higher score which translated to a better match. For the quick list and forgotten foods steps, broad food group category matches were identified. For example, the following responses were considered a match: if "milk" was recalled and "low-fat milk" was served, if "a turkey sandwich" was recalled and a "turkey sandwich with wheat bread and mayonnaise" was served. A score of 2 was assigned for a match, 1 for a partial match and 0 for an omission. For the time and eating occasion step, the food or beverage recalled needed to be identified as being consumed at the correct meal or snack and correct time. Matching in the detail step was split into the description and portion size matching. To be scored as a complete match, the food items needed to be recalled in detail. For example, in the turkey sandwich, single items needed to be recalled such as sliced turkey, wheat bread and mayonnaise to achieve a maximum score of 2. Foods were classified as partial matches when the recalled item was in the same family of foods. For example, if chicken was recalled instead of turkey a score of 1 was assigned. When the foods recalled could not be matched within the same food grouping, they were considered a mismatch and scored 0. For example, milk was recalled and orange juice was served. The food and beverage items that matched on portion size within $\pm10\%$ of the weight or household measure were scored as a match (score = 3); within 10%–25% a partial match (score = 2), 25% or more was scored as a mismatch (score = 1) and missing or an omission scored as 0. The score for each step were summed, divided by the total possible score and expressed as a percentage, where a score of 100% indicated a perfect match for that particular step.

Omission and intrusion rates were assessed separately for the quick list and forgotten foods steps for the first and second recall. Food or beverages recalled by the participant but not served were classified as "intrusions" and foods or beverages served that were not recalled were classified as "omissions". As only a few food or beverage items were recalled in the final probe these were included in the 'forgotten food steps' calculations. Weighted intrusion and omission rates were calculated according to the method outlined by Baxter *et al.* [15] and were calculated as follows: Omission rate = (sum of weighted omissions/[sum of weighted omissions + sum of weighted matches]) × 100%. Values range from 0% (no omissions) to 100% (no food or beverage items reported eaten). A weight was assigned to each item according to importance by meal component. For example turkey sandwich = 2; condiment such as jam, margarine = 0.33; other meal/snack single items = 1. Intrusion rate (percentage of items reported eaten but not served) was calculated as (sum of weight intrusions/[sum of weighted intrusions + sum of weighted matches]) × 100%. Values range from 0% (no intrusions) to 100%. Means and standard deviations for omission and intrusion rates expressed as percentages were determined for the first and second dietary recall for the quick list and the forgotten foods steps. The score for each defined component for four of the five steps were expressed as a percentage, as well as the omission rate and the intrusion rate. Non-parametric statistics were used to test the difference in scores and rates between the recalled days. Wilcoxon Signed Rank Test (with exact test option) were used to assess if there were significant differences in the components and rates comparing the first and second recall.

The participants' 24-h recalls and the known food and beverage items for the days recalled, were analyzed using the Nutrition Coordinating Center food and nutrient database. Data coding and entry were performed by staff trained in the use of the Nutrition Data System for Research (NDS-R) Database Version v5.0/35 (© Regents of the University of Minnesota). Accuracy of the 24-h recalls was assessed by comparing the items recalled by the adolescents with the known food and beverage items. A paired sample t-test was used to test differences between the known food and beverage items and foods recalled.

## 3. Results

There were 24 participants who completed two 24-h recalls. The 11 boys mean (±standard deviation) ages were 13.9 ± 1.2 years with a mean body mass index (BMI) of 20.0 ± 4.1. For the 13 girls, these same parameters were 13.2 ± 1.3 years old and 19.2 ± 2 for BMI.

The number of participants who reported omissions for each menu item is shown in Table 1. For the first recall, the most frequently omitted item was margarine, where 13 participants (out of 24) did not recall the item. In the second recall, milk was omitted by 18 participants (75%).

Table 2 shows the individual details of the intrusions (food or beverages recalled but not served). Ten participants reported intrusions on the first recall compared with 16 intrusions on the second recall. There were five children out of 24, who reported no intrusions for either the first or the second recall.

**Table 2.** Details of food and beverage intrusions reported by participants ($n = 24$) in either the first, second, or both 24-h dietary recalls. Intrusions were food or beverage items recalled but not served.

| | Intrusions | |
|---|---|---|
| Participant | 1st recall | 2nd recall |
| 1 | 0 | 0 |
| 2 | 0 | orange juice |
| 3 | 0 | butter, milk, orange juice |
| 4 | 0 | orange juice |
| 5 | orange juice | 0 |
| 6 | 0 | 0 |
| 7 | apples | 0 |
| 8 | 0 | 0 |
| 9 | shrimp chips, orange juice | orange juice, pears |
| 10 | orange juice, apples | orange juice, orange juice, catsup |
| 11 | 0 | 0 |
| 12 | 0 | milk |
| 13 | 0 | 0 |
| 14 | peanut butter sandwich, jam | peaches |
| 15 | milk | butter, jelly, biscuit |
| 16 | milk | milk |
| 17 | 0 | milk |
| 18 | 0 | orange juice |
| 19 | orange juice | juice box |
| 20 | orange juice, popsicle | peanut butter, crackers, popsicle |
| 21 | soup | 0 |
| 22 | 0 | orange juice |
| 23 | 0 | orange juice |
| 24 | 0 | Juice box |
| Participants reporting intrusions | 10 | 16 |

Table 3 shows the component scores for the first four steps of the 24-h recall expressed as a percentage where a higher score indicates a better food and beverage match. Examination of the scores for each component comparing the first recall with the second recall showed significant differences in the matching for the time and occasion step ($p < 0.01$), detailed description ($p < 0.05$) and portion size matching ($p < 0.05$), but not for the first (quick list) or second (forgotten foods) step.

Table 3. Data from 24-h dietary recalls collected from adolescents ($n = 24$): The component scores of the first four steps of the 5-step multiple-pass method by first and second day of recall. For Step 4, the description and portion size are presented separately. A higher score indicates a better match between foods and beverages recalled and the known foods and beverages consumed.

| | Step 1: Quick List | Step 2: Forgotten Foods | Step 3 : Time and Eating Occasion | Step 4: Detail Cycle | |
|---|---|---|---|---|---|
| | | | | Description | Portion Size |
| | ← | Mean ± Standard Deviation (%) | | | → |
| First recall | 75 ± 15 | 84 ± 10 | 84 ± 11 | 79 ± 10 | 61 ± 10 |
| Second recall | 71 ± 20 | 80 ± 12 | 76 ± 13 ** | 72 ± 11 * | 55 ± 9 * |

$* p < 0.05; ** p < 0.01$ comparing the first recall with the second recall.

The rate of omissions and intrusions were compared between the first and second recall for the first two steps of the 24-h recall (Table 4). For both the first and second recalls, the omission rate decreased significantly from the 'quick list' to the 'forgotten foods' step, *i.e.*, first recall was 21.9 ± 13.9% to 12.9 ± 8.3% ($p < 0.001$) and the second recall was 28.9 ± 21.3% to 20.5 ± 14.1% ($p < 0.001$). This indicates the importance of the second step in the 24-h recall for improving recalled items. Lower omission rates were observed for the first recall compared with the second recall, for both the 'quick list' ($p < 0.05$) and the 'forgotten foods' step ($p < 0.01$). In the second recall, intrusion rate increased from the first to the second step (2.8 ± 4.4% to 6.4 ± 5.5% respectively; $p < 0.001$), indicating more errors occurred with food and beverages recalled but not served. The time taken to complete the first recall was longer compared to the second recall (51 ± 13 min to 35 ± 11 min respectively; $p < 0.01$).

Table 5 shows the differences between the nutrient composition of the known food and beverage items consumed and the 24-h dietary recall for the first and second day of recall. For energy intake the adolescents were able to accurately recall food and beverage items. For the first recall there was an over-estimate of energy (11.3 ± 22.5%; $p < 0.05$), protein (17.2 ± 29.4%; $p < 0.05$) and fat intake (35.9 ± 45.9%; $p < 0.01$) compared with the known food and beverage items. There were also significant differences in calcium ($p < 0.001$), fiber ($p < 0.01$), and iron ($p < 0.01$), between the known food and beverage items and the first recall. In the second recall, there were differences between the known food and beverage items and the interviewer-conducted recall for calcium (22.1 ± 48.9%; $p < 0.05$) and folate (39.2 ± 32.5%; $p < 0.001$) only. The standard deviation for first recall and second recall, respectively, for energy was 375 kcal and 413 kcal. The standard deviation for the mean of the energy from first and second recall was 317 kcal consistent with the use of two recalls reducing the variability of the data.

**Table 4.** Omission and intrusion rates by the first and second day of recall for the Quick List and Forgotten Foods Steps of the 5-step multiple-pass method completed by 24 adolescents.

| Recall | Step | Omission Rate (%) [a] $n = 24$ | Intrusion Rate (%) [b] $n = 24$ |
|--------|------|-------------------------------|--------------------------------|
| | | Mean ± Standard Deviation | |
| First Recall | Quick List | 21.9 ± 13.9 | 2.8 ± 5.4 |
| | Forgotten Foods | 12.9 ± 8.3 *** | 4.3 ± 6.2 |
| Second Recall | Quick List | 28.9 ± 21.3 * | 2.8 ± 4.4 |
| | Forgotten Foods | 20.5 ± 14.1 ***, ** | 6.4 ± 5.5 *** |

[a]: Omission rate = (sum of weighted omissions/[sum of weighted omissions + sum of weighted matches]) × 100%. Values range from 0% (no omissions) to 100% (no food or beverage items reported eaten); [b]: Intrusion rate (percentage of items reported eaten but not served) was calculated as (sum of weight intrusions/[sum of weighted intrusions + sum of weighted matches]) × 100%. Values range from 0% (no intrusions) to 100%; ***: $p < 0.001$ comparing Quick List with Forgotten Foods; *: $p < 0.05$ comparing first recall with the second recall for Quick List; **: $p < 0.01$ comparing first recall with the second recall for Forgotten Foods.

**Table 5.** Mean differences between the nutrient composition of the food and beverages consumed (actual intake) and the 24-h dietary recall by the first and Second day of recall among adolescents participating in a controlled feeding study ($n = 24$). A negative value for % difference indicates an underestimation by the recall; a positive value indicates an overestimation by the recall.

| | 1st Recalled Day | | | 2nd Recalled Day | | |
|---|---|---|---|---|---|---|
| | Actual intake | Recalled intake | % Difference | Actual intake | Recalled intake | % Difference |
| Energy (kcal/day) | 1699 ± 236 | 1877 ± 375 | 11.3 ± 22.5 * | 1744 ± 194 | 1870 ± 413 | 10.1 ± 20.8 |
| Protein (g/day) | 58 ± 10 | 67 ± 18 | 17.2 ± 29.4 * | 56 ± 7 | 54 ± 18 | −2.9 ± 30.4 |
| Carbohydrate (g/day) | 294 ± 36 | 300 ± 62 | 2.9 ± 22.7 | 305 ± 28 | 333 ± 79 | 9.2 ± 23.9 |
| Fat (g/day) | 36 ± 6 | 48 ± 17 | 35.9 ± 45.9 ** | 39 ± 7 | 40 ± 15 | 4.2 ± 38.7 |
| Calcium (mg) | 538 ± 32 | 889 ± 401 | 65.6 ± 71.7 *** | 655 ± 5 | 801 ± 326 | 22.1 ± 48.9 * |
| Vitamin C (mg) | 399 ± 16 | 381 ± 156 | −4.5 ± 39.1 | 426 ± 10 | 428 ± 141 | 0.5 ± 33.5 |
| Total dietary fibre | 16.8 ± 1.4 | 13.7 ± 3.8 | −17.7 ± 24.7 ** | 13.3 ± 1.4 | 12.4 ± 4.8 | −7.1 ± 35.6 |
| Total folate (mcg) | 660 ± 38 | 534 ± 193 | −19.2 ± 28.4 ** | 732 ± 37 | 747 ± 160 | 1.9 ± 21 |
| Iron (mg) | 10.4 ± 1.7 | 10.2 ± 3.0 | −1.6 ± 27.5 | 11.3 ± 1.0 | 15.8 ± 3.9 | 39.2 ± 32.5 *** |
| Zinc (mg) | 6.4 ± 1.5 | 6.2 ± 1.7 | −1.2 ± 26.1 | 5.9 ± 0.7 | 7.1 ± 3.2 | 19.6 ± 49 |
| | Macronutrient energy distribution | | | | | |
| Protein (%) | 13.6 ± 0.7 | 14.4 ± 3.1 | 5.7 ± 20.8 | 12.7 ± 0.6 | 11.2 ± 2.8 | −11.9 ± 22.7 * |
| Carbohydrate (%) | 69.3 ± 1.9 | 63.0 ± 5.4 | −9.2 ± 7.6 *** | 70.1 ± 1.1 | 69.9 ± 7.9 | −0.3 ± 11 |
| Fat (%) | 19.0 ± 0.8 | 22.6 ± 5.0 | 19.6 ± 26.8 ** | 19.9 ± 1.4 | 18.9 ± 5.9 | −4.4 ± 30.7 |

*: $p < 0.05$ between recall and actual intake; **: $p < 0.01$; ***: $p < 0.001$.

157

## 4. Discussion

This study showed that that adolescents' accuracy of recall did not improve when a 24-h recall was repeated. Accuracy was assessed by direct comparison of the known food and beverage items consumed with those recalled by the adolescents. However, the combined standard deviation for the mean of the energy of the two days indicates the overall variability in the estimates of energy intake would be reduced by the inclusion of a second recall. A unique aspect of this study was all food and beverage items were weighed prior to being offered. Thus the food and beverages recalled were known by the investigators, thus eliminating potential biases associated with observers. Overall, the omission rate was greater in the second recall compared to the first recall, which was offset by a significantly higher rate of intrusions. This partially explains the energy estimates from the two recalls being nearly identical (1877 ± 375 kcal and 1870 ± 413 kcal). The comparisons between the reported and known food and beverage items were statistically significantly different for only the first recall at 11% higher ($p < 0.05$) and 10% higher (NS) for the second recall. Thus, despite the errors (either omissions or intrusions) made by the adolescents, these had only a minor effect on the accuracy of estimated energy intake. However, although the overall energy intake may appear acceptable, the adolescents made reporting errors in foods omitted (Table 1), additional items recalled but not served (intrusions, Table 2) as well as errors in portion size estimation (Table 3) that affected the accuracy of the energy and nutrient intake. By using a controlled feeding study where the amount of food and beverage items served was known we were able to identify these errors. Of importance, these errors would not be detected with biomarkers such as doubly labelled water or urine nitrogen or by direct observation where the exact weight of the food or beverage was not known.

The omission rate, where foods were not recalled by the participant but were consumed, was shown to improve from the quick list (first step) to the forgotten foods (second step) on both recalls. This consistent improvement demonstrates the importance of these sequential steps in the multi-pass method. The omission rate for the second step increased from 13% in the first recall to 20% in the second recall. Intrusions (food or beverages recalled by the participant but not consumed) showed a significant increase from the first to the second step on the second recall. However, overall the rate of intrusions and omissions were lower than reported by Baxter et al. [15] who showed in 10 and 11 year olds an intrusion rate of 24% and an omission rate of 34% for recalls conducted on school lunches. Intrusions may be based on specific memories of foods consumed during the recording period or at a previous time [16]. As the 24-h recalls were conducted during a metabolic study, some of the foods or beverages may have been unfamiliar to the participants and the children would have been cognizant of the absence of their usual foods. The study design in the current study may be a similar situation to school lunches at the beginning of the school year or when menus items are changed. Thus, if there is a desire to assess children's intakes at these times, these results would be most relevant. Further, the possibility exists that the recalls may have improved if the 24-h dietary recalls were conducted at the end of camp. On the other hand, frequency of foods being served didn't necessarily help as demonstrated by the errors that occurred with the recall of milk and orange juice.

In meal observation studies, trained observers record the food and beverage items and estimate the portion sizes [11,17]. For a reference standard, these studies rely on the dietitian being able to unobtrusively assess the food type and quantity accurately. In the current study the dietitians conducting the 24-h recall did not observe the adolescents during meal and snack times, as the food and beverage items served were known and weighed, making accurate comparison to the recalled food and beverage items possible. Thus, some of the differences between this study and others regarding omission and intrusion rates may be due to study design and implementation.

There was poorer matching of portion size with the second recall (55% matching) compared to the first recall (61% matching; $p < 0.05$). Standard food models were used in the current study however, estimation accuracy of portion size decreased from the first recall to the second recall, indicating that repeating the task did not improve the estimation accuracy of portion sizes. Further, the more detailed description of foods and beverages declined between the first and the second recall (79% compared to 72%, $p < 0.05$). The participants' scores, indicating better matches, did not improve for any of the steps with the second 24-h recall. The adolescents took significantly less time to complete the second recall which perhaps reflects less attention to detail instead of becoming more skilled with the process.

Ironically, despite the increase in the number of foods not matching the actual foods served for the second recall, the energy/nutrient profile better matched the energy/nutrient profile of the foods associated with the second recall than occurred with the first recall where there was a better food match. In a study among adults using an objective biomarker for energy [18], the second administration of the 24-h recall showed greater underreporting. Thus, the results among the adolescents in this study reflect the same observations made among adults of some sort of waning of enthusiasm to provide consistent quality data. On the other hand, the increase in intrusions, could reflect a desire among the adolescents to guess in order to provide a "right" answer [3]. In addition, the time taken to complete the second recall was shorter, perhaps indicating declining interest in the process. The observed decrease in time taken to complete the second recall compared to first was also observed among the adults in the OPEN study [18]. Although the adolescents in this study were able to complete the second recall more quickly they made more errors in recalling the food and beverage items and started to recall items they didn't consume.

This latter observation may reflect a social desirability bias [19]. Other possible factors proposed to influence reporting accuracy of the recalls have been noted by Baxter *et al.* [20] in (fourth-grade) 9 to 10 year old children, who found the retention interval between when the recall was conducted to be important. When the recall was conducted on the previous day's intake errors (intrusions and omissions) were higher for the afternoon and evening. In the current study, the recall was conducted on the previous day's intake and the interview undertaken at the same time for both recalls. Baxter *et al.* [20] also suggested that efforts to improve children's accuracy should focus on the reporting food items as they found that when children accurately recall, the amounts reported are quite accurate. Milk and orange juice (Table 2) were common intrusions in the current study. As both of these items were served on several occasions on the menu, it may have led to more mistakes in recalling the items.

There are several limitations of the current study that may limit the generalizability of the findings. The relatively small sample size reduces the statistical power of the study. However, as the participants were part of a metabolic study, we were limited by the constraints of the primary study in the sample size. Future studies should seek to replicate these findings in a larger sample. Further the adolescents in the current study were of one ethnic group and part of a metabolic study where they were required to eat everything, which may not reflect what would occur in a community-dwelling situation. Finally, there may have been an order effect observed with the second recall, due to factors related to the camp environment. Focus group data suggests that adolescents find dietary recalls 'pointless' and 'boring' [3]. It may well be that dietary recalls were of less interest to the adolescents, as they took part in a variety of educational and recreational activities coordinated as a summer-camp environment and these may have had greater appeal.

## 5. Conclusions

These results of this study show that the adolescents' accuracy to recall food items declined with a second recall. Our hypothesis was that adolescents' accuracy would improve when the 24-h recall was repeated. This was not the case and errors occurred due to omissions, intrusions and portion size estimation. These results indicate that adolescents' accuracy to recall food items declined when the 24-h recall was repeated over two non-consecutive days. Due to the limitations of the study, no recommendation can be made on whether a second recall will improve accuracy, but our findings suggest that further research in this age group is needed to insure accurate results. Dietary assessment methods need to continue to evolve to address these challenges as further improvements will enhance the consistency and strength of the association of diet with disease risk, especially in light of the current obesity epidemic among youth.

**Acknowledgments:** We wish to thank Connie Weaver and Berdine Martin for facilitating access to the participants, as well as the study participants.

**Author Contributions:** Deborah A Kerr Janine L Wright and Carol J. Boushey designed the study and took part in data collection. Satvinder S. Dhaliwal advised on statistical analysis. All authors read and contributed to the final manuscript.

**Conflicts of Interest:** The authors declare no conflict of interest.

## References

1. Ogden, C.L.; Carroll, M.D.; Kit, B.K.; Flegal, K.M. Prevalence of obesity and trends in body mass index among us children and adolescents, 1999–2010. *JAMA* **2012**, *307*, 483–490.

2. Nimptsch, K.; Malik, V.S.; Fung, T.T.; Pischon, T.; Hu, F.B.; Willett, W.C.; Fuchs, C.S.; Ogino, S.; Chan, A.T.; Giovannucci, E.; *et al.* Dietary patterns during high school and risk of colorectal adenoma in a cohort of middle-aged women. *Int. J. Cancer* **2014**, *134*, 2458–2467.

3. Boushey, C.J.; Kerr, D.A.; Wright, J.; Lutes, K.D.; Ebert, D.S.; Delp, E.J. Use of technology in children's dietary assessment. *Eur. J. Clin. Nutr.* **2009**, *63*, S50–S57.

4. Livingstone, M.B.; Black, A.E. Markers of the validity of reported energy intake. *J. Nutr.* **2003**, *133* (Suppl. 3), 895S–920S.

5. Andersen, L.F.; Lioret, S.; Brants, H.; Kaic-Rak, A.; de Boer, E.J.; Amiano, P.; Trolle, E. Recommendations for a trans-european dietary assessment method in children between 4 and 14 years. *Eur. J. Clin. Nutr.* **2011**, *65* (Suppl. 1), S58–S64.

6. Conway, J.M.; Ingwersen, L.A.; Moshfegh, A.J. Accuracy of dietary recall using the USDA five-step multiple-pass method in men: An observational validation study. *J. Am. Diet. Assoc.* **2004**, *104*, 595–603.

7. Burrows, T.L.; Martin, R.J.; Collins, C.E. A systematic review of the validity of dietary assessment methods in children when compared with the method of doubly labeled water. *J. Am. Diet. Assoc.* **2010**, *110*, 1501–1510.

8. Fisher, J.O.; Johnson, R.K.; Lindquist, C.; Birch, L.L.; Goran, M.I. Influence of body composition on the accuracy of reported energy intake in children. *Obes. Res.* **2000**, *8*, 597–603.

9. Johnson, R.K.; Driscoll, P.; Goran, M.I. Comparison of multiple-pass 24-hour recall estimates of energy intake with total energy expenditure determined by the doubly labeled water method in young children. *J. Am. Diet. Assoc.* **1996**, *96*, 1140–1144.

10. Baranowski, T.; Islam, N.; Baranowski, J.; Martin, S.; Beltran, A.; Dadabhoy, H.; Adame, S.H.; Watson, K.B.; Thompson, D.; Cullen, K.W.; *et al.* Comparison of a web-based *versus* traditional diet recall among children. *J. Acad. Nutr. Diet.* **2012**, *112*, 527–532.

11. Baranowski, T.; Islam, N.; Baranowski, J.; Cullen, K.W.; Myres, D.; Marsh, T.; de Moor, C. The food intake recording software system is valid among fourth-grade children. *J. Am. Diet. Assoc.* **2002**, *102*, 380–385.

12.	Baxter, S.D.; Hardin, J.W.; Smith, A.F.; Royer, J.A.; Guinn, C.H.; Mackelprang, A.J. Twenty-four hour dietary recalls by fourth-grade children were not influenced by observations of school meals. *J. Clin. Epidemiol.* **2009**, *62*, 878–885.

13.	Wu, L.; Martin, B.R.; Braun, M.M.; Wastney, M.E.; McCabe, G.P.; McCabe, L.D.; DiMeglio, L.A.; Peacock, M.; Weaver, C.M. Calcium requirements and metabolism in Chinese-American boys and girls. *J. Bone Miner. Res.* **2010**, *25*, 1842–1849.

14.	Conway, J.M.; Ingwersen, L.A.; Vinyard, B.T.; Moshfegh, A.J. Effectiveness of the us department of agriculture 5-step multiple-pass method in assessing food intake in obese and nonobese women. *Am. J. Clin. Nutr.* **2003**, *77*, 1171–1178.

15.	Baxter, S.D.; Hitchcock, D.B.; Guinn, C.H.; Royer, J.A.; Wilson, D.K.; Pate, R.R.; McIver, K.L.; Dowda, M. A pilot study of the effects of interview content, retention interval, and grade on accuracy of dietary information from children. *J. Nutr. Educ. Behav.* **2013**, *45*, 368–373.

16.	Smith, A.F.; Baxter, S.D.; Hardin, J.W.; Royer, J.A.; Guinn, C.H. Some intrusions in dietary reports by fourth-grade children are based on specific memories: Data from a validation study of the effect of interview modality. *Nutr. Res.* **2008**, *28*, 600–608.

17.	Baxter, S.D.; Thompson, W.O.; Litaker, M.S.; Guinn, C.H.; Frye, F.H.A.; Baglio, M.L.; Shaffer, N.M. Accuracy of fourth-graders' dietary recalls of school breakfast and school lunch validated with observations: In-person *versus* telephone interviews. *J. Nutr. Educ. Behav.* **2003**, *35*, 124.

18.	Subar, A.F.; Kipnis, V.; Troiano, R.P.; Midthune, D.; Schoeller, D.A.; Bingham, S.; Sharbaugh, C.O.; Trabulsi, J.; Runswick, S.; Ballard-Barbash, R.; *et al.* Using intake biomarkers to evaluate the extent of dietary misreporting in a large sample of adults: The open study. *Am. J. Epidemiol.* **2003**, *158*, 1–13.

19.	Guinn, C.H.; Baxter, S.D.; Royer, J.A.; Hardin, J.W.; Mackelprang, A.J.; Smith, A.F. Fourth-grade children's dietary recall accuracy for energy intake at school meals differs by social desirability and body mass index percentile in a study concerning retention interval. *J. Health Psychol.* **2010**, *15*, 505–514.

20.	Baxter, S.D.; Hardin, J.W.; Guinn, C.H.; Royer, J.A.; Mackelprang, A.J.; Smith, A.F. Fourth-grade children's dietary recall accuracy is influenced by retention interval (target period and interview time). *J. Am. Diet. Assoc.* **2009**, *109*, 846–856.

# Section 2:
# Advances in Biomarkers and Metabolomics

# Urinary Sugars—A Biomarker of Total Sugars Intake

Natasha Tasevska

**Abstract:** Measurement error in self-reported sugars intake may explain the lack of consistency in the epidemiologic evidence on the association between sugars and disease risk. This review describes the development and applications of a biomarker of sugars intake, informs its future use and recommends directions for future research. Recently, 24 h urinary sucrose and fructose were suggested as a predictive biomarker for total sugars intake, based on findings from three highly controlled feeding studies conducted in the United Kingdom. From this work, a calibration equation for the biomarker that provides an unbiased measure of sugars intake was generated that has since been used in two US-based studies with free-living individuals to assess measurement error in dietary self-reports and to develop regression calibration equations that could be used in future diet-disease analyses. Further applications of the biomarker include its use as a surrogate measure of intake in diet-disease association studies. Although this biomarker has great potential and exhibits favorable characteristics, available data come from a few controlled studies with limited sample sizes conducted in the UK. Larger feeding studies conducted in different populations are needed to further explore biomarker characteristics and stability of its biases, compare its performance, and generate a unique, or population-specific biomarker calibration equations to be applied in future studies. A validated sugars biomarker is critical for informed interpretation of sugars-disease association studies.

Reprinted from *Nutrients*. Cite as: Tasevska, N. Urinary Sugars—A Biomarker of Total Sugars Intake. *Nutrients* **2015**, *7*, 5816–5833.

## 1. Introduction

Measurement error (ME) in self-reported diet has been a long-standing obstacle for determining the true association between sugars and chronic disease risk. While the evidence for sugars' association with dental caries [1] and weight gain [2–4] has been rather consistent, the link to cardiovascular disease (CVD) [5–8], type 2 diabetes [9,10] and cancer [6,11–15] has been ambiguous and inconclusive. Although added sugars consumption in the United States (US) has declined over the last ten years, it still remains high, particularly among children (17% of energy intake [EI]) and young adults (16% EI) [16,17]. However, despite the high prevalence of this behavior and its implicated adverse effects on health, the inconsistency in evidence obtained from large prospective studies and randomized controlled trials has hindered the setting of a specific and unique recommendation on sugars intake in the US [18–20]. Sugars comprise monosaccharides (glucose, fructose, galactose) and disaccharides (sucrose, maltose, lactose), and their sum is known as "total sugars." Sugars that are naturally occurring in fruits, vegetables, and dairy products only partly account for total sugars intake, whereas sugars from highly processed food and drinks, added during food processing and preparation or at the table, have become more significant contributors of total sugars intake [21]. As a source of empty calories and a common ingredient of unhealthy foods, sugars are among the nutrients that are frequently misreported [22,23]. It is highly plausible that ME in self-reported sugars may be obscuring the true relationship between sugars and disease risk and may explain the lack of consistency in the epidemiologic evidence. Development of novel approaches for obtaining more accurate estimates of intake, independent of self-reported diet, is crucial for attaining more valid and reliable risk estimates for sugars in relation to chronic disease risk. Until then, it is uncertain whether the lack of association is due to our inability to measure sugars accurately or to a genuine lack of an association between sugars and disease risk.

Dietary biomarkers hold a lot of promise as objective measures of intake in diet-related studies. Thus far, four categories have been described based on biomarkers' characteristics: recovery, predictive, concentration, and replacement biomarkers [24]. They have multiple applications, including (1) in dietary validation studies, to characterize ME in dietary self-reports [25,26]; (2) in calibration studies nested within prospective cohorts, to develop calibration equations for "correcting" self-reported intake in the main studies [27–29]; (3) in population studies with available biological samples, as measures of dietary exposure, either alone [30–33] or in combination with self-reports [34,35]; and (4) in dietary intervention studies as measures of compliance [36].

## 2. Development of the 24 h Urinary Sucrose and Fructose Biomarker

### 2.1. Preliminary Work

Early work has shown that under physiological conditions, small amounts of dietary sucrose [37] and fructose [38] are excreted in the urine. During digestion, sucrase hydrolyzes sucrose into glucose and fructose in the brush border of the duodenum. Although healthy gastrointestinal mucosa is relatively impermeable to disaccharides, under physiological conditions, very small amounts of unhydrolyzed dietary sucrose may pass the intact intestinal wall, probably by a process of non-mediated diffusion [37], and once in the circulation, sucrose is readily excreted in urine [39]. Fructose is absorbed unchanged in the lower part of duodenum and jejunum; it is passively transported by a fructose-specific facilitative transporter

(GLUT5) across the apical membrane of the intestinal epithelial cells and by a facilitative transporter for glucose and fructose (GLUT2) across the basolateral membrane into the circulation [40,41]. The amount of fructose occurring in urine is probably a fraction of the dietary fructose or fructose derived from sucrose that escapes the uptake by the liver, as the main site of fructose metabolism, and by other tissues, such as kidneys, adipose tissue and skeletal muscle [42,43], and that escapes the reabsorption in the renal tubules [41]. Considerable amounts of fructose were detected in urine after ingesting sucrose in a bolus [38]. Although some amount of glucose can be measured in urine, it appears to be person-specific and is not reflective of dietary intake due to insulin-controlled glucose reabsorption occurring in the kidneys.

The preliminary work on sucrose and fructose as potential biomarkers of sucrose intake was conducted by Luceri *et al.* [44], based on data from nine participants consuming a "regular Italian" diet for a week and a low-sucrose diet for three days. Sucrose and fructose were measured in spot urine samples collected within 2 h of breakfast, lunch, and dinner on the last day of each study diet. Sucrose and fructose excretion during the low-sucrose diet was significantly lower compared than the excretion during the regular diet. Furthermore, the sucrose content of both the low-sucrose and regular diet, as assessed by a food diary, was significantly associated with the post-meal urinary excretion of sucrose and fructose. As the slopes of the regression lines calculated from the regression models for the low-sucrose and regular diet were similar, a common slope for the association between sucrose intake from low-sucrose or regular diet and sucrose excretion was calculated ($\beta = 0.26$; SE = 0.08). Similarly, a common slope for the association between sucrose intake from low-sucrose or regular diet and fructose excretion was reported ($\beta = 0.15$; SE = 0.05). No correlation was found between the urinary excretion of glucose and intake of sucrose. The findings from this study implied that sucrose and fructose may have the potential to be used as biomarkers of sugars consumption, however further work was needed to study the characteristics of the biomarker and to develop prediction equations based on a daily diet and against true intake.

## 2.2. Development of the Urinary Sugars Biomarker under Controlled Conditions

Urinary sugars as potential sugars biomarkers were then rigorously investigated under highly controlled conditions in two feeding studies conducted in the United Kingdom [45]. All dietary intake in these studies was known, and multiple 24 h urine samples were collected and verified for completeness using the para-amino benzoic acid (PABA) test [46]. The first study was a 30-day randomized cross-over design study involving 12 healthy males aged 25–77 years. In randomized order, all participants consumed low (63 g), medium (143 g), and high (264 g) total sugars diet over three 10 day dietary periods, respectively; this level of intake corresponded to the lower and upper 2.5 percentiles and median total sugars intake for the adult UK population [47]. All foods consumed by the participants were prepared in a metabolic kitchen, and no foods or drinks obtained outside the metabolic suite were allowed to be consumed. On Days 4–7 during each 10-d dietary period, participants collected 24 h urine samples, which were analyzed for sucrose and fructose. Although the within-subject variability of sucrose and fructose excretion was rather high in these 12 participants at the same level of total sugars intake, the mean urinary sucrose and fructose increased across the increasing levels of sugars consumption over the three dietary periods, and there was a significant difference in the mean excretion of both sucrose ($p < 0.001$) and fructose ($p < 0.001$) between the three diets. Given that the dose-response association between the diet and sugars excretion improved after combining urinary sucrose and fructose, their sum was further investigated as a potential biomarker.

The 2nd feeding study assessed the performance of the biomarker in subjects consuming their usual diets over an extended period of time, *i.e.*, simulating normal dietary behavior under controlled conditions [45]. Seven male and six female participants aged 23–66 years consumed their habitual diet (previously assessed by four consecutive 7-day diet records), and collected 24 h urine samples daily over 30 days while residing in a metabolic suite. All the foods consumed by the participants were prepared in the metabolic kitchen, where the foods were weighed to the nearest gram and left-overs weighed out upon return. The group 30 day mean sum of the 24 h urinary sucrose and fructose (24uSF) was 98 mg/day (range 25.4–267.5 mg/day), which represented a very low proportion of their 30 day mean total sugars intake (approximately 0.05%), yet, the two were highly correlated ($r = 0.84$; $p < 0.001$). The 24uSF was also highly correlated to sucrose intake ($r = 0.77$; $p = 0.002$). In the linear regression of urinary to dietary sugars, true total sugars intake explained 72% of the variability in the sucrose and fructose excretion, revealing sugars intake as a strong determinant of sucrose and fructose excretion [45]. The mean correlation between 24uSF measured from single 24 h urine and the "usual" total sugars intake was 0.71 [48]. In this study, the 30 day mean 24uSF was significantly correlated to the 30 day mean intake of extrinsic sugars (*i.e.*, any sugars or syrups added during processing and preparation of foods and drinks or added at the table, including sugars from fruit juices and honey.) ($r = 0.84$; $p < 0.001$) but not intrinsic sugars (*i.e.*, any sugars from fruits and vegetables (excluding fruit juices) and cereal and cereal products (excluding breakfast cereals, biscuits, cakes, sweet buns, pies, flans, pastries, scones, and cereal-based puddings)) ($r = 0.43$; $p = 0.144$) [49]. Nonetheless, this study was not designed to investigate the performance of urinary sugars as dietary biomarkers of extrinsic *vs.* intrinsic sugars. The stronger correlation observed with extrinsic sugars may have been due to the fact that the intake of intrinsic sugars in these 13 subjects was lower and narrower in range ($68 \pm 23$ (SD) g/day) than was their extrinsic sugars intake ($123 \pm 41$ (SD) g/day).

To investigate the effect of body mass index (BMI) on the performance and validity of the biomarker, Joosen *et al.* [50] compared the biomarker's response to diets providing 13%, 30%, and 50% energy from total sugars, in a randomized cross-over design under controlled conditions, in 10 normal-weight and nine obese participants living in a metabolic suite over 12 days. The excretion of both sucrose and fructose in urine increased to a similar degree in both the normal-weight and obese participants with the increase in total sugars intake; no significant interaction effect of BMI on urinary sucrose ($p = 0.65$) or fructose ($p = 0.55$) was observed. These findings have lent support to the application of this biomarker as a valid measure of intake in participants regardless of their BMI, as well as to investigations of the relationship between the consumption of sugars and the risk of obesity.

Given that the sugars biomarker exhibited a high correlation to "true" intake and was related to intake in a dose-response and time-sensitive manner, yet was recovered in a very low proportion in urine, 24uSF was categorized into a new class called "*predictive*" biomarkers [45]. Unlike recovery biomarkers, which are gold standard reference instruments, free of bias [51], predictive biomarkers contain a certain level of person-specific, intake-related, and covariate-related bias [52]. However, for these measures to qualify as predictive biomarkers, their biases should not explain a significant proportion of the variability in the biomarker, should be stable between individuals and across populations, and be estimable from a feeding study. Once those biases have been estimated, they can be applied to "correct" or "calibrate" the biomarker that can then serve as a reference instrument [52]. Such an equation for "calibrating" the 24uSF biomarker was generated from the 2nd UK feeding study [45,52]. The equation describes the association between the 24uSF and "true" total sugars intake, quantifies the biases associated with the 24uSF biomarker, and "calibrates" the biomarker to provide an unbiased measure of intake: $M_{ij}^* = M_{ij} - 1.67 - 0.02 \times S_i + 0.71 \times A_i$ (*Equation (1)*); where $M_{ij}^*$ is the log-transformed calibrated sugars biomarker, $M_{ij}$ is the log-transformed biomarker, $S_i$ is an indicator variable that equals 0 for men and 1 for women, and $A_i$ is the log-transformed age in years. The calibrated biomarker $M_{ij}^*$ satisfies the following *ME model for predictive biomarkers*: $M_{ij}^* = T_i + u_{M_i} + \varepsilon_{M_{ij}}$, where $T_i$ is the log-transformed true usual intake of total sugars, $u_{M_i}$ is a person-specific bias, and $\varepsilon_{M_{ij}}$ is a within-person random error [52]. Assuming that these biases are similar between individuals and across populations, this biomarker calibration equation can be applied in other studies with available 24 h urine collections to "calibrate" the sugars biomarker to be used as a reference instrument for total sugars intake. If spot urines, rather than 24 h urine collections, are available in population studies, the biomarker "calibration" equation cannot be applied to provide an unbiased measure of intake, however, the biomarker can be used as a correlate to intake, *i.e.,* concentration biomarker.

### 2.3. Investigation of Urinary Fructose as a Biomarker against Self-Report in Children

Johner *et al.* [53] investigated the use of urinary fructose as a biomarker of sugars intake among children in a subsample from the Dortmund Nutritional and Anthropometric Longitudinally Designed (DONALD) study. The analysis included 58 boys and 56 girls with mean age of 9.3 ± 0.8 and 7.9 ± 0.7 years, respectively, with available 24 h urinary fructose and self-reported diet data. Total sugars intake assessed by a three day weighed food record was significantly associated with fructose excretion from a single 24 h urine ($r = 0.43$; $p < 0.001$); each gram of total sugars intake was associated with a 0.9% increase in the amount of 24 h urinary fructose. The $R^2$ for the observed association was low ($R^2 = 0.18$), most probably due to the availability of a single-day urinary measurement, which would have introduced considerable random error in the biomarker, and to the use of a self-reported diet. Based on the authors' preliminary data, in which a less consistent dose-response relationship between sucrose intake and excretion was found, urinary sucrose was omitted from the analysis [53]. In contrast to previous studies [44,45], no preservative was used to preserve the 24 h urine collection but the urine was only refrigerated, which may have led to sucrose hydrolysis and thus to unreliability of the sucrose data. The lower correlation for fructose excretion observed by Johner *et al.* [53] may also have been partly due to fructose degradation or uptake by bacteria in preservative-free urine, in case of noncompliance with the storage instructions of their 24 h urine collection protocol.

## 3. Application of the Urinary Sugars Biomarker in Validation and Calibration Studies with Free-Living Individuals

Acknowledging the impact of ME, researchers have started conducting dietary validation studies with available biomarkers to assess ME in dietary self-reports [25,54]. They have also begun incorporating calibration substudies within their cohorts to develop regression calibration equations [27–29] that could then be applied to calibrate self-reported intake, *i.e.,* predict unbiased intake in all cohort participants to obtain more reliable risk estimates in diet-disease analyses [55–60].

The urinary sugars biomarker has recently been applied in two US biomarker-based studies, the Observing Protein and Energy Nutrition (OPEN) study [52] and the Nutrition and Physical Activity Assessment Study (NPAAS) [61]. The OPEN study involved 484 participants aged 40–69 years recruited from Montgomery County, MD, in 1999 and 2000 [62]. The NPAAS is a biomarker study embedded in the Women's Health Initiative (WHI) Observational Study ($n = 93,676$), involving 450 postmenopausal women aged 50–79 years at baseline, recruited from nine WHI centers between 2007 and 2009 [27]. Participants from both studies completed a food frequency questionnaire (FFQ) and at least two 24 h dietary recalls (24HR), and the NPAAS participants additionally completed a four-day food record (4DFR). The 24uSF biomarker and doubly-labeled water, a biomarker for energy intake, were measured in both studies, with an aim to investigate ME in self-reported total sugars (g/day) and total sugars density (g/1000 kcal). Given that the 24uSF biomarker has been found to contain a certain amount of bias that has been estimated in a feeding study, the biomarker was first "calibrated," using the biomarker "calibration" equation (Equation(1)) previously described [52], to provide an unbiased measure of total sugars intake. These applications assume that the biases in the biomarker are stable across different populations. Once "calibrated," the biomarker was applied to the OPEN and the NPAAS data as a reference instrument to assess the ME in self-report instruments by estimating the Attenuation Factor (AF) and the correlation between true and self-reported intake. AF represents the slope in the regression of true on reported intake and measures the attenuation (underestimation) of the disease risk due to ME in self-reported intake, where observed relative risk (RR) = true $RR^{AF}$ [63]. AF can have values between 0 and 1; AF = 1 would indicate no attenuation, whereas as AF gets closer to 0, the extent of attenuation increases. Table 1 reports the AFs for the instruments used in the OPEN and NPAAS, and the observed disease RR associated with self-reported sugars measured with error when true RR = 2. For absolute sugars, the AF for the FFQ was lower (less favorable) than the AFs for the average of two or three 24HRs, and, in the OPEN study, for both the 24HR and FFQ, the AFs were lower in women than in men. For sugars density, the AF for the FFQ was somewhat lower than for the 24HR and was lowest (least favorable) for the 4DFR.

Another estimate of ME in dietary self-report is the correlation between true and self-reported intake, calculated based on the ME model parameters of the biomarker and self-reports [63]. The correlation between the true and self-reported total sugars density in the OPEN participants was 0.5 for the FFQ and a single 24HR, and 0.6 for the average of two 24HRs in men, and 0.2 and 0.3 in women respectively [52]. The correlation between the true and self-reported total sugars density in the NPAAS women was of a similar magnitude to the correlation observed in the OPEN women, and was 0.3 for the FFQ, a single 24HR, and the average of two 24HRs, 0.4 for average of three 24HRs, and 0.2 for the 4DFR [61]. Based on the ME estimates from these two studies, women misreported sugars consumption more than men, and even though all investigated self-reporting instruments were associated with substantial ME, the average of multiple 24HRs was found to perform the best [52,61].

**Table 1.** Attenuation factors (AF) for self-reported total sugars in the OPEN and NPAAS studies from a measurement error model with urinary sugars biomarker as a reference instrument and observed relative risk (RR) for true RR = 2 [52,61].

| | | OPEN | | | | NPAAS | | |
|---|---|---|---|---|---|---|---|---|
| | | Men | | Women | | Women | | |
| | | FFQ | 24HR [†] | FFQ | 24HR [†] | FFQ | 24HR [‡] | 4DFR |
| Total sugars (g/day) | AF | 0.28 | 0.41 | 0.17 | 0.29 | 0.22 | 0.34 | 0.33 |
| | Obs RR (true RR = 2) | 1.21 | 1.33 | 1.13 | 1.22 | 1.16 | 1.27 | 1.26 |
| Total sugars density (g/1000 kcal) | AF | 0.39 | 0.41 | 0.33 | 0.35 | 0.48 | 0.57 | 0.32 |
| | Obs RR (true RR = 2) | 1.31 | 1.33 | 1.26 | 1.27 | 1.39 | 1.48 | 1.25 |

Obs—Observed; FFQ—Food frequency questionnaire; 24HR—24 h dietary recall; 4DFR—4 day food record; [†]: The average of two 24HRs; [‡]: The average of three 24HRs.

Next, using the 24uSF biomarker in the NPAAS, regression calibration equations for total sugars (g/day) and total sugars density (g/1000 kcal) were derived by regressing the "calibrated" 24uSF biomarker, *i.e.*, unbiased intake, on the FFQ-reported total sugars intake and the baseline characteristics, which were found to be significant predictors of unbiased intake [61]. These calibration equations also allow an investigation of various baseline characteristics, known to be associated with dietary misreporting, as potential predictors of true intake, given the ME in the self-report [27,28]. These regression calibration equations can be used to "correct" the FFQ sugars and sugars density intake for ME in all WHI participants in future WHI association studies of sugars and disease risk to obtain more reliable risk estimates. The derived equations are as follows: regression calibration equation for total sugars, g/day: log-true intake = $3.51 + 0.23 \times \log$ FFQ + $0.17 \times \log$ Age $- 0.11 \times \log$ BMI $- 0.64 \times$ current smoker + $0.55 \times <$ high school (HS) graduate + $0.30 \times$ HS graduate + $0.16 \times$ some college + $0.04 \times$ square-root metabolic equivalents/week; regression calibration equation for total sugars density, g/1000 kcal: log-true density = $0.49 + 0.44 \times \log$ FFQ + $0.77 \times \log$ Age $- 0.37 \times \log$ BMI $- 0.56 \times$ current smoker + $0.64 \times <$ HS graduate + $0.43 \times$ HS graduate + $0.18 \times$ some college.

## 4. Application of the Urinary Sugars Biomarker as a Measure of Dietary Exposure in Diet-Disease Association Studies

The urinary sugars biomarker has so far been used as a surrogate measure of intake in two analyses of the Norfolk arm of the European Prospective Investigation into Cancer (EPIC) investigating the effect of sugars consumption on obesity risk [32,33]. Given only spot urine samples were collected in this study population, the biomarker calibration equation could not be applied to obtain unbiased estimates of total sugars intake. Therefore, the biomarker was used as a concentration biomarker.

The first analysis was a cross-sectional investigation involving 404 obese (BMI > 30 kg/m$^2$) and 471 normal-weight (BMI < 25 kg/m$^2$) participants from the EPIC-Norfolk aged 45–75 years [32]. Participants in the highest $vs.$ lowest quintile for the biomarker ($i.e.$, the ratio of urinary sucrose to fructose measured in spot urine) were at 2.4 times higher risk of being obese (age- and gender-adjusted OR = 2.44, 95% CI = 1.54–3.86; $p_{trend}$ < 0.001). The risk of obesity was also positively associated with sucrose measured in spot urine (OR$_{Q5\ vs.\ Q1}$ = 1.82, 95% CI = 1.26–2.85; $p_{trend}$ = 0.02). A non-significant inverse association between sugars intake and obesity risk was observed when FFQ-measured total sugars (OR$_{Q5\ vs.\ Q1}$ = 0.89, 95% CI = 0.54–1.43; $p_{trend}$ = 0.4) or the ratio of FFQ-measured sucrose to fructose (OR$_{Q5\ vs.\ Q1}$ = 0.77, 95% CI = 0.48–1.25; $p_{trend}$ = 0.3) were used as measures of sugars intake. Given that creatinine was highly correlated with BMI, and could not be used to adjust for urine concentration, the authors used the ratio of sucrose to fructose in urine as a measure of intake.

In the second more recent analysis involving 1734 participants from the EPIC-Norfolk aged 39–77 years, the BMI measured at baseline and after 3 years of follow-up was positively associated with urinary sucrose from spot urine, and inversely associated with self-reported sucrose intake assessed by a seven day diet record (7DR), FFQ or 24HR collected at baseline [33]. Participants in the highest $vs.$ lowest quintile of urinary sucrose were 1.54 times more likely to become overweight or obese (OR$_{Q5\ vs.\ Q1}$ = 1.54, 95% CI = 1.12–2.12; $p_{trend}$ = 0.008), whereas those in the highest $vs.$ lowest quintile of 7DR-based sucrose intake were at 44% lower risk of becoming overweight or obese (OR$_{Q5\ vs.\ Q1}$ = 0.56, 95% CI = 0.40–0.77; $p_{trend}$ < 0.0001) after three years of follow-up. The authors used urinary sucrose per specific gravity to control for urine concentration, rather than the ratio of urinary sucrose to fructose, due to their having fewer available samples with both sucrose and fructose values within the acceptable analytical range. However, in sensitivity analyses in a reduced sample that used the sucrose to fructose ratio as a biomarker, all risk estimates remained virtually unchanged. Available evidence has consistently linked increased sugars consumption with an increase in obesity risk [2–4]. In this population, such an association was detected when using urinary sugars from spot urine as a concentration biomarker but not when using self-reported intake.

## 5. Summary and Future Research

Applying a sugars biomarker in future diet-disease association studies is crucial for detecting unbiased disease-risk estimates for sugars consumption. Biomarkers have been successful in revealing diet and disease associations that otherwise have been difficult to ascertain. Energy intake has been found to be associated with increased risk of breast cancer [58], all-cancer [56], CVD [57] and type 2 diabetes [60]; and protein intake with risk of type 2 diabetes [60] and frailty [64]; using biomarker-calibrated self-report estimates but not using un-calibrated instruments. When biomarkers are collected for all participants, they can also be used as surrogate measures of intake in relation to disease, either alone [30–32] or in combination with self-reports [34,35]. High sugars consumption was associated with statistically significant increased risk of obesity when the urinary sugars biomarker was used as a measure of dietary exposure [32,33], whereas no association [32] or inverse association [33] was found when using self-reported intake.

Although the 24uSF biomarker has been developed under highly controlled conditions, has great potential, and exhibits considerably favorable characteristics for a biomarker, available data come from only a few controlled studies with limited sample sizes ($n = 12$, $n = 13$, $n = 19$) [45,50]. Data from these feeding studies showed that the biomarker contains bias, which may originate from the between-subject variability in sucrose and fructose absorption, fructose uptake by individual tissues or reabsorption in the kidneys, and may be determined by genetic, dietary or lifestyle factors, or physiological or medical conditions. Some variability may be due to the analytical methods or issues related to urine collection, processing or storage. Increased sucrose excretion has long been used as a marker of altered gastrointestinal permeability [65,66], attributed to either structurally damaged or inflamed mucosa occurring in gastroduodenal, celiac [67] or inflammatory bowel disease [68], or the presence of congenital sucrose-isomaltose deficiency, which is considered to be particularly rare [69,70]. The intake of certain medications (e.g., non-steroid anti-inflammatory drugs [NSAID] [71], proton pump inhibitors [72]) and alcohol have also been associated with increased gastrointestinal permeability [73], while smoking has been found to decrease permeability, and to reduce the adverse effect of NSAID and alcohol on the gastrointestinal mucosa during simultaneous exposure, possibly by protecting the intercellular tight junctions of the epithelium [73,74]. Intestinal inflammation and infection leads to decreased expression of GLUT5, a fructose-specific transporter in the brush border membrane, and thus may impair fructose absorption [41]. Although, GLUT5 is acutely and efficiently upregulated by fructose concentration in the intestinal lumen and facilitates absorption, fructose malabsorption has been shown to occur among healthy individuals at fructose doses higher than 15 g, particularly in presence of low luminal glucose concentration, as glucose significantly improves fructose transport through enterocyte [41,75].

In the applications of the biomarker "calibration" equation in the US-based studies [52,61], an assumption was made that the biomarker's biases are stable across participants and across different populations, which may not hold and needs to be further investigated. The original feeding study, the source of the urinary sugars "calibration" equation, was conducted in the UK [45]. Total sugars composition in the UK diet differs from sugars composition in the diet in the US and other countries. In the UK, table sugar or disaccharide sucrose is the main caloric sweetener, while in the US, monosaccharide sweeteners (e.g., fructose, glucose, dextrose) derived primarily from corn represent more than half of the caloric sweeteners used in the food supply [76,77]. A significantly different sucrose to fructose ratio in the US diet may result in different levels of sucrose and fructose measured in urine. The presence of glucose in the intestinal lumen enhances fructose absorption [75]. Hence, consuming fructose as part of sucrose or from a diet with a similar content of glucose may result in higher fructose absorption and thus excretion. Therefore, the performance and applicability of the calibration equation for the 24uSF developed with the UK diet requires further investigation and validation among US participants. We need further highly-controlled studies conducted in different populations across geographical regions to further explore biomarker characteristics and the stability of its biases, compare its performance, and validate the existing calibration equation for the 24uSF, or, if more applicable, generate population-specific biomarker calibration equations to be applied in future studies. Obtaining large sample sizes ($n > 100$) in future controlled studies will be crucial for achieving precision in estimating the biases arising from between-subject variability and for reliably investigating their effect on biomarker performance (personal communications, L. Freedman). Preparing and analyzing duplicate diets in such studies will avoid introducing ME from food composition tables in the estimate of "true intake" and will further increase the precision of the biomarker calibration equations. Although ensuring completeness of urine collections may not be necessary in population-based biomarker studies [78], it is essential in controlled feeding studies. Misestimation of the 24 h urinary biomarker excretion due to incomplete urine collections may affect the biomarker calibration equation and thus may lead to errors in the estimation of unbiased sugars intake in future biomarker studies. Preserving 24 h urine during collection is required for maintaining the stability of the sucrose and fructose [48], and boric acid in a concentration of $\leq 2$ g/L has so far been used [45]. Among the analytical methods applied to measure sucrose and fructose in urine, liquid chromatography and gas chromatography with mass spectrometry (LC/MS and GC/MS) techniques use low-cost consumables, however, require expensive instrumentation and technical expertise [79]. In addition, for the GC and GC/MS analytical approaches, the sample-preparation step is labor intensive and time consuming [79,80], whereas the colorimetric method can be easily set up in most laboratories and is compatible with boric acid as a preservative [45].

Due to large participant burden, complex logistics, and high costs, collection of 24 h urine samples is not always feasible in large population studies. Investigation of the utility of spot urines in assessment of sugars intake is much needed and would undoubtedly lead to findings that could have major practical implications for epidemiologic studies. The urinary sucrose and fructose biomarker is a short-term measure of intake excreted 2–6 h after ingestion [44], and so when measured in spot urine, the biomarker (besides its inherent biases) will also contain a certain amount of ME, depending on the timing of the spot urine collection relative to intake. In the scenario of a population study, these errors will be expected to attenuate the association between true intake and the biomarker and to make it unstable. Hence, when measured in spot urine, this biomarker may possibly be used as a concentration, rather than as a predictive biomarker. Further investigation under controlled conditions, and identification of determinants of errors associated with the sugars biomarker measured in spot urine, will inform its future applications as an unbiased instrument. The concentration of sucrose and fructose in partial collections has been shown to correlate well with total sugars intake [44] and has been used previously as surrogate measures of intake, showing a positive association with obesity risk in a population study [32,33], consistent with the current evidence [2–4].

Recently, the carbon stable isotope ratio ($^{13}C/^{12}C$, expressed as $\delta^{13}C$) was proposed as a biomarker of sugars intake in populations consuming sugars abundant with $^{13}C$, such as corn-based sugars and sugar cane [81–83]. Although measuring component-specific $\delta^{13}C$, such as $\delta^{13}C$ in red blood cell alanine, has shown much promise [84], this biomarker has never been investigated under highly-controlled conditions of a feeding study. Investigating the comparative performance of the urinary sugars biomarker and $\delta^{13}C$ in relevant populations under controlled conditions would be particularly useful. Furthermore, a panel of four urinary biomarkers (formate, citrulline, taurine and isocitrate) indicative of sugar-sweetened beverage consumption has been identified using a metabolomics-based approach, and further work needs to be conducted to define their use in population-based research [85].

The urinary sugars biomarker has so far been used in observational studies only. One of the critical limitations of intervention studies investigating the effect of sugars consumption has been the reliance on self-reported measures [5], thus application of the sugars biomarker as a measure of intervention compliance will inform the interpretation of findings and help obtain valid estimates of the intervention effect.

Methodologically rigorous development of the urinary sugars biomarker and its applications in population-based studies has shown that this biomarker exhibits favorable characteristics for a biomarker and has great potential, yet further investigation is needed to better characterize and inform its application in different populations. A validated sugars biomarker that can be applied in available and future observational and intervention studies with biological samples will serve as an instrumental resource that would allow correction for ME in self-reported sugars and detection of unbiased sugars-disease associations. Until strong and consistent evidence for adverse health effects of sugars is found, no firm advice can be given to the general public.

**Acknowledgments:** The author would like to thank the late Sheila A. Bingham (Dunn Human Nutrition Unit, Medical Research Council, Cambridge, UK), Victor Kipnis (National Cancer Institute (NCI)), Nancy Potischman (NCI), Douglas Midthune (NCI), Gunter G. Kuhnle (University of Reading, UK) and Shirley A. Runswick (Dunn Human Nutrition Unit, Medical Research Council, Cambridge, UK) for their contribution, valuable discussions, and expert advice on this work, and Dr. Laurence Freedman for sharing unpublished analysis.

**Conflicts of Interest:** The author declares no conflict of interest.

## References

1. Moynihan, P.J.; Kelly, S.A. Effect on caries of restricting sugars intake: Systematic review to inform WHO guidelines. *J. Dent. Res.* **2014**, *93*, 8–18.

2. Te Morenga, L.; Mallard, S.; Mann, J. Dietary sugars and body weight: Systematic review and meta-analyses of randomised controlled trials and cohort studies. *BMJ* **2013**, *346*, e7492.

3. Malik, V.S.; Pan, A.; Willett, W.C.; Hu, F.B. Sugar-sweetened beverages and weight gain in children and adults: A systematic review and meta-analysis. *Am. J. Clin. Nutr.* **2013**, *98*, 1084–1102.

4. Hu, F.B. Resolved: There is sufficient scientific evidence that decreasing sugar-sweetened beverage consumption will reduce the prevalence of obesity and obesity-related diseases. *Obes. Rev.* **2013**, *14*, 606–619.

5. Sonestedt, E.; Overby, N.C.; Laaksonen, D.E.; Birgisdottir, B.E. Does high sugar consumption exacerbate cardiometabolic risk factors and increase the risk of type 2 diabetes and cardiovascular disease? *Food Nutr. Res.* **2012**, *56*.

6. Tasevska, N.; Park, Y.; Jiao, L.; Hollenbeck, A.; Subar, A.F.; Potischman, N. Sugars and risk of mortality in the NIH-AARP Diet and Health Study. *Am. J. Clin. Nutr.* **2014**, *99*, 1077–1088.

7. Yang, Q.; Zhang, Z.; Gregg, E.W.; Flanders, W.D.; Merritt, R.; Hu, F.B. Added sugar intake and cardiovascular diseases mortality among US adults. *JAMA Intern. Med.* **2014**, *174*, 516–524.

8. Te Morenga, L.A.; Howatson, A.J.; Jones, R.M.; Mann, J. Dietary sugars and cardiometabolic risk: Systematic review and meta-analyses of randomized controlled trials of the effects on blood pressure and lipids. *Am. J. Clin. Nutr.* **2014**, *100*, 65–79.

9. Malik, V.S.; Popkin, B.M.; Bray, G.A.; Despres, J.P.; Hu, F.B. Sugar-sweetened beverages, obesity, type 2 diabetes mellitus, and cardiovascular disease risk. *Circulation* **2010**, *121*, 1356–1364.

10. Malik, V.S.; Hu, F.B. Sweeteners and Risk of Obesity and Type 2 Diabetes: The Role of Sugar-Sweetened Beverages. *Curr. Diabetes Rep.* **2012**, *12*, 195–203.

11. World Cancer Research Fund; American Institute for Cancer Research. *Food, Nutrition and the Prevention of Cancer: A Global Perspective*; American Institute for Cancer Research: Washington, DC, USA, 1997.

12. Tasevska, N.; Jiao, L.; Cross, A.J.; Kipnis, V.; Subar, A.F.; Hollenbeck, A.; Schatzkin, A.; Potischman, N. Sugars in diet and risk of cancer in the NIH-AARP Diet and Health Study. *Int. J. Cancer* **2012**, *130*, 159–169.

13. World Cancer Research Fund; American Institute for Cancer Research. Food, Nutrition, Physical Activity, and the Prevention of Colorectal Cancer. Available online: http://www.dietandcancerreport.org/cancer_resource_center/downloads/cu/Colorectal-Cancer-2011-Report.pdf (accessed on 1 April 2015).

14. World Cancer Research Fund; American Institute for Cancer Research. Food, Nutrition, Physical Activity, and the Prevention of Endometrial Cancer. Available online: http://www.dietandcancerreport.org/cancer_resource_center/downloads/cu/Endometrial-Cancer-2013-Report.pdf (accessed on 1 April 2015).

15. World Cancer Research Fund; American Institute for Cancer Research. Food, Nutrition, Physical Activity, and the Prevention of Pancreatic Cancer. Available online: http://www.dietandcancerreport.org/cancer_resource_center/downloads/cu/Pancreatic-Cancer-2012-Report.pdf (accessed on 1 April 2015).

16. Welsh, J.A.; Sharma, A.J.; Grellinger, L.; Vos, M.B. Consumption of added sugars is decreasing in the United States. *Am. J. Clin. Nutr.* **2011**, *94*, 726–734.

17. McGuire, S.; Ervin, R.B.; Kit, B.K.; Carroll, M.D.; Ogden, C.L. *Consumption of Added Sugar among U.S. Children and Adolescents, 2005–2008*; NCHS Data Brief No. 87; National Center for Health Statistics: Hyattsville, MD, USA, 2012.

18. Johnson, R.K.; Appel, L.J.; Brands, M.; Howard, B.V.; Lefevre, M.; Lustig, R.H.; Sacks, F.; Steffen, L.M.; Wylie-Rosett, J. Dietary sugars intake and cardiovascular health: A scientific statement from the American Heart Association. *Circulation* **2009**, *120*, 1011–1020.

19. Institute of Medicine; Food and Nutrition Board. *Dietary Reference Intakes for Energy, Carbohydrates, Fiber, Fat, Fatty Acids, Cholsterol, Protein, and Amino Acids*; The National Academies Press: Washington, DC, USA, 2005.

20. U.S. Department of Agriculture; U.S. Department of Health and Human Services. *Dietary Guidelines for Americans, 2010*, 7th ed.U.S. Government Printing Office: Washington, DC, USA, 2010.

21. Popkin, B.M.; Nielsen, S.J. The sweetening of the world's diet. *Obes. Res.* **2003**, *11*, 1325–1332.

22. Price, G.M.; Paul, A.A.; Cole, T.J.; Wadsworth, M.E. Characteristics of the low-energy reporters in a longitudinal national dietary survey. *Br. J. Nutr.* **1997**, *77*, 833–851.

23. Krebs-Smith, S.M.; Graubard, B.I.; Kahle, L.L.; Subar, A.F.; Cleveland, L.E.; Ballard-Barbash, R. Low energy reporters vs others: A comparison of reported food intakes. *Eur. J. Clin. Nutr.* **2000**, *54*, 281–287.

24. Jenab, M.; Slimani, N.; Bictash, M.; Ferrari, P.; Bingham, S.A. Biomarkers in nutritional epidemiology: Applications, needs and new horizons. *Hum. Genet.* **2009**, *125*, 507–525.

25. Schatzkin, A.; Kipnis, V.; Carroll, R.J.; Midthune, D.; Subar, A.F.; Bingham, S.; Schoeller, D.A.; Troiano, R.P.; Freedman, L.S. A comparison of a food frequency questionnaire with a 24 hour recall for use in an epidemiological cohort study: Results from the biomarker-based Observing Protein and Energy Nutrition (OPEN) study. *Int. J. Epidemiol.* **2003**, *32*, 1054–1062.

26. Bingham, S.A.; Gill, C.; Welch, A.; Cassidy, A.; Runswick, S.A.; Oakes, S.; Lubin, R.; Thurnham, D.I.; Key, T.J.; Roe, L.; *et al.* Validation of dietary assessment methods in the UK arm of EPIC using weighed records, and 24-hour urinary nitrogen and potassium and serum vitamin C and carotenoids as biomarkers. *Int. J. Epidemiol.* **1997**, *26* (Suppl. 1), S137–S151.

27. Prentice, R.L.; Mossavar-Rahmani, Y.; Huang, Y.; van Horn, L.; Beresford, S.A.; Caan, B.; Tinker, L.; Schoeller, D.; Bingham, S.; Eaton, C.B.; *et al.* Evaluation and comparison of food records, recalls, and frequencies for energy and protein assessment by using recovery biomarkers. *Am. J. Epidemiol.* **2011**, *174*, 591–603.

28. Neuhouser, M.L.; Tinker, L.; Shaw, P.A.; Schoeller, D.; Bingham, S.A.; Horn, L.V.; Beresford, S.A.; Caan, B.; Thomson, C.; Satterfield, S.; *et al.* Use of recovery biomarkers to calibrate nutrient consumption self-reports in the Women's Health Initiative. *Am. J. Epidemiol.* **2008**, *167*, 1247–1259.

29. Huang, Y.; van Horn, L.; Tinker, L.F.; Neuhouser, M.L.; Carbone, L.; Mossavar-Rahmani, Y.; Thomas, F.; Prentice, R.L. Measurement error corrected sodium and potassium intake estimation using 24-hour urinary excretion. *Hypertension* **2014**, *63*, 238–244.

30. Kyrø, C.; Olsen, A.; Landberg, R.; Skeie, G.; Loft, S.; Åman, P.; Leenders, M.; Dik, V.K.; Siersema, P.D.; Pischon, T.; *et al.* Plasma alkylresorcinols, biomarkers of whole-grain wheat and rye intake, and incidence of colorectal cancer. *J. Natl. Cancer Inst.* **2014**, *106*, djt352.

31. Cottet, V.; Collin, M.; Gross, A.S.; Boutron-Ruault, M.C.; Morois, S.; Clavel-Chapelon, F.; Chajès, V. Erythrocyte membrane phospholipid fatty acid concentrations and risk of colorectal adenomas: A case-control nested in the French E3N-EPIC cohort study. *Cancer Epidemiol. Biomark. Prev.* **2013**, *22*, 1417–1427.

32. Bingham, S.; Luben, R.; Welch, A.; Tasevska, N.; Wareham, N.; Khaw, K.T. Epidemiologic assessment of sugars consumption using biomarkers: Comparisons of obese and nonobese individuals in the European Prospective Investigation of Cancer Norfolk. *Cancer Epidemiol. Biomark. Prev.* **2007**, *16*, 1651–1654.

33. Kuhnle, G.G.; Tasevska, N.; Lentjes, M.A.; Griffin, J.L.; Sims, M.A.; Richardson, L.; Aspinall, S.M.; Mulligan, A.A.; Luben, R.N.; Khaw, K.T. Association between sucrose intake and risk of overweight and obesity in a prospective sub-cohort of the European Prospective Investigation into Cancer in Norfolk (EPIC-Norfolk). *Public Health Nutr.* **2015**, 1–10.

34. Knudsen, M.D.; Kyrø, C.; Olsen, A.; Dragsted, L.O.; Skeie, G.; Lund, E.; Aman, P.; Nilsson, L.M.; Bueno-de-Mesquita, H.B.; Tjønneland, A.; *et al.* Self-reported whole-grain intake and plasma alkylresorcinol concentrations in combination in relation to the incidence of colorectal cancer. *Am. J. Epidemiol.* **2014**, *179*, 1188–1196.

35. Freedman, L.S.; Tasevska, N.; Kipnis, V.; Schatzkin, A.; Mares, J.; Tinker, L.; Potischman, N. Gains in statistical power from using a dietary biomarker in combination with self-reported intake to strengthen the analysis of a diet-disease association: An example from CAREDS. *Am. J. Epidemiol.* **2010**, *172*, 836–842.

36. Marklund, M.; Magnusdottir, O.K.; Rosqvist, F.; Cloetens, L.; Landberg, R.; Kolehmainen, M.; Brader, L.; Hermansen, K.; Poutanen, K.S.; Herzig, K.H.; *et al.* A dietary biomarker approach captures compliance and cardiometabolic effects of a healthy Nordic diet in individuals with metabolic syndrome. *J. Nutr.* **2014**, *144*, 1642–1649.

37. Menzies, I.S. Absorption of intact oligosaccharide in health and disease. *Biochem. Soc. Trans.* **1974**, *2*, 1042–1047.

38. Nakamura, H.; Tamura, Z. Gas chromatographic analysis of mono- and disaccharides in human blood and urine after oral administration of disaccharides. *Clin. Chim. Acta* **1972**, *39*, 367–381.

39. Deane, N.; Smith, H.W. Fate of inulin and sucrose in normal subjects as determined by a urine reinfusion technique. *J. Clin. Investig.* **1955**, *34*, 681–684.

40. Sun, S.Z.; Empie, M.W. Fructose metabolism in humans—What isotopic tracer studies tell us. *Nutr. Metab. Lond.* **2012**, *9*, 89.

41. Douard, V.; Ferraris, R.P. Regulation of the fructose transporter GLUT5 in health and disease. *Am. J. Physiol. Endocrinol. Metab.* **2008**, *295*, E227–E237.

42. Mayes, P.A. Intermediary metabolism of fructose. *Am. J. Clin. Nutr.* **1993**, *58* (Suppl. 5), 754S–765S.

43. Björkman, O.; Felig, P. Role of the kidney in the metabolism of fructose in 60-hour fasted humans. *Diabetes* **1982**, *31*, 516–520.

44. Luceri, C.; Caderni, G.; Lodovici, M.; Spagnesi, M.T.; Monserrat, C.; Lancioni, L.; Dolara, P. Urinary excretion of sucrose and fructose as a predictor of sucrose intake in dietary intervention studies. *Cancer Epidemiol. Biomark. Prev.* **1996**, *5*, 167–171.

45. Tasevska, N.; Runswick, S.A.; McTaggart, A.; Bingham, S.A. Urinary sucrose and fructose as biomarkers for sugar consumption. *Cancer Epidemiol. Biomark. Prev.* **2005**, *14*, 1287–1294.

46. Bingham, S.A.; Cummings, J.H. Creatinine and PABA as markers for completeness of collection of 24-hour urine samples. *Hum. Nutr. Clin. Nutr.* **1986**, *40*, 473–476.

47. Gregory, J.; Foster, K.; Tyler, H.; Wiseman, M. *The Dietary and Nutritional Survey of British Adults—A Survey Carried Out by the Social Survey Division of OPCS with Dietary and Nutritional Evaluations by the Ministry of Agriculture, Fisheries and Food and the Department of Health*; HMSO: London, UK, 1990; p. 75.

48. Tasevska, N. *Biomarkers for Validation of Dietary Exposure Assessments in Nutritional Epidemiology (Doctoral disseration)*; University of Cambridge: Cambridge, UK, 2005.

49. Tasevska, N.; Runswick, S.A.; Welch, A.A.; McTaggart, A.; Bingham, S.A. Urinary sugars biomarker relates better to extrinsic than to intrinsic sugars intake in a metabolic study with volunteers consuming their normal diet. *Eur. J. Clin. Nutr.* **2008**, *63*, 653–659.

50. Joosen, A.M.; Kuhnle, G.G.; Runswick, S.A.; Bingham, S.A. Urinary sucrose and fructose as biomarkers of sugar consumption: Comparison of normal weight and obese volunteers. *Int. J. Obes. Lond.* **2008**, *32*, 1736–1740.

51. Kaaks, R.; Riboli, E.; Sinha, R. Biochemical markers of dietary intake. *IARC Sci. Publ.* **1997**, *142*, 103–126.

52. Tasevska, N.; Midthune, D.; Potischman, N.; Subar, A.F.; Cross, A.J.; Bingham, S.A.; Schatzkin, A.; Kipnis, V. Use of the predictive sugars biomarker to evaluate self-reported total sugars intake in the Observing Protein and Energy Nutrition (OPEN) study. *Cancer Epidemiol. Biomark. Prev.* **2011**, *20*, 490–500.

53. Johner, S.A.; Libuda, L.; Shi, L.; Retzlaff, A.; Joslowski, G.; Remer, T. Urinary fructose: A potential biomarker for dietary fructose intake in children. *Eur. J. Clin. Nutr.* **2010**, *64*, 1365–1370.

54. Day, N.; McKeown, N.; Wong, M.; Welch, A.; Bingham, S. Epidemiological assessment of diet: A comparison of a 7-day diary with a food frequency questionnaire using urinary markers of nitrogen, potassium and sodium. *Int. J. Epidemiol.* **2001**, *30*, 309–317.

55. Prentice, R.L.; Tinker, L.F.; Huang, Y.; Neuhouser, M.L. Calibration of self-reported dietary measures using biomarkers: An approach to enhancing nutritional epidemiology reliability. *Curr. Atheroscler. Rep.* **2013**, *15*, 353.

56. Prentice, R.L.; Shaw, P.A.; Bingham, S.A.; Beresford, S.A.; Caan, B.; Neuhouser, M.L.; Patterson, R.E.; Stefanick, M.L.; Satterfield, S.; Thomson, C.A.; *et al.* Biomarker-calibrated energy and protein consumption and increased cancer risk among postmenopausal women. *Am. J. Epidemiol.* **2009**, *169*, 977–989.

57. Prentice, R.L.; Huang, Y.; Kuller, L.H.; Tinker, L.F.; Horn, L.V.; Stefanick, M.L.; Sarto, G.; Ockene, J.; Johnson, K.C. Biomarker-calibrated energy and protein consumption and cardiovascular disease risk among postmenopausal women. *Epidemiology* **2011**, *22*, 170–179.

58. Prentice, R.L.; Pettinger, M.; Tinker, L.F.; Huang, Y.; Thomson, C.A.; Johnson, K.C.; Beasley, J.; Anderson, G.; Shikany, J.M.; Chlebowski, R.T.; *et al.* Regression calibration in nutritional epidemiology: Example of fat density and total energy in relationship to postmenopausal breast cancer. *Am. J. Epidemiol.* **2013**, *178*, 1663–1672.

59. Beasley, J.M.; Lacroix, A.Z.; Larson, J.C.; Huang, Y.; Neuhouser, M.L.; Tinker, L.F.; Jackson, R.; Snetselaar, L.; Johnson, K.C.; Eaton, C.B.; *et al.* Biomarker-calibrated protein intake and bone health in the Women's Health Initiative clinical trials and observational study. *Am. J. Clin. Nutr.* **2014**, *99*, 934–940.

60. Tinker, L.F.; Sarto, G.E.; Howard, B.V.; Huang, Y.; Neuhouser, M.L.; Mossavar-Rahmani, Y.; Beasley, J.M.; Margolis, K.L.; Eaton, C.B.; Phillips, L.S.; *et al.* Biomarker-calibrated dietary energy and protein intake associations with diabetes risk among postmenopausal women from the Women's Health Initiative. *Am. J. Clin. Nutr.* **2011**, *94*, 1600–1606.

61. Tasevska, N.; Midthune, D.; Tinker, L.F.; Potischman, N.; Lampe, J.W.; Neuhouser, M.L.; Beasley, J.M.; van Horn, L.; Prentice, R.; Kipnis, V. Use of a urinary sugars biomarker to assess measurement error in self-reported sugars intake in the Nutrition and Physical Activity Assessment Study (NPAAS). *Cancer Epidemiol. Biomark. Prev.* **2014**, *23*, 2874–2883.

62. Subar, A.F.; Kipnis, V.; Troiano, R.P.; Midthune, D.; Schoeller, D.A.; Bingham, S.; Sharbaugh, C.O.; Trabulsi, J.; Runswick, S.; Ballard-Barbash, R.; *et al.* Using intake biomarkers to evaluate the extent of dietary misreporting in a large sample of adults: The OPEN study. *Am. J. Epidemiol.* **2003**, *158*, 1–13.

63. Kipnis, V.; Subar, A.F.; Midthune, D.; Freedman, L.S.; Ballard-Barbash, R.; Troiano, R.P.; Bingham, S.; Schoeller, D.A.; Schatzkin, A.; Carroll, R.J. Structure of dietary measurement error: Results of the OPEN biomarker study. *Am. J. Epidemio.* **2003**, *158*, 14–21.

64. Beasley, J.M.; LaCroix, A.Z.; Neuhouser, M.L.; Huang, Y.; Tinker, L.; Woods, N.; Michael, Y.; Curb, J.D.; Prentice, R.L. Protein intake and incident frailty in the Women's Health Initiative observational study. *J. Am. Geriatr. Soc.* **2010**, *58*, 1063–1071.

65. Sutherland, L.R.; Verhoef, M.; Wallace, J.L.; van Rosendaal, G.; Crutcher, R.; Meddings, J.B. A simple, non-invasive marker of gastric damage: Sucrose permeability. *Lancet* **1994**, *343*, 998–1000.

66. Van Wijck, K.; Verlinden, T.J.; van Eijk, H.M.; Dekker, J.; Buurman, W.A.; Dejong, C.H.; Lenaerts, K. Novel multi-sugar assay for site-specific gastrointestinal permeability analysis: A randomized controlled crossover trial. *Clin. Nutr.* **2013**, *32*, 245–251.

67. Cobden, I.; Rothwell, J.; Axon, A.T. Intestinal permeability and screening tests for coeliac disease. *Gut* **1980**, *21*, 512–518.

68. Dastych, M.; Novotná, H.; Cíhalová, J. Lactulose/mannitol test and specificity, sensitivity, and area under curve of intestinal permeability parameters in patients with liver cirrhosis and Crohn's disease. *Dig. Dis. Sci.* **2008**, *53*, 2789–2792.

69. Sander, P.; Alfalah, M.; Keiser, M.; Korponay-Szabo, I.; Kovács, J.B.; Leeb, T.; Naim, H.Y. Novel mutations in the human sucrase-isomaltase gene (SI) that cause congenital carbohydrate malabsorption. *Hum. Mutat.* **2006**, *27*.

70. Nichols, B.L.; Adams, B.; Roach, C.M.; Ma, C.X.; Baker, S.S. Frequency of sucrase deficiency in mucosal biopsies. *J. Pediatr. Gastroenterol. Nutr.* **2012**, *55* (Suppl. 2), S28–S30.

71. Kerckhoffs, A.P.; Akkermans, L.M.; de Smet, M.B.; Besselink, M.G.; Hietbrink, F.; Bartelink, I.H.; Busschers, W.B.; Samsom, M.; Renooij, W. Intestinal permeability in irritable bowel syndrome patients: Effects of NSAIDs. *Dig. Dis. Sci.* **2010**, *55*, 716–723.

72. Mullin, J.M.; Valenzano, M.C.; Whitby, M.; Lurie, D.; Schmidt, J.D.; Jain, V.; Tully, O.; Kearney, K.; Lazowick, D.; Mercogliano, G.; *et al.* Esomeprazole induces upper gastrointestinal tract transmucosal permeability increase. *Aliment. Pharmacol. Ther.* **2008**, *28*, 1317–1325.

73. Gotteland, M.; Cruchet, S.; Frau, V.; Wegner, M.E.; Lopez, R.; Herrera, T.; Sanchez, A.; Urrutia, C.; Brunser, O. Effect of acute cigarette smoking, alone or with alcohol, on gastric barrier function in healthy volunteers. *Dig. Liver Dis.* **2002**, *34*, 702–706.

74. Suenaert, P.; Bulteel, V.; den Hond, E.; Hiele, M.; Peeters, M.; Monsuur, F.; Ghoos, Y.; Rutgeerts, P. The effects of smoking and indomethacin on small intestinal permeability. *Aliment. Pharmacol. Ther.* **2000**, *14*, 819–822.

75. Jones, H.F.; Butler, R.N.; Brooks, D.A. Intestinal fructose transport and malabsorption in humans. *Am. J. Physiol. Gastrointest. Liver Physiol.* **2011**, *300*, G202–G206.

76. Haley, S.; Reed, J.; Lin, B.-H.; Cook, A. *Sweetener Consumption in the United States: Distribution by Demographic and Product Characteristics*; Electronic Outlook Report from the Economic Research Service, SSS-243–01; U.S. Department of Agriculture, Economic Research Service: Washington, DC, USA, 2005.

77. Ng, S.W.; Slining, M.M.; Popkin, B.M. Use of caloric and noncaloric sweeteners in US consumer packaged foods, 2005–2009. *J. Acad. Nutr. Diet.* **2012**, *112*, 1828–1834.

78. Subar, A.F.; Midthune, D.; Tasevska, N.; Kipnis, V.; Freedman, L.S. Checking for completeness of 24-h urine collection using para-amino benzoic acid not necessary in the Observing Protein and Energy Nutrition study. *Eur. J. Clin. Nutr.* **2013**, *67*, 863–867.

79. Kuhnle, G.G.; Joosen, A.M.; Wood, T.R.; Runswick, S.A.; Griffin, J.L.; Bingham, S.A. Detection and quantification of sucrose as dietary biomarker using gas chromatography and liquid chromatography with mass spectrometry. *Rapid Commun. Mass Spectrom.* **2008**, *22*, 279–282.

80. Song, X.; Navarro, S.L.; Diep, P.; Thomas, W.K.; Razmpoosh, E.C.; Schwarz, Y.; Wang, C.Y.; Kratz, M.; Neuhouser, M.L.; Lampe, J.W. Comparison and validation of 2 analytical methods for measurement of urinary sucrose and fructose excretion. *Nutr. Res.* **2013**, *33*, 696–703.

81. Yeung, E.H.; Saudek, C.D.; Jahren, A.H.; Kao, W.H.; Islas, M.; Kraft, R.; Coresh, J.; Anderson, C.A. Evaluation of a novel isotope biomarker for dietary consumption of sweets. *Am. J. Epidemiol.* **2010**, *172*, 1045–1052.

82. Cook, C.M.; Alvig, A.L.; Liu, Y.Q.; Schoeller, D.A. The natural 13C abundance of plasma glucose is a useful biomarker of recent dietary caloric sweetener intake. *J. Nutr.* **2010**, *140*, 333–337.

83. Nash, S.H.; Kristal, A.R.; Bersamin, A.; Hopkins, S.E.; Boyer, B.B.; O'Brien, D.M. Carbon and nitrogen stable isotope ratios predict intake of sweeteners in a Yup'ik study population. *J. Nutr.* **2013**, *143*, 161–165.

84. Choy, K.; Nash, S.H.; Kristal, A.R.; Hopkins, S.; Boyer, B.B.; O'Brien, D.M. The carbon isotope ratio of alanine in red blood cells is a new candidate biomarker of sugar-sweetened beverage intake. *J. Nutr.* **2013**, *143*, 878–884.

85. Gibbons, H.; McNulty, B.A.; Nugent, A.P.; Walton, J.; Flynn, A.; Gibney, M.J.; Brennan, L. A metabolomics approach to the identification of biomarkers of sugar-sweetened beverage intake. *Am. J. Clin. Nutr.* **2015**, *101*, 471–477.

# Metabolomics to Explore Impact of Dairy Intake

Hong Zheng, Morten R. Clausen, Trine K. Dalsgaard and Hanne C. Bertram

**Abstract:** Dairy products are an important component in the Western diet and represent a valuable source of nutrients for humans. However, a reliable dairy intake assessment in nutrition research is crucial to correctly elucidate the link between dairy intake and human health. Metabolomics is considered a potential tool for assessment of dietary intake instead of traditional methods, such as food frequency questionnaires, food records, and 24-h recalls. Metabolomics has been successfully applied to discriminate between consumption of different dairy products under different experimental conditions. Moreover, potential metabolites related to dairy intake were identified, although these metabolites need to be further validated in other intervention studies before they can be used as valid biomarkers of dairy consumption. Therefore, this review provides an overview of metabolomics for assessment of dairy intake in order to better clarify the role of dairy products in human nutrition and health.

Reprinted from *Nutrients*. Cite as: Zheng, H.; Clausen, M.R.; Dalsgaard, T.K.; Bertram, H.C. Metabolomics to Explore Impact of Dairy Intake. *Nutrients* **2015**, *7*, 4875–4896.

## 1. Introduction

Cow's milk is a good source of nutrients for humans and its health benefits have been appreciated since the Middle Ages [1]. Currently, cow's milk plays an important role in human nutrition, spanning the entire age range from infants to elderly, especially in Western countries but also increasingly in Asia and Africa. Cow's milk can be processed into different types of dairy products, such as butter, cheese, cream, and yogurt. Due to the different dairy processes, nutritional characteristics may differ among dairy products, which results in different impacts on human health [2]. Therefore, it is of great importance to qualitatively and quantitatively evaluate consumption of different dairy products in order to better correlate the effect of dairy intake to human health. Metabolomics aims at profiling all low-molecular-weight metabolites in a biological system and has been used as a promising tool to discriminate different dietary patterns [3], and also to identify dietary biomarkers [4]. Therefore, metabolomics could potentially be used as tool to assess dietary intake of specific food items in an unbiased way and thereby reduce human error and subjective bias, such as misremembering, under-reporting and misclassification of a specific diet, from traditional dietary assessment methods [5]. However, application of metabolomics for assessment of dairy intake is still in its infancy and solid markers for dairy intake still need to be identified and models that can quantify dairy intake based on analysis of bio fluids, such as urine, are still warranted.

Therefore, the main aim of this review is to emphasize state-of-the-art assessment of dairy intake using metabolomics and encourage its application in this area. The present review consists of (i) a short introduction of dairy processing and nutrients; (ii) a brief description on the association between dairy intake and human health; (iii) a mini review of the application of metabolomics for assessment of dairy consumption; and (iv) concluding remarks and future perspectives.

## 2. Dairy Products and Composition

Cow's milk is a liquid formed in the mammary glands of dairy cows during lactation and it is composed of water, protein (approximately 80% casein and 20% whey), fat (approximately 98% triglycerides), lactose, vitamins, and minerals [6]. Milk is often consumed after minimal processing including removal of varying amounts of fat and heat treatment, but milk is also to a large extent processed to other dairy products. Figure 1 displays an overview of the main dairy product categories. The milk fat can be concentrated from raw milk (4.0% fat) by centrifugation to obtain cream (up to 48% fat) and low-fat (1.0%–2.0% fat) or skim milk (< 0.5% fat) [6]. Thus, fat-soluble vitamins (e.g., vitamins A and D) in low-fat or skim milk are reduced or removed with the fat. In order to be compensated for this vitamin reduction, low-fat milk can be fortified with the fat-soluble vitamins, especially vitamin D. Butter is produced by churning cream to achieve a phase inversion from oil-in-water to water-in-oil emulsion [6]. In addition, fermented milk represents a large proportion of dairy products. Cheese, as a popular fermented product, is formed after coagulation of casein micelles using the enzyme chymosin, starter bacteria or heat treatment [7]. Numerous different varieties of cheese exist and their nutrients differ with the cheese type. In general, cheese consists of casein, saturated fat, fat-soluble vitamins, calcium, and bioactive peptides [7]. Yogurt is also a fermented dairy product obtained from a fermentation process by lactic acid bacteria, which produces lactic acid from lactose. The composition of yogurt is comparable to the original milk, while many nutrients in yogurt are more concentrated [8]. Whey protein can be concentrated as a by-product from cheese production and used as an additive in food to enhance specific physical properties or improve its nutritional value. Moreover, water can be removed from milk or other dairy products by evaporation to produce dry dairy products.

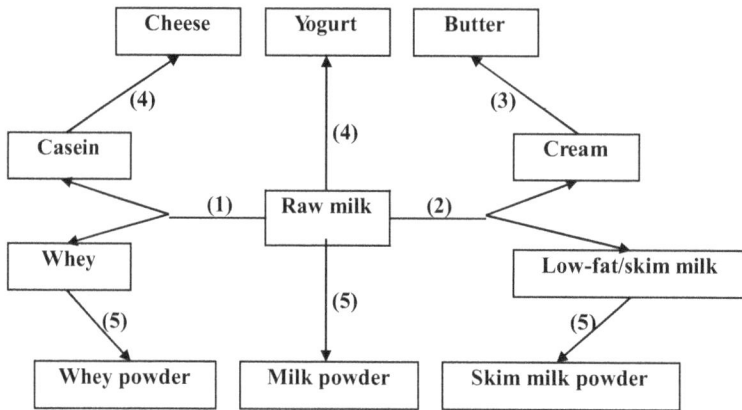

**Figure 1.** Overview of milk and various dairy products obtained from different processing schemes: (1) coagulation; (2) separation; (3) churning; (4) fermentation; (5) evaporation.

## 3. Dairy Intake and Human Health

Dairy products as nutrient-rich sources have been recommended as an important component in human nutrition and associated with potential health benefits.

### 3.1. Overweight and Obesity

Overweight and obesity are becoming more and more common health issues and their prevalence is rapidly growing in the world [9]. Many studies have examined the relationship between dairy consumption and body weight regulation. A systematic review based on prospective cohort studies revealed that the weight-lowering effect of dairy intake is suggestive but not consistent [10]. A meta-analysis from Abargouei *et al.* [11] reported that the effect of dairy intake on body weight depended on the energy intake; without energy restriction no effect of dairy intake was observed, but with energy restriction a beneficial effect of dairy intake on body weight was observed. Similarly, Chen *et al.* [12] found that dairy intake only attenuated body weight gain in the short-term or in energy-restricted studies, but not in the long-term or in non-energy-restricted studies. Dairy products have traditionally been considered to have an undesirable effect with respect to overweight and obesity due to a high content of saturated fat. Yet, in a recent systematic review the intake of high-fat dairy products was inversely linked with adiposity in 11 of 16 studies and adverse effects of high intake of dairy fat [13] could not be supported. Mechanisms explaining the potential weight-lowering effects of dairy intake have been suggested. The high calcium content in dairy products may facilitate a weight loss: firstly, calcium can suppress lipogenesis and stimulate lipolysis [14]; secondly, calcium can increase fecal fat excretion by combining with fatty acids and thereby forming insoluble soaps in the gut [15]; thirdly, calcium may increase fat oxidation [16]. Recently, milk and primary its medium chain fatty acids showed an up-regulating effect of the *ANGPTL4*-gene [17,18]. The *ANGPTL4*-gene increases the production of the ANGPTL4 protein, which has great impact on the uptake of fat from the blood stream to the adipose tissue by inhibition of lipoprotein lipase, but which recently also was shown to inhibit the pancreatic lipase in the gut [19], thus potentially also reducing the uptake of dietary fat. In addition, milk protein, especially whey, may regulate body weight: firstly, whey increases satiety and reduces energy intake [20]; secondly, whey enhances the thermic effect of food, resulting in higher post-meal energy expenditure [21]; thirdly, whey suppresses lipogenic enzyme in the adipose tissue [22]. In addition, fermented dairy products have been shown to result in increased gut bacterial content in humans [23], which must be considered an intriguing finding as there is increasing attention to the role of gut microbiota on the development of obesity [24].

## 3.2. Diabetes

Diabetes is a growing challenge for human health. Interestingly, an inverse correlation between dairy intake and the incidence of type 2 diabetes (T2D) has been established. In a meta-analysis performed by Pittas *et al.* [25], a lower T2D risk was found in the highest dairy intake group (3–5 servings/day) compared with the lowest dairy intake group (1.5 servings/day). Elwood *et al.* [26] also reported that the relative risk of T2D is almost 10% lower after high milk intake. Moreover, several meta-analyses found that low-fat or fermented dairy products protect against T2D [27–30]. Yet, a recent systematic review based on short- and long-term intervention studies did not show a consistent association between dairy intake and insulin sensitivity [31]. The mechanism behind the impact of dairy consumption on T2D can likely be explained partly by the weight-lowering effect of dairy intake (Section 3.1). In addition, several components in dairy products are suggested to protect against T2D. Dairy minerals, such as calcium and magnesium, have a potential for improving insulin sensitivity [32,33]. Intake of vitamin D has been associated with a lower risk of T2D by reducing insulin resistance [34]. Insulinotropic and glucose-lowering properties of whey protein have been reported in healthy subjects and patients with T2D [35]. Free fatty acids have been shown to increase insulin secretion from pancreatic β cells by activating G-protein-coupled receptor, GPR40 [36]. *trans*-Palmitoleate, primarily from dairy fat, may also reduce insulin resistance and incident diabetes [37].

## 3.3. Hypertension

Intake of milk and low-fat dairy products has been reported to hold an inverse correlation with hypertension risk [38,39]. A meta-analysis based on randomized controlled trials revealed that probiotic fermented milk protects against hypertension [40]. Several mechanisms behind the association between dairy intake and hypertension have been proposed. Firstly, the weight-lowering effect of dairy consumption is responsible for a lower risk of hypertension according to a meta-analysis performed by Neter *et al.* [41], where they found that systolic and diastolic blood pressure decreased by 1.1 and 0.9 mm Hg, respectively, with a decrease in body weight of 1 kg. Secondly, calcium intake from dairy products can maintain smooth muscle tone in blood vessels [42,43]. Other dairy minerals including magnesium [44], calcium [45], and potassium [46] may also contribute to a hypotensive effect. Thirdly, casein hydrolysates containing Val-Pro-Pro and Ile-Pro-Pro peptides have been observed to lower blood pressure in intervention studies [47–49], which is attributed to an inhibition of angiotensin converting enzyme (ACE). Several other possible peptide inhibitors of ACE have also been identified from milk, such as casokinins [50], C12 peptide [51], lactotripeptides [52], and lactokinins [53]. Moreover, milk peptides, such as lactokinin, may also regulate the release of endothelin-1, which can raise blood pressure by constricting blood vessels [54,55].

## 3.4. Cancer

Meta-analyses show an inverse correlation between dairy intake and colorectal cancer [56], a direct correlation between dairy ingestion and prostate cancer [57], while the correlations between dairy consumption and breast cancer [58], pancreatic cancer [59] and ovarian cancer [60] are inconclusive. For bladder cancer, the link varied with different types of dairy products [61,62]. The risk of cancer has been associated with obesity and T2D, which may be attributed to a high IGF-I level, insulin resistance and hyperinsulinemia [63,64]. Therefore, the effect of dairy intake on obesity and T2D may partly have contributed to the link between dairy consumption and cancer risk (Sections 3.1 and 3.2). Yet, milk consumption may increase the IGF-I level, indicating an adverse effect of milk intake on cancer development [65]. An inadequate intake of calcium and vitamin D is associated with an increased risk of cancer [66]. Whey protein exerts anticancer properties by increasing the level of glutathione, which can reduce reactive oxygen species and carcinogens [67]. Bovine lactoferrin also plays a role in cancer prevention by induction of apoptosis and regulation of carcinogen-metabolizing enzymes [68]. Dairy fat like conjugated linoleic acid may also protect against cancer [69]. In addition, Lampe [70] suggested that the associations between fermented dairy products, gut microbiota, and cancer risk needs further exploration. Overall, due to the complexity of cancer, the mechanisms behind the effect of dairy intake on cancer risk remain unresolved.

## 3.5. Stroke

A recent meta-analysis revealed that low-fat or fermented dairy products were significantly related to low risk of stroke [71]. Moreover, a non-linear dose dependency was established between milk intake and relative stroke risk, in which the highest protective effect was found at approx. 200 mL/day and such an effect remained up to 700 mL/day. The correlation between dairy intake and stroke can most likely be attributed to the weight-lowering effect of dairy consumption [72]. Another possible mechanism might be that dairy consumption can reduce platelet aggregation and insulin resistance [73]. In addition, dairy minerals such as K, Ca, and Mg potentially contribute to reduce stroke risk [73].

## 3.6. Bone Health

Dairy product intake plays an important role in bone development during childhood and adolescence and prevention of bone loss in the elderly, which is attributed to the high contents of calcium, vitamin D, potassium, and phosphorus in dairy products [74,75].

## 4. Dairy Intake Assessment

### 4.1. Significance of Dairy Intake Assessment

Epidemiological evidence for a role of dairy products on human health has been comprehensively reported, yet their correlations differed with different types of dairy products, human diseases, and dietary regime (Section 3). A possible explanation for this discrepancy sometimes observed could be the different compositions of various dairy products. In addition, a poor or incorrect assessment of dairy intake may be another reason for this discrepancy. Thus, one of the greatest challenges for achieving a better understanding of dairy health in humans relies on the ability to obtain trustworthy information on dairy intake. Dietary assessment can be classified into two levels; qualitative and quantitative assessment. The former aims at discriminating between different diet groups, while the latter attempts to evaluate the amount of dietary intake. Food frequency questionnaires (FFQ), food records, and 24-h recalls are traditionally used to quantitatively assess dietary intake. However, these methods have several limitations, such as misremembering, under-reporting, and misclassification of the specific food items [76], which may mask important or make incorrect links between dietary intake and human health. Therefore, finding a reliable assessment method, such as biomarker utilization, is of great importance. Biomarkers, as measurable indicators of biological features, are categorized into exogenous and endogenous markers based on their origin [77]. Exogenous biomarkers can be applied to evaluate potential exposure to a specific diet, while endogenous markers are directly associated with metabolic changes in response to dietary ingestion. Thus, using exogenous biomarkers to evaluate dairy consumption may reduce the limitations of traditional assessment methods, improve the reliability and accuracy of dairy intake data, and thereby better elucidate the impact of dairy intake on human health.

### 4.2. Assessment of Dairy Fat Intake

By correlating the level of fatty acids in biological samples with the dietary data from traditional methods, several biomarkers for assessment of dairy fat intake have been identified. Wolk *et al.* [78] found that pentadecanoic (15:0) and heptadecanoic (17:0) acids in adipose tissue might be validated as exogenous biomarkers of long-term milk fat intake. The content of 15:0 in serum was also identified as a marker of dairy fat intake [79–81]. Wolk *et al.* [80] identified a new marker, myristic acid (14:0), in adipose tissue for dairy fat intake. Biong *et al.* [82] confirmed that the levels of 14:0, 15:0, and 17:0 in adipose tissue can be regarded as valid biomarkers of dairy fat intake. Moreover, 14:1 and 17:1 could be two new potential markers and serum 15:0 cholesteryl esters is the best alternative if adipose tissue is not obtainable [82]. Moreover, plasma and erythrocyte levels of 15:0 and *trans*-16:1n-7 might be indicators to assess dairy fat consumption [83].

Furthermore, there have been attempts to associate these biomarkers with human diseases for exploring the health benefits of dairy intake. A higher plasma level of 15:0 was linked to a higher risk of ischemic heart disease in women [83]. Warensjö *et al.* [84] established an inverse correlation between the level of milk fat biomarkers (15:0 and 17:0) in plasma and risk of developing a first myocardial infarction. Yet, the levels of 15:0 and 17:0 in adipose tissue were not associated with myocardial infarction risk, probably due to the influence of other nutrients [85]. The plasma *trans*-16:1n-7 level was inversely correlated with blood pressure and T2D incidence [37]. The content of 15:0 but not 14:0 and *trans*-16:1n-7 in plasma was observed to have an inverse correlation with cardiovascular disease and coronary heart disease [86]. Moreover, Santaren *et al.* [87] found that the serum 15:0 level was inversely correlated with T2D risk. Plasma 14:0, 15:0, 17:0, and *trans*-16:1n-7 levels were not significantly associated with stroke risk [88].

However, recently Ratnayake [89] raised concern in relation to the use of these fatty acids as biomarkers of dairy fat intake. This concern is related to the fact that the fatty acids 15:0, 17:0, and *trans*-16:1n-7 may also be derived from other food sources than dairy fat, and *trans*-16:1n-7 may also be endogenously synthesized from $\beta$-oxidation of dietary vaccenic acid. In addition, analytical challenges exist as these fatty acids need to be identified carefully due to small amounts in samples and co-elution with other fatty acids during GC analysis. Lankinen & Schwab [90] also suggested that 15:0 and 17:0 might be used as valid biomarkers of dairy fat intake if subjects consume a high amount of dairy fat and a low amount of fish. Overall, care must be taken to use these fatty acids in dietary assessment studies of dairy intake, and dietary origin and the analytical method should be taken into account.

Dairy fat in different matrices may possess different health effects. For instance, cheese fat lowers LDL-cholesterol level more than butter fat [91,92]. Therefore, the discrimination between consumption of different types of dairy products is also of great interest and important for elucidating the impact of dairy fat on human health.

### 4.3. Principle in Assessment of Dairy Intake by Metabolomics

Metabolomics aims to provide a comprehensive profile of all low-molecular-weight metabolites in the biological system under a particular condition, such as a dietary intervention. Metabolites can be regarded as exposure markers or metabolic products after consumption of a specific food. The basic procedure of metabolomics is shown in Figure 2: Firstly, biological samples typically urine, blood and/or feces are collected from subjects consuming a specific food; secondly, metabolite profiles of the samples are measured by analytical techniques such as nuclear magnetic resonance (NMR), liquid chromatography-mass spectrometry (LC-MS) and gas chromatography-mass spectrometry (GC-MS); thirdly, multivariate and univariate analyses are applied to analyze data in order to identify potential metabolites related to dietary intake; and finally, potential markers are validated in further studies. However, the validation of candidate biomarkers is rarely performed in most published metabolomics studies on dietary intake evaluation, which hampers the use of these biomarkers in clinical studies.

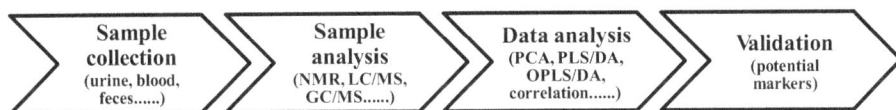

| Sample collection (urine, blood, feces......) | Sample analysis (NMR, LC/MS, GC/MS......) | Data analysis (PCA, PLS/DA, OPLS/DA, correlation......) | Validation (potential markers) |

**Figure 2.** The basic procedure of metabolomics for dietary intake assessment.

Metabolomics provides a good opportunity in dietary intervention studies to identify biomarkers for assessment of dietary intake [3,5]. Yet, metabolomics is also facing many challenges, such as metabolite identification and efficient data analysis of the comprehensive data sets [93]. Except technical challenges, intrinsic (e.g., genotype, gender, age, health status) and extrinsic (e.g., diet, drug, physical activity) factors that influence the metabolome also challenge the development of metabolomics in dietary nutrition studies [94].

*4.4. Metabolomics Applied to Identify Biomarkers Related to Dairy Intake*

Metabolomics in combination with data analysis can potentially identify biomarkers, fingerprints, and associated models that can assess dairy intake quantitatively. However, only a few studies have applied metabolomics with main focus on the identification of biomarkers related to the intake of dairy products. In order to review current metabolomics studies on dairy products intake, we did a systematic literature search using the databases, PubMed [95], EMBASE [96] and SCOPUS [97], from 1995 to May 2015 by using the following search terms: ("dairy" OR "milk" OR "cheese" OR "butter" OR "casein" OR "whey") AND ("metabolomic" OR "metabonomic" OR "metabolic profiling" OR "metabolite" OR "metabolomic" OR "mass spectrometry" OR "nuclear magnetic resonance" OR "LC MS" OR "GC MS" OR "NMR") AND ("random" OR "andomly" OR "randomized" OR "control" OR "controlled" OR "cross over" OR "intervention" OR "trial") AND ("urine" OR "urinary" OR "blood" OR "plasma" OR "serum" OR "feces" OR "faeces" OR "fecal"). The selected literature was published in English and conducted in human subjects.

Metabolomics was applied to identify dietary biomarkers in an epidemiologic study by Guertin *et al.* [98]. In this study, serum metabolites were measured using MS-based metabolomics and intake of 36 different dietary groups was recorded through the FFQ method. Using a correlation analysis between the MS-based metabolome and the FFQ data, Guertin *et al.* [98] found that serum 15:0, 16:0, and 10-undecenoate levels were directly correlated with butter consumption. However, the disadvantage of the FFQ such as under- or over-reporting of food consumption should be taken into account in this study.

*4.5. Metabolomics Applied to Elucidate Metabolic Impact of Dairy Intake*

Metabolomics has been applied for the assessment of both whole product and dairy protein intake under different experimental designs. Table 1 shows changes in metabolites detected as a function of dairy intake by metabolomics. These metabolites may be potential markers for quantitative assessment of dairy consumption. Metabolomics has also been applied to examine the change of metabolites after dairy intake in controlled intervention trials. Bertram *et al.* [99] investigated the metabolic response of milk and meat intake in 8-year-old boys for seven days using NMR-based metabolomics and found that milk consumption reduced urinary hippurate excretion and increased serum SCFA level. Both GC-MS and NMR-based serum metabolomics failed to discriminate between intake of probiotic and non-probiotic acidified milk in the subjects aged from 18–79 years, while an increase in lactate, glutamine, proline, creatinine/creatine, aspartic acid, and 3-hydroxybutyrate, as well as a reduced glucose level were observed after the 8-week intervention of both acidified milk drinks [100,101]. Moreover, NMR-based urine metabolomics was applied to elucidate the different responses to casein and whey consumption in 12–15 year old overweight adolescents during a 12-week intervention period and a significant increase in urinary urea excretion was found after casein intake but not after whey intake [102]. Piccolo *et al.* [103] revealed that whey protein supplementation in obese women resulted in a unique plasma metabolic pattern during an 8-week weight loss intervention by GC-MS-based metabolomics and decreased Pro- and Cys-related metabolites, as compared with a gelatin-based protein supplementation. Using an NMR-based metabolomics approach, we found that high dairy intake (4–5 dairy products/day) had a significant impact on urinary metabolite profiles in overweight/obese women (age: 18–60 years old) relative to low dairy intake (0–1 dairy products/day) during a 24-week energy-restricted intervention [unpublished data]. The 24-week intervention with high dairy consumption increased urinary citrate excretion and decreased TMAO levels significantly.

In a crossover study, subjects consumed each diet at different time periods, which means that the influence of individual variation is minimized. Hjerpsted *et al.* [104] applied LC-MS metabolomics on urine to evaluate the difference between cheese and butter consumption in the subjects aged from 22–70 years during a 6-week crossover intervention, yet no separation was obtained by multivariate data analysis. However, by using univariate data analysis, the increases in urinary indoxyl sulfate, xanthurenic acid, tyramine sulfate, 4-hydroxyphenylacetic acid, isovalerylglutamic acid, isovalerylglycine, tiglylglycine, and isobutyrylglycine levels were identified after cheese intake. Intriguingly, in a 2-week crossover study, an NMR-based metabolomics approach based on urine and feces samples was able to successfully discriminate between intake of cheese and milk in 18–50 year old healthy men [105]. Cheese intake resulted in increased urinary prolinebetaine, tyrosine and hippurate as well as fecal butyrate and malonate, while reduced levels of citrate, creatine and creatinine in urine and glycerol in feces.

Yde *et al.* [106] investigated the impact of dairy protein (whey and calcium caseinate) on post-exercise plasma metabolism in young male subjects (age: 28 $\pm$ 2 years old) using NMR-based metabolomics. No difference in low-molecular-weight metabolites was found between the two dairy proteins. However, whey protein increased VLDL and reduced LDL, while an increase in both VLDL and LDL levels in plasma was observed after intake of caseinate protein [106].

**Table 1.** Change of metabolites as determined by metabolomics after intake of dairy products.

| Reference | Dairy Product | Design | Subject | N | Age | Time | Sample | Technique | Metabolite |
|---|---|---|---|---|---|---|---|---|---|
| Guertin et al. [98] | Butter | E [a] | Women (44%) | 502 | 64 ± 5 | 1 year | Serum | UPLC/GC-MS | Methyl palmitate (16:0)↑; 15:0↑; 10-undecenoate↑ |
| Bertram et al. [99] | Milk | R [b] | Boy (100%) | 24 | 8 | 7 days | Urine, plasma | NMR | Urinary hippurate↑; plasma SCFA↑ |
| Pedersen et al. [100] | Probiotic/non-probiotic acidified milk | R | Women (74%) | 61 | 19–79 | 8 weeks | Serum | NMR | Lactate↑; 3-hydroxybutyrate↑ |
| Pedersen et al. [101] | Probiotic/non-probiotic acidified milk | R | Women (74%) | 61 | 19–79 | 8 weeks | Serum | GC-MS | Lactate↑; glutamine↑ proline↑; creatinine/creatine↑; aspartic acid↑; glucose↓ |
| Zheng et al. [102] | Casein, whey, skim milk | R | Overweight adolescents (Girl, 62%) | 192 | 12–15 | 12 weeks | Urine | NMR | **Casein/skim milk:** urea↑ |
| Piccolo et al. [103] | Whey | R | Obese women (100%) | 27 | - | 8 weeks | Plasma | GC-MS | **Whey vs. gelatin protein:** Pro-/Cys-related metabolites↓ |
| Zheng et al. [104] | Low or high dairy product | R | Women (100%) | 38 | 18–60 | 24 weeks | Urine | NMR | **High vs. low dairy intake:** citrate↑; TMAO↓ |
| Hjerpsted et al. [105] | Cheese, butter | C [c] | Women (43%) | 23 | 22–70 | 6 weeks | Urine | UPLC-MS | **Cheese:** indoxyl sulfate↑; xanthurenic acid↑; tyramine sulfate↑; 4-hydroxyphenylacetic acid↑; isovalerylglutamic acid↑; isovalerylglycine↑; tiglylglycine↑; isobutyrylglycine↑ |
| Zheng et al. [106] | Cheese, milk | C | Men (100%) | 15 | 18–50 | 2 weeks | Urine | NMR | **Cheese vs. control:** creatine↓; creatinine↓; prolinebetaine↑; choline↓; TMAO↓; tyrosine↑ **Milk vs. control:** citrate↑; prolinebetaine↓; TMAO↓; hippurate↓; urea↑ **Cheese vs. milk:** citrate↓; creatine↓; creatinine↓; prolinebetaine↑; tyrosine↑; hippurate↑ |

194

Table 1. Cont.

| Reference | Dairy Product | Design | Subject | N | Age | Time | Sample | Technique | Metabolite |
|---|---|---|---|---|---|---|---|---|---|
| Zheng et al. [106] | Cheese, milk | C | Men (100%) | 15 | 18–50 | 2 weeks | Feces | NMR | **Cheese vs. control:** propionate↑; butyrate↑; malonate↓; fecal lipid↑ **Milk vs. control:** propionate↑; acetate↑; glycerol↑; malonate↓; choline↓; fecal lipid↑ **Cheese vs. milk:** butyrate↑; malonate↑; glycerol↓ |
| Yde et al. [107] | Whey, calcium caseinate | C | Men (100%) | 12 | 28 ± 2 | Postexercise 70–330 min | Plasma | NMR | **Whey:** VLDL↑; LDL↓ **Caseinate:** VLDL↓; LDL↑ |
| Stanstrup et al. [108] | Whey isolate (WI), whey hydrolysate (WH), α-lactalbumin, caseinoglycomacropeptide | C | Obese, nondiabetic subjects | 11 | 44–74 | Postprandial 1–8 h | Plasma | LC-MS | **WH:** methionine sulfoxide↑; cyclo(Pro-Thr)↑; cyclo(Phe-Val)↑; cyclo(Ile-Val)/cyclo(Leu-Val)↑; β-Asp-Leu↑; pGlu-Pro↑; Cyclo(Ala-Ile)↑; pGlu-Leu↑; pGlu-Val↑; N-phenylacetylmethionine↑; methionine↓; hydroxyphenyllactic acid↓; N-phenylacetylmethionine sulfoxide↑; glutamic acid↑ **WI:** threonine↓; indolelactic acid↑; γ-glutamyl-leucine↑; phenylalanine↑; γ-glutamyl-leucine↑; kynurenine↑ |
| Stanstrup et al. [109] | Whey isolate (WI), casein | C | Obese, nondiabetic subjects | 11 | 40–68 | Postprandial 1–8 h | Plasma | LC-MS | **WI:** leucine/isoleucine↑; γ-glutamyl-leucine↑; tryptophan↑; isoleucine↑; paracetamol↓; threonine↑; γ-glutamyl-methionine↑; lysine↑; β-hydroxyisobutyric acid↑; methionine↑; γ-glutamyl-valine↑; paracetamol sulfate↓; kynurenine↑; paracetamol glucuronide↓; α-keto-3-methylvaleric acid↑; valine↑; citrulline↑; 3-hydroxy-2-methylbutyric acid↑; glutamic acid↑; propionylcarnitine↑; α-hydroxydecanoic acid↓; lauric acid↓; myristic acid↓; hydroxybutyric acid↑ **Casein:** methionine sulfoxide↑; N-phenylacetyl-methionine↑ |

[a] epidemiologic study; [b] randomized study; [c] crossover study.

Furthermore, the postprandial effect of dairy protein intake was assessed by metabolomics. Stanstrup *et al.* [107] used a LC-MS-based metabolomics approach to discriminate between different whey protein fractions consumption on plasma metabolite profiles of obese/non-diabetic subjects (age: 44–74 years old) and found that the levels of amino acids and their derivatives were directly correlated with the composition of whey proteins. Moreover, increased cyclic dipeptides were identified after intake of hydrolysed whey, which is probably associated with its insulinotropic effect [107]. Stanstrup *et al.* [108] also observed that intake of whey isolate caused a postprandial increase in amino acids and a reduction in fatty acids in plasma of obese/non-diabetic subjects (age: 40–68 years old).

Overall, metabolomics has been applied for qualitative assessment of dairy intake under different experimental conditions, where many factors including individual difference, intervention dose and duration as well as daily diet and physical activity may affect the human metabolome. Thus, care should be taken when comparing the results from different studies. In addition, the potential of these metabolites as biomarkers needs to be further established in other intervention or cohort studies before they can be used as valid markers for quantitatively evaluating dairy consumption and for exploring the association between dairy intake and human health.

## 5. Conclusions

A reliable dairy intake assessment method is essential to better explore the impact of dairy products on human health. Metabolomics as a qualitative assessment tool has shown a potential to discriminate between consumption of different dairy products. Furthermore, metabolomics identified several potential metabolites related to dairy intake, but further validations are required to establish valid biomarkers for quantitative assessment of dairy consumption. Currently the most prominent biomarkers candidates include the 14:1 and 17:1 fatty acids and serum 15:0 cholesteryl esters [83].

Metabolomics could be used as an assessment tool of dairy intake, yet further studies are needed to confirm its usefulness and to expand its application in this research area. In addition, a number of suggestions need to be addressed. Metabolomics studies related to dairy consumption have primarily focused on discriminating between intake of different dairy products, but the quantitative association between metabolite profiles and dairy intake have still not been examined. Since different dairy products have different compositions and therefore may exert different metabolic effects, it would be attractive to investigate different types of dairy products separately when evaluating their consumption. Measuring the composition of dairy products may facilitate identification and analysis of exogenous biomarkers in metabolomics datasets obtained from biological samples. It is suggested to further identify and validate exogenous biomarkers, especially more specific biomarkers, as indicators of dairy intake instead of the FFQ method in the dairy nutrition research. Combined biomarkers could be more reliable and valid for dairy intake assessment than a single marker. Finally, biomarkers need to be validated in clinical trials.

**Acknowledgments:** The authors would like to thank the Danish Council for Strategic Research, Arla Foods, and the Danish Dairy Research Foundation for financial support through the project "FIAF-Milk in regulating lipid metabolism and overweight; Uncovering milk's ability to increase expression and activity of fasting-induced adipose factor".

**Author Contributions:** Hong Zheng and Hanne C. Bertram designed and wrote the manuscript. All authors read, revised, and approved the final manuscript.

**Conflicts of Interest:** The authors declare no conflict of interest.

# References

1.  Miller, G.D.; Jarvis, J.K.; McBean, L.D. *Handbook of Dairy Foods and Nutrition*, 3rd ed.; CRC Press: Boca Raton, FL, USA, 2007.
2.  Visioli, F.; Strata, A. Milk, dairy products, and their functional effects in humans: A narrative review of recent evidence. *Adv. Nutr.* **2014**, *5*, 131–143.
3.  O'Sullivan, A.; Gibney, M.J.; Brennan, L. Dietary intake patterns are reflected in metabolomic profiles: Potential role in dietary assessment studies. *Am. J. Clin. Nutr.* **2011**, *93*, 314–321.
4.  O'Gorman, A.; Gibbons, H.; Brennan, L. Metabolomics in the identification of biomarkers of dietary intake. *Comput. Struct. Biotechnol. J.* **2013**, *4*, 1–7.
5.  Favé, G.; Beckmann, M.E.; Draper, J.H.; Mathers, J.C. Measurement of dietary exposure: A challenging problem which may be overcome thanks to metabolomics? *Genes Nutr.* **2009**, *4*, 135–141.
6.  Walstra, P.; Wouters, J.T.M.; Geurts, T.J. *Dairy Science and Technology*, 2nd ed.; CRC Press: Boca Raton, FL, USA, 2006.
7.  Henning, D.R.; Baer, R.J.; Hassan, A.N.; Dave, R. Major advances in concentrated and dry milk products, cheese, and milk fat-based spreads 1. *J. Dairy Sci.* **2006**, *89*, 1179–1188.
8.  Adolfsson, O.; Meydani, S.N.; Russell, R.M. Yogurt and gut function. *Am. J. Clin. Nutr.* **2004**, *80*, 245–256.
9.  Stevens, G.A.; Singh, G.M.; Lu, Y.; Danaei, G.; Lin, J.K.; Finucane, M.M.; Bahalim, A.N.; McIntire, R.K.; Gutierrez, H.R.; Cowan, M.; *et al.* National, regional, and global trends in adult overweight and obesity prevalences. *Popul. Health Metr.* **2012**, *10*, 22.
10. Louie, J.C.Y.; Flood, V.M.; Hector, D.J.; Rangan, A.M.; Gill, T.P. Dairy consumption and overweight and obesity: A systematic review of prospective cohort studies. *Obes. Rev.* **2011**, *12*, e582–e592.
11. Abargouei, A.S.; Janghorbani, M.; Salehi-Marzijarani, M.; Esmaillzadeh, A. Effect of dairy consumption on weight and body composition in adults: A systematic review and meta-analysis of randomized controlled clinical trials. *Int. J. Obes.* **2012**, *36*, 1485–1493.

12. Chen, M.; Pan, A.; Malik, V.S.; Hu, F.B. Effects of dairy intake on body weight and fat: A meta-analysis of randomized controlled trials. *Am. J. Clin. Nutr.* **2012**, *96*, 735–747.

13. Kratz, M.; Baars, T.; Guyenet, S. The relationship between high-fat dairy consumption and obesity, cardiovascular, and metabolic disease. *Eur. J. Nutr.* **2013**, *52*, 1–24.

14. Zemel, M.B. The role of dairy foods in weight management. *J. Am. Coll. Nutr.* **2005**, *24*, 537S–546S.

15. Christensen, R.; Lorenzen, J.K.; Svith, C.R.; Bartels, E.M.; Melanson, E.L.; Saris, W.H.; Tremblay, A.; Astrup, A. Effect of calcium from dairy and dietary supplements on faecal fat excretion: A meta-analysis of randomized controlled trials. *Obes. Rev.* **2009**, *10*, 475–486.

16. Melanson, E.L.; Sharp, T.A.; Schneider, J.; Donahoo, W.T.; Grunwald, G.K.; Hill, J.O. Relation between calcium intake and fat oxidation in adult humans. *Int. J. Obes. Relat. Metab. Disord.* **2003**, *27*, 196–203.

17. Nielsen, S.D.; Young, J.F.; Mortensen, G.; Petersen, R.K.; Kristiansen, K.; Dalsgaard, T.K. Activation of the angiopoietin-like 4 (ANGPLT4) gene by milk fat and casein. *Int. Dairy J.* **2014**, *36*, 136–142.

18. Nielsen, S.D.; Amer, B.; Young, J.F.; Mortensen, G.; Petersen, R.K.; Kristiansen, K.; Dalsgaard, T.K. Medium chain fatty acids from milk induce angiopoietin-like 4 (ANGPTL4) gene expression. *Int. Dairy J.* **2015**, *42*, 34–41.

19. Mattijssen, F.; Alex, S.; Swarts, H.J.; Groen, A.K.; van Schothorst, E.M.; Kersten, S. Angptl4 serves as an endogenous inhibitor of intestinal lipid digestion. *Mol. Metable* **2014**, *3*, 135–144.

20. Luhovyy, B.L.; Akhavan, T.; Anderson, G.H. Whey proteins in the regulation of food intake and satiety. *J. Am. Coll. Nutr.* **2007**, *26*, 704S–712S.

21. Brehm, B.J.; Spang, S.E.; Lattin, B.L.; Seeley, R.J.; Daniels, S.R.; D'Alessio, D.A. The role of energy expenditure in the differential weight joss in obese women on low-fat and low-carbohydrate diets. *J. Clin. Endocrinol. Metable* **2005**, *90*, 1475–1482.

22. Morifuji, M.; Sakai, K.; Sanbongi, C.; Sugiura, K. Dietary whey protein down regulates fatty acid synthesis in the liver, but up regulates it in skeletal muscle of exercise-trained rats. *Nutrition* **2005**, *21*, 1052–1058.

23. St-Onge, M.P.; Farnworth, E.R.; Jones, P.J. Consumption of fermented and nonfermented dairy products: Effects on cholesterol concentrations and metabolism. *Am. J. Clin. Nutr.* **2000**, *71*, 674–681.

24. DiBaise, J.K.; Zhang, H.; Crowell, M.D.; Krajmalnik-Brown, R.; Decker, G.A.; Rittmann, B.E. Gut microbiota and its possible relationship with obesity. *Mayo Clin. Proc.* **2008**, *83*, 460–469.

25. Pittas, A.G.; Lau, J.; Hu, F.B.; Dawson-Hughes, B. The role of vitamin D and calcium in type 2 diabetes. A systematic review and meta-analysis. *J. Clin. Endocrinol. Metable* **2007**, *92*, 2017–2029.

26. Elwood, P.C.; Givens, D.I.; Beswick, A.D.; Fehily, A.M.; Pickering, J.E.; Gallacher, J. The survival advantage of milk and dairy consumption: An overview of evidence from cohort studies of vascular diseases, diabetes and cancer. *J. Am. Coll. Nutr.* **2008**, *27*, 723S–734S.

27. Tong, X.; Dong, J.Y.; Wu, Z.W.; Li, W.; Qin, L.Q. Dairy consumption and risk of type 2 diabetes mellitus: A meta-analysis of cohort studies. *Eur. J. Clin. Nutr.* **2011**, *65*, 1027–1031.

28. Aune, D.; Norat, T.; Romundstad, P.; Vatten, L.J. Dairy products and the risk of type 2 diabetes: A systematic review and dose-response meta-analysis of cohort studies. *Am. J. Clin. Nutr.* **2013**.

29. Gao, D.; Ning, N.; Wang, C.; Wang, Y.; Li, Q.; Meng, Z.; Liu, Y.; Li, Q. Dairy products consumption and risk of type 2 diabetes: Systematic review and dose-response meta-analysis. *PLoS ONE* **2013**, *8*, e73965.

30. Chen, M.; Sun, Q.; Giovannucci, E.; Mozaffarian, D.; Manson, J.E.; Willett, W.C.; Hu, F.B. Dairy consumption and risk of type 2 diabetes: 3 cohorts of US adults and an updated meta-analysis. *BMC Med.* **2014**, *12*, 215.

31. Turner, K.M.; Keogh, J.B.; Clifton, P.M. Dairy consumption and insulin sensitivity: A systematic review of short-and long-term intervention studies. *Nutr. Metab. Cardiovasc. Dis.* **2015**, *25*, 3–8.

32. Ma, B.; Lawson, A.B.; Liese, A.D.; Bell, R.A.; Mayer-Davis, E.J. Dairy, magnesium, and calcium intake in relation to insulin sensitivity: approaches to modeling a dose-dependent association. *Am. J. Epidemiol.* **2006**, *164*, 449–458.

33. Larsson, S.C.; Wolk, A. Magnesium intake and risk of type 2 diabetes: A meta-analysis. *J. Intern. Med.* **2007**, *262*, 208–214.

34. George, P.S.; Pearson, E.R.; Witham, M.D. Effect of vitamin D supplementation on glycaemic control and insulin resistance: A systematic review and meta-analysis. *Diabetic Med.* **2012**, *29*, e142–e150.

35. Jakubowicz, D.; Froy, O. Biochemical and metabolic mechanisms by which dietary whey protein may combat obesity and Type 2 diabetes. *J. Nutr. Biochem.* **2013**, *24*, 1–5.

36. Itoh, Y.; Kawamata, Y.; Harada, M.; Kobayashi, M.; Fujii, R.; Fukusumi, S.; Ogi, K.; Hosoya, M.; Tanaka, Y.; Uejima, H.; *et al.* Free fatty acids regulate insulin secretion from pancreatic β cells through GPR40. *Nature* **2003**, *422*, 173–176.

37. Mozaffarian, D.; de Oliveira Otto, M.C.; Lemaitre, R.N.; Fretts, A.M.; Hotamisligil, G.; Tsai, M.Y.; Siscovick, D.S.; Nettleton, J.A. *trans*-Palmitoleic acid, other dairy fat biomarkers, and incident diabetes: The Multi-Ethnic Study of Atherosclerosis (MESA). *Am. J. Clin. Nutr.* **2013**, *97*, 854–861.

38. Ralston, R.A.; Lee, J.H.; Truby, H.; Palermo, C.E.; Walker, K.Z. A systematic review and meta-analysis of elevated blood pressure and consumption of dairy foods. *J. Hum. Hypertens.* **2012**, *26*, 3–13.

39. Soedamah-Muthu, S.S.; Verberne, L.D.; Ding, E.L.; Engberink, M.F.; Geleijnse, J.M. Dairy consumption and incidence of hypertension a dose-response meta-analysis of prospective cohort studies. *Hypertension* **2012**, *60*, 1131–1137.

40. Dong, J.Y.; Szeto, I.M.Y.; Makinen, K.; Gao, Q.; Wang, J.; Qin, L.Q.; Zhao, Y. Effect of probiotic fermented milk on blood pressure: A meta-analysis of randomised controlled trials. *Br. J. Nutr.* **2013**, *110*, 1188–1194.

41. Neter, J.E.; Stam, B.E.; Kok, F.J.; Grobbee, D.E.; Geleijnse, J.M. Influence of weight reduction on blood pressure a meta-analysis of randomized controlled trials. *Hypertension* **2003**, *42*, 878–884.

42. Allender, P.S.; Cutler, J.A.; Follmann, D.; Cappuccio, F.P.; Pryer, J.; Elliott, P. Dietary calcium and blood pressure: A meta-analysis of randomized clinical trials. *Ann. Intern. Med.* **1996**, *124*, 825–831.

43. Bucher, H.C.; Cook, R.J.; Guyatt, G.H.; Lang, J.D.; Cook, D.J.; Hatala, R.; Hunt, D.L. Effects of dietary calcium supplementation on blood pressure: A meta-analysis of randomized controlled trials. *JAMA* **1996**, *275*, 1016–1022.

44. Mizushima, S.; Cappuccio, F.P.; Nichols, R.; Elliott, P. Dietary magnesium intake and blood pressure: A qualitative overview of the observational studies. *J. Hum. Hypertens.* **1998**, *12*, 447–453.

45. Griffith, L.E.; Guyatt, G.H.; Cook, R.J.; Bucher, H.C.; Cook, D.J. The influence of dietary and nondietary calcium supplementation on blood pressure: An updated metaanalysis of randomized controlled trials. *Am. J. Hypertens.* **1999**, *12*, 84–92.

46. Geleijnse, J.M.; Kok, F.J.; Grobbee, D.E. Blood pressure response to changes in sodium and potassium intake: A metaregression analysis of randomised trials. *J. Hum. Hypertens.* **2003**, *17*, 471–480.

47. Nakamura, T.; Mizutani, J.; Sasaki, K.; Yamamoto, N.; Takazawa, K. Beneficial potential of casein hydrolysate containing Val-Pro-Pro and Ile-Pro-Pro on central blood pressure and hemodynamic index: A preliminary study. *J. Med. Food* **2009**, *12*, 1221–1226.

48. Nakamura, T.; Mizutani, J.; Ohki, K.; Yamada, K.; Yamamoto, N.; Takeshi, M.; Takazawa, K. Casein hydrolysate containing Val-Pro-Pro and Ile-Pro-Pro improves central blood pressure and arterial stiffness in hypertensive subjects: A randomized, double-blind, placebo-controlled trial. *Atherosclerosis* **2011**, *219*, 298–303.

49. Ishida, Y.; Shibata, Y.; Fukuhara, I.; Yano, Y.; Takehara, I.; Kaneko, K. Effect of an excess intake of casein hydrolysate containing Val-Pro-Pro and Ile-Pro-Pro in subjects with normal blood pressure, high-normal blood pressure, or mild hypertension. *Biosci. Biotechnol. Biochem.* **2011**, *75*, 427–433.

50. Meisel, H.; Schlimme, E. Inhibitors of angiotensinconverting-enzyme derived from bovine casein (casokinins). In β-*Casomorphins and Related Peptides: Recent Developments*; Wiley-Blackwell: Weinheim, Germany, 1994.

51. Cadée, J.A.; Chang, C.Y.; Chen, C.W.; Huang, C.N.; Chen, S.L.; Wang, C.K. Bovine casein hydrolysate (C12 peptide) reduces blood pressure in prehypertensive subjects. *Am. J. Hypertens.* **2007**, *20*, 1–5.

52. Cicero, A.F.G.; Gerocarni, B.; Laghi, L.; Borghi, C. Blood pressure lowering effect of lactotripeptides assumed as functional foods: A meta-analysis of current available clinical trials. *J. Hum. Hypertens.* **2011**, *25*, 425–436.

53. FitzGerald, R.J.; Meisel, H. Lactokinins: Whey protein-derived ACE inhibitory peptides. *Food/Nahrung* **1999**, *43*, 165–167.

54. Maes, W.; van Camp, J.; Vermeirssen, V.; Hemeryck, M.; Ketelslegers, J.M.; Schrezenmeir, J.; Oostveldt, P.V.; Huyghebaert, A. Influence of the lactokinin Ala-Leu-Pro-Met-His-Ile-Arg (ALPMHIR) on the release of endothelin-1 by endothelial cells. *Reg. Peptides* **2004**, *118*, 105.

55. Alonso, A.; Nettleton, J.A.; Ix, J.H.; de Boer, I.H.; Folsom, A.R.; Bidulescu, A.; Kestenbaum, B.R.; Chambless, L.E.; Jacobs, D.R., Jr. Dietary phosphorus, blood pressure, and incidence of hypertension in the atherosclerosis risk in communities study and the multi-ethnic study of atherosclerosis. *Hypertension* **2010**, *55*, 776–784.

56. Aune, D.; Lau, R.; Chan, D.S.M.; Vieira, R.; Greenwood, D.C.; Kampman, E.; Norat, T. Dairy products and colorectal cancer risk: A systematic review and meta-analysis of cohort studies. *Ann. Oncol.* **2012**, *23*, 37–45.

57. Aune, D.; Navarro Rosenblatt, D.A.; Chan, D.S.; Vieira, A.R.; Vieira, R.; Greenwood, D.C.; Vatten, L.J.; Norat, T. Dairy products, calcium, and prostate cancer risk: A systematic review and meta-analysis of cohort studies. *Am. J. Clin. Nutr.* **2015**.

58. Dong, J.Y.; Zhang, L.; He, K.; Qin, L.Q. Dairy consumption and risk of breast cancer: A meta-analysis of prospective cohort studies. *Breast Cancer Res. Treat.* **2011**, *127*, 23–31.

59. Genkinger, J.M.; Wang, M.; Li, R.; Albanes, D.; Anderson, K.E.; Bernstein, L.; van den Brandt, P.A.; English, D.R.; Freudenheim, J.L.; Fuchs, C.S.; *et al.* Dairy products and pancreatic cancer risk: A pooled analysis of 14 cohort studies. *Ann. Oncol.* **2014**, *25*, 1106–1115.

60. Liu, J.; Tang, W.; Sang, L.; Dai, X.; Wei, D.; Luo, Y.; Zhang, J. Milk, yogurt, and lactose intake and ovarian cancer risk: A meta-analysis. *Nutr. Cancer* **2014**, *67*, 68–72.

61. Li, F.; An, S.L.; Zhou, Y.; Liang, Z.K.; Jiao, Z.J.; Jing, Y.M.; Wan, P.; Shi, X.J.; Tan, W.L. Milk and dairy consumption and risk of bladder cancer: A meta-analysis. *Urology* **2011**, *78*, 1298–1305.

62. Mao, Q.Q.; Dai, Y.; Lin, Y.W.; Qin, J.; Xie, L.P.; Zheng, X.Y. Milk consumption and bladder cancer risk: A meta-analysis of published epidemiological studies. *Nutr. Cancer* **2011**, *63*, 1263–1271.

63. Gallagher, E.J.; LeRoith, D. Minireview: IGF, insulin, and cancer. *Endocrinology* **2011**, *152*, 2546–2551.

64. Cohen, D.H.; LeRoith, D. Obesity, type 2 diabetes, and cancer: The insulin and IGF connection. *Endocr. Relat. Cancer* **2012**, *19*, F27–F45.

65. Qin, L.Q.; He, K.; Xu, J.Y. Milk consumption and circulating insulin-like growth factor-I level: A systematic literature review. *Int. J. Food Sci. Nutr.* **2009**, *60*, 330–340.

66. Peterlik, M.; Grant, W.B.; Cross, H.S. Calcium, vitamin D and cancer. *Anticancer Res.* **2009**, *29*, 3687–3698.

67. Parodi, P.W. A role for milk proteins and their peptides in cancer prevention. *Curr. Pharm. Des.* **2007**, *13*, 813–828.

68. Tsuda, H.; Sekine, K.; Ushida, Y.; Kuhara, T.; Takasuka, N.; Iigo, M.; Han, B.S.; Moore, M.A. Milk and dairy products in cancer prevention: Focus on bovine lactoferrin. *Mutation Res.* **2000**, *462*, 227–233.

69. Lee, K.W.; Lee, H.J.; Cho, H.Y.; Kim, Y.J. Role of the conjugated linoleic acid in the prevention of cancer. *Crit. Rev. Food Sci. Nutr.* **2005**, *45*, 135–144.

70. Lampe, J.W. Dairy products and cancer. *J. Am. Coll. Nutr.* **2011**, *30*, 464S–470S.

71. Hu, D.; Huang, J.; Wang, Y.; Zhang, D.; Qu, Y. Dairy foods and risk of stroke: A meta-analysis of prospective cohort studies. *Nutr. Metab. Cardiovasc. Dis.* **2014**, *24*, 460–469.

72. Strazzullo, P.; D'Elia, L.; Cairella, G.; Garbagnati, F.; Cappuccio, F.P.; Scalfi, L. Excess body weight and incidence of stroke meta-analysis of prospective studies with 2 million participants. *Stroke* **2010**, *41*, e418–e426.

73. Massey, L.K. Dairy food consumption, blood pressure and stroke. *J. Nutr.* **2001**, *131*, 1875–1878.

74. Caroli, A.; Poli, A.; Ricotta, D.; Banfi, G.; Cocchi, D. Invited review: Dairy intake and bone health: A viewpoint from the state of the art. *J. Dairy Sci.* **2011**, *94*, 5249–5262.

75. Rizzoli, R. Dairy products, yogurts, and bone health. *Am. J. Clin. Nutr.* **2014**, *99*, 1256S–1262S.

76. Hedrick, V.E.; Dietrich, A.M.; Estabrooks, P.A.; Savla, J.; Serrano, E.; Davy, B.M. Dietary biomarkers: Advances, limitations and future directions. *Nutr. J.* **2012**, *11*, 109.

77. Strimbu, K.; Tavel, J.A. What are biomarkers? *Curr. Opin. HIV/AIDS* **2010**, *5*, 463–466.

78. Wolk, A.; Vessby, B.; Ljung, H.; Barrefors, P. Evaluation of a biological marker of dairy fat intake. *Am. J. Clin. Nutr.* **1998**, *68*, 291–295.

79. Smedman, A.E.; Gustafsson, I.B.; Berglund, L.G.; Vessby, B.O. Pentadecanoic acid in serum as a marker for intake of milk fat: Relations between intake of milk fat and metabolic risk factors. *Am. J. Clin. Nutr.* **1999**, *69*, 22–29.

80. Wolk, A.; Furuheim, M.; Vessby, B. Fatty acid composition of adipose tissue and serum lipids are valid biological markers of dairy fat intake in men. *J. Nutr.* **2001**, *131*, 828–833.

81. Brevik, A.; Veierod, M.B.; Drevon, C.A.; Andersen, L.F. Evaluation of the odd fatty acids 15:0 and 17:0 in serum and adipose tissue as markers of intake of milk and dairy fat. *Eur. J. Clin. Nutr.* **2005**, *59*, 1417–1422.

82. Biong, A.S.; Berstad, P.; Pedersen, J.I. Biomarkers for intake of dairy fat and dairy products. *Eur. J. Lipid Sci. Technol.* **2006**, *108*, 827–834.

83. Sun, Q.; Ma, J.; Campos, H.; Hu, F.B. Plasma and erythrocyte biomarkers of dairy fat intake and risk of ischemic heart disease. *Am. J. Clin. Nutr.* **2007**, *86*, 929–937.

84. Warensjö, E.; Jansson, J.H.; Cederholm, T.; Boman, K.; Eliasson, M.; Hallmans, G.; Johansson, I.; Sjögren, P. Biomarkers of milk fat and the risk of myocardial infarction in men and women: A prospective, matched case-control study. *Am. J. Clin. Nutr.* **2010**, *92*, 194–202.

85. Aslibekyan, S.; Campos, H.; Baylin, A. Biomarkers of dairy intake and the risk of heart disease. *Nutr. Metab. Cardiovasc. Dis.* **2012**, *22*, 1039–1045.

86. de Oliveira Otto, M.C.; Nettleton, J.A.; Lemaitre, R.N.; M. Steffen, L.; Kromhout, D.; Rich, S.S.; Tsai, M.Y.; Jacobs, D.R.; Mozaffarian, D. Biomarkers of dairy fatty acids and risk of cardiovascular disease in the multi-ethnic study of atherosclerosis. *J. Am. Heart Assoc.* **2013**, *2*, e000092.

87. Santaren, I.D.; Watkins, S.M.; Liese, A.D.; Wagenknecht, L.E.; Rewers, M.J.; Haffner, S.M.; Lorenzo, C.; Hanley, A.J. Serum pentadecanoic acid (15:0), a short-term marker of dairy food intake, is inversely associated with incident type 2 diabetes and its underlying disorders. *Am. J. Clin. Nutr.* **2014**, *100*, 1532–1540.

88. Yakoob, M.Y.; Shi, P.; Hu, F.B.; Campos, H.; Rexrode, K.M.; Orav, E.J.; Willett, W.C.; Mozaffarian, D. Circulating biomarkers of dairy fat and risk of incident stroke in U.S. men and women in 2 large prospective cohorts. *Am. J. Clin. Nutr.* **2014**, *100*, 1437–1447.

89. Ratnayake, W.N. Concerns about the use of 15:0, 17:0, and *trans*-16:1n-7 as biomarkers of dairy fat intake in recent observational studies that suggest beneficial effects of dairy food on incidence of diabetes and stroke. *Am. J. Clin. Nutr.* **2015**, *101*, 1102–1103.

90. Lankinen, M.; Schwab, U. Biomarkers of dairy fat. *Am. J. Clin. Nutr.* **2015**, *101*, 1101–1102.

91. Tholstrup, T.; Høy, C.E.; Andersen, L.N.; Christensen, R.D.K.; Sandström, B. Does fat in milk, butter and cheese affect blood lipids and cholesterol differently? *J. Am. Coll. Nutr.* **2004**, *23*, 169–176.

92. Hjerpsted, J.; Leedo, E.; Tholstrup, T. Cheese intake in large amounts lowers LDL-cholesterol concentrations compared with butter intake of equal fat content. *Am. J. Clin. Nutr.* **2011**, *94*, 1479–1484.

93. Gibney, M.J.; Walsh, M.; Brennan, L.; Roche, H.M.; German, B.; van Ommen, B. Metabolomics in human nutrition: Opportunities and challenges. *Am. J. Clin. Nutr.* **2005**, *82*, 497–503.

94. Zheng, H.; Yde, C.C.; Arnberg, K.; Mølgaard, C.; Michaelsen, K.F.; Larnkjær, A.; Bertram, H.C. NMR-based metabolomic profiling of overweight adolescents: An elucidation of the effects of inter-/intraindividual differences, gender, and pubertal development. *BioMed. Res. Int.* **2014**.

95. PubMed. Available online: http://www.ncbi.nlm.nih.gov-pubmed (accessed on 7 May 2015).

96. EMBASE. Available online: http://www.embase.com (accessed on 7 May 2015).

97. SCOPUS. Available online: http://www.scopus.com (accessed on 7 May 2015).

98. Guertin, K.A.; Moore, S.C.; Sampson, J.N.; Huang, W.Y.; Xiao, Q.; Stolzenberg-Solomon, R.Z.; Sinha, R.; Cross, A.J. Metabolomics in nutritional epidemiology: Identifying metabolites associated with diet and quantifying their potential to uncover diet-disease relations in populations. *Am. J. Clin. Nutr.* **2014**.

99. Bertram, H.C.; Hoppe, C.; Petersen, B.O.; Duus, J.Ø.; Mølgaard, C.; Michaelsen, K.F. An NMR-based metabonomic investigation on effects of milk and meat protein diets given to 8-year-old boys. *Br. J. Nutr.* **2007**, *97*, 758–763.

100. Pedersen, S.M.; Nielsen, N.C.; Andersen, H.J.; Olsson, J.; Simrén, M.; Öhman, L.; Svensson, U.; Malmendal, A.; Bertram, H.C. The serum metabolite response to diet intervention with probiotic acidified milk in irritable bowel syndrome patients is indistinguishable from that of non-probiotic acidified milk by $^1$H NMR-based metabonomic analysis. *Nutrients* **2010**, *2*, 1141–1155.

101. Pedersen, S.M.M.; Nebel, C.; Nielsen, N.C.; Andersen, H.J.; Olsson, J.; Simrén, M.; Öhman, L.; Svensson, U.; Bertram, H.C.; Malmendal, A. A GC-MS-based metabonomic investigation of blood serum from irritable bowel syndrome patients undergoing intervention with acidified milk products. *Eur. Food Res. Technol.* **2011**, *233*, 1013–1021.

102. Zheng, H.; Yde, C.C.; Dalsgaard, T.K.; Arnberg, K.; Mølgaard, C.; Michaelsen, K.; Larnkjær, A.; Bertram, H.C. Nuclear magnetic resonance-based metabolomics reveals that dairy protein fractions affect urinary urea excretion differently in overweight adolescents. *Eur. Food Res. Technol.* **2015**, *240*, 489–497.

103. Piccolo, B.D.; Comerford, K.B.; Karakas, S.E.; Knotts, T.A.; Fiehn, O.; Adams, S.H. Whey protein supplementation does not alter plasma branched-chained amino acid profiles but results in unique metabolomics patterns in obese women enrolled in an 8-week weight loss trial. *J. Nutr.* **2015**, *145*, 691–700.

104. Zheng, H.; Lorenzen, J.K.; Astrup, A.; Larsen, L.H.; Yde, C.C.; Clausen, M.R.; Bertram, H.C.; Aarhus University, Aarslev, Denmark. Unpublished work. 2015.

105. Hjerpsted, J.; Ritz, C.; Schou, S.; Tholstrup, T.; Dragsted, L. Effect of cheese and butter intake on metabolites in urine using an untargeted metabolomics approach. *Metabolomics* **2014**, *10*, 1176–1185.

106. Zheng, H.; Yde, C.C.; Clausen, M.R.; Kristensen, M.; Lorenzen, J.; Astrup, A.; Bertram, H.C. Metabolomics investigation to shed light on cheese as a possible piece in the French paradox puzzle. *J. Agric. Food Chem.* **2015**, *63*, 2830–2839.

107. Yde, C.C.; Ditlev, D.B.; Reitelseder, S.; Bertram, H.C. Metabonomic response to milk proteins after a single bout of heavy resistance exercise elucidated by $^1$H nuclear magnetic resonance spectroscopy. *Metabolites* **2013**, *3*, 33–46.

108. Stanstrup, J.; Rasmussen, J.; Ritz, C.; Holmer-Jensen, J.; Hermansen, K.; Dragsted, L. Intakes of whey protein hydrolysate and whole whey proteins are discriminated by LC-MS metabolomics. *Metabolomics* **2014**, *10*, 719–736.

109. Stanstrup, J.; Schou, S.S.; Holmer-Jensen, J.; Hermansen, K.; Dragsted, L.O. Whey protein delays gastric emptying and suppresses plasma fatty acids and their metabolites compared to casein, gluten, and fish protein. *J. Proteome Res.* **2014**, *13*, 2396–2408.

# Section 3:
# Comparisons of Food Consumption Data and Statistical Methods

# Cross-Continental Comparison of National Food Consumption Survey Methods—A Narrative Review

Willem De Keyzer, Tatiana Bracke, Sarah A. McNaughton, Winsome Parnell, Alanna J. Moshfegh, Rosangela A. Pereira, Haeng-Shin Lee, Pieter van't Veer, Stefaan De Henauw and Inge Huybrechts

Abstract: Food consumption surveys are performed in many countries. Comparison of results from those surveys across nations is difficult because of differences in methodological approaches. While consensus about the preferred methodology associated with national food consumption surveys is increasing, no inventory of methodological aspects across continents is available. The aims of the present review are (1) to develop a framework of key methodological elements related to national food consumption surveys, (2) to create an inventory of these properties of surveys performed in the continents North-America, South-America, Asia and Australasia, and (3) to discuss and compare these methodological properties cross-continentally. A literature search was performed using a fixed set of search terms in different databases. The inventory was completed with all accessible information from all retrieved publications and corresponding authors were requested to provide additional information where missing. Surveys from ten individual countries, originating from four continents are listed in the inventory. The results are presented according to six major aspects of food consumption surveys. The most common dietary intake assessment method used in food consumption surveys worldwide is the 24-HDR (24 h dietary recall), occasionally administered repeatedly, mostly using interview software. Only three countries have incorporated their national food consumption surveys into continuous national health and nutrition examination surveys.

Reprinted from *Nutrients*. Cite as: De Keyzer, W.; Bracke, T.; McNaughton, S.A.; Parnell, W.; Moshfegh, A.J.; Pereira, R.A.; Lee, H.-S.; van't Veer, P.; De Henauw, S.; Huybrechts, I. Cross-Continental Comparison of National Food Consumption Survey Methods—A Narrative Review. *Nutrients* **2015**, *7*, 3587–3620.

## 1. Introduction

Food consumption surveys (FCS) are used to estimate intakes of foods and nutrients by a certain target population from a specified region. Usually, they are initiated by governmental organizations to (1) identify deficient or excessive intakes of nutrients, (2) assess accordance with food-based dietary guidelines, or (3) estimate food safety related risks (e.g., contaminant exposures), using national representative samples. However, in light of comparability of results cross-continentally, a thorough overview and comparison of methodological aspects associated with these surveys in each continent is requested and has therefore been initiated in this cross-continental comparison of national food consumption survey methods.

In Europe, efforts have been made to harmonize methodological aspects related to dietary intake assessment (DIA) in the context of national nutrition surveys. Briefly, in the European Food Consumption Survey Method project (EFCOSUM), it was agreed that two non-consecutive 24-HDR (24 h dietary recall), are the most suitable to get internationally comparable data on population means and distributions of actual intake [1]. In addition, the menu-driven standardized 24-HDR program EPIC-Soft (IARC, Lyon, France) was considered to be the most appropriate software for standardized data collection in a pan-European survey. Following the EFCOSUM project, in the European Food Consumption Validation (EFCOVAL) project, EPIC-Soft was upgraded and adapted, and the two non-consecutive 24-HDRs using EPIC-Soft were validated using urinary biomarkers [2]. The software was further evaluated for use in the European Union (EU) Menu project [3], a pan-European food consumption survey among EU member states led by EFSA via the feasibility studies EMP-PANEU (Food Consumption Data Collection Methodology for the EU Menu Survey) and PANCAKE (Pilot study for Assessment of Nutrient intake and food Consumption Among Kids in Europe) [4–6]. In 2014, an EFSA report was published aiming to identify and evaluate available European data collection protocols and tools for capturing food consumption information [7]. Previously, Huybrechts *et al.* reported on the experiences from European national or regional dietary monitoring surveys using the standardized EPIC-Soft program [8], making a further inventory on this standardized methodology used in Europe redundant and leading to the decision to exclude Europe from this cross-continental inventory.

Within the framework of the African Study on Physical Activity and Dietary Assessment Methods (AS-PADAM) project, an inventory questionnaire on the availability of dietary assessment methods was developed and results from eighteen African countries were presented [9]. In contrast to Europe, the inventory showed that for the African continent, high quality, validated and standardized tools are currently lacking, making it difficult to monitor the different phases and speed of the nutrition transition across its countries. Due to this in depth inventory published in the framework of the AS-PADAM project, it was decided to exclude Africa as well from this cross-continental inventory.

As mentioned before, in light of comparability of results cross-continentally, a thorough overview and comparison of methodological aspects associated with these surveys in each continent is requested. Therefore, the aims of the present paper are (1) to develop a framework of key parameters describing methodological aspects of FCS, (2) to create an inventory of methodological properties of national food consumption surveys performed on the continents North-America, South-America, Asia and Australasia, and the remaining continents for which such in depth inventory is still missing, and (3) to discuss and compare these methodological properties cross-continentally.

## 2. Experimental Section

### 2.1. Development of the Inventory Framework

First, key methodological properties of FCS were identified in order to construct a framework available for developing the inventory. This framework was based on the one used by Huybrechts and co-workers [8]. After author debate, it was decided to categorize the properties into six aspects of conducting an FCS: (1) target population, survey design and sampling, (2) dietary intake and other assessments, (3) recruitment of participants, (4) fieldwork characteristics, (5) data/nutrient analyses, and (6) recruitment and training of the interviewers. The framework was designed as a table listing FCS in the rows and property fields in the columns. In total, twenty-nine fields were created. The fields to be completed per survey are presented in Table 1.

**Table 1.** Overview of inventory framework.

| General items | Recruitment of participants | Recruitment and training of interviewers |
|---|---|---|
| Continent | Invitation type | Recruitment criteria interviewers |
| Country | Incentives | Number of interviewers |
| Survey | Number of participants ($n$) | Training material/Training topics |
| **Target population, survey design and sampling** | Participation rate (%) | Training duration |
| Sex | Problems in recruitment | |
| Age (years) | **Fieldwork characteristics and data controls** | |
| Sampling method and design | Place of DIA administration | |
| Sampling frame | Time-span fieldwork | |
| **Dietary intake and other assessments** | Intermediate controls | |
| Method | Final data controls | |
| Total recalls ($n$) | **Food linking and analysis** | |
| Administration | Food classification system | |
| Portion size estimation | Food composition databases | |
| Interview aids/software | Statistical procedures/ adjustment (software) | |
| Measured anthropometrics | Methods for calculating under- or overreporters | |
| Biological samples | | |

DIA: dietary intake assessment.

As proposed by Blanquer *et al.* [10], a combined strategy for data acquisition was used. Firstly, a systematic literature search was performed and subsequently, experts were contacted to complete missing information which could not be found in the literature. We used the electronic database MEDLINE (PubMed) and Web of Science to identify studies reporting on food consumption surveys from 1985 to December 2011. Text terms with appropriate truncations, Boolean operators and relevant indexing terms were used. The reference lists in the articles, reviews and textbooks retrieved were also investigated for additional publications yielding a substantial amount of grey literature like reports available on websites of governmental bodies. The key words used in the search were: "national nutrition survey"; "food and nutrition survey"; "dietary consumption survey"; "dietary intake"; "nutrition examination"; "nutrition survey"; and "dietary intake assessment". Additional terms referring to a country or continent were added to this search query for obtaining region-specific information. The selection of continents was based on the seven-continent model excluding Europe (pan-European methodology and inventory of experiences are reported elsewhere [7,8,11]), Africa (availability of dietary assessment tools in Africa have been reported previously by Gavrieli *et al.* [7]) and Antarctica (no permanent habitation).

The exclusion criteria that were used to withdraw retrieved surveys were: (1) age (nutrition surveys in children only were excluded given their age-specific approach in terms of dietary intake assessment); (2) indirect or ecological measurement of food intake (e.g., food balance sheets or household budget surveys); (3) absence of dietary intake assessment (e.g., nutritional assessment based on anthropometric or clinical measurements), and (4) publications or reports not available in English and/or not accessible online.

Once the table was completed based on the information available from the retrieved publications, it was e-mailed to principal investigators or corresponding authors of studies reporting on the food consumption survey with an accompanying request to fill in the blanks. This additional information was then merged with the tables and the inventory was distributed to all collaborators for final review.

## 3. Results

The first step of the search strategy yielded a total of 12,605 articles. From this, 4,511 articles met at least one of the exclusion criteria. In the remaining articles, single surveys from individual countries were identified. A total of ten countries from four continents were retained: North-America: Canada, United States (US), Mexico; South-America: Brazil; Asia: China, Japan, Korea (South), Malaysia; Australasia: Australia, New Zealand. In total, data from 28 FCS are presented in the overview.

## 3.1. Target Population, Survey Design and Sampling Method

Table 2 summarizes the study design aspects and methods of the selected surveys. The ages of the target populations ranged from less than 1 year of age to over 80 years. Surveys including all age categories were from Canada, US, Mexico (MHNS-06), China (1991 and onwards), Japan, Korea and Australia. In all surveys, both genders were included except for Mexico (NNS-1999) that included women only. In all surveys, a multistage sampling design was used to select study participants. The sampling frames used for selection of sampling units were based either on census data (US, Mexico, Brazil, Korea and New Zealand), a combination of frames like healthcare registries and labour force data (Canada), strata from counties (China), or enumeration blocks (geographical areas which are artificially created to have about 80 to 120 living quarters (Malaysia)). For Canada, the US, Mexico, China, Korea and Australia the national food consumption survey was also part of a health (examination) survey. The dietary monitoring surveys were cross-sectional, some of which have a continuing character since they are repeated annually or biennially (the US, China, Japan and Korea). For the US and China, participants are included in a cohort for tracking over time.

## 3.2. Numbers of Participants and Participation Rates

In Table 3, recruitment aspects of all selected surveys are listed. Sample sizes of single surveys ranged from 2,596 (Mexico; NNS-1999) to over 30,000 (Canada and Brazil). This latter figure was larger when taking into account the totals of all samples in the continuous programs in the US, China and Korea. Participation rates were above 90% in Korea (KNHANES 1998) and Malaysia; between 80.0%–89.9% in the US (NHANES 2001, 2005), Mexico (NNS-1999), Brazil, China and Korea; between 70.0%–79.9% in Canada, the US (NHANES 2003, 2007 and 2009), and Australia (for the FFQ); and below 70% in Japan, Australia (for the 24-HDR) and New Zealand.

211

**Table 2.** Target population, survey design and sampling method of national nutrition surveys per continent.

| Continent Country [Ref.] | Survey name | Institution | Year(s) | Sex | Age (years) | Sampling method and design | Sampling frame |
|---|---|---|---|---|---|---|---|
| North-America | | | | | | | |
| Canada [12,13] | Canadian Community Health Survey - Nutrition (CCHS) | Statistics Canada | 2004 | M and F | All age categories (<1–71+) | Two-step strategy: 1) 80 units in 14 age/sex groups per province 2) power allocation scheme for remaining anticipated units | 4 frames: Labour Force Survey (LFS) area frame, CCHS 2.1 dwellings, Prince Edward Island and Manitoba Healthcare registries |
| US [14,15] | What we Eat in America (WWEIA), National Health and Nutrition Examination Survey (Continuous NHANES) | National Center for Health Statistics (NCHS) from the Centers for Disease Control and Prevention (CDC) | 2001–2002 | M and F | All age categories (< 1–80+) | Stratified, multistage probability sample: Primary Sampling Units (PSUs) (counties) > segments within PSUs (blocks containing a cluster of households) > households within segments > one or more participants within households | PSU samples were selected from a frame of all U.S. counties, using the 2000 census data and associated estimates and projections |
| | | | 2003–2004 | " | " | " | " |
| | | | 2005–2006 | " | " | " | " |
| | | | 2007–2008 | " | " | " | " |
| | | | 2009–2010 | " | " | " | " |
| Mexico [16–20] | National Nutrition Survey 1999 (NNS-1999) | Instituto Nacional de Salud Pública (INSP) | 1998–1999 | Adolescents and adults: F Children: M and F | 12–49  <12 | Probabilistic, multistage, stratified cluster sample: basic geographical statistical area (BGSA) > household block > household | Census data (1995), stratification of BGSA by socioeconomic status index |

212

**Table 2.** *Cont.*

| Continent Country [Ref.] | Survey name | Institution | Year(s) | Sex | Age (years) | Sampling method and design | Sampling frame |
|---|---|---|---|---|---|---|---|
| | Encuesta Nacional de Salud y Nutrición 2006 (ENSANUT 2006), Mexican Health and Nutrition Survey 2006 (MHNS-06) | Instituto Nacional de Salud Pública (INSP) | 2005–2006 | Children: M and F Adults: M and F | <19 ≥19 | Multistage, stratified cluster sample | n/a |
| South-America | | | | | | | |
| *Brazil* [21] | Brazilian Individual Dietary Survey (IDS 2008-2009) | Instituto Brasileiro de Geografia e Estatística (IBGE) | 2008–2009 | M and F | ≥10 | Probabilistic two-stage complex cluster sampling: census tracts > households | Census data (2000), a subsample (25%) of households selected in the Household Budget Survey was randomly selected to participate in the IDS |
| Asia | | | | | | | |
| *China* [22,23] | China Health and Nutrition Survey (CHNS) | National Institute of Nutrition and Food Safety (NINFS) from the China Center for Disease Control and Prevention (CCDC) | 1989 | Children: M and F Adults: M and F | 1–6 20–45 | Multistage, random cluster sample: province > county > PSUs (n = 190) > household | Stratification of counties by income (low, middle, and high), four counties per province were selected, PSUs are urban neighborhoods, suburban neighborhoods, towns, and rural villages |
| | | | 1991 | M and F | All age categories | // | // |
| | | | 1993 | // | // | // | // |
| | | | 1997 | // | // | // | // |
| | | | 2000 | // | // | Multistage, random cluster sample: province > county > PSUs (n = 216) > household | // |
| | | | 2004 | // | // | // | // |
| | | | 2006 | // | // | // | // |
| | | | 2009 | // | // | // | // |

Table 2. Cont.

| Continent Country [Ref.] | Survey name | Institution | Year(s) | Sex | Age (years) | Sampling method and design | Sampling frame |
|---|---|---|---|---|---|---|---|
| Japan [24,25] | National Nutrition Survey in Japan (NNS-J) | National Institute of Health and Nutrition (NIHN) | 2004–2007 | M and F | ≥1–70+ | Stratified random sample:survey district units (n = 300) > households | n/a |
| Korea [26,27] | Korean National Health and Nutrition Examination Survey (KNHANES) | Korean Institute for Health and Social Affairs (KIHASA) and the Korea Health Industry Development Institute (KHIDI) | 1998 | M and F | ≥1 – 70+ | Stratified, multistage probability sample: PSUs (n = 600) > households | Census data, population register |
| | | " | 2001 | " | " | " | " |
| | | KIHASA, KHIDI and the Korean Centers for Disease Control and Prevention (KCDC) | 2005 | " | " | " | " |
| | | KCDC | 2007 | " | " | " | " |
| | | " | 2008 | " | " | " | " |
| | | " | 2009 | " | " | " | " |
| Malaysia [28,29] | Malaysian Adult Nutrition Survey (MANS) | Ministry of Health Malaysia (MOH-M) | 2004 | M and F | 18–59 | Stratified random sample with proportional allocation | Enumeration Blocks (EB) and Living Quarters (LQ) were sampled proportionate to population size |
| Australasia | | | | | | | |
| Australia [30–33] | National Nutrition Survey (NNS) | Australian Bureau of Statistics (ABS) and Commonwealth Department of Health and Family Services (HFS) | 1995 | M and F | ≥ 2 | Multistage, area-based sample | Householders in private dwellings in 8 states and territories; Area-based selection using census collector districts from the 1991 Population Census |

**Table 2.** *Cont.*

| Continent Country [Ref.] | Survey name | Institution | Year(s) | Sex | Age (years) | Sampling method and design | Sampling frame |
|---|---|---|---|---|---|---|---|
| *New Zealand* [34–36] | New Zealand National Nutrition Survey (NNS97) | New Zealand Ministry of Health (MOH-NZ) | 1996–1997 | M and F | ≥ 15 | Multistage, stratified sample: PSUs ($n = 18,000$) > households > participant | Area based, census data (1991) |
| | New Zealand Adult Nutrition Survey (NZANS) | // | 2008–2009 | // | // | Multistage, stratified, probability-proportional-to-size (PPS) sample | Area based, New Zealand census meshblocks (2006) |

M: male; F: female; //: ditto; n/a: not available

**Table 3.** Dietary intake and other assessments of national nutrition surveys per continent.

| Continent Country [Ref.] | Survey name | Year(s) | Dietary intake assessment | | | | | Interview aids/software | Measured anthropometrics | Biological samples |
|---|---|---|---|---|---|---|---|---|---|---|
| | | | Method | Total recalls (n) | Administration of method | Portion size estimation | | | | |
| **North-America** | | | | | | | | | | |
| *Canada* [12,13] | Canadian Community Health Survey - Nutrition (CCHS) | 2004 | 24-HDR (children: 6–11 years assisted by parents; <6 years reported by parents)/ FFQ (past year, fruit and vegetables only) | 1 (70% of sample) 2 (30% of sample) | Face-to-face (first interview) Telephone (recall)/ Paper-pencil | Food model booklet, volume measures (tablespoon, cup, etc.), weight measures (ounce, gram, etc.), dimensions (length, width, etc.), general measures (relative sizes, container units) Three-dimensional food models for first interview. | | CAI software, developed by Statistics Canada (adopted from AMPM, USDA) | Weight and height | n/a |
| *US* [14,15] | What we Eat in America (WWEIA), National Health and Nutrition Examination Survey (Continuous NHANES) | 2001–2002 | 24-HDR (children < 16 years proxy provided information)/ FFQ (past year, 124 items) | 1 | Face-to-face/ Paper-pencil | Three-dimensional food models for first interview. | | CAI software, developed by USDA: Automated Multiple-Pass Method (AMPM) | Body composition and bone density (Dual energy x-ray absorptiometry), body measurements. | For a complete list of laboratory components of NHANES 1999–2012 visit http://www.cdc.gov/nchs/nhanes/about_nhanes.htm. |
| | | 2003–2004 | " | 2 (3–10 day interval) | Face-to-face (first interview) Telephone (recall) | Three-dimensional food models for first interview. USDA's Food Model Booklet (two-dimensional drawings of glasses, mugs, bowls, mounds, circles, *etc.*) and three-dimensional models (measuring cups and spoons, a ruler, and two household spoons) for telephone interview. | | " | " | " |

**Table 3.** *Cont.*

| Continent Country [Ref.] | Survey name | Year(s) | Dietary intake assessment Method | Total recalls (n) | Administration of method | Portion size estimation | Interview aids/software | Measured anthropometrics | Biological samples |
|---|---|---|---|---|---|---|---|---|---|
| *Mexico* [16–20] | National Nutrition Survey 1999 (NNS-1999) | 2005–2006 | ″ | ″ | ″ | ″ | ″ | ″ | ″ |
| | | 2007–2008 | ″ | ″ | ″ | ″ | ″ | ″ | ″ |
| | | 2009–2010 | ″ | ″ | ″ | ″ | ″ | ″ | ″ |
| | | 1998–1999 | 24-HDR | 1 | n/a | n/a | n/a | Weight and height (in women, waist and hip circumferences) | Capillary blood: concentration of hemoglobin Venous blood and urine: assessment of micronutrient status |
| | Encuesta Nacional de Salud y Nutrición 2006 (ENSANUT 2006), Mexican Health and Nutrition Survey 2006 (MHNS-06) | 2005–2006 | Semi-quantitative FFQ (past 7 days, 101 foods, 14 food groups) | | n/a | n/a | n/a | | |
| South-America *Brazil* [21] | Brazilian Individual Dietary Survey (IDS 2008-2009) | 2008–2009 | 2-day EDR (non-consecutive on pre-determined days spanning one week) | | Paper pencil, face-to-face interview to review food records | Picture book (pictures of plates, glasses, bottles and cutlery) | CAPI software | Weight and height | n/a |
| Asia *China* [22,23] | China Health and Nutrition Survey (CHNS) | 1989 | 24-HDR (children < 12 years proxy provided information) | 3 (consecutive on pre-determined days spanning one week) | Paper pencil, face-to-face interview | Food models and picture aids | n/a | Weight and height, head circumference, arm circumference, and waist-hip ratio | None |
| | | 1991 | ″ | ″ | ″ | ″ | ″ | ″ | ″ |
| | | 1993 | ″ | ″ | ″ | ″ | ″ | ″ | ″ |
| | | 1997 | ″ | ″ | ″ | ″ | ″ | ″ | ″ |
| | | 2000 | ″ | ″ | ″ | ″ | ″ | ″ | ″ |

217

Table 3. Cont.

| Continent Country [Ref.] | Survey name | Year(s) | Dietary intake assessment | | | | | | |
|---|---|---|---|---|---|---|---|---|---|
| | | | Method | Total recalls (n) | Administration of method | Portion size estimation | Interview aids/software | Measured anthropometrics | Biological samples |
| Japan [24,25] | National Nutrition Survey in Japan (NNS-J) | 2004 | " | " | " | " | " | " | " |
| | | 2006 | " | " | " | " | " | " | " |
| | | 2009 | " | " | " | " | " | " | Blood collection |
| | | 2004–2007 | 1- or 3-day semi-weighed DR/ FFQ (≥20 years/ past 2 months, 122 foods and composite dishes) | | Paper pencil, face-to-face interview to review food records/ Paper-pencil | Kitchen scale | n/a | Weight and height (subjects aged 1 year or older), abdominal circumference (subjects aged 6 year or older) | Blood collection (subjects aged 20 years or older) |
| Korea [26,27] | Korean National Health and Nutrition Examination Survey (KNHANES) | 1998 | 24-HDR (in 200 PSUs)/ FFQ (past year, 109 food items) | 1 | Face-to-face/ Paper-pencil | Three-dimensional food models and a picture book with color photographs of foods | n/a | Weight and height | Blood and urine collection |
| | | 2001 | " | " | " | " | n/a | " | " |
| | | 2005 | " | " | " | " | n/a | " | " |
| | | 2007 | " | " | " | " | n/a | " | " |
| | | 2008 | " | " | " | " | n/a | " | " |
| | | 2009 | " | " | " | " | n/a | " | " |
| Malaysia [28,29] | Malaysian Adult Nutrition Survey (MANS) | 2004 | 24-HDR/ FFQ (past year, 126 foods, 15 food groups) | 1 | Face-to-face/ Paper-pencil | Album of food pictures and household measures | Nutritionist Pro™ Nutrition Analysis Software (for data entry) | Weight and height | n/a |
| Australasia Australia [30–33] | National Nutrition Survey (NNS) | 1995 | 24-HDR (children: 2-4 years reported by adult; 5-11 yrs assisted by adult)/ FFQ (≥ 12 years/ past year, 107 foods) | 1 (90% of sample)2 (10% of sample) | Face-to-face/ Paper-pencil | Measuring cups and spoons, grids and ruler | Food instruction booklet with types of foods and quantities of 15 food groups | Weight and height, waist and hip circumference | n/a |

**Table 3.** *Cont.*

| Continent Country [Ref.] | Survey name | Year(s) | Dietary intake assessment | | | | Measured anthropometrics | Biological samples |
|---|---|---|---|---|---|---|---|---|
| | | | Method | Total recalls (*n*) | Administration of method | Portion size estimation | Interview aids/software | | |

| Continent Country [Ref.] | Survey name | Year(s) | Method | Total recalls (*n*) | Administration of method | Portion size estimation | Interview aids/software | Measured anthropometrics | Biological samples |
|---|---|---|---|---|---|---|---|---|---|
| *New Zealand [34–36]* | New Zealand National Nutrition Survey (NNS97) | 1996–1997 | 24-HDR/ FFQ (past year, 9 food categories) | 1 2 (*n* = 695) | Face-to-face/ Paper-pencil | Cups, spoons, thickness sticks (thickness of meat, fish, poultry and cheese), photographs, grids and concentric circles, balls (to estimate apples and oranges), beans bags (to describe mashed potato and rice), standard serving sizes of foods and weights | CAPI software, LINZ24© (analogous to AMPM, USDA) | Weight and height, circumference of waist, hip and arm, waist-hip ratio, triceps and subscapular skinfold thickness, elbow breadth | Non-fasting blood sample: cellular evaluation, blood lipids, iron |
| | New Zealand Adult Nutrition Survey (NZANS) | 2008–2009 | 24-HDR/ dietary habits questionnaire | 1 (75% of sample) 2 (25% of sample) | Face-to-face/ Paper-pencil | Food photographs, shape dimensions, food portion assessment aids (e.g. dried beans) and packaging information | " | Weight and height, waist circumference | Non-fasting blood sample: cellular evaluation, blood lipids, iron, HbA1c Spot urine sample: sodium, potassium, iodine, creatinine |

*"*: ditto; n/a: not available; EDR: Estimated dietary record; CAI: computer assisted interview; CAPI: computer assisted personal interview; AMPM: Automated Multiple-Pass Method.

### 3.3. Dietary Intake Assessment Methods

Most surveys used 24-HDR as the principal DIA method (Table 4). Multiple recalls for all participants were available in the US (2 recalls in NHANES 2003 and onwards) and China (3 recalls). In some countries, duplicate recalls were available in a subsample only (Canada, Korea, Australia and New Zealand). A computer-assisted personal interview (CAPI) was performed in the US (NHANES 2001), Malaysia and New Zealand. In Canada and the US (NHANES 2003 and onwards), a CAPI was performed during the first recall and a computer assisted telephone interview (CATI) during the second recall. In the surveys from China and Australia, the 24-HDR was performed with paper and pencil in a face-to-face interview. In Korea, a face-to-face interview was performed, no interview software was reported, and in Mexico, the administration of the 24-HDR was also not reported in the study report. A prospective DIA method was only used in Brazil and Japan (2-day EDR and 1- or 3-day semi-weighed DR respectively). Finally, Mexico (MHNS-06) used only a semi-quantitative FFQ to report on frequencies of intake during the past seven days. An FFQ (formerly called Food Propensity Questionnaire) was also used in addition to a principal DIA method to identify frequencies of consumption and non-consumers of various food groups in Canada, the US, Japan, Korea, Malaysia, Australia and New Zealand (NNS97).

### 3.4. Fieldwork Characteristics and Data Controls

In Table 5, the fieldwork aspects of the nutrition surveys are presented. All surveys reported that at least one interview was conducted when the participant was at home. For surveys with multiple interviews, at least one was conducted at home. Interviews could either be a face-to-face or a telephone interview. In cases where the DIA was a dietary record, interviews were performed to review the participant's records and to check for completeness (Brazil and Japan). Another place for administrating the DIA was at mobile examination centres (MEC) (the US, NHANES). The time-span of the fieldwork was at least one year (all seasons) in Canada, the US, Brazil, Korea (KNHANES 2008 and onwards), Malaysia, Australia and New Zealand.

**Table 4.** Recruitment of the participants in national nutrition surveys per continent.

| Continent Country [Ref.] | Survey name | Year(s) | Invitation type | Incentives | Number of participants (n) | Participation rate (%) | Problems in recruitment/ recruitment notes |
|---|---|---|---|---|---|---|---|
| **North-America** | | | | | | | |
| Canada [12,13] | Canadian Community Health Survey-Nutrition (CCHS) | 2004 | Invitation letter and telephone invitation | None | 35.107 | 76.5 | Difficulties in approaching target population, participation was experienced as burdensome |
| US [14,15] | What we Eat in America (WWEIA), National Health and Nutrition Examination Survey (Continuous NHANES) | 2001–2002 | Invitation letter, personal visit at home | Participants receive remuneration as well as reimbursement for transportation and child/elder care expenses | 11.039 | 84.0 | NHANES is designed to sample larger numbers of certain subgroups of particular public health interest. Oversampling is done to increase the reliability and precision of estimates of health status indicators for these population subgroups. |
| | | 2003–2004 | ″ | ″ | 10.122 | 79.0 | ″ |
| | | 2005–2006 | ″ | ″ | 10.348 | 80.5 | ″ |
| | | 2007–2008 | ″ | ″ | 10.149 | 78.4 | ″ |
| | | 2009–2010 | ″ | ″ | 10.537 | 79.4 | ″ |
| Mexico [16–20] | National Nutrition Survey 1999 (NNS-1999) | 1998–1999 | n/a | n/a | Adolescent F: 416 Adult F: 2,596 | 82.4 | n/a |
| | Encuesta Nacional de Salud y Nutrición 2006 (ENSANUT 2006), Mexican Health and Nutrition Survey 2006 (MHNS-06) | 2005–2006 | n/a | n/a | Adolescents: 7,464 Adults: 21,113 | n/a | n/a |

**Table 4.** *Cont.*

| Continent Country [Ref.] | Survey name | Year(s) | Invitation type | Incentives | Number of participants (n) | Participation rate (%) | Problems in recruitment/ recruitment notes |
|---|---|---|---|---|---|---|---|
| **South-America** | | | | | | | |
| *Brazil* [21] | Brazilian Individual Dietary Survey (IDS 2008-2009) | 2008–2009 | Personal visit at home | None | 34.032 | 81.0 | The burden of participating in a survey was reported as a recruitment problem |
| **Asia** | | | | | | | |
| *China* [22,23] | China Health and Nutrition Survey (CHNS) | 1989 | Personal visit at home | n/a | 15.927 | n/a | Participants leaving in one survey and moving back in a later year, migration of participants, natural disasters and major redevelopment of housing in all large urban centres |
| | | 1991 | ʺ | ʺ | 14.789 | 88.1 | ʺ |
| | | 1993 | ʺ | ʺ | 13.893 | 88.2 | ʺ |
| | | 1997 | ʺ | ʺ | 15.874 | 80.9 | ʺ |
| | | 2000 | ʺ | ʺ | 17.054 | 83.0 | ʺ |
| | | 2004 | ʺ | ʺ | 16.129 | 80.2 | ʺ |
| | | 2006 | ʺ | ʺ | 18.764 | 88.0 | ʺ |
| | | 2009 | ʺ | ʺ | n/a | n/a | ʺ |
| *Japan* [24,25] | National Nutrition Survey in Japan (NNS-J) | 2004–2007 | n/a | n/a | 8,762 (2004) 8,885 (2007) | ≈60.0 (a) | n/a |
| *Korea* [26,27] | Korean National Health and Nutrition Examination Survey (KNHANES) | 1998 | Invitation letter | Small present | 11.525 | 95.9 | n/a |
| | | 2001 | ʺ | ʺ | 10.051 | 81.0 | n/a |

Table 4. *Cont.*

| Continent<br>Country<br>[Ref.] | Survey name | Year(s) | Invitation type | Incentives | Number of participants (n) | Participation rate (%) | Problems in recruitment/ recruitment notes |
|---|---|---|---|---|---|---|---|
| | | 2005 | " | Small present and a letter with individual results from examination | 9.047 | 80.5 | The burden of participating in a survey and motivation of participants were reported as recruitment problems |
| | | 2007<br>2008<br>2009 | "<br>"<br>" | "<br>"<br>" | 4.099<br>8.641<br>9.397 | 80.6<br>82.0<br>82.2 | "<br>"<br>" |
| *Malaysia*<br>*[28,29]* | Malaysian Adult Nutrition Survey (MANS) | 2004 | n/a | n/a | 6.886 | 93.6 (24-HDR)<br>92.0 (FFQ) | n/a |
| Australasia<br>*Australia*<br>*[30–33]* | National Nutrition Survey (NNS) | 1995 | Invitation letter | None | 13.858 | 61.4 (24-HDR)<br>76.0 (FFQ) | n/a |
| *New Zealand*<br>*[34–36]* | New Zealand National Nutrition Survey (NNS97) | 1996–1997 | Telephone invitation and/or personal visit at home | Small present | 4.636 | 50.1 | Participants of the Health Survey were asked if they would further consent to the Nutrition Survey which badly affected the response rate since added respondent burden and time lapse between both surveys |
| | New Zealand Adult Nutrition Survey (NZANS) | 2008–2009 | Personal visit at home | Grocery voucher (if blood collected) and a letter with individual results from examination | 4.721 | 61.0 | " |

F: female; ": ditto; n/a: not available

**Table 5.** Fieldwork characteristics and data controls of national nutrition surveys per continent.

| Country [Ref.] | Survey name | Year(s) | Place of DIA administration | Time-span fieldwork | Intermediate controls | Final data controls |
|---|---|---|---|---|---|---|
| **North-America** | | | | | | |
| Canada [12,13] | Canadian Community Health Survey-Nutrition (CCHS) | 2004 | Participant's home | Jan 2004–Jan 2005 | Quality control at data entry, checking completeness and accuracy of collected data, regular meetings to review the progress of fieldwork and interviewers. | Identification of extreme values of nutrients and food groups. Calculation of misreporting (see Table 6). |
| US [14,15] | What we Eat in America (WWEIA), National Health and Nutrition Examination Survey (Continuous NHANES) | 2001–2002 | First interview: Mobile Examination Center (MEC) | Jan 2001–Dec 2002 | The CAPI software program has built-in data edit and consistency checks to reduce data entry errors. Interviewers were alerted the when unusual or potentially erroneous data values were recorded. | Interview records were reviewed by the NHANES field office staff for accuracy and completeness. A subset of the household interviews was verified by re-contacting the survey participants. Periodically, interviews were audio-taped and reviewed by NCHS and contractor staff. |
| | | 2003–2004 | First interview: MEC Second interview: participant's home | Jan 2003–Dec 2004 | " | " |
| | | 2005–2006 | " | Jan 2005–Dec 2006 | " | " |
| | | 2007–2008 | " | Jan 2007–Dec2008 | " | " |
| | | 2009–2010 | " | Jan 2009–Dec2010 | " | " |
| Mexico [16–20] | National Nutrition Survey 1999 (NNS-1999) | 1998–1999 | n/a | Oct 1998–Mar1999 | n/a | n/a |
| | Encuesta Nacional de Salud y Nutrición 2006 (ENSANUT 2006), Mexican Health and Nutrition Survey 2006 (MHNS-06) | 2005–2006 | n/a | Oct 2005–May 2006 | n/a | n/a |

**Table 5.** *Cont.*

| Country [Ref.] | Survey name | Year(s) | Place of DIA administration | Time-span fieldwork | Intermediate controls | Final data controls |
|---|---|---|---|---|---|---|
| South-America | | | | | | |
| Brazil [21] | Brazilian Individual Dietary Survey (IDS 2008–2009) | 2008–2009 | Participant's home | May 2008–May 2009 | Cross-check data, quality control during data entry, completeness and accuracy checks of collected data, regular meetings to review the progress of fieldwork and make adjustments as required | Calculation of misreporting (see Table 6). |
| Asia | | | | | | |
| China [22,23] | China Health and Nutrition Survey (CHNS) | 1989 | Participant's home | n/a | Internal controls on quality measures have been based on collecting measures of selected factors from multiple perspectives and then using these data to refine measurements. | Individual's average daily dietary intake, calculated from the household survey, was compared with dietary intake based on 24-h recall data. In case of discrepancies, households were revisited. |
| | | 1991 | " | " | " | " |
| | | 1993 | " | " | " | " |
| | | 1997 | " | " | " | " |
| | | 2000 | " | " | " | " |
| | | 2004 | " | " | " | " |
| | | 2006 | " | " | " | " |
| | | 2009 | " | " | " | " |
| Japan [24,25] | National Nutrition Survey in Japan (NNS-J) | 2004–2007 | Participant's home | n/a | Interview with participant to review food records and check for completeness | n/a |
| Korea [26,27] | Korean National Health and Nutrition Examination Survey (KNHANES) | 1998 | Participant's home | Nov 1998–Dec 1998 | Cross-check of data, participants were re-contacted to provide extra information when the data is incomplete or possibly wrong | Extreme values for some nutrients and food groups were calculated |
| | | 2001 | " | Nov 2001–Dec 2001 | " | " |
| | | 2005 | " | Apr 2005–May 2005 | " | " |
| | | 2007 | " | Jul 2007–Dec 2007 | " | " |

225

**Table 5.** *Cont.*

| Country [Ref.] | Survey name | Year(s) | Place of DIA administration | Time-span fieldwork | Intermediate controls | Final data controls |
|---|---|---|---|---|---|---|
| | | 2008 | ” | Jan 2008–Dec 2008 | ” | ” |
| | | 2009 | ” | Jan 2009–Dec 2009 | ” | ” |
| Malaysia [28,29] | Malaysian Adult Nutrition Survey (MANS) | 2004 | Participant's home | Oct 2002–Dec 2003 | Data entry clerks trained to identify, describe foods and recipes and performed quality control checks, interviewers reviewed the recall with the respondent to check for completeness and accuracy | Calculation of misreporting (see Table 6). |
| Australasia | | | | | | |
| Australia [30–33] | National Nutrition Survey (NNS) | 1995 | Participant's home | Feb 1995–Mar 1996 | Data was checked immediately after collection using standardised checklists. During data entry, all data was scrutinized and quality control checks for extreme quantities were built-in to the data entry computer system. | Extreme values for for energy, macro-nutrients and micro-nutrients by age and sex were checked. Calculation of misreporting (see Table 6). |
| New Zealand [34–36] | New Zealand National Nutrition Survey (NNS97) | 1996–1997 | Participant's home | Dec 1996–Nov 1997 | Interviewers sent diet recalls to project office within 24 hours of collection so the project office could check each recall for accuracy and completeness which enabled interviewers to go back to participants, and/or clarify data with project office | Extreme values for nutrient intakes were scrutinised after conversion of food to nutrients |
| | New Zealand Adult Nutrition Survey (NZANS) | 2008–2009 | Participant's home | Oct 2008–Oct 2009 | ” | ” |

*”*: ditto; n/a: not available

226

**Table 6.** Food linking and analysis of national nutrition surveys per continent.

| Continent Country [Ref.] | Survey name | Year(s) | Food classification system | Food composition databases | Statistical procedures/adjustment (software) | Methods for calculating under- or overreporting |
|---|---|---|---|---|---|---|
| **North-America** | | | | | | |
| Canada [12,13] | Canadian Community Health Survey—Nutrition (CCHS) | 2004 | Bureau of Nutritional Sciences (BNS) food groups, based on British and American food group systems | Nutrition Survey System (NSS) | Nusser method using SIDE (Iowa State University) | Equations by Black and Cole |
| US [14,15] | What we Eat in America (WWEIA), National Health and Nutrition Examination Survey (Continuous NHANES) | 2001–2002 | Food Surveys Research Group (FSRG) defined food groups | USDA Food and Nutrient Database (FNDDS), 1.0 | SUDAAN was used to adjust for survey design effects resulting from NHANES' complex, multistage, probability sampling | Calculation of EI:BMRest |
| | | 2003–2004 | " | USDA Food and Nutrient Database (FNDDS), 2.0 | Nusser method using C-SIDE (Iowa State University) | " |
| | | 2005–2006 | " | USDA Food and Nutrient Database (FNDDS), 3.0 | NCI method | " |
| | | 2007–2008 | " | USDA Food and Nutrient Database (FNDDS), 4.1 | " | " |
| | | 2009–2010 | " | USDA Food and Nutrient Database (FNDDS), 5.0 | " | " |
| Mexico [16–20] | National Nutrition Survey 1999 (NNS-1999) | 1998–1999 | n/a | USDA Nutrient database for standard reference, University of California Food composition database, Tabla de composición de alimentos para uso en América Latina (PAHO, INCAP), Tablas de composición de alimentos mexicanos del Instituto Nacional de Ciencias Médicas y Nutrición Salvador Zubirán, Tablas de valor nutritivo de los alimentos de mayor consumo en México, Food composition and nutrition tables (Souci, Fachmann & Kraut) | n/a | n/a |

227

**Table 6.** *Cont.*

| Continent Country [Ref.] | Survey name | Year(s) | Food classification system | Food composition databases | Statistical procedures/adjustment (software) | Methods for calculating under- or overreporting |
|---|---|---|---|---|---|---|
| | Encuesta Nacional de Salud y Nutrición 2006 (ENSANUT 2006), Mexican Health and Nutrition Survey 2006 (MHNS-06) | 2005–2006 | n/a | n/a | n/a | n/a |
| South-America | | | | | | |
| *Brazil* [21] | Brazilian Individual Dietary Survey (IDS 2008–2009) | 2008–2009 | National food classification system | Nutrition Coordination Center Nutrient Databank (Nutrition Data System for Research—NDSR, Minneapolis), Brazilian Food Composition Table (TACO) | NCI method | Calculation of EI:BMRest |
| Asia | | | | | | |
| *China* [22,23] | China Health and Nutrition Survey (CHNS) | 1989 | n/a | Food Composition Table for China (ed. 1991) | n/a | n/a |
| | | 1991 | ″ | ″ | ″ | ″ |
| | | 1993 | ″ | ″ | ″ | ″ |
| | | 1997 | ″ | ″ | ″ | ″ |
| | | 2000 | ″ | ″ | ″ | ″ |
| | | 2004 | ″ | Food Composition Table for China (ed. 2002) | ″ | ″ |
| | | 2006 | ″ | Food Composition Table for China (ed. 2004) | ″ | ″ |
| | | 2009 | ″ | ″ | ″ | ″ |
| *Japan* [24,25] | National Nutrition Survey in Japan (NNS-J) | 2004-2007 | n/a | Standard Tables of Food Composition in Japan | n/a | n/a |
| *Korea* [26,27] | Korean National Health and Nutrition Examination Survey (KNHANES) | 1998 | National food classification system | Food composition table from the National Rural Living Science Institute | Nusser method using C-SIDE (Iowa State University) | Not applied |
| | | 2001 | ″ | ″ | ″ | ″ |
| | | 2005 | ″ | ″ | ″ | ″ |
| | | 2007 | ″ | ″ | ″ | ″ |
| | | 2008 | ″ | ″ | ″ | ″ |
| | | 2009 | ″ | ″ | ″ | ″ |

228

Table 6. *Cont.*

| Continent Country [Ref.] | Survey name | Year(s) | Food classification system | Food composition databases | Statistical procedures/adjustment (software) | Methods for calculating under- or overreporting |
|---|---|---|---|---|---|---|
| *Malaysia* [28,29] | Malaysian Adult Nutrition Survey (MANS) | 2004 | n/a | USDA Food Database, Canadian Food Database, Mexico Food Database, Malaysian Food Composition Tables (all available in Nutritionist Pro), Singapore Food Composition Guide, ASEAN Food Composition Tables, and The China Food Composition Tables | n/a | Calculation of EI:BMRest |
| *Australasia* | | | | | | |
| *Australia* [30–33] | National Nutrition Survey (NNS) | 1995 | National food classification system developed by ANZFA | NNS nutrient composition database AUSNUT (1999) developed by the Australia New Zealand Food Authority (ANZFA). Food and beverage intake data were coded using the Australian Nutrition Survey System (ANSURS). | Adjustment for within-person variability using the equation put forward by the US National Academy of Science (NAS) Subcommittee on Criteria for Dietary Evaluation (1986) | Calculation of EI:BMRest |
| *New Zealand* [34–36] | New Zealand National Nutrition Survey (NNS97) | 1996–1997 | National food classification system | New Zealand Food Composition Database (NZFCD), FOODfiles electronic subset of data from the NZFCD, NUTTAB Food Composition Tables (Australia), McCance and Widdowson's Composition of Foods and other international data as required | Nusser method using C-SIDE (Iowa State University) | Not applied |
| | New Zealand Adult Nutrition Survey (NZANS) | 2008–2009 | *"* | *"* | *"* | *"* |

*"*: ditto; n/a: not available.

229

**Table 7.** Recruitment and training of the interviewers in national nutrition surveys per continent.

| Continent Country [Ref.] | Survey name | Year(s) | Recruitment criteria interviewers | Number of interviewers (n) | Training material/ Training topics | Training duration | Remarks |
|---|---|---|---|---|---|---|---|
| **North-America** | | | | | | | |
| *Canada* [12,13] | Canadian Community Health Survey - Nutrition (CCHS) | 2004 | Professional interviewers who work on a variety of surveys, full-time and part-time | 600 | Software training, interview training | 3, 5 days | |
| *US* [14,15] | What we Eat in America (WWEIA), National Health and Nutrition Examination Survey (Continuous NHANES) | 2001–2002 | High School diploma required/BA preferred | n/a | Intensive training course and supervised practice interviews, periodic and annual retraining sessions | 2 weeks | |
| | | 2003–2004 | ″ | ″ | ″ | ″ | |
| | | 2005–2006 | ″ | ″ | ″ | ″ | |
| | | 2007–2008 | ″ | ″ | ″ | ″ | |
| | | 2009–2010 | ″ | ″ | ″ | ″ | |
| *Mexico* [16–20] | Mexican Health and Nutrition Survey 2006 (MHNS-06) Encuesta Nacional de Salud y Nutrición 2006 (ENSANUT 2006), Mexican Health and Nutrition Survey 2006 (MHNS-06) | 2005–2006 | n/a | n/a | n/a | n/a | |
| | | 2005–2006 | n/a | n/a | n/a | n/a | |
| **South-America** | | | | | | | |
| *Brazil* [21] | Brazilian Individual Dietary Survey (IDS 2008-2009) | 2008–2009 | n/a | n/a | Software training, training on contacting participants, interview training, data-collection skills | 1 week | |

**Table 7.** *Cont.*

| Continent Country [Ref.] | Survey name | Year(s) | Recruitment criteria interviewers | Number of interviewers (*n*) | Training material/ Training topics | Training duration | Remarks |
|---|---|---|---|---|---|---|---|
| Asia | | | | | | | |
| *China* [22,23] | China Health and Nutrition Survey (CHNS) | 1989 | Trained nutritionists | 160 | Specific training in the collection of dietary data for field staff and office staff | 3 days | |
| | | 1991 | " | " | " | " | |
| | | 1993 | " | " | " | " | |
| | | 1997 | " | " | " | " | |
| | | 2000 | " | " | " | " | |
| | | 2004 | " | " | " | " | |
| | | 2006 | " | " | " | " | |
| | | 2009 | " | " | " | " | |
| *Japan* [24,25] | National Nutrition Survey in Japan (NNS-J) | 2004–2007 | Registered dietitians and dietitians for nutrition component of health survey | n/a | n/a | n/a | |
| *Korea* [26,27] | Korean National Health and Nutrition Examination Survey (KNHANES) | 1998 | Trained dietitians/nutritionists | 160 | Training on contacting participants, interview training, data-collection skills | 5 days | |
| | | 2001 | " | 100 | " | 3 days | |
| | | 2005 | " | 150 | " | 4 days | |
| | | 2007 | " | 10 | " | 11 days | A smaller number of well-trained dietitians were used after changing to the annual survey |
| | | 2008 | " | 12 | " | 10 days | |
| | | 2009 | " | 12 | " | 15 days | |

231

**Table 7.** *Cont.*

| Continent Country [Ref.] | Survey name | Year(s) | Recruitment criteria interviewers | Number of interviewers (*n*) | Training material/ Training topics | Training duration | Remarks |
|---|---|---|---|---|---|---|---|
| *Malaysia* [28,29] | Malaysian Adult Nutrition Survey (MANS) | 2004 | Nutritionists familiar with local food customs | n/a | Training on interviewing and probing skills, quantification of portion sizes of foods | n/a | |
| **Australasia** | | | | | | | |
| *Australia* [30–33] | National Nutrition Survey (NNS) | 1995 | Qualified dietitians and nutritionists | n/a | Intensive training and supervision of interviewers to reduce non-sampling errors | 2 weeks | |
| *New Zealand* [34–36] | New Zealand National Nutrition Survey (NNS97) | 1996–1997 | Trained interviewers familiar with local food customs passing an admission test | n/a (every interviewer was assisted by one assistant) | Software training, training on contacting participants, interview training, data-collection skills and training on the use of the survey tools. | Interviewer: 2 weeks Assistant: 2 days | Additional training was provided at the regional level every two months. Pacific interviewers and assistants were trained to survey non-English speaking Pacific and Asian immigrant groups. |
| | New Zealand Adult Nutrition Survey (NZANS) | 2008–2009 | ″ | 22 | ″ | 2 weeks | Additional training was provided at the regional level every three months. Pacific interviewers and assistants were trained to survey non-English speaking Pacific and Asian immigrant groups. |

### 3.5. Food Linking and Analysis

Table 6 summarizes features related to data analyses of the nutrition surveys. Surveys using multiple measures of intake are able to correct for within-person variability. Most surveys used the Nusser method (using Software for Intake Distribution Estimation SIDE or C-SIDE) developed at the Iowa State University (ISU) to calculate distributions of usual intake (Canada, US NHANES 2003, Brazil, Korea and New Zealand). For the US, from NHANES 2005 and onwards, the NCI method developed by the National Cancer Institute was used. Finally, in the Australian survey, an equation by the US National Academy of Science (NAS) was used to adjust for within-person variance [33]. Furthermore, misreporting of energy intake was assessed using either the Goldberg method [37] (EI:BMR$_{est}$) (the US, Brazil, Malaysia and Australia) or the equations by Black and Cole [38] (Canada). Two surveys indicated that no calculation of misreporting was performed (Korea and New Zealand).

### 3.6. Recruitment and Training of Field Staff

In Table 7, recruitment and training of the interviewers and field staff in the nutrition surveys are listed. In China, Japan, Korea, Malaysia and Australia, it was mandatory that the interviewers be nutritionists or dietitians. In other countries, interviews were performed by trained interviewers, who were familiar with local food customs (New Zealand), or professional interviewers working on a variety of surveys (Canada). For interviewers in the US, a high school diploma was considered to be the minimum education requirement, as this is necessary for government jobs. Training was provided on a variety of topics like interviewing (and probing) skills (Canada, the US, Brazil, China, Korea, Malaysia, Australia and New Zealand), training on contacting participants, and software training. The duration of these training sessions ranged from three days (China) to fifteen days (Korea, KNHANES 2009). The average duration of reported training programs for interviewers was around seven days.

### 4. Discussion

This review presents an inventory of methodological aspects related to the performance of national food consumption surveys in different continents for which an in depth inventory on the dietary intake assessment methods used was still missing. Inventories covering both standardized and non-standardized data collection protocols and tools for capturing food consumption information on the European and African continent have been published before [7–9]. The present inventory comprises a total of twenty-eight food consumption surveys performed in ten countries from four continents: North-America, South-America, Asia and

Australasia. In six countries (Canada, the US, Mexico, China, Korea and Australia), the FCS was part of a larger health examination survey from which three (the US, China and Korea) have been continuous programs. When surveys were not part of a larger health examination survey, the overview shows that questionnaires on health and physical activity were often still included.

The most common approach to assess dietary intake was the use of replicate 24-HDR in combination with an FFQ. In most countries, replicate 24-HDR interviews were administered to subsamples ranging from <10% to 30% of the total sample. For instance, in 2002, the Korean National Nutrition Survey by Season (KNNSS) was conducted and an additional 24-HDR was administered to a subsample of KNHANES over three subsequent seasons to offset seasonal variation in food intake [27]. Duplicate and triplicate 24-HDR were administered to all participants in the US and China respectively. A single 24-HDR without additional FFQ was used in Mexico (NNS-1999). In the more recent Mexican Health and Nutrition survey (MHNS-06), the 24-HDR was replaced by a semi-quantitative FFQ that was used to assess frequencies of consumption during the past seven days [17]. This FFQ included the 95% most consumed foods reported in the 24-HDR collected in the previous survey (MNS-99) [16]. Two countries used a dietary record to assess intakes (Brazil and Japan). However, a research group under the auspices of the Japanese Ministry of Health, Labour and Welfare suggested transferring the method currently in use from a semi-weighed dietary record combined with an FFQ to the 24-HDR making international comparisons possible [25]. Regardless of the DIA methods used, administration took place most often in the participants' homes, providing the major advantage for interviewers to verify food packages or household measures in their home if this could help them to obtain more detailed information. In a study performed by Huybrechts *et al.* [8], participants of the EFCOVAL project were asked to indicate their preferred location for a future 24-HDR interview. Forty-nine percent of the subjects would prefer the study centre (*versus* 22% at home and 10% at work) if the interview was face-to-face and 63% would prefer to be at home for a telephone interview (compared with 11% at work). The high number of subjects that preferred the study centre for face-to-face interview might be explained because the EFCOVAL protocol required a visit to the study centre to collect blood samples and to provide participants with material for 24 h urine collections.

A large variety of portion size estimation tools was used in the different surveys ranging from three-dimensional aids like food models, cups, spoons and thickness sticks to two-dimensional albums or booklets depicting either photographs of foods, plates and glasses, or drawings of glasses, mugs and bowls (United States Department of Agriculture (USDA) food model booklet). The USDA Food Model Booklet was also adapted to create the USDA Food Models for Estimating Portions available for nutrition educators, consumers, and researchers to use outside of the context of the fully computerized Automated Multiple-Pass Method (AMPM) [39]. The AMPM is a validated five-step computerized dietary recall instrument developed by USDA and used in the "What We Eat in America" survey, the dietary intake interview component of the U.S. National Health and Nutrition Examination Survey (NHANES) [40,41]. Computer Assisted Interview (CAI) software is frequently used in national nutrition surveys because it allows structured and standardized collection of dietary intake data. The present overview shows that several countries use USDA-based CAI software and food classification. The leading role of this department is not surprising given its long history that goes back to 1892 [42]. Like North America, Europe has standardized its CAI software for future pan-European food consumption surveys [43]. The EPIC-Soft program, originally developed for the EPIC Study by the International Agency for research on Cancer (IARC), has been validated [44,45] and adapted to fit the purpose of pan-European food consumption surveys [46]. Recently, a name change of EPIC-Soft to GloboDiet software was announced, since this better suits the current and anticipated use of the increasingly widespread application of the tool worldwide [47].

Given that individual quantitative dietary intake surveys are expensive and difficult to implement, the Food and Agriculture Organization (FAO) Dietary Diversity questionnaire has been developed as a simple proxy to measure access to food at the household level [48] and micronutrient adequacy in women's and children's diets at the individual level [49,50].

Recruitment criteria for interviewers in national nutrition surveys are different between Asia and North America. In all Asian countries presented in the overview and Australia, interviews were conducted by either qualified/registered dietitians or nutritionists. In Japan, no interview was performed since dietary records were used; however, dietitians were recruited for data entry. In Canada and the US, it was not mandatory that the interviewers be dietitians or nutritionists. Both surveys rely either on professional interviewers involved in a variety of surveys or survey staff with a given minimal educational qualification, complemented with specific software and interview training. The duration of the training provided to interviewers varied across all available surveys from 2 days to 15 days (median duration: 7.5 days).

The current overview is the first of its kind to present a wide range of methodological aspects associated with national food consumption surveys across multiple continents. Although substantial efforts have been made to undertake a comprehensive overview, it is inevitable that some surveys were not captured. The present review qualifies as a narrative review and not a systematic review for a number of reasons. During the past decades, editors of scientific journals adopted reporting guidelines for producing systematic reviews. This was initiated in the medical research area enabling evidence-based decision making and improved health care. With the advent of these guidelines, publications on randomized (clinical) trials and intervention studies adhere to these criteria for inclusion in future systematic reviews. First, the time window of the present review including studies from 1985 exceeds the initiation of reporting guidelines by a decade so at that time, such guidelines were not yet available. Second, both guidelines for reporting as protocols to perform systematic reviews are not well adopted to studies using observational designs. Just recently, efforts have been made to adapt existing guidelines like the STROBE checklist (STrengthening the Reporting of OBservational studies in Epidemiology) to fit nutritional epidemiology studies (STROBE-NUT, reference equator). Third, a major source for information on methodological aspects of food consumptions surveys like details on sampling, instruments and training of staff are reports, information on websites of public agencies, both qualified as grey literature, and personal communications. These sources of information are sometimes not indexed in scientific databases and are, therefore, difficult to obtain using reproducible search strategies. Therefore, narrative reviews can be criticized because of their limited reproducibility. However, for reasons mentioned before, the two-step approach using both available literature and expert consultation, was the best method available to create the comprehensive overview presented.

This overview shows that the methods used for dietary intake assessment in national nutrition surveys are relatively similar across continents. The most frequently used method is the 24-HDR, sometimes administered repeatedly to correct for within-person variability, and mostly using interview software. Nevertheless, caution is still warranted when comparing results from food surveys between countries because of differences in conversion factors used for calculating nutrients (e.g., energy, protein, *etc.*). A variety of errors are introduced because many national or regional food composition tables or databases contain incomplete, outdated and unreliable data, or, countries borrow data from publicly available databases and neighbouring countries when such tables or databases are unavailable or inadequate [51].

Notwithstanding the growing consensus about the use of the 24-HDR methodology in food consumption surveys, the assessment remains self-reported. The most accurate and precise method for measuring energy expenditure is the doubly labeled water (DLW) method [52]. In weight stable conditions, one can expect that energy intake equals energy expenditure; hence, DLW is used in studies examining the validity of energy intake assessment. Such validation studies have indicated that the prevalence of energy underreporting in self-reported methods was about 30% (range: 12%–67%), and the magnitude of underestimation of energy intake was roughly 15% (range: 7%–20%) [53–55]. These reporting errors vary between men and women and are generally higher among overweight and obese subjects [41].

## 5. Conclusions

The 24-HDR was the most frequently used method in national food consumption surveys worldwide. Although this method is probably the most optimal to monitor dietary intakes of free-living subjects in large samples, it also has limitations and requires in depth training of the interviewers. In addition, future research is still necessary to explore and develop innovative methods that help us to measure dietary intake of populations and subgroups. For national FCS, it is recommended to combine different DIA methods like replicate 24-HDR and FFQs. For purposes of comparability of surveys, standardized procedures for data collection are required and a detailed description of the methods used should be included when reporting results. The inventory used in this review can serve as a guide to check if all methodological aspects related to the performance of a FCS are stated in such reports.

**Acknowledgments:** The authors gratefully acknowledge the contributions of the Health Statistics Division of Statistics Canada, Simón Barquera, Barry Popkin, Chris Killick-Moran and Shufa Du. The work presented was part of the PhD dissertation of W.D.K., who was financially supported by the Research Fund of University College Ghent. S.A.M. is funded by an Australian Research Council Future Fellowship (FT100100581).

**Author Contributions:** W.D.K. and T.B. performed the search for literature. W.D.K. made the inventory and wrote the manuscript. I.H. and S.D.H. were involved in the conception of the review. All authors reviewed, commented on and approved the final version.

**Conflicts of Interest:** The authors declare no conflict of interest.

## References

1. Brussaard, J.H.; Lowik, M.R.; Steingrimsdottir, L.; Moller, A.; Kearney, J.; de Henauw, S.; Becker, W.; Group, E. A European food consumption survey method—Conclusions and recommendations. *Eur. J. Clin. Nutr.* **2002**, *56*, S89–S94.

2. de Boer, E.J.; Slimani, N.; van 't Veer, P.; Boeing, H.; Feinberg, M.; Leclercq, C.; Trolle, E.; Amiano, P.; Andersen, L.F.; Freisling, H.; *et al.* Rationale and methods of the European Food Consumption Validation (EFCOVAL) Project. *Eur. J. Clin. Nutr.* **2011**, *65* (Suppl. 1), S1–S4.

3. EFSA. *Declaration of the Advisory Forum on the Pan-European Food Consumption Survey*; EFSA: Seville, Spain, 2010.

4. European Food Safety Authority (EFSA). Guidance on the EU Menu methodology. *EFSA J.* **2014**, *12*, 77.

5. Ocke, M.; Brants, H.; Dofkova, M.; Freisling, H.; van Rossum, C.; Ruprich, J.; Slimani, N.; Temme, E.; Trolle, E.; Vandevijvere, S.; *et al.* Feasibility of dietary assessment methods, other tools and procedures for a pan-European food consumption survey among infants, toddlers and children. *Eur. J. Nutr.* **2014**.

6. Freisling, H.; Ocke, M.C.; Casagrande, C.; Nicolas, G.; Crispim, S.P.; Niekerk, M.; van der Laan, J.; de Boer, E.; Vandevijvere, S.; de Maeyer, M.; *et al.* Comparison of two food record-based dietary assessment methods for a pan-European food consumption survey among infants, toddlers, and children using data quality indicators. *Eur. J. Nutr.* **2015**, *54*, 437–445.

7. Gavrieli, A.; Naska, A.; Berry, R.; Roe, M.; Harvey, L.; Finglas, P.; Glibetic, M.; Gurinovic, M.; Trichopoulou, A. *Dietary Monitoring Tools for Risk Assessment*; EFSA supporting publication: Parma, Italy, 2014; p. 287.

8. Huybrechts, I.; Casagrande, C.; Nicolas, G.; Geelen, A.; Crispim, S.P.; de Keyzer, W.; Freisling, H.; de Henauw, S.; de Maeyer, M.; Krems, C.; *et al.* Inventory of experiences from national/regional dietary monitoring surveys using EPIC-Soft. *Eur. J. Clin. Nutr.* **2011**, *65*, S16–S28.

9. Pisa, P.T.; Landais, E.; Margetts, B.; Vorster, H.H.; Friedenreich, C.M.; Huybrechts, I.; Martin-Prevel, Y.; Branca, F.; Lee, W.T.; Leclercq, C.; *et al.* Inventory on the dietary assessment tools available and needed in Africa: A prerequisite for setting up a common methodological research infrastructure for nutritional surveillance, research and prevention of diet-related non-communicable diseases. *Crit. Rev. Food Sci. Nutr.* **2014**.

10. Blanquer, M.; Garcia-Alvarez, A.; Ribas-Barba, L.; Wijnhoven, T.M.; Tabacchi, G.; Gurinovic, M.; Serra-Majem, L. How to find information on national food and nutrient consumption surveys across Europe: systematic literature review and questionnaires to selected country experts are both good strategies. *Br. J. Nutr.* **2009**, *101*, S37–S50.

11. European Food Safety Authority. General principles for the collection of national food consumption data in the view of a pan-European dietary survey. *EFSA J.* **2009**, *7*, 51.

12. Statistics Canada. Canadian Community Health Survey-Nutrition (CCHS). Available online: http://www.statcan.gc.ca/cgi-bin/imdb/p2SV.pl?Function=getSurvey&SDDS=5049&lang=en&db=imdb&adm=8&dis=2 (accessed on 5 November 2012).

13. Health and Statistics Division Canada. *Inventory of Food Consumption Surveys—Request for Information*; Health and Statistics Division Canada: Ottawa, Canada, 2012.

14. USDA. What We Eat in America, NHANES. Available online: http://www.ars.usda.gov/Services/docs.htm?docid=13793 (accessed on 24 October 2012).

15. Centers for Disease Control and Prevention. National Health and Nutrition Examination Survey. Available online: http://www.cdc.gov/nchs/nhanes.htm (accessed on 13 October 2012).

16. Barquera, S.; Campirano, F.; Bonvecchio, A.; Hernandez-Barrera, L.; Rivera, J.A.; Popkin, B.M. Caloric beverage consumption patterns in Mexican children. *Nutr. J.* **2010**, *9*, 47.

17. Barquera, S.; Hernandez-Barrera, L.; Tolentino, M.L.; Espinosa, J.; Ng, S.W.; Rivera, J.A.; Popkin, B.M. Energy intake from beverages is increasing among Mexican adolescents and adults. *J. Nutr.* **2008**, *138*, 2454–2461.

18. Barquera, S.; Rivera, J.A.; Espinosa-Montero, J.; Safdie, M.; Campirano, F.; Monterrubio, E.A. Energy and nutrient consumption in Mexican women 12–49 years of age: Analysis of the National Nutrition Survey 1999. *Salud Pública Méx.* **2003**, *45*, 530–539.

19. Resano-Pérez, E.; Méndez-Ramírez, I.; Shamah-Levy, T.; Rivera, J.A.; Sepúlveda-Amor, J. Methods of the National Nutrition Survey, 1999. *Salud Pública Méx.* **2003**, *45*, 558–564.

20. Rivera, J.A.; Sepúlveda Amor, J. Conclusions from the Mexican National Nutrition Survey 1999: Translating results into nutrition policy. *Salud Pública de Méx.* **2003**, *45*, 565–575.

21. Pereira, R.A.; Duffey, K.J.; Sichieri, R.; Popkin, B.M. Sources of excessive saturated fat, *trans* fat and sugar consumption in Brazil: an analysis of the first Brazilian nationwide individual dietary survey. *Public Health Nutr.* **2014**, *17*, 113–121.

22. Popkin, B.M.; Du, S.; Zhai, F.; Zhang, B. Cohort Profile: The China Health and Nutrition Survey—Monitoring and understanding socio-economic and health change in China, 1989–2011. *Int. J. Epidemiol.* **2010**, *39*, 1435–1440.

23. Chinese Center for Disease Control and Prevention. China Health and Nutrition Survey. Available online: http://www.cpc.unc.edu/projects/china (accessed on 13 November 2012).

24. National Institute of Health and Nutrition Japan. Available online: http://www0.nih.go.jp/eiken/english/ (accessed on 15 October 2012).

25. Tokudome, S.; Nishi, N.; Tanaka, H. Towards a better National Health and Nutrition Survey in Japan. *Lancet* **2012**, *379*, E44.

26. Korea Health Industry Development Institute. *Inventory of Food Consumption Surveys—Request for Information*; Nutrition Management Service and Policy Team: Chungbuk, Korea, 2012.

27. Kim, D.W.; Shim, J.E.; Paik, H.Y.; Song, W.O.; Joung, H. Nutritional intake of Korean population before and after adjusting for within-individual variations: 2001 Korean National Health and Nutrition Survey Data. *Nutr. Res. Pract.* **2011**, *5*, 266–274.

28. Mirnalini, K.; Zalilah, M.; Safiah, M.; Tahir, A.; Siti Haslinda, M.; Siti Rohana, D.; Khairul Zarina, M.; Mohd Hasyami, S.; Normah, H. Energy and Nutrient Intakes: Findings from the Malaysian Adult Nutrition Survey (MANS). *Malays. J. Nutr.* **2008**, *14*, 1–24.

29. Norimah, A.; Safiah, M.; Jamal, K.; Siti Haslinda, M.; Zuhaida, H.; Rohida, S.; Fatimah, S.; Siti Norazlin, N.; Poh, B.; Kandiah, M.; *et al.* Food Consumption Patterns: Findings from the Malaysian Adult Nutrition Survey (MANS). *Malays. J. Nutr.* **2008**, *14*, 25–39.

30. Cook, T.; Rutishauser, I.; Seelig, M. *Comparable Data on Food and Nutrient Intake and Physical Measurements from the 1983, 1985 and 1995 National Nutrition Surveys*; 3057; National Food and Nutrition Monitoring and Surveillance Project—Commonwealth Department of Health and Aged Care: Canberra, Australia, 2001.

31. McLennan, W.; Podger, A. *National Nutrition Survey Selected Highlights Australia 1995*; Australian Bureau of Statistics Commonwealth Department of Health and Family Services: Canberra, Australia, 1997.

32. Rutishauser, I.H. *Getting It Right: How to Use the Data from the 1995 National Nutrition Survey*; Commonwealth Department of Health and Aged Care: Canberra, Australia, 2000.

33. Mackerras, D.; Rutishauser, I. 24-Hour national dietary survey data: How do we interpret them most effectively? *Public Health Nutr.* **2005**, *8*, 657–665.

34. Ministry of Health. Nutrition Survey (New-Zealand). Available online: http://www.health.govt.nz/nz-health-statistics/national-collections-and-surveys/surveys/current-recent-surveys/nutrition-survey (accessed on 12 October 2012).

35. Parnell, W.R.; Wilson, N.C.; Russell, D.G. Methodology of the 1997 New Zealand National Nutrition Survey. *N. Z. Med. J.* **2001**, *114*, 123–126.

36. Quigley, R.; Watts, C. *Food Comes First: Methodologies for the National Nutrition Survey of New Zealand*; Public Health Group: Wellington, New Zealand, 1997.

37. Goldberg, G.R.; Black, A.E.; Jebb, S.A.; Cole, T.J.; Murgatroyd, P.R.; Coward, W.A.; Prentice, A.M. Critical evaluation of energy intake data using fundamental principles of energy physiology: 1. Derivation of cut-off limits to identify under-recording. *Eur. J. Clin. Nutr.* **1991**, *45*, 569–581.

38. Black, A.E.; Cole, T.J. Biased over- or under-reporting is characteristic of individuals whether over time or by different assessment methods. *J. Am. Diet. Assoc.* **2001**, *101*, 70–80.

39. U.S. Department of Agriculture. *Using the USDA Food Models for Estimating Portions*; Agricultural Research Service, Beltsville Human Nutrition Research Center, Food Surveys Research Group: Beltsville, MD, USA, 2007.

40. Blanton, C.A.; Moshfegh, A.J.; Baer, D.J.; Kretsch, M.J. The USDA Automated Multiple-Pass Method accurately estimates group total energy and nutrient intake. *J. Nutr.* **2006**, *136*, 2594–2599.

41. Moshfegh, A.J.; Rhodes, D.G.; Baer, D.J.; Murayi, T.; Clemens, J.C.; Rumpler, W.V.; Paul, D.R.; Sebastian, R.S.; Kuczynski, K.J.; Ingwersen, L.A.; *et al.* The US Department of Agriculture Automated Multiple-Pass Method reduces bias in the collection of energy intakes. *Am. J. Clin. Nutr.* **2008**, *88*, 324–332.

42. Ahuja, J.K.; Moshfegh, A.J.; Holden, J.M.; Harris, E. USDA food and nutrient databases provide the infrastructure for food and nutrition research, policy, and practice. *J. Nutr.* **2013**, *143*, 241S–249S.

43. Ocke, M.C.; Slimani, N.; Brants, H.; Buurma-Rethans, E.; Casagrande, C.; Nicolas, G.; Dofkova, M.; le Donne, C.; Freisling, H.; Geelen, A.; *et al.* Potential and requirements for a standardized pan-European food consumption survey using the EPIC-Soft software. *Eur. J. Clin. Nutr.* **2011**, *65*, S48–S57.

44. Crispim, S.P.; de Vries, J.H.M.; Geelen, A.; Souverein, O.W.; Hulshof, P.J.M.; Lafay, L.; Rousseau, A.-S.; Lillegaard, I.T.L.; Andersen, L.F.; Huybrechts, I.; *et al.* Two non-consecutive 24 h recalls using EPIC-Soft software are sufficiently valid for comparing protein and potassium intake between five European centres—Results from the European Food Consumption Validation (EFCOVAL) study. *Br. J. Nutr.* **2011**, *105*, 447–458.

45. Crispim, S.P.; Geelen, A.; Souverein, O.W.; Hulshof, P.J.M.; Ruprich, J.; Dofkova, M.; Huybrechts, I.; De Keyzer, W.; Lillegaard, I.T.; Andersen, L.F.; *et al.* Biomarker-based evaluation of two 24-h recalls for comparing usual fish, fruit and vegetable intakes across European centers in the EFCOVAL Study. *Eur. J. Clin. Nutr.* **2011**, *65*, S38–S47.

46. Slimani, N.; Casagrande, C.; Nicolas, G.; Freisling, H.; Huybrechts, I.; Ocke, M.C.; Niekerk, E.M.; van Rossum, C.; Bellemans, M.; De Maeyer, M.; *et al.* The standardized computerized 24-h dietary recall method EPIC-Soft adapted for pan-European dietary monitoring. *Eur. J. Clin. Nutr.* **2011**, *65*, S5–S15.

47. IARC. *Formal Announcement of the Name Change from EPIC-Soft®to GloboDiet®Software*; Communications Group: Lyon, France, 2014.

48. Hoddinott, J.; Yisehac, Y. *Dietary Diversity as a Food Security Indicator. Food and Nutrition Technical Assistance Project (FANTA)*; Academy for Educational Development (AED): Washington, DC, USA, 2002.

49. Working Group on Infant and Young Child Feeding Indicators. *Developing and Validating Simple Indicators of Dietary Quality and Energy Intake of Infants and Young Children in Developing Countries: Summary of Findings from Analysis of 10 Data Sets. Food and Nutrition Technical Assistance (FANTA) Project*; Academy for Educational Development (AED): Washington, DC, USA, 2006.

50. Arimond, M.; Wiesmann, D.; Becquey, E.; Carriquiry, A.; Daniels, M.C.; Deitchler, M.; Fanou-Fogny, N.; Joseph, M.L.; Kennedy, G.; Martin-Prevel, Y.; *et al.* Simple food group diversity indicators predict micronutrient adequacy of women's diets in 5 diverse, resource-poor settings. *J. Nutr.* **2010**, *140*, 2059S–2069S.

51. FAO. Food Composition Challenges. Available online: http://www.fao.org/infoods/infoods/food-composition-challenges (accessed on 21 May 2013).

52. Schoeller, D.A. Validation of habitual energy intake. *Public Health Nutr.* **2002**, *5*, 883–888.

53. Poslusna, K.; Ruprich, J.; de Vries, J.H.; Jakubikova, M.; van't Veer, P. Misreporting of energy and micronutrient intake estimated by food records and 24 hour recalls, control and adjustment methods in practice. *Br. J. Nutr.* **2009**, *101*, S73–S85.

54. Hill, R.J.; Davies, P.S. The validity of self-reported energy intake as determined using the doubly labelled water technique. *Br. J. Nutr.* **2001**, *85*, 415–430.

55. Trabulsi, J.; Schoeller, D.A. Evaluation of dietary assessment instruments against doubly labeled water, a biomarker of habitual energy intake. *Am. J. Physiol. Endocrinol. Metab.* **2001**, *281*, E891–E899.

# Comparison of the ISU, NCI, MSM, and SPADE Methods for Estimating Usual Intake: A Simulation Study of Nutrients Consumed Daily

Greice H. C. Laureano, Vanessa B. L. Torman, Sandra P. Crispim, Arnold L. M. Dekkers and Suzi A. Camey

**Abstract:** Various methods are available for estimating usual dietary intake distributions. Hence, there is a need for simulation studies to compare them. The methods Iowa State University (ISU), National Cancer Institute (NCI), Multiple Source Method (MSM) and Statistical Program to Assess Dietary Exposure (SPADE) were previously compared in another study, but some results were inconclusive due to the small number of replications used in the simulation. Seeking to overcome this limitation, the present study used 1000 simulated samples for 12 different scenarios to compare the accuracy of estimates yielded by the aforementioned methods. The focus is on scenarios that exhibited the most uncertainty in the conclusions of the mentioned study above, *i.e.*, scenarios with small sample sizes, skewed intake distributions, and large ratios of the between- and within-person variances. Bias was used as a measure of accuracy. For scenarios with small sample sizes ($n = 150$), the ISU, MSM and SPADE methods generally achieved more accurate estimates than the NCI method, particularly for the 10th and 90th percentiles. The differences between methods became smaller with larger sample sizes ($n = 300$ and $n = 500$). With few exceptions, the methods were found to perform similarly.

Reprinted from *Nutrients*. Cite as: Laureano, G.H.C.; Torman, V.B.L.; Crispim, S.P.; Dekkers, A.L.M.; Camey, S.A. Comparison of the ISU, NCI, MSM, and SPADE Methods for Estimating Usual Intake: A Simulation Study of Nutrients Consumed Daily. *Nutrients* **2016**, *8*, 166.

## 1. Introduction

The assessment of usual dietary intake (*i.e.*, long-term average intake) is a topic of current interest in the field of nutrition, as many diseases are influenced or even caused by individual dietary habits [1]. In particular, the study of usual intake distributions can help us to identify population groups who are at risk of having an inadequate dietary intake, either for insufficient or excessive consumption. The methods that are currently applied for estimating usual intake distributions use data that assess dietary intake over at least two independent days for each subject. It bears stressing that there is no gold-standard method for dietary intake

242

assessment, although the most widely used include 24-h dietary recalls (24-HDRs), food frequency questionnaires (FFQs), and dietary records. However, when assessing the long-term average intake from short-term measurements, the data derived from such measurements require statistical modeling in order to take into account between-person and within-person variations. The main reason for using statistical modeling for estimating usual intake distributions is to handle skewed data and to distinguish and remove the day-to-day (short-term) variation (within-person variation) from the total variation.

Various statistical methodologies have been proposed for estimating usual intake distributions [2–21]. Although the same general approach is used, the methods may differ when it comes to details such as the numerical methods used, software implementation, or differences in underlying assumptions. In this regard, some questions are still unanswered in the literature: What is the accuracy and precision of such methods? How should they be compared with real or simulated data? Some efforts have been made in this direction [6,7,9,16,19,21–23].

Souverein *et al.* [22] compared the Iowa State University (ISU), the National Cancer Institute (NCI), the Multiple Source Method (MSM) and the Statistical Program to Assess Dietary Exposure (SPADE) methods by assessing the influence of sample size, ratio of the within- and between-person variances, and Box-Cox transformation parameter values on the quality of their estimates [24]. Souverein *et al.* [22] concluded that the various methods generated similar estimates for most scenarios, but estimates diverged and bias increased when the variance ratio increased above 4 and the sample size decreased below 500. However, this study used only 100 replicates per scenario and used three samples sizes, which can be considered somewhat extreme. In fact, an intermediate sample size (between 150 and 500) should be more interesting because results were consistent for sample sizes greater than 500. These limitations prevented solid conclusions from being drawn as to the quality of the methods tested in some scenarios and percentiles, particularly the 90th percentile.

Therefore, the present paper reports on a simulation study conducted using the same approach as Souverein *et al.* [22], comparing once again the ISU, NCI, MSM and SPADE methods for daily-consumed nutrient intakes. Our study was focused on those scenarios that exhibited the most uncertainty in the conclusions of Souverein *et al.* [22]. We used a greater number of replicates (1000), small to moderate sample sizes ($n = 150, 300 \text{ and } 500$), and diversified the values of the within- and between-person variances in the simulation, with large ratios of the between- and within-person variances.

## 2. Materials and Methods

The ISU method was proposed by the Iowa State University [6,7,18] and has two different implementations: one in SAS [25], which was used in this study, and a menu driven stand-alone version, which can be obtained from the authors upon request at the ISU-SIDE website [26]. To estimate the usual intake distribution for daily-consumed nutrients, the ISU method follows four steps:

1. The ratio of the shifted, power-transformed observed intakes is adjusted to take into account nuisance effects, such as day of the week and interview mode (telephone or in-person). Construct smoothed daily intakes by undoing the initial power transformation and shifting for the adjusted observations.
2. A grafted polynomial function is fit to the normal probability plot of the smoothed intakes using least-squares. The inverse of the fitted function is used to transform the smoothed intakes to normality.
3. Moment estimates of variance components are computed for the transformed intakes, and an estimate of the normal-scale usual intake distribution is obtained,
4. A grafted cubic and a 9-point approximation to use to transform the normal-scale usual intake distribution to original scale.

The NCI method, as its name implies, was proposed by the U.S. National Cancer Institute [10,11,15,16]. It has been implemented with SAS macros [25] and is available [27]. In this study, version 2.1 of the SAS macros was used. To estimate the usual intake distribution of daily-consumed nutrients, the NCI method follows four steps:

1. The observed intakes are transformed to improve normality by means of a one-parameter Box-Cox transformation, indicated by $\lambda$ in this paper.
2. A linear mixed effects model on the transformed intake data is fit to estimate the mean and the within- and between-person variances.
3. $k$ (value to be set) pseudo-person intakes from a normal distribution is simulated with mean equal to the estimated mean and variance equal to the between-person variance.
4. The simulated values by a 9-point approximation is back-transformed, which involves the estimated Box-Cox parameter and the within-person variation.

The MSM was proposed for use in Europe by a German team [17,28] within the European Food Consumption Validation (EFCOVAL) consortium and is available through an online interface [29]. To estimate the usual intake distribution for daily-consumed nutrients, the MSM method proposes five steps:

1. A linear regression model is applied to the data and the residuals are used for the shrinkage part of the MSM method.

2. The fitted model residuals are transformed to normality by means of a two-parameter Box-Cox transformation, with $\lambda$ restricted to $1/\lambda = 1, 2, 3 \ldots$.

3. The within- and between-person variances are estimated by means of the transformed residuals.

4. The back-transformation is defined by a closed formula, involving the estimated $\lambda$ and the within-person variance.

5. The distribution is estimated by the inverse regression model after the back-transformation to the original scale of the residuals.

The SPADE [19,21,22] method is implemented in R software [30] and is based on the AGEMODE [13] model, where intake estimates are modeled with age as a covariate. However, although SPADE considers the model as a function of age, this information can be omitted after minor adjustments to the software, which enables the comparison with the other methods. SPADE is freely available as an R-package called SPADE.RIVM [31]. To estimate the usual intake distribution for daily-consumed nutrients, the SPADE method follows four steps:

1. The observed intakes are transformed by means of a one-parameter Box-Cox transformation.

2. A linear mixed effects model on the transformed scale is used to estimate the mean and within-person and between-person variances.

3. The mean on the transformed scale is directly back-transformed by Gaussian Quadrature, using the total variance of the model and the Box-Cox transformation parameter $\lambda$.

4. The percentiles on the transformed scale correspond exactly with the percentiles on the original scale, and their back-transformation by Gaussian Quadrature involves the within-person variance and $\lambda$ [19]. The distribution is calculated directly in the back-transformation step.

*Simulations*

Data simulation was used for the intake of daily-consumed nutrients with a Box-Cox distribution. For this purpose, we defined the following parameters on the transformed scale: overall mean intake ($\mu$), between-person standard deviation ($\sigma_u$), within-person standard deviation ($\sigma_\varepsilon$), the ratio of within- and between-person variances $\left( r_{var} = \left( \sigma_\varepsilon^2 / \sigma_u^2 \right) \right)$, and the Box-Cox transformation parameter ($\lambda$).

Twelve scenarios were generated based on the simulation results of Souverein *et al.* [22]. We explored the scenarios that had the most uncertainty in the results of this study, including sample sizes of 150, 300 and 500 and $r_{var}$ values of 4 and 9. Because Souverein *et al.* [22] did not provide the values for the variances, we decided to use different combinations of variance values. Box 1 shows the chosen parameter values for each scenario.

245

**Box 1.** Simulation scenarios.

| Scenario | $n$ | Within-Person Variance $(\sigma_\varepsilon^2)$ | Between-Person Variance $(\sigma_u^2)$ | Variance Ratio $(r_{var})$ |
|----------|-----|------------------------|-------------------------|-------------------|
| I  | 150 |     | 0.25 | 4 |
| II |     |     | 0.11 | 9 |
| III | 300 | 1  | 0.25 | 4 |
| IV  |     |    | 0.11 | 9 |
| V   | 500 |    | 0.25 | 4 |
| VI  |     |    | 0.11 | 9 |
| VII  | 150 | 1.2 |     | 4 |
| VIII |     | 2.7 |     | 9 |
| IX | 300 | 1.2 | 0.3 | 4 |
| X  |     | 2.7 |     | 9 |
| XI  | 500 | 1.2 |     | 4 |
| XII |     | 2.7 |     | 9 |

Souverein *et al.* [21] discussed in their study that, although an $r_{var}$ equal or higher to 9 is rare, there are cases where this has been reported [1,32] for nutrients: zinc in women, vitamin B-12 in men, and vitamin A in women and men.

The simulated data for intake of daily-consumed nutrients were generated as follows:

First, we generated for each scenario $n$ individual means from a normal distribution with mean $\mu = 7.5$ and the between-person variance as described in Box 1. We then generated two daily intake observations per subject on the transformed scale, using a normal distribution with the individual mean intake generated in the previous step and the within-person variance as described in Box 1. Finally, we applied the Box-Cox back-transformation ($\lambda = 0.2$) to transform the two intakes back to the original scale. These definitions generated a mean intake on the original scale equal to 105.56 for scenarios I, III, and V, equal to 104.67 for scenarios II, IV, and VI, equal to 107.17 for scenarios VII, IX, and XI, and equal to 116.95 for scenarios VIII, X, and XII.

The software environments employed for simulation were R to generate data and run the SPADE method, SAS to run the ISU and NCI methods, and AutoHotkey [33] to automate the MSM method.

To compare estimates, we calculated mean bias B for each method,

$$B(\hat{\theta}) = \frac{\sum_{i=1}^{N}(\hat{\theta}_j - \theta)}{N} \tag{1}$$

relative (percent) bias RB,

$$RB(\hat{\theta}) = \left| \frac{B(\hat{\theta})}{\theta} \right| \times 100 \tag{2}$$

and mean squared error MSE,

$$MSE(\hat{\theta}) = \frac{\sum_{i=1}^{N} (\hat{\theta}_j - \theta)^2}{N} \tag{3}$$

where $\hat{\theta}_j$ is the estimated value of the parameter for the replicate $j$, $\theta$ is the true value of the parameter, and $N$ is the number of replicates in the simulation. Bonferroni confidence intervals for the mean bias with 95% confidence level were also calculated to compare the methods.

To calculate these measures, we calculated the true mean and percentiles through Gaussian quadrature (obtained with the *f.gauss.quad* function implemented in the R-library SPADE.RIVM). This function enables the calculation of the mean and percentiles on the original scale using the parameters $\mu$, the between- and within-person variances (all in transformed scale), and $\lambda$, if all the model assumptions are fulfilled [19].

The code for generating the data is provided as supplementary material to this article.

## 3. Results

In this study, the ISU, NCI and SPADE methods were not able to yield estimates for some simulated samples, per scenario. When the ISU and NCI methods estimated the between-person variance as zero, they were unable to complete the estimations. SPADE completed the estimations, but all percentiles were equal, indicating an estimated between-person variance equal to zero. When this happened with at least one of the methods, the sample was excluded from the analysis for all methods.

Figures 1–3 show boxplots of the biases in each scenario with sample sizes of 150, 300, and 500 respectively, confirming similar results between the methods. However, it is clear that all methods were less accurate for estimation of the 10th and 90th percentiles across all scenarios. As expected, accuracy was lower in scenarios with a smaller sample size ($n = 150$). It is interesting to note that, in the first six scenarios with between-person variance equal to one (the upper plots in Figures 1–3), the differences in the spread of the bias are much fewer than in the scenarios VII–XII (the lower plots in Figures 1–3).

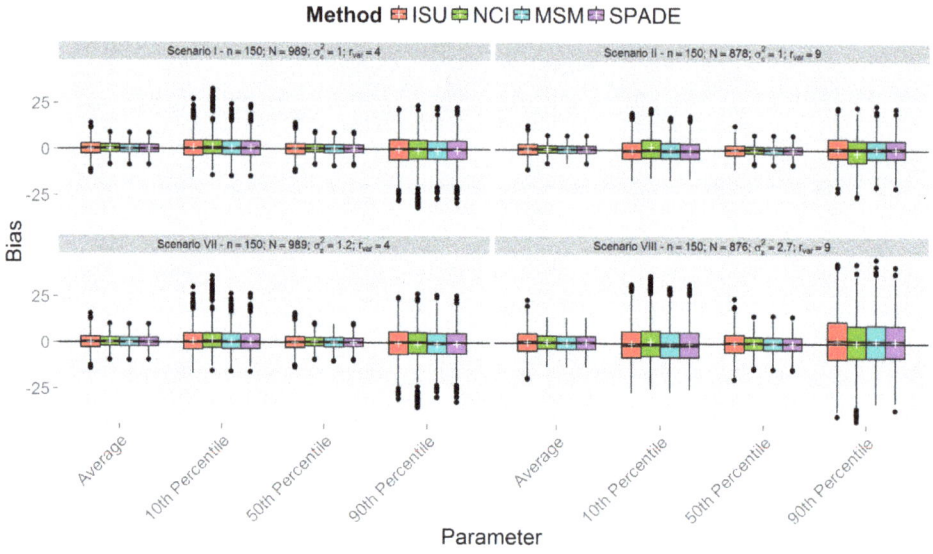

**Figure 1.** Boxplot of biases calculated for each method and scenarios with $n = 150$ for samples with estimated between-person variance different from zero for all methods (N denotes the number of usable samples).

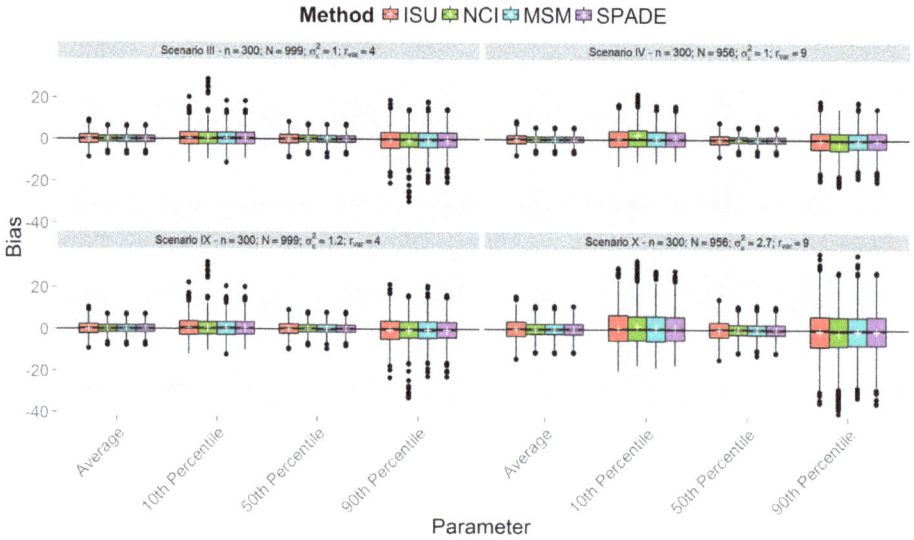

**Figure 2.** Boxplot of biases calculated for each method and scenarios with $n = 300$ for samples with estimated between-person variance different from zero for all methods (N denotes the number of usable samples).

Figures 1–3 show that the methods tend to overestimate the 10th percentile and to underestimate the 90th percentile, indicating a greater shrinkage of the data than expected. Figure 4 shows that the biases for the mean and the median are not statistically significant, except for the NCI method in scenario XII. There is a statistically significant overestimation of the 10th percentile in all methods except in scenarios II and VIII, whereas the 90th percentile is sometimes overestimated (scenarios II and VIII) and underestimated to a statistically significant degree by all methods in scenario VI. The NCI method showed a statistically significant larger bias than the ISU, SPADE, and MSM methods for the percentiles 10th and 90th in scenarios II, IV, and VI.

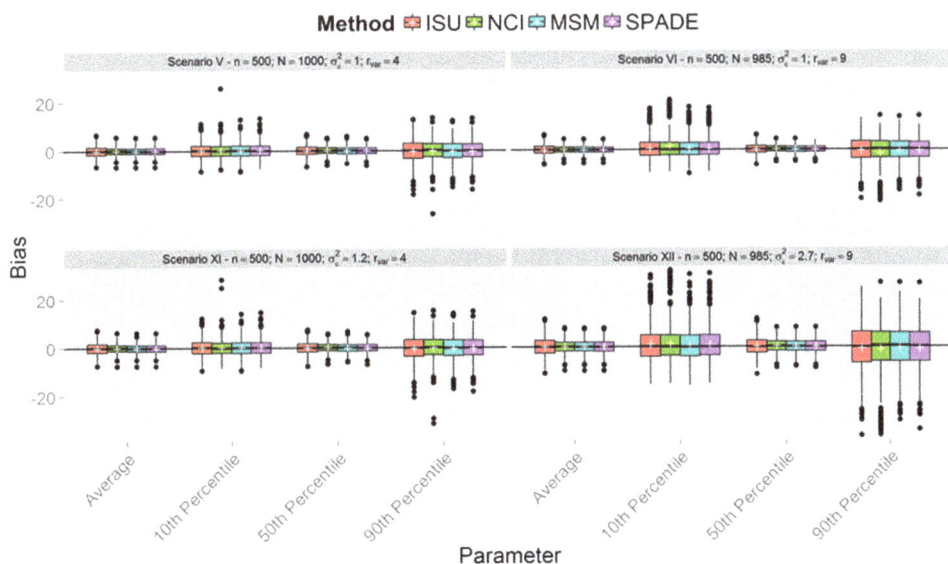

**Figure 3.** Boxplot of biases calculated for each method and scenarios with $n = 500$ for samples with estimated between-person variance different from zero for all methods (N denotes the number of usable samples).

More results are presented in the supplementary material, including: the number of simulated samples for which the between-person variance was estimated as zero; the bias and relative bias of estimates in the 5th, 10th, 25th, 50th, 75th, 90th, and 95th percentiles for each scenario; the Mean Square Error (MSE) of estimates for each scenario; the boxplot of biases calculated for each method with more percentiles; as well as two tables with the bias (relative bias) and the MSE for each method with all available results—without excluding samples when other methods estimated between-person variance equal to zero.

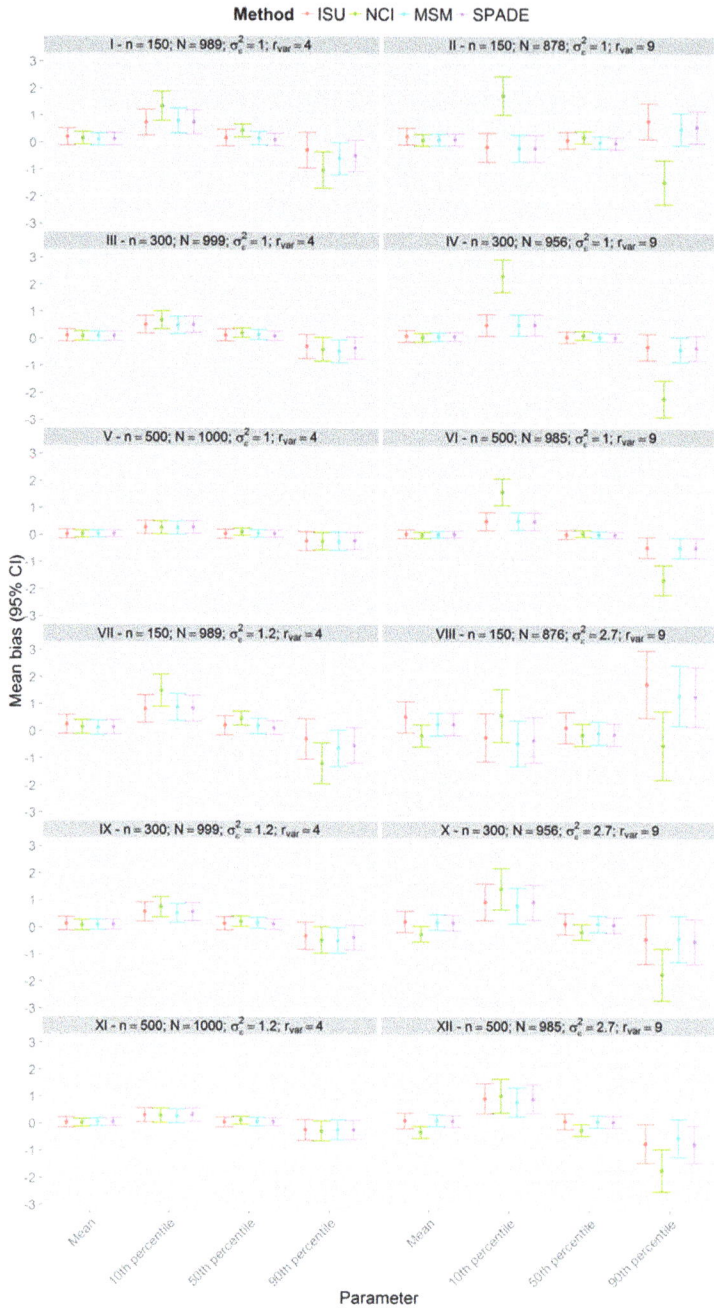

**Figure 4.** Bonferroni confidence interval for the mean bias with 95% confidence level for each scenario for samples with estimated between-person variance different from zero for all methods (n indicates the sample size and N the number of usable simulated samples).

## 4. Discussion

This paper reports the results of a simulation study that compared four methods employed for estimation of usual dietary intake distributions of daily-consumed nutrients, suggesting that, with a few exceptions, they performed similarly. The results obtained from the simulated scenarios showed that the bias of estimated mean and percentiles of all methods decreased when sample sizes increased and the ratio of variances was fixed. Furthermore, the ratio of variances had a small impact on the bias of the mean and median, although the variation in the bias increased for larger ratio of variances in the last six scenarios (compare in Figures 1–3 each lower plot, representing one of the last six scenarios, with the plot above). Other percentiles showed a larger bias for larger ratios. Indeed, the further the percentiles are from the median, the larger the biases.

Results also showed a poorer quality of estimation with all methods with respect to the 10th and 90th percentiles. Since one of the interests of estimating usual intake distributions in a population is to assess whether they have nutritional inadequacies in deficit or excess [34], a valid estimation of these percentiles is of the utmost importance and of concern.

In terms of accuracy, all four methods were similar with relatively low bias, but the behavior of the methods was different for the estimation of the mean usual intake and for the estimation of the percentiles. The methods use different numerical procedures to estimate the within- and between-person variances, which may cause numerical problems like an estimated between-person variance close to zero. These estimated values lead to unusable results such as unrealistically small differences between the estimated 10th and 90th percentiles. This happened for all methods, except the MSM.

In most of the scenarios, all methods seemed to shrink the intake distributions more than expected, resulting in overestimation of the low percentiles and underestimation of the high percentiles. For the NCI, when the sample size was small and the ratio was greater, the within-person variance seemed to be overestimated. This probably resulted in shrinkage greater than expected, which can be seen in the estimates of the percentiles. In fact, the NCI method showed only comparable results for scenarios V and XI, with $n = 500$ and $r_{var} = 4$.

The behavior of the MSM and SPADE methods was similar for almost all scenarios. ISU seemed to perform better for scenarios I and VII and worse for II and VIII compared to MSM and SPADE for higher percentiles. This may indicate that, for lower ratio values, the ISU method is better than MSM and SPADE for small sample sizes, but worse for small sample sizes ($n = 150$) and a higher ratio. These differences disappeared for simulations with $n = 300$ and $n = 500$.

It is noteworthy that the NCI method had larger or equal bias compared to the other methods for the estimate of the mean habitual intake in all scenarios. When the within-person variance is larger than the between-person variance, Tooze et al. [16] advise that the NCI method should use the same back-transformation used by the ISU method. In this paper, we used version 2.1 of the NCI with ISU back-transformation implemented (Bethesda, MD, USA); however, as was the case for Souverein et al. [22], the NCI method had the worst results in scenarios where the ratio-variance was equal to 9.

It bears stressing that this study did not address the influence of covariates or episodically consumed foods, as well as all possible combinations of sample sizes and parameters that could relate to existent daily consumed nutrients of different populations. For that, the results may differ as it depends on other aspects of the diet. However, further studies are needed to draw any conclusions on this matter.

In this study, a similar approach to the one reported by Souverein et al. [22] was proposed, but with a larger number of replications, a greater sample size, and some extra statistics for checking the results. As we used a larger number of replications, the results showed that unstable behavior of estimations not only happened because of the number of replications, but also depended on the sample size and the variance ratio.

## 5. Conclusions

In conclusion, this study showed the importance of the sample size and variance ratio for the quality of the estimation of usual intake distributions of daily consumed nutrients. It showed some limitations to the numerical solutions used in the various methods. Furthermore, the models almost behaved the same, as shown by Souverein et al. [22] and Dekkers et al. [19–21], but the NCI was less accurate for sample sizes of 150 and 300 than the other three methods. We agree with Souverein et al. [22] that people can choose their favorite method for practical reasons such as user-friendliness or assessment of the results for making plots, simulations, or a bootstrap. However, we also recommend that, in the case of small sample sizes and/or large within- and between-person variances, one should also use the SPADE or MSM methods to corroborate the results.

**Supplementary Materials:** The following are available online at http://www.mdpi.com/2072-6643/8/3/166/s1, Table S1: the number of simulated samples for which the between-person variance was estimated as zero; Table S2: Bias and relative bias of estimates obtained with each method for each scenario ($\lambda = 0.2$); Table S3: MSEs of estimates obtained with each method for each scenario ($\lambda = 0.2$) and Figure S1: Boxplot of biases calculated for each method and scenario, all results for the methods that had a positive estimate for the between-person variance. Table S4: Bias and relative bias of estimates obtained with each method for each scenario ($\lambda = 0.2$) and Table S5: MSEs of estimates obtained with each method for each scenario ($\lambda = 0.2$), both for each method without excluded samples when other methods estimated between-person variance equal to zero. All supplementary tables and figures had more percentile results than in the article (5th, 25th, 75th, and 95th).

**Author Contributions:** Greice H.C. Laureano, Vanessa B.L. Torman, Arnold L.M. Dekkers and Suzi A. Camey conceived and designed the simulation, analyzed the data and wrote the paper, Sandra P. Crispim wrote the paper.

**Conflicts of Interest:** The authors declare no conflict of interest.

## References

1.  Willett, W. *Nutritional Epidemiology, Monographs in Epidemiology and Biostatistics*, 3rd ed.; Oxford University Press: Oxford, UK; New York, NY, USA, 2013.
2.  Slob, W. Modeling long-term exposure of the whole population to chemicals in food. *Risk Anal. Off. Publ. Soc. Risk Anal.* **1993**, *13*, 525–530.
3.  Gay, C. Estimation of population distributions of habitual nutrient intake based on a short-run weighed food diary. *Br. J. Nutr.* **2000**, *83*, 287–293.
4.  Wallace, L.A.; Duan, N.; Ziegenfus, R. Can Long-Term Exposure Distributions Be Predicted from Short-Term Measurements? *Risk Anal.* **1994**, *14*, 75–85.
5.  Buck, R.J.; Hammerstrom, K.A.; Ryan, P.B. Estimating long-term exposures from short-term measurements. *J. Expo. Anal. Environ. Epidemiol.* **1995**, *5*, 359–373.
6.  Nusser, S.M.; Carriquiry, A.L.; Dodd, K.W.; Fuller, W.A. A Semiparametric Transformation Approach to Estimating Usual Daily Intake Distributions. *J. Am. Stat. Assoc.* **1996**, *91*, 1440–1449.
7.  Guenther, P.M.; Kott, P.S.; Carriquiry, A.L. Development of an approach for estimating usual nutrient intake distributions at the population level. *J. Nutr.* **1997**, *127*, 1106–1112.
8.  Chang, H.-Y.; Suchindran, C.M.; Pan, W.-H. Using the overdispersed exponential family to estimate the distribution of usual daily intakes of people aged between 18 and 28 in Taiwan. *Stat. Med.* **2001**, *20*, 2337–2350.
9.  Hoffmann, K.; Boeing, H.; Dufour, A.; Volatier, J.L.; Telman, J.; Virtanen, M.; Becker, W.; De Henauw, S.; EFCOSUM Group. Estimating the distribution of usual dietary intake by short-term measurements. *Eur. J. Clin. Nutr.* **2002**, *56* (Suppl. 2), S53–S62.
10. Tooze, J.A.; Grunwald, G.K.; Jones, R.H. Analysis of repeated measures data with clumping at zero. *Stat. Methods Med. Res.* **2002**, *11*, 341–355.
11. Tooze, J.A.; Midthune, D.; Dodd, K.W.; Freedman, L.S.; Krebs-Smith, S.M.; Subar, A.F.; Guenther, P.M.; Carroll, R.J.; Kipnis, V. A new statistical method for estimating the usual intake of episodically consumed foods with application to their distribution. *J. Am. Diet. Assoc.* **2006**, *106*, 1575–1587.
12. Slob, W. Probabilistic dietary exposure assessment taking into account variability in both amount and frequency of consumption. *Food Chem. Toxicol. Int. J. Publ. Br. Ind. Biol. Res. Assoc.* **2006**, *44*, 933–951.
13. Waijers, P.M.C.M.; Dekkers, A.L.M.; Boer, J.M.A.; Boshuizen, H.C.; van Rossum, C.T.M. The potential of AGE MODE, an age-dependent model, to estimate usual intakes and prevalences of inadequate intakes in a population. *J. Nutr.* **2006**, *136*, 2916–2920.
14. Staudenmayer, J.; Ruppert, D.; Buonaccorsi, J.P. Density Estimation in the Presence of Heteroscedastic Measurement Error. *J. Am. Stat. Assoc.* **2008**, *103*, 726–736.

15. Kipnis, V.; Midthune, D.; Buckman, D.W.; Dodd, K.W.; Guenther, P.M.; Krebs-Smith, S.M.; Subar, A.F.; Tooze, J.A.; Carroll, R.J.; Freedman, L.S. Modeling data with excess zeros and measurement error: application to evaluating relationships between episodically consumed foods and health outcomes. *Biometrics* **2009**, *65*, 1003–1010.

16. Tooze, J.A.; Kipnis, V.; Buckman, D.W.; Carroll, R.J.; Freedman, L.S.; Guenther, P.M.; Krebs-Smith, S.M.; Subar, A.F.; Dodd, K.W. A mixed-effects model approach for estimating the distribution of usual intake of nutrients: The NCI method. *Stat. Med.* **2010**, *29*, 2857–2868.

17. Haubrock, J.; Nöthlings, U.; Volatier, J.-L.; Dekkers, A.; Ocké, M.; Harttig, U.; Illner, A.-K.; Knüppel, S.; Andersen, L.F.; Boeing, H. European Food Consumption Validation Consortium Estimating usual food intake distributions by using the multiple source method in the EPIC-Potsdam Calibration Study. *J. Nutr.* **2011**, *141*, 914–920.

18. Nusser, S.M.; Fuller, W.A.; Guenther, P.M. Estimating Usual Dietary Intake Distributions: Adjusting for Measurement Error and Nonnormality in 24-Hour Food Intake Data. In *Survey Measurement and Process Quality*; Lyberg, L., Biemer, P., Collins, M., De Leeuw, E., Dippo, C., Schwarz, N., Trewin, D., Eds.; John Wiley & Sons, Inc.: Hoboken, NJ, USA, 2012; pp. 689–709.

19. Dekkers, A.L.M.; Slob, W. Gaussian Quadrature is an efficient method for the back-transformation in estimating the usual intake distribution when assessing dietary exposure. *Food Chem. Toxicol.* **2012**, *50*, 3853–3861.

20. Goedhart, P.W.; Voet, H.; Knüppel, S.; Dekkers, A.L.M.; Dodd, K.W.; Boeing, H.; Klaveren, J. *A Comparison by Simulation of Different Methods to Estimate the Usual Intake Distribution for Episodically Consumed Foods*; European Food Safety Authority: Parma, Italy, 2012.

21. Dekkers, A.L.; Verkaik-Kloosterman, J.; van Rossum, C.T.; Ocke, M.C. SPADE, a New Statistical Program to Estimate Habitual Dietary Intake from Multiple Food Sources and Dietary Supplements. *J. Nutr.* **2014**, *144*, 2083–2091.

22. Souverein, O.W.; Dekkers, A.L.; Geelen, A.; Haubrock, J.; de Vries, J.H.; Ocké, M.C.; Harttig, U.; Boeing, H.; van't Veer, P.; EFCOVAL Consortium. Comparing four methods to estimate usual intake distributions. *Eur. J. Clin. Nutr.* **2011**, *65* (Suppl. 1), S92–S101.

23. Freedman, L.S.; Midthune, D.; Carroll, R.J.; Krebs-Smith, S.; Subar, A.F.; Troiano, R.P.; Dodd, K.; Schatzkin, A.; Bingham, S.A.; Ferrari, P.; *et al.* Adjustments to improve the estimation of usual dietary intake distributions in the population. *J. Nutr.* **2004**, *134*, 1836–1843.

24. Box, G.E.P.; Cox, D.R. An Analysis of Transformations. *J. R. Stat. Soc. Ser. B Methodol.* **1964**, *26*, 211–252.

25. SAS|Business Analytics and Business Intelligence Software. Available online: http://www.sas.com/ (accessed on 9 March 2016).

26. Iowa State University. Available online: http://www.side.stat.iastate.edu/pc-side.php/ (accessed on 9 March 2016).

27. National Cancer Institute. Available online: http://www.riskfactor.cancer.gov/diet/ usualintakes/ (accessed on 9 March 2016).

28. Harttig, U.; Haubrock, J.; Knüppel, S.; Boeing, H. EFCOVAL Consortium the MSM program: Web-based statistics package for estimating usual dietary intake using the Multiple Source Method. *Eur. J. Clin. Nutr.* **2011**, *65* (Suppl. 1), S87–S91.

29. The Multiple Source Method (MSM). Available online: https://msm.dife.de (accessed on 9 March 2016).

30. R Core Team. *R: A Language and Environment for Statistical Computing*; R Foundation for Statistical Computing: Vienna, Austria, 2015.

31. National Institute for Public Health and the Environment. Available online: https://rivm.nl/en/Topics/SPADE (accessed on 9 March 2016).

32. McAvay, G.; Rodin, J. Interindividual and intraindividual variation in repeated measures of 24-hour dietary recall in the elderly. *Appetite* **1988**, *11*, 97–110.

33. AutoHotkey. Available online: http://www.autohotkey.com/ (accessed on 9 March 2016).

34. National Research Council (U.S.). *Nutrient Adequacy: Assessment Using Food Consumption Surveys*; National Academy Press: Washington, DC, USA, 1986.

# Section 4:
# Application of Dietary Assessment Methods to Enhance Our Understanding of Dietary Intakes among Populations

# Folate and Nutrients Involved in the 1-Carbon Cycle in the Pretreatment of Patients for Colorectal Cancer

Ariana Ferrari, Aline Martins de Carvalho, Josiane Steluti, Juliana Teixeira, Dirce Maria Lobo Marchioni and Samuel Aguiar Jr.

**Abstract:** To assess the ingestion of folate and nutrients involved in the 1-carbon cycle in non-treated patients with colorectal adenocarcinoma in a reference center for oncology in southeastern Brazil. In total, 195 new cases with colorectal adenocarcinoma completed a clinical evaluation questionnaire and a Food Frequency Questionnaire (FFQ). Blood samples from 161 patients were drawn for the assessment of serum folate. A moderate correlation was found between serum concentrations of folate, folate intake and the dietary folate equivalent (DFE) of synthetic supplements. Mulatto or black male patients with a primary educational level had a higher intake of dietary folate. Of patients obtaining folate from the diet alone or from dietary supplements, 11.00% and 0.10%, respectively, had intake below the recommended level. Of the patients using dietary supplements, 35% to 50% showed high levels of folic acid intake. There was a prevalence of inadequacy for vitamins B2, B6 and B12, ranging from 12.10% to 20.18%, while 13.76% to 22.55% of patients were likely to have adequate choline intake. The considerable percentage of patients with folate intake above the recommended levels deserves attention because of the harmful effects that this nutrient may have in the presence of established neoplastic lesions.

Reprinted from *Nutrients*. Cite as: Ferrari, A.; de Carvalho, A.M.; Steluti, J.; Teixeira, J.; Maria, D.; Marchioni, L.; Aguiar, S., Jr. Folate and Nutrients Involved in the 1-Carbon Cycle in the Pretreatment of Patients for Colorectal Cancer. *Nutrients* **2015**, *7*, 4318–4335.

## 1. Introduction

The incidence of colorectal cancer (CRC) is increasing in Brazil, especially in the major metropolitan regions of the Southeast, probably due to modifications in lifestyle habits [1]. The populations in emerging countries have complex patterns of nutritional status, with some areas acquiring the lifestyle and nutrition patterns of developed countries and others maintaining the nutritional characteristics associated with developing countries.

Epidemiological studies have shown the importance of folate in colorectal carcinogenesis due to its key role in the methylation and synthesis of nucleotides [2]. B-complex vitamins, such as vitamins B2, B6 and B12 [3], choline, and betaine [4] act as cofactors in the reactions of 1-carbon metabolism and are therefore essential for the metabolic processes involving folate.

Because folate intake has a controversial but important association with colorectal carcinogenesis, we investigated the pattern of folate intake and other associated nutrients in a cohort of CRC patients from a single institution in Southeast Brazil.

The objectives of this study were to assess the ingestion of folate and other nutrients involved in the 1-carbon cycle in untreated patients with colorectal adenocarcinoma at an oncology referral center in southeastern Brazil and to identify clinical variables that are associated with folate serum levels and intake.

## 2. Methodology

### 2.1. Study Design

This was an observational, cross-sectional study with prospective data collection of new cases of patients diagnosed with adenocarcinoma of the colon and rectum at the Colorectal Tumor Center of A.C. Camargo Cancer Center from May 2011 to May 2012. The inclusion criteria included patients with adenocarcinoma of the colon or rectum, at any stage of the disease and with an indication for surgical intervention at the primary site, or patients with adenomatous lesions and an indication for surgical intervention. Patients who had previously undergone surgery, radiotherapy and/or chemotherapy for colorectal tumor; patients with colon or rectal tumor recurrence; patients previously treated with chemotherapy for another malignancy in the last 3 months; or patients who, during the interview, did not present clinical conditions and/or an understanding when completing the questionnaires were excluded.

### 2.2. Clinical Evaluation Questionnaire

The questionnaire consisted of sociodemographic (sex, age, race, and educational level) and clinical (tumor site, clinicopathological staging) questions. In total, 195 patients were evaluated. The system used for clinicopathological staging was based on the Cancer Staging Manual published by the American Joint Committee on Cancer (AJCC) [5].

### 2.3. Dietary Assessment

A dietary assessment was conducted for alcohol, folate, vitamin B2, vitamin B6, vitamin B12, choline, betaine, methionine, energy, carbohydrate, protein and lipid using a validated Food Frequency Questionnaire (FFQ) by LAMEZA (2010) [6]. Of the 195 patients who participated in the study, 189 were included based on their dietary intake, with 169 patients obtaining folate from their diet alone and 20 patients using supplements containing folic acid. The values obtained from the FFQ were converted to energy and nutrient intake values through the software *Nutrition Data System for Research-NDSR* [7] and were considered unadjusted habitual food intake values (the raw data). Dietary synthetic folate values were corrected according to a mandatory fortification of wheat flour and corn (150 µg of folic acid $(100 \text{ g})^{-1}$ of flour) that has been implemented in Brazil since 2004 [8]. In addition, corrections were made for the differences in the additive amount of folic acid in fortified foods (150 µg $(100 \text{ g})^{-1}$ of flour in Brazil and 140 µg $(100 \text{ g})^{-1}$ of flour in the United States). After these corrections, and taking into account the differences in the bioavailability of folate found naturally in food and folic acid in fortified foods (1 µg synthetic folate = 1.70 µg folate) [9], DFE was calculated. In addition to the DFE values from diet, the values of folic acid intake through supplementation (synthetic folate supplement) were evaluated. In this case, the patients were asked whether they consumed multivitamins. If yes, the value of folic acid was calculated for each supplement. Only the amount of folic acid in the supplements was considered. From this value, we calculated the DFE for the supplements, assuming that every 1 µg of folic acid supplement on an empty stomach provides 2.0 µg of DFE [10]. The overall DFE was calculated from the sum of DFE from the diet and DFE from supplements. In total, 20 patients used supplements with folic acid. After calculating the unadjusted values, the data were calibrated. For calibration, we used three 24-h dietary recalls and a second FFQ collected in a previous study [6]. The R24 data were used as a reference and subjected to linear regression, with β1 values used as a calibration factor for the FFQ data collected. To assess the prevalence of folate inadequacy, patients were divided into two groups. The first group was composed of patients who ingested this nutrient from diet alone ($n$ = 169), and the second group consisted of patients who ingested folate through diet and supplementation ($n$ = 20). For patients who ingested folate from diet alone, an Estimated Average Requirement (EAR) cutoff value of 20 µg day$^{-1}$ and a Tolerable Upper Intake Levels (UL) of 1000 µg day$^{-1}$ were used, according to equations proposed by FISBERG *et al.* (2005) [11]. Patients on a diet with folic acid supplementation ($n$ = 20) were treated individually. In this case, we assessed whether there were any patients with food intake below the RDA cutoff point of 400 µg day$^{-1}$. For intake above the UL, a qualitative interpretation was performed and the percentage of patients above or below the UL was calculated [12]. For all patients, the prevalence of inadequate intake and the unadjusted and calibrated values for vitamin B2, vitamin B6 and vitamin B12 were also based on the EAR cutoff value [10]. There are no EAR recommendations for choline, therefore all values were considered [13].

## 2.4. Determination of Serum Folate

After 4 h of fasting, 10-mL blood samples were drawn from the patients by preoperative venipuncture. For patient candidates who were eligible for neoadjuvant treatment, samples were drawn from peripheral blood before radiochemotherapy. As previously described by Pufulete *et al.* [14], the competitive enzyme immunoassay technique was used for the analysis of the serum folic acid concentration. Of the 195 patients who participated in the study, 161 were examined for serum folic acid.

## 2.5. Ethical Aspects

This study was approved by the research ethics committee of Fundação Antonio Prudente under number 1542/11.

## 3. Results

The median age was 61 years (Quartile interval $_{25\%-75\%}$: 53–71 years). Of the 195 patients interviewed, 94 (48.21%) were female and 101 (51.79%) were male. Of the patients evaluated, 63 (32.31%) completed their primary education, 59 (30.26%) attained a high school/college incomplete level of education and 73 (37.44%) were at a college graduate/postgraduate level of education. There was a predominance of white patients (70.26%), followed by Asian (17.95%) and mulatto/black (11.79%). There was a higher incidence of colon tumors (66.67%) compared with rectal tumors (33.33%). In clinicopathological staging, 50.77% of the patients conformed to staging I and II and 47.69% to staging III and IV.

Of the 195 patients interviewed, 189 were included in the dietary analysis. Table 1 presents the mean, standard deviation and minimum and maximum nutrient values obtained from the unadjusted and calibrated FFQ.

One-hundred and sixty-one patients were examined for serum folate levels. The mean serum folate was 10.89 ng mL$^{-1}$. When the median serum folate concentrations were compared according to sociodemographic variables, there was a significant difference ($p$ = 0.001) between females (12.95 ng mL$^{-1}$) and males (10.10 ng mL$^{-1}$). In addition, patients aged less than 61 years had a median serum folate concentration that was significantly lower than the group of patients $\geq$61 years (10.45 *vs.* 11.60 ng mL$^{-1}$), with a $p$-value = 0.04. The concentrations of serum folate showed no significant differences in relation to race, education level, tumor site and staging.

To evaluate the correlation between the values of folate intake and the level of serum folate, Spearman's rank correlation coefficient test was used, as shown in Table 2. Of the 189 patients who were included in the dietary analysis, 156 were examined for serum folate levels. Of the 20 patients who consumed folic acid supplements, 17 were examined for serum folate levels. We observed a moderate correlation between the intake of synthetic folate supplement and serum folate levels. The same moderate correlation was observed between DFE supplement values and serum folate; both showed a significant difference ($p$ = 0.02). There was a fair correlation between the total calibrated DFE values and serum folate levels, but this was not significant ($p = 0.06$). There was no correlation between the serum folate and intake values for vitamin B2, B6, and B12; methionine; choline; betaine; and alcohol.

**Table 1.** Mean, standard deviation and minimum and maximum nutrient values from the unadjusted and calibrated FFQ in the pretreatment of patients for colorectal adenocarcinoma.

| Nutrients FFQ ($n = 189$) | | Mean | SD | Minimum | Maximum |
|---|---|---|---|---|---|
| Energy (Kcal) | unadjusted | 3144.58 | 1119.22 | 1120.72 | 6312.25 |
| | calibrated | 1766.32 | 171.13 | 1351.40 | 2160.68 |
| Lipid (g) | unadjusted | 103.35 | 40.29 | 38.48 | 242.95 |
| | calibrated | 68.46 | 8.92 | 49.60 | 93.22 |
| Carbohydrate (g) | unadjusted | 434.48 | 208.84 | 69.28 | 1280.54 |
| | calibrated | 204.79 | 20.54 | 140.09 | 263.48 |
| Protein (g) | unadjusted | 122.31 | 50.06 | 50.29 | 304.53 |
| | calibrated | 79.33 | 6.60 | 66.56 | 97.49 |
| Alcohol (g) | unadjusted | 8.41 | 21.90 | 0.00 | 214.99 |
| | calibrated | 0.41 | 0.41 | 0.00 | 2.42 |
| Vitamin B2 (mg) | unadjusted | 2.46 | 0.89 | 0.78 | 5.46 |
| | calibrated | 1.55 | 0.09 | 1.29 | 1.79 |
| Vitamin B6 (mg) | unadjusted | 2.95 | 1.70 | 0.78 | 12.28 |
| | calibrated | 1.51 | 0.22 | 1.02 | 2.41 |
| Vitamin B12 (µg) | unadjusted | 7.75 | 3.90 | 1.38 | 22.14 |
| | calibrated | 4.40 | 0.81 | 2.37 | 6.71 |
| Methionine (g) | unadjusted | 2.71 | 1.22 | 1.02 | 7.22 |
| | calibrated | 1.81 | 0.19 | 1.43 | 2.37 |
| Natural folate (µg) | unadjusted | 376.18 | 167.80 | 95.59 | 1075.83 |
| | calibrated | 215.65 | 24.60 | 151.51 | 291.54 |
| Synthetic folate (µg) | unadjusted | 146.61 | 90.52 | 10.77 | 549.99 |
| | calibrated | 76.86 | 12.70 | 40.23 | 112.61 |
| DFE diet (µg) | unadjusted | 625.43 | 257.29 | 116.26 | 1584.56 |
| | calibrated | 361.25 | 13.58 | 311.79 | 396.00 |
| Choline (mg) | unadjusted | 449.85 | 184.52 | 178.73 | 1140.15 |
| | calibrated | 284.54 | 25.22 | 233.95 | 356.02 |
| Betaine (mg) | unadjusted | 255.58 | 198.69 | 23.98 | 1692.13 |
| | calibrated | 130.63 | 9.50 | 100.38 | 167.31 |

DFE—Dietary Folate Equivalent.

Table 3 shows a comparison of the median DFE from unadjusted and calibrated diet data according to the sociodemographic and clinical characteristics. Women had a significantly lower intake of DFE compared with men, with a median unadjusted diet DFE for women and men of 537.09 µg and 610.29 µg, respectively ($p = 0.03$). The same $p$-value was found in the comparison of median calibrated diet DFE among women (358.67 µg) and men (362.89 µg). The unadjusted and calibrated DFE values were highest among the mulatto/black race, followed by the white and Asian races. The difference was significant between the Asian and white races and between the Asian and mulatto/black races ($p = 0.03$). Regarding the educational level, patients completing their primary education had an unadjusted and calibrated DFE intake that was significantly higher than those at the college graduate/postgraduate level ($p = 0.01$). The unadjusted and calibrated DFE values showed no significant difference in relation to age.

Table 2. Spearman's rank correlation coefficient of folate intake with the dosage of serum folate in the pretreatment of patients for colorectal adenocarcinoma.

| | Serum Folate (ng mL$^{-1}$) | | |
|---|---|---|---|
| | $N$ | Spearman correlation coefficient (rho) | $p$ |
| Unadjusted DFE diet [1] ($\mu$g) | 156 | 0.05 | 0.53 |
| Calibrated DFE diet [1] ($\mu$g) | 156 | 0.05 | 0.53 |
| Synthetic folate supplement | 17 | 0.54 | 0.02 * |
| DFE supplement [2] ($\mu$g) | 17 | 0.54 | 0.02 * |
| Total unadjusted DFE [3] ($\mu$g) | 17 | 0.40 | 0.10 |
| Total calibrated DFE [3] ($\mu$g) | 17 | 0.45 | 0.06 |

DFE—Dietary Folate Equivalent; [1] DFE diet = natural folate + 1.7 × (dietetic synthetic folate); [2] DFE supplement = synthetic folate supplement × 2; [3] Total DFE = DFE diet + DFE supplement; * $p < 0.05$.

Regarding the intake of folic acid supplements, a comparison of the medians of supplement, total unadjusted and total calibrated DFE is shown in Table 4, according to the sociodemographic characteristics. DFE supplement intake was significantly higher among women (1750.00 $\mu$g) compared to men (440.00 $\mu$g). DFE supplement values showed no significant difference in relation to age, race and education level. Similar results were obtained for the total unadjusted and calibrated DFE, where the median values showed no significant difference in relation to sociodemographic variables. As previously mentioned, of the 189 patients evaluated, 10.58% received folic acid supplementation, and 8.46% of these had colon cancer and 2.12% had rectal cancer. There was an association between total unadjusted and calibrated DFE with the tumor site. The median total unadjusted DFE intake of patients with colon cancer was 1177.18 $\mu$g vs. 845.60 $\mu$g for rectal tumor patients ($p = 0.001$). The total calibrated DFE intake was also higher among colon tumor patients when compared with individuals with rectal tumors, with a median intake of 845.81 $\mu$g in patients with colon tumors and 702.72 $\mu$g in patients with rectal cancer ($p = 0.02$) (Table 5).

Regarding the prevalence of folate inadequacy in patients with intake from diet alone, 11.00% had intakes below the EAR according to the unadjusted FFQ. However, according to the calibrated FFQ, only 0.10% of individuals had intakes below the recommended EAR level. When evaluating the prevalence of inadequacy above the UL, 6.06% of patients had a dietary folate intake above the UL according to the unadjusted FFQ, while the calibrated FFQ showed no cases of inadequacy.

**Table 3.** Median comparison of DFE from unadjusted diet data and calibrated diet DFE according to sociodemographic and clinical characteristics in the pretreatment of patients for colorectal adenocarcinoma.

| | DFE Diet [1] Unadjusted (µg) (n = 189) | | | DFE Diet [1] Calibrated (µg) (n = 189) | | |
|---|---|---|---|---|---|---|
| | N | Median | p | N | Median | p |
| **Sex** | | | | | | |
| Female | 93 | 537.09 | 0.03 * | 93 | 358.67 | 0.03 * |
| Male | 96 | 610.29 | | 96 | 362.89 | |
| **Age** | | | | | | |
| <61 years | 86 | 615.20 | 0.17 | 86 | 363.15 | 0.17 |
| ≥61 years | 103 | 560.96 | | 103 | 360.10 | |
| **Race** | | | | | | |
| Asian (a) | 35 | 495.93 | | 35 | 356.06 | |
| White (b) | 135 | 591.95 | 0.03 *ab,ac | 135 | 361.88 | 0.03 *ab,ac |
| Mulatto/Black (c) | 19 | 620.98 | | 19 | 363.47 | |
| **Education level** | | | | | | |
| Primary education (a) | 62 | 633.04 | | 62 | 364.10 | |
| High school/college incomplete level (b) | 55 | 598.83 | 0.01 *ac | 55 | 362.26 | 0.01 *ac |
| College graduate/postgraduate level (c) | 72 | 524.09 | | 72 | 357.86 | |
| **Tumor site** | | | | | | |
| Colon | 125 | 584.12 | 0.42 | 125 | 361.44 | 0.42 |
| Rectal | 64 | 610.29 | | 64 | 362.89 | |
| **Staging** | | | | | | |
| I e II | 97 | 584.70 | 0.41 | 97 | 361.47 | 0.41 |
| III e IV | 89 | 589.11 | | 89 | 361.72 | |

DFE—Dietary Folate Equivalent; [1] DFE diet = natural folate + 1.7 × (dietetic synthetic folate); * $p < 0.05$; In race, "a" is Asian, "b" is white and "c" is mulatto/black; In Education level, "a" is primary education, "b" is high school and "c" is college graduate.

Of the patients on diets with folic acid supplementation, no patient had an intake below the cutoff points of the Recommended Dietary Allowances (RDA). However, when considering the values of the UL through a qualitative interpretation of the adequacy of folate intake, the FFQ evaluates the usual intake and thus corresponds to a survey over a large number of days. According to unadjusted and calibrated FFQ, 50.00% and 35.00% of patients, respectively, had a greater intake up to the UL, which is a potential risk for adverse effects.

The prevalence of inadequacy of vitamins B2, B6 and B12 was calculated using the values of EAR and is presented in Table 6. We observed a higher prevalence of inadequate intake of vitamin B6, followed by vitamin B12, and B2. For the evaluation of inadequate choline, a qualitative evaluation was used, which considered that the FFQ takes into account a greater number of days. When evaluated as the unadjusted FFQ, 22.55% of female patients and 13.76% of males had intake values of choline above the levels stated by the AI. This indicates that the mean intake in these individuals is likely adequate. Nevertheless, when analyzed using the calibrated FFQ, no patient had a dietary intake above the AI and the adequacy of intake could not be determined.

## 4. Discussion and Conclusion

This study is one of the few published studies that present the dietary intake of folate and nutrients involved in the 1-carbon cycle in CRC patients without any previous treatment.

A study conducted with 196 patients with CRC, which used a FFQ validated for Portuguese individuals, found a mean intake of vitamin B6, vitamin B12, folate, methionine and alcohol of 2.80 mg day$^{-1}$ (SD = 1.06), 14.50 µg day$^{-1}$ (SD = 9.10), 401.60 µg day$^{-1}$ (SD = 161.9) 2.85 mg day$^{-1}$ (SD = 1.28) and 25.17 g day$^{-1}$ (SD = 39.80), respectively [15]. These results are consistent with the present study with regard to the unadjusted data for B6 and methionine and the calibrated data for folate. Jiang $et$ $al.$ [16] assessed the relationship between folate, methionine and alcohol and a genetic polymorphism and found a mean folate intake similar to the unadjusted data found in this study, 634 µg day$^{-1}$ (SD = 307) for patients with colon cancer and 638 µg day$^{-1}$ (SD = 334) for rectal tumors. In the same study, patients with colon cancer had a mean energy intake of 4260 Kcal day$^{-1}$ (SD = 2220) and methionine of 2047 mg day$^{-1}$ (SD = 939). In patients with rectal cancer, the mean energy intake was 4321 Kcal day$^{-1}$ (SD = 1669) and methionine was 2117 mg day$^{-1}$ (SD = 801). In another study conducted with 787 patients with colorectal tumors, the mean energy intake was 1588.6 Kcal (SD = 449.5) and folate was 248.1 µg day$^{-1}$ (SD = 111.1). Furthermore, 54.5% of these patients consumed <5 g day$^{-1}$ of alcohol, 19.10% consumed from 5 to <30 g day$^{-1}$ and 26.40% consumed alcohol in quantities greater than 30 g day$^{-1}$ [17]. Laso $et$ $al.$ [18] evaluated the dietary intake of 246 patients with CRC and found a mean intake of vitamin B2 of 1.91 mg day$^{-1}$ (SD = 0.6), vitamin B6 of 1.98 mg day$^{-1}$ (SD = 0.5), vitamin B12 of 7.67 mg day$^{-1}$ (SD = 4.7), folate of 288.1 µg day$^{-1}$ (SD = 89.1) and alcohol of 9.94 g day$^{-1}$ (SD = 18.4). These data are similar to the unadjusted data found in this study in relation to vitamin B12 and alcohol. Al-ghnaniem $et$ $al.$ [19] described in their study a mean alcohol intake of 13 g day$^{-1}$ and a mean folate intake of 289 µg day$^{-1}$. The mean folate intake in the study of Pufulete $et$ $al.$ [14] was 304 µg day$^{-1}$.

An important difference between this study and previous studies is that folate intake in this study was assessed by several methods, including an assessment of the values from the diet (DFE diet), from supplementation by fortification and supplements (DFE supplement), and from dietary folate plus supplemental folate (DFE total). We found only one study in the literature that considered these three types of folate. This study suggests that the best way to assess folate intake is through the total DFE because it encompasses the 19 different sources of folate [20].

FFQ are one of the most commonly used methods for evaluating habitual dietary intake in large-scale epidemiological studies, given their low cost and ease of application [21,22]. However, the errors present in the measurements of the questionnaire may attenuate the estimates of the relative risks that are found, and thus diminish the statistical power of studies evaluating the relationship between diet and disease [22,23]. Knowing that error is inherent in food intake measurements, methodological strategies have been used in an attempt to make the measurements obtained through the FFQ closer to the quantities actually consumed, which are the calibration. To assess the folate intake FFQ was used and fasting serum folate levels. FFQ relies on reported food intake and although it is a validated tool, it is prone to error, using the 24h as reference method only partly removes this error; indeed it is easier to accurately estimate folate intake in subjects who use supplements (as evidenced by the results presented in Table 2).

Biochemical markers are more sensitive and specific when compared to methods of dietary intake assessment through questionnaires and/or dietary recalls [11]. The study of Al-ghnaniem et al. [19] showed a mean serum folate of 12.30 ng mL$^{-1}$, a mean level greater than that found in the present study. In contrast, some studies have shown lower plasma levels compared to this study. For example, Pufulete et al. [14] found a mean serum folate value of 5.40 ng mL$^{-1}$ and Chang et al. [24] found a level of 5.02 ng mL$^{-1}$ (SD = 4.43 ng mL$^{-1}$).

**Table 4.** Comparison of the medians of supplement, total unadjusted and total calibrated DFE according to sociodemographic characteristics in the pretreatment of patients for colorectal adenocarcinoma.

| | DFE Supplement [1] (µg) (n = 20) | | | Total Unadjusted DFE [2] (µg) (n = 20) | | | Total Calibrated DFE [2] (µg) (n = 20) | | |
|---|---|---|---|---|---|---|---|---|---|
| | N | Median | p | N | Median | p | N | Median | p |
| **Sex** | | | | | | | | | |
| Female | 12 | 1750.00 | 0.01 * | 12 | 2724.50 | 0.44 | 12 | 2128.77 | 0.05 |
| Male | 8 | 440.00 | | 8 | 969.77 | | 8 | 794.31 | |
| **Age** | | | | | | | | | |
| <61 years | 3 | 304.00 | 0.55 | 3 | 900.26 | 0.63 | 3 | 659.87 | 0.49 |
| ≥61 years | 17 | 480.00 | | 17 | 1069.11 | | 17 | 837.44 | |
| **Race** | | | | | | | | | |
| Asian | 6 | 480.00 | 0.22 | 6 | 984.68 | 0.16 | 6 | 835.98 | 0.22 |
| White | 13 | 480.00 | | 13 | 997.18 | | 13 | 831.99 | |
| Mulatto/Black | 1 | 20,000.00 | | 1 | 21,079.60 | | 1 | 20,382.30 | |
| **Education level** | | | | | | | | | |
| Primary education High | 8 | 8000.00 | 0.07 | 8 | 9150.01 | 0.06 | 8 | 8382.11 | 0.09 |
| school/college incomplete level College | 4 | 480.00 | | 4 | 956.48 | | 4 | 834.66 | |
| graduate/postgraduate level | 8 | 440.00 | | 8 | 910.92 | | 8 | 793.44 | |

DFE—Dietary Folate Equivalent; [1] DFE supplement = synthetic folate supplement × 2; [2] Total DFE = DFE diet + DFE supplement.

**Table 5.** Comparison of the medians of supplement, total unadjusted and total calibrated DFE according to clinical characteristics in the pretreatment of patients for colorectal adenocarcinoma.

| | DFE Supplement [1] (µg) (n = 20) | | | Total Unadjusted DFE [2] (µg) (n = 20) | | | Total Calibrated DFE [2] (µg) (n = 20) | | |
|---|---|---|---|---|---|---|---|---|---|
| | N | Median | p | N | Median | p | N | Median | p |
| **Tumor site** | | | | | | | | | |
| Colon | 16 | 480.00 | | 16 | 1177.18 | | 16 | 845.81 | |
| Rectal | 4 | 352.00 | 0.06 | 4 | 845.60 | 0.001 * | 4 | 702.72 | 0.02 * |
| **Staging** | | | | | | | | | |
| I e II | 12 | 480.00 | | 12 | 1059.72 | | 12 | 834.71 | |
| III e IV | 8 | 440.00 | 0.96 | 8 | 1005.74 | 0.58 | 8 | 799.17 | 0.93 |

DFE—Dietary Folate Equivalent; [1] DFE supplement = synthetic folate supplement × 2; [2] Total DFE = DFE diet + DFE supplement; * p < 0.05.

**Table 6.** The prevalence of inadequacy of vitamins B2, B6, B12 and folate in the pretreatment of patients for colorectal adenocarcinoma.

| | % Bellow of EAR (n = 189) |
|---|---|
| **Unadjusted FFQ** | |
| Vitamin B2 | 4.00 |
| Vitamin B6 | 14.86 |
| Vitamin B12 | 7.00 |
| Folate | 11.00 |
| **Calibrated FFQ** | |
| Vitamin B2 | 0.00 |
| Vitamin B6 | 20.18 |
| Vitamin B12 | 0.10 |
| Folate | 0.10 |

FFQ—Food Frequency Questionnaire; EAR—Estimated Average Requirement.

In the present study, there was a significant difference in plasma levels of folate in relation to sex and age, but no studies have been found in the literature that evaluated this relationship. Furthermore, when assessing the correlation of serum folate concentrations with folate intake, a significant difference was found in relation to a synthetic folate from supplement as well as a DFE supplement. Additionally, there were no verified studies that assessed the correlation between the ingestion of supplements with plasma folate levels.

The present study also evaluated the correlation between serum folate with other nutrients involved in the 1-carbon cycle, but significant differences were not found. Studies were not found in the literature that assessed this correlation. However, in relation to dietary data, one study showed a moderate correlation between vitamin B2 and B6 (rho = 0.44) and folate (rho = 0.45). In that study, vitamin B6 showed a moderate correlation with vitamin B12 (rho = 0.38) and folate (rho = 0.48). Vitamin B12 also showed a moderate correlation with folate (rho = 0.34) [25].

In this study, men ingested significantly more folate (unadjusted and calibrated) than women. In addition, Asian participants ingested less folate, both unadjusted and calibrated, than the participants of any other race. The difference was significant between the Asian and white races and between the Asian and mulatto/black races. Regarding education, patients with up to a primary school education had an unadjusted and calibrated folate intake that was significantly higher than patients with higher education at the college graduate/postgraduate level. We found no studies in the literature that showed a correlation between folate intake with the variables mentioned here.

The prevalence of the inadequacy of a particular nutrient has been a target of interest among researchers because this information allows for the development of healthcare strategies, such as planning and monitoring actions that are specific to a group of individuals [26]. Folate, vitamins B2, B6, B12, and choline are part of numerous biochemical reactions that are involved in the 1-carbon cycle, which is essential for the synthesis and methylation of DNA, the synthesis of RNA precursors and the conversion of homocysteine in methionine [14,27–29]. A deficiency of nutrients in this group can lead to decreased levels S-adenosylmethionine (SAM), chromosomal instability, changes in transcriptional regulation, poor incorporation of uracil into DNA, *DNA* hypomethylation and increased risk of colorectal tumors [30–35]. When analyzing the prevalence of folate inadequacy in patients with intake from diet alone, 11.00% and 0.10% had intakes below the EAR according to the unadjusted and calibrated FFQ, respectively. One of the mechanisms by which folate deficiency can lead to CRC is related to the synthesis of purines and thymidylate. Thus, adequate levels are essential for the synthesis, stability, integrity and adequate repair of DNA [29,36]. In some studies, a dietary intake of 400 $\mu$g day$^{-1}$ of folate for 10 weeks increased DNA methylation in lymphocytes and in the colonic mucosa of patients with colorectal adenomas [37,38]. One study that evaluated the colon in 609 cases showed that an intake of <200 µg day$^{-1}$ of folate was related to increased hypomethylation of LINE-1 regulatory sequences in contrast to a dietary intake of folate ≥400 µg day$^{-1}$, which showed a decrease in hypomethylation. The consumption of ethanol ≥15 g day$^{-1}$ was associated with an increased risk of LINE-1 hypomethylation [39].

Regarding vitamin B6, the prevalence of inadequacy according to unadjusted and calibrated FFQ was 14.86% and 20.18%, respectively. Vitamin B6 acts as an enzyme cofactor for serine hydroxy-methyltransferase (SHMT) and cystathionine b-synthase (CBS). Vitamin B6 is responsible for the formation of glycine and 5,10-methylenetetrahydrofolate and allows for the irreversible reaction of homocysteine to cystathionine [40]. It is known that vitamin B6 deficiency can lead to hyperhomocysteinemia, weakness, nervous disorders, irritability, insomnia and difficulty walking [41].

The prevalence of inadequate dietary intake of vitamin B12 was 7.00% and 0.10% according to unadjusted and calibrated FFQ, respectively. During the methylation of homocysteine to methionine, vitamin B12 acts as a cofactor for the enzyme methionine synthase [42,43]. Additionally, this vitamin plays an important role during the isomerization of L-methylmalonyl-CoA to succinyl-CoA [44].

Regarding vitamin B2, the prevalence of inadequacy was 4%, assessed by the FFQ unadjusted data only. Vitamin B2, besides taking part in the remethylation of homocysteine to methionine, acts as a cofactor for methylenetetrahydrofolate reductase (MTHFR) and pyridoxine 5′-phosphate oxidase [45].

The prevalence of the inadequacy of choline could only be assessed by the unadjusted FFQ and was 22.55% in female patients. Of these female patients, 13.76% likely had adequate intake. This nutrient participates as a cofactor for SAM-dependent transmethylation reactions [46].

A low proportion of patients showed folate deficiency in this sample. On the other hand, a high proportion of patients showed folate intake above the recommended levels. Female patients and patients less than 61 years old presented significantly lower serum folate levels.

In the present study, we found a considerable number of patients who had a folate intake above the UL, both those who only ingested this nutrient from the diet and, in many cases, those patients with supplementation. Food fortification with folic acid has been deployed in several countries around the world to prevent embryonic neural tube defects and some diseases, such as cancer [47], and is likely the most important action in the field of nutrition and public health [48]. After fortification in the U.S. and Canada, considerable increases have been seen both in the intake and serum concentration of folic acid [49,50]. However, folate fortification or folic acid supplementation may negatively interfere with the 1-carbon cycle and thus could

271

become an important issue for extrapolation [51]. Folate intake above the UL, in addition to not diminishing the risk for CRC, increases the risk that an individual may develop this type of tumor [52]. Studies using animal models have shown that before the presence of neoplastic foci, a moderate deficiency of dietary folate increased the onset and progression of adenomas, whereas supplementation with 4 to 10 times above the basal daily requirement for folic acid suppressed the onset and progression of these adenomas. However, when such folate intervention was performed after the establishment of preneoplastic lesions, a moderate deficiency of dietary folate suppressed tumor growth and progression in addition to promoting the regression of the tumor [53,54]. A study conducted by Lindzon *et al.* which aimed to evaluate the effects of folic acid supplementation in aberrant crypt foci and CCR, used 152 male rats at weaning that received supplementation of 2 mg folic acid (kg day)$^{-1}$. Six weeks after the induction of the aberrant crypt foci, the rats were randomized into four groups. In these groups, the rodents received 0, 2, 5 or 8 mg (kg day)$^{-1}$ of folic acid. The rats were sacrificed after 34 weeks to assess the result of supplementation. The number of aberrant crypt foci increased with increasing amounts of supplementation. Furthermore, although the tumor incidence was significantly different among the four groups from the tumor multiplicity, the tumor load and rectal epithelial proliferation were positively correlated with the folate levels and inversely correlated with the concentration of homocysteine [55]. Thus, studies in animals have evaluated the effects of supplements [56,57]. For this reason, recent studies in humans suggest that in normal mucosa, folic acid can prevent the onset of CRC. Despite not being completely understood because of its dual role, folate intake in a previously established preneoplastic lesion can accelerate the growth of tumor cells [36,58–61]. Thus, it is stressed that careful assessment should be given with regards to the dose and when to start folate intervention, while observing the presence or absence of preneoplastic lesions [36,59]. This is because folate appears to have a dual modulating role in colorectal cancer (CCR), which involves the onset and progression of this tumor and depends on the dose and start of intervention [36]. The mechanisms by which this occurs include the provision of precursors for DNA synthesis and hypermethylation of tumor suppressor genes [29].

In the study by Kim *et al.* [17], 18.00% of the patients used multivitamin supplements. Two other studies that evaluated 28 and 18 patients with colorectal tumors found that 93% [19] and 7% [20] of these patients ingested supplementation, respectively. Corroborating the present work, one study reported a higher intake of multivitamins for patients with colon cancer, 6.20% of patients with rectal cancer and 9.10% of patients with colon cancer [62].

Recent studies have shown that folate deficiency in normal intestinal mucosa can lead to the instability and incorporation of uracil in the DNA molecule. Therefore, adequate nutritional intake of folate can act as a protective agent against cancer in the carcinogenesis of the colon and rectum. However, in preneoplastic lesions, with intense cell division, folate deficiency appears to disrupt this process, thus inhibiting tumor growth and even tumor regression [57]. This occurs because folic acid can act as a substrate for tumor growth and replication, increasing the chances of disease progression [29,63,64].

Several authors have shown no or positive associations between folate supplementation and the recurrence of adenomas [25,63,65,66]. In study by Cole *et al.* [65], the participants were randomly chosen and 516 received 1 mg day$^{-1}$ of folic acid and 505 received placebo. They also were separately randomized to receive aspirin (81 or 325 mg day$^{-1}$) or placebo. Follow-up consisted of two colonoscopic surveillance cycles, the first after three years and the second between three and five years, and found that patients who received folic acid at 1 mg day$^{-1}$ did not have reduced colorectal adenoma risk. Logan *et al.* [66], in a randomized study, noted that aspirin (300 mg day$^{-1}$) but not folate (0.5 mg day$^{-1}$) use was found to reduce the risk of colorectal adenoma recurrence. Sauer *et al.* [51], notes that fortification or supplementation with folic acid can interfere negatively in the carbon-1 cycle and thus becomes an important issue for extrapolation. According to Bollheimer *et al.* [52], folate intake above the UL, in addition to not reducing the risk for CRC, increases the risk that the individual will develop this type of tumor [52].

After mandatory fortification in Brazil, dietary folate intake probably increased in the population. Steluti *et al.* (2011) conducted a study in Brazil in order to investigate serum concentrations and the prevalence of inadequate folate intake and also vitamin B6 and vitamin B12 intakes. The study showed low prevalence rates of inadequate folate; vitamin B6 and vitamin B12 intakes were low, which is possibly the result of improved access to and availability of foods that are dietary sources of these vitamins [67]. In addition, a recent study in Brazil, analyzed folic acid intake before and since mandatory fortification and showed that prevalence of inadequate folic acid intake mainly decreased in adolescents and adult males. The paper also discusses that while folate has been associated with decreased risk of certain chronic diseases, there is strong evidence that the excess of nutrients may increase DNA synthesis, stimulating cell proliferation and participate in tumor progression [68]. Furthermore, because current evidence of the benefits of regular use and risk of excessive consumption of supplements containing folic acid, it is necessary to monitor use of supplements [69,70].

## 5. Conclusions

The purchase of multivitamins by the population is often performed without guidance. Moreover, due to the difficulty of the early diagnosis of CRC, the medical professional and/or nutritionist cannot adequately guide the patient in the use of nutritional supplements. Thus, because of the increased supply of folic acid through foods, in combination with the use of multivitamin supplements, a part of the population may far exceed the intake of folic acid recommended by the DRIs, which established a tolerable UL of 1 mg day$^{-1}$. More studies are needed to understand the impact of high folic acid intake through food fortification and use of dietary supplements, as well as other nutrients involved in the 1-carbon cycle, and whether high intake promotes adverse health effects, especially in cancer patients. We also suggest further studies to identify potential polymorphisms in the MTHFR enzyme, which is involved in the metabolic pathways that degrade homocysteine, in order to determine whether changes in this enzyme can effectively interfere with folate metabolism.

**Author Contributions:** Study conception and design: Ariana Ferrari and Samuel Aguiar Junior; Acquisition of data: Ariana Ferrari; Analysis and interpretation of data: Ariana Ferrari, Aline Martins de Carvalho, Josiane Steluti, Juliana Teixeira, Dirce Maria Marchioni and Samuel Aguiar Junior; Drafting of manuscript: Ariana Ferrari; Critical revision: Ariana Ferrari, Aline Martins de Carvalho, Josiane Steluti, Juliana Teixeira, Dirce Maria Marchioni and Samuel Aguiar Junior; Financial support: FAPESP.

**Conflicts of Interest:** The authors declare no conflict of interest.

# References

1. Ministério da Saúde; Instituto Nacional do Câncer. *Estimativa/2012 Incidência de Câncer no Brasil*; INCA: Rio de Janeiro, Brazil, 2011.

2. Mason, J.B.; Choi, S.W.; Liu, Z. Other one-carbon micronutrients and age modulate the effects of folate on colorectal carcinogenesis. *Nutr. Rev.* **2008**, *66*, S15–S17.

3. Xu, X.; Chen, J. One-carbon metabolism and breast cancer: An epidemiological perspective. *J. Genet. Genomics* **2009**, *36*, 203–214.

4. Ueland, P.M. Choline and betaine in health and disease. *J. Inherit. Metab. Dis.* **2011**, *34*, 3–15.

5. Edge, S.B.; Byrd, D.R.; Compton, C.C.; Fritz, A.G.; Greene, F.L.; Trotti, A. *AJCC Cancer Staging Manual*, 7th ed.; Springer: New York, NY, USA, 2010; pp. 143–159.

6. Lameza, M.M.S. Validação de Questionário de Frequência Alimentar para Pacientes Tratados de Câncer Colorretal. Master's Thesis, Fundação Antônio Prudente, São Paulo, Brazil, September 2010.

7. *Nutrition Data System for Research*; Version 2007; University of Minnesota: Minneapolis, MN, USA, 2007.

8. Agência Nacional de Vigilância Sanitária. *Resolução no. 344, de 13 de Dezembro de 2002. Aprova o Regulamento Técnico para a Fortificação das Farinhas de Trigo e das Farinhas de Milho com Ferro e Ácido Fólico, Constante no Anexo Desta Resolução*; Diário Oficial da União: Brasília, Brazil, 2002. Available online: http://www.anvisa.gov.br/legis/resol/2002/344_02rdc.htm (accessed on 12 May 2012).

9. Suitor, C.W.; Bailey, L.B. Dietary folate equivalents: Interpretation and application. *J. Am. Diet. Assoc.* **2000**, *100*, 88–94.

10. Summary Table: Estimated Average Requirements. In *Dietary Reference Intakes: Applications in Dietary Assessment (2000)*; National Academies Press: Washington, DC, USA, 2000; pp. 282–283.

11. Fisberg, R.M.; Slater, B.; Marchioni, D.M.L.; Martini, L.A. *Inquéritos Alimentares: Métodos e Bases Científicas*; Manole: Barueri, Brazil, 2005.

12. Fisberg, R.M.; Marchioni, D.M.L.; Villar, B.S. Planejamento e avaliação da ingestão de energia e nutrientes para indivíduos. In *Guia de Nutrição: Nutrição Clínica no Adulto*, 2nd ed.; Cuppari, L., Ed.; Manole: Barueri, Brazil, 2007; pp. 51–62.

13. Dietary Reference Intakes for Thiamin, Riboflavin, Niacin, Vitamin B6, Folate, Vitamin B12, Pantothenic Acid, Biotin, and Choline. 1998. Available online: http://www.nap.edu/catalog/6015.html (accessed on 12 May 2012).

14. Pufulete, M.; Al-Ghnaniem, R.; Leather, A.J.; Appleby, P.; Gout, S.; Terry, C.; Emery, P.W.; Sanders, T.A. Folate status, genomic DNA hypomethylation, and risk of colorectal adenoma and cancer: A case control study. *Gastroenterology* **2003**, *124*, 1240–1248.

15. Guerreiro, C.S.; Carmona, B.; Gonçalves, S.; Carolino, E.; Fidalgo, P.; Brito, M.; Leitão, C.N.; Cravo, M. Risk of colorectal cancer associated with the C677T polymorphism in 5,10-methylenetetrahydrofolate reductase in Portuguese patients depends on the intake of methyl-donor nutrients. *Am. J. Clin. Nutr.* **2008**, *88*, 1413–1418.

16. Jiang, Q.; Chen, K.; Ma, X.; Li, Q.; Yu, W.; Shu, G.; Yao, K. Diets, polymorphisms of methylenetetrahydrofolate reductase, and the susceptibility of colon cancer and rectal cancer. *Cancer Detect. Prev.* **2005**, *29*, 146–154.

17. Kim, J.; Cho, Y.A.; Kim, D.H.; Lee, B.H.; Hwang, D.Y.; Jeong, J.; Lee, H.J.; Matsuo, K.; Tajima, K.; Ahn, Y.O. Dietary intake of folate and alcohol, MTHFR C677T polymorphism, and colorectal cancer risk in Korea. *Am. J. Clin. Nutr.* **2012**, *95*, 405–412.

18. Laso, N.; Mas, S.; Jose Lafuente, M.; Casterad, X.; Trias, M.; Ballesta, A.; Molina, R.; Salas, J.; Ascaso, C.; Zheng, S.; *et al.* Decrease in specific micronutrient intake in colorectal cancer patients with tumors presenting Ki-*ras* mutation. *Anticancer Res.* **2004**, *24*, 2011–2020.

19. Al-Ghnaniem, R.; Peters, J.; Foresti, R.; Heaton, N.; Pufulete, M. Methylation of estrogen receptor alpha and mutL homolog 1 in normal colonic mucosa: Association with folate and vitamin B-12 status in subjects with and without colorectal neoplasia. *Am. J. Clin. Nutr.* **2007**, *86*, 1064–1072.

20. Stevens, V.L.; McCullough, M.L.; Sun, J.; Jacobs, E.J.; Campbell, P.T.; Gapstur, S.M. High levels of folate from supplements and fortification are not associated with increased risk of colorectal cancer. *Gastroenterology* **2011**, *141*, 98–105.

21. Bingham, S.A.; Luben, R.; Welch, A.; Wareham, N.; Khaw, K.; Day, N. Are imprecise methods obscuring a relation between fat and breast cancer? *Lancet* **2003**, *362*, 212–214.

22. Kaaks, R.; Ferrari, P. Dietary intake assessment in epidemiology: Can we know what we are measuring? *Ann. Epidemiol.* **2006**, *16*, 377–380.

23. Rosner, B.; Willett, W.C.; Spiegelman, D. Correction of logistic regression relative risk estimates and confidence intervals for systematic within-person measurement error. *Stat. Med.* **1989**, *8*, 1051–1069.

24. Chang, S.C.; Lin, P.C.; Lin, J.K.; Yang, S.H.; Wang, H.S.; Li, A.F. Role of MTHFR polymorphisms and folate levels in different phenotypes of sporadic colorectal cancers. *Int. J. Colorectal Dis.* **2007**, *22*, 483–489.

25. Figueiredo, J.C.; Levine, A.J.; Grau, M.V.; Midttun, O.; Ueland, P.M.; Ahnen, D.J.; Barry, E.L.; Tsang, S.; Munroe, D.; Ali, I.; *et al.* Vitamins B2, B6, and B12 and risk of new colorectal adenomas in a randomized trial of aspirin use and folic acid supplementation. *Cancer Epidemiol. Biomark. Prev.* **2008**, *17*, 2136–2145.

26. Slater, B.; Marchioni, D.L.; Fisberg, R.M. Estimando a prevalência da ingestão inadequada de nutrientes. *Rev. Saúde Pública* **2004**, *38*, 599–605. (In Portuguese)

27. Kim, Y.I. Folate and DNA methylation: A mechanistic link between folate deficiency and colorectal cancer? *Cancer Epidemiol. Biomark. Prev.* **2004**, *13*, 511–519.

28. Kim, Y.I. Nutritional epigenetics: Impact of folate deficiency on DNA methylation and colon cancer susceptibility. *J. Nutr.* **2005**, *135*, 2703–2709.

29. Migheli, F.; Migliore, L. Epigenetics of colorectal cancer. *Clin. Genet.* **2012**, *81*, 312–318.

30. Bailey, L.B.; Gregory, J.F. Folate metabolism and requirements. *J. Nutr.* **1999**, *129*, 779–782.

31. Fenech, M. The role of folic acid and Vitamin B12 in genomic stability of human cells. *Mutat. Res.* **2001**, *475*, 57–67.

32. Choi, S.W.; Mason, J.B. Folate status: Effects on pathways of colorectal carcinogenesis. *J. Nutr.* **2002**, *132*, 2413S–2418S.

33. Lamprecht, S.A.; Lipkin, M. Chemoprevention of colon cancer by calcium, vitamin D and folate: Molecular mechanisms. *Nat. Rev. Cancer* **2003**, *3*, 601–614.

34. Cabelof, D.C.; Raffoul, J.J.; Nakamura, J.; Kapoor, D.; Abdalla, H.; Heydari, A.R. Imbalanced base excision repair in response to folate deficiency is accelerated by polymerase beta haploinsufficiency. *J. Biol. Chem.* **2004**, *279*, 36504–36513.

35. Davis, C.D.; Uthus, E.O. DNA methylation, cancer susceptibility, and nutrient interactions. *Exp. Biol. Med.* **2004**, *229*, 988–995.

36. Kim, Y.I. Folate and colorectal cancer: An evidence-based critical review. *Mol. Nutr. Food Res.* **2007**, *51*, 267–292.

37. Pufulete, M.; Al-Ghnaniem, R.; Khushal, A.; Appleby, P.; Harris, N.; Gout, S.; Emery, P.W.; Sanders, T.A. Effect of folic acid supplementation on genomic DNA methylation in patients with colorectal adenoma. *Gut* **2005**, *54*, 648–653.

38. Pufulete, M.; Al-Ghnaniem, R.; Rennie, J.A.; Appleby, P.; Harris, N.; Gout, S.; Emery, P.W.; Sanders, T.A. Influence of folate status on genomic DNA methylation in colonic mucosa of subjects without colorectal adenoma or cancer. *Br. J. Cancer* **2005**, *92*, 838–842.

39. Schernhammer, E.S.; Giovannucci, E.; Kawasaki, T.; Rosner, B.; Fuchs, C.S.; Ogino, S. Dietary folate, alcohol and B vitamins in relation to LINE-1 hypomethylation in colon cancer. *Gut* **2010**, *59*, 794–799.

40. Yi, P.; Melnyk, S.; Pogribna, M.; Pogribny, I.P.; Hine, R.J.; James, S.J. Increase in plasma homocysteine associated with parallel increases in plasma S-adenosylhomocysteine and lymphocyte DNA hypomethylation. *J. Biol. Chem.* **2000**, *275*, 29318–29323.

41. Clayton, P.T. B6-responsive disorders: A model of vitamin dependency. *J. Inherit. Metab. Dis.* **2006**, *29*, 317–326.

42. McNulty, H.; Pentieva, K.; Hoey, L.; Ward, M. Homocysteine, B-vitamins and CVD. *Proc. Nutr. Soc.* **2008**, *67*, 232–237.

43. Gruber, K.; Puffer, B.; Kräutler, B. Vitamin B12-derivatives-enzyme cofactors and ligands of proteins and nucleic acids. *Chem. Soc. Rev.* **2011**, *40*, 4346–4363.

44. Scott, J.M. Folate and vitamin B12. *Proc. Nutr. Soc.* **1999**, *58*, 441–448.

45. Hoey, L.; McNulty, H.; Strain, J.J. Studies of biomarker responses to intervention with riboflavin: A systematic review. *Am. J. Clin. Nutr.* **2009**, *89*, 1960S–1980S.

46. Ueland, P.M.; Holm, P.I.; Hustad, S. Betaine: A key modulator of one-carbon metabolism and homocysteine status. *Clin. Chem. Lab. Med.* **2005**, *43*, 1069–1075.

47. Porcelli, L.; Assaraf, Y.G.; Azzariti, A.; Paradiso, A.; Jansen, G.; Peters, G.J. The impact of folate status on the efficacy of colorectal cancer treatment. *Curr. Drug Metab.* **2011**, *12*, 975–984.

48. Rosenberg, I.H. Science-based micronutrient fortification: Which nutrients, how much, and how to know? *Am. J. Clin. Nutr.* **2005**, *2005*, 279–280.

49. Pfeiffer, C.M.; Caudill, S.P.; Gunter, E.W.; Osterloh, J.; Sampson, E.J. Biochemical indicators of B vitamin status in the US population after folic acid fortification: Results from the National Health and Nutrition Examination Survey 1999–2000. *Am. J. Clin. Nutr.* **2005**, *82*, 442–450.

50. Pfeiffer, C.M.; Johnson, C.L.; Jain, R.B.; Yetley, E.A.; Picciano, M.F.; Rader, J.I.; Fisher, K.D.; Mulinare, J.; Osterloh, J.D. Trends in blood folate and vitamin B-12 concentrations in the United States, 1988–2004. *Am. J. Clin. Nutr.* **2007**, *86*, 718–727.

51. Sauer, J.; Mason, J.B.; Choi, S.W. Too much folate: A risk factor for cancer and cardiovascular disease? *Curr. Opin. Clin. Nutr. Metab. Care* **2009**, *12*, 30–36.

52. Bollheimer, L.C.; Buettner, R.; Kullmann, A.; Kullmann, F. Folate and its preventive potential in colorectal carcinogenesis. How strong is the biological and epidemiological evidence? *Crit. Rev. Oncol. Hematol.* **2005**, *55*, 13–36.

53. Song, J.; Medline, A.; Mason, J.B.; Gallinger, S.; Kim, Y.I. Effects of dietary folate on intestinal tumorigenesis in the apcMin mouse. *Cancer Res.* **2000**, *60*, 5434–5440.

54. Song, J.; Sohn, K.J.; Medline, A.; Ash, C.; Gallinger, S.; Kim, Y.I. Chemopreventive effects of dietary folate on intestinal polyps in Apc+/-Msh2-/- mice. *Cancer Res.* **2000**, *60*, 3191–3199.

55. Lindzon, G.M.; Medline, A.; Sohn, K.J.; Depeint, F.; Croxford, R.; Kim, Y.I. Effect of folic acid supplementation on the progression of colorectal aberrant crypt foci. *Carcinogenesis* **2009**, *30*, 1536–1543.

56. Kim, Y.I. Will mandatory folic acid fortification prevent or promote cancer? *Am. J. Clin. Nutr.* **2004**, *80*, 1123–1128.

57. Ulrich, C.M.; Potter, J.D. Folate supplementation: Too much of a good thing? *Cancer Epidemiol. Biomark. Prev.* **2006**, *15*, 189–193.

58. Giovannucci, E. Epidemiologic studies of folate and colorectal neoplasia: A review. *J. Nutr.* **2002**, *132*, 2350S–2355S.

59. Kim, Y.I. Role of folate in colon cancer development and progression. *J. Nutr.* **2003**, *133*, 3731S–3739S.

60. Kim, Y.I. Folate: A magic bullet or a double edged sword for colorectal cancer prevention? *Gut* **2006**, *55*, 1387–1389.

61. Kim, Y.I. Folic acid supplementation and cancer risk: Point. *Cancer Epidemiol. Biomark. Prev.* **2008**, *17*, 2220–2225.

62. Wakai, K.; Hirose, K.; Matsuo, K.; Ito, H.; Kuriki, K.; Suzuki, T.; Kato, T.; Hirai, T.; Kanemitsu, Y.; Tajima, K. Dietary risk factors for colon and rectal cancers: A comparative case-control study. *J. Epidemiol.* **2006**, *16*, 125–135.

63. Wei, E.K.; Wolin, K.Y.; Colditz, G.A. Time course of risk factors in cancer etiologyand progression. *J. Clin. Oncol.* **2010**, *28*, 4052–4057.

64. Lee, J.E.; Chan, A.T. Fruit, vegetables, and folate: Cultivating the evidence forcancer prevention. *Gastroenterology* **2011**, *141*, 16–20.

65. Cole, B.F.; Baron, J.A.; Sandler, R.S.; Haile, R.W.; Ahnen, D.J.; Bresalier, R.S.; McKeown-Eyssen, G.; Summers, R.W.; Rothstein, R.I.; Burke, C.A.; *et al.* Folic acid for the prevention ofcolorectal adenomas: A randomized clinical trial. *JAMA* **2007**, *297*, 2351–2359.

66. Logan, R.F.; Grainge, M.J.; Shepherd, V.C.; Armitage, N.C.; Muir, K.R.; ukCAP TrialGroup. Aspirin and folic acid for the prevention of recurrent colorectal adenomas. *Gastroenterology* **2008**, *134*, 29–38.

67. Steluti, J.; Martini, L.A.; Peters, B.S.; Marchioni, D.M. Folate, vitamin B6 and vitamin B12 in adolescence: Serum concentrations, prevalence of inadequate intakes and sources in food. *J. Pediatr.* **2011**, *87*, 43–49.

68. Marchioni, D.M.; Verly, E., Jr.; Steluti, J.; Cesar, C.L.; Fisberg, R.M. Folic acid intake before and after mandatory fortification: A population-based study in São Paulo, Brazil. *Cad. Saude Publica* **2013**, *29*, 2083–2092.

69. Brunacio, K.H.; Verly-Jr, E.; Cesar, C.L.; Fisberg, R.M.; Marchioni, D.M. Use of dietary supplements among inhabitants of the city of São Paulo, Brazil. *Cad. Saude Publica* **2013**, *29*, 1467–1472.

70. Santos, Q.; Sichieri, R.; Marchioni, D.M.; Verly, E. Evaluation of the safety of different doses of folic acid supplements in women in Brazil. *Rev. Saude Publica* **2013**, *47*, 952–957.

# Assessment of Pre-Pregnancy Dietary Intake with a Food Frequency Questionnaire in Alberta Women

Stephanie M. Ramage, Linda J. McCargar, Casey Berglund, Vicki Harber, Rhonda C. Bell and the APrON Study Team

**Abstract:** Purpose: Pre-pregnancy is an under-examined and potentially important time to optimize dietary intake to support fetal growth and development as well as maternal health. The purpose of the study was to determine the extent to which dietary intake reported by non-pregnant women is similar to pre-pregnancy dietary intake reported by pregnant women using the same assessment tool. Methods: The self-administered, semi-quantitative food frequency questionnaire (FFQ) was adapted from the Canadian version of the Diet History Questionnaire, originally developed by the National Cancer Institute in the United States. Pregnant women ($n$ = 98) completed the FFQ which assessed dietary intake for the year prior to pregnancy. Non-pregnant women ($n$ = 103) completed the same FFQ which assessed dietary intake for the previous year. Energy, macronutrients, and key micronutrients: long-chain omega-3 fatty acids, folate, vitamin $B_6$, vitamin $B_{12}$, calcium, vitamin D and iron were examined. Results: Dietary intake between groups; reported with the FFQ; was similar except for saturated fat; *trans* fat; calcium; and alcohol. Pregnant women reported significantly higher intakes of saturated fat; *trans* fat; and calcium and lower intake of alcohol in the year prior to pregnancy compared to non-pregnant women who reported intake in the previous year. Conclusions: Despite limitations; a FFQ may be used to assist with retrospective assessment of pre-pregnancy dietary intake.

Reprinted from *Nutrients*. Cite as: Ramage, S.M.; McCargar, L.J.; Berglund, C.; Harber, V.; Bell, R.C.; the APrON Study Team Assessment of Pre-Pregnancy Dietary Intake with a Food Frequency Questionnaire in Alberta Women. *Nutrients* **2015**, *7*, 6155–6166.

## 1. Introduction

It is well known that dietary intake during pregnancy impacts fetal growth and development as well as maternal health. However, a woman's weight status and dietary intake over the course of her life and particularly before becoming pregnant may also affect fetal growth and development and long-term maternal health [1,2]. Maternal obesity prior to pregnancy has been associated with negative maternal outcomes including increased risk of miscarriage, gestational diabetes, pregnancy-induced hypertension, venous thrombo-embolism, induction of labour, caesarean delivery, excessive gestational weight gain, and post-partum weight retention [3–6]. Pre-pregnancy maternal obesity is also associated with increased risk of poor infant outcomes including fetal macrosomia, childhood obesity and increased risk of diabetes later in life [3,5,6]. Due to its importance for both maternal and infant outcomes, weight status of women prior to pregnancy has been emphasized as a key variable in the United States Institute of Medicine gestational weight gain guidelines published in 2009 [7].

While the effects of pre-pregnancy dietary intake are not well characterized, improvements prior to pregnancy may decrease the risk of poor maternal and fetal outcomes. Maternal nutrition status prior to conception and during the peri-implantation phase is believed to affect embryonic and fetal growth [8]. Recent research from the Nurses' Health Study indicated that increased intake of fried foods prior to pregnancy was associated with increased risk of gestational diabetes even after adjusting for multiple factors including age, body mass index (BMI), family history of diabetes, total energy intake and diet quality [9]. Results from studies in animal models are consistent with these results in humans. For example, an animal model fed a high-fat diet prior to pregnancy demonstrated negative effects in offspring including increased insulin like growth factor 2 receptor mRNA, smaller offspring that undergo catch-up growth, and in males, increased cholesterol, increased percent body fat, and glucose intolerance in later life [10]. Another animal model that utilized a high-fat diet prior to pregnancy found the offspring had increased lipid droplet storage in hepatocytes and increased body weight compared to controls fed standard chow during pre-pregnancy as well as pregnancy and lactation [11]. Liver tissue in offspring also had a unique up-regulation of Acacb and Scd1 gene expression in those mice fed a high-fat diet during the pre-pregnancy period only [11].

In addition to high dietary fat intake, maternal nutrient deficiencies prior to pregnancy have also been linked with fetal developmental defects. The most commonly known defect related to pre-pregnancy nutrition is the increased risk of neural tube defects (NTDs) with low levels of maternal folate [12]. Other nutrient insufficiencies or deficiencies may also be important. One study found that after adjusting for energy intake, low maternal dietary intake of vegetable protein, fibre, beta-carotene, vitamin C, vitamin D, iron and magnesium were linked to an increased risk of orofacial clefts in newborns [13].

Determining an appropriate method of dietary intake assessment during the pre-pregnancy period is important to support future interventions. For example, it has been found that women who received pre-conception advice from a health professional were more likely than other women to make positive behavior changes prior to pregnancy including taking supplementary folic acid and consuming a healthier diet [2]. A pre-pregnancy dietary intake assessment tool that has the potential to track changes could assist in determining the impact of interventions in creating positive diet changes during this critical period. However, recruitment of women before pregnancy is difficult, thus a tool that examines dietary intake retrospectively would be important.

This study was completed as a pilot project to support an ongoing cohort study: Alberta Pregnancy Outcomes and Nutrition (APrON) [14]. The APrON study is exploring the relationship of maternal dietary intake and nutrient status during pregnancy with maternal mental health, birth outcomes and child neurodevelopment up to three years of age. Women were enrolled in the APrON study once they became pregnant, however, as described above, it was important to assess dietary intake prior to pregnancy. The purpose of the study was to determine the extent to which dietary intake reported by non-pregnant women is similar to pre-pregnancy dietary intake reported by pregnant women using the same assessment tool.

## 2. Methods

### 2.1. Participants

Pregnant and non-pregnant women were recruited from Edmonton, Alberta, Canada. For the pregnant group, any woman who was currently pregnant was eligible to participate in the study. There were no restrictions placed on number of weeks gestation. For the non-pregnant group, women who had not been pregnant during the past 12 months and were aged 17–45 years were eligible to participate. We have no information as to whether any of the participants were planning a pregnancy. Women in both groups were excluded if they were unable to speak, read, or write in English.

A sample size of 100 participants in each group was chosen in order to allow for comparison between groups; this sample size has been identified as appropriate for assessment of validity of FFQs [15]. Although this study did not directly assess validity of the FFQ, other aspects of the study beyond the scope of this short report did examine relative validity.

Different recruitment strategies were utilized for the pregnant and non-pregnant groups. Recruitment of pregnant participants was also completed as a pilot test for one of the APrON study recruitment strategies. This was organized in conjunction with the Women and Children's Health Research Institute (WCHRI) at the University of Alberta along with two other studies also recruiting pregnant women. Upon having pregnancy confirmed at a medical clinic, potential participants were asked if they would be interested in participating in pregnancy research. If the individual was interested, her name and telephone number was forwarded to the WCHRI office. Names were randomly assigned between the three studies. Once names and telephone numbers were received from WCHRI, potential participants were called to invite the woman to participate in the study. It was made clear to participants that they would be taking part in a pilot study to test questionnaires for a larger study. Pregnant women in the present study were not APrON participants.

Non-pregnant participants were recruited through a variety of other methods as there was no affiliation with medical clinics to recruit these women. These methods included recruitment tables, posters, advertisements in newsletters and word-of-mouth at a variety of locations including the University of Alberta community and City of Edmonton recreation facilities.

This research was approved by the Health Research Ethics Board at the University of Alberta, Human Research Ethics Study Number Pro00003163. All participants provided informed consent prior to participation.

## 2.2. Demographic Assessment

All participants reported age, height, marital status, parity, ethnicity, chronic illness, education level, employment status, and annual household income. Pregnant participants reported their weight immediately prior to pregnancy, and number of week's gestation. Non-pregnant participants reported their current weight. Body mass index (BMI) was calculated by dividing weight (in kilograms) by height (in metres) squared.

## 2.3. The Food Frequency Questionnaire

The FFQ was adapted from the Canadian version of the Diet History Questionnaire (DHQ) [16] which was originally developed by the National Cancer Institute in the United States [17]. The original DHQ utilized the United States Department of Agriculture (USDA) Nutrient Database for Standard Reference (SR11) [17]. Csizmadi *et al.* [16] adapted the FFQ for use in Canada to reflect differences in Canadian nutrient fortification practices and food availability. The changes made utilized the Canadian Nutrient File 2007b [18] nutrient database for analyses. The FFQ was further adapted for the APrON study to address nutrients of concern prior to pregnancy [8] as well as incorporating culturally appropriate foods. Changes included the addition of foods fortified with omega-3 fatty acids (eggs, juice, margarine, milk, soymilk, and yogurt), an expanded fish section, and more multigrain/flax grain products. Additionally, some questions were re-ordered or combined. The nutrient profiles of additional foods were added using the Canadian Nutrient File 2007b [18].

The FFQ was a self-administered, semi-quantitative, retrospective questionnaire that asked about dietary intake over the 12 months prior to pregnancy for pregnant women or the past 12 months for non-pregnant women. Since women were recruited over an 18 month time frame, and "past 12 months" was used as the time over which diet was reported, differences that occur in dietary intake according to seasonality were minimized [15].

## 2.4. Comparison between Groups

Pregnant and non-pregnant women both completed the same FFQ. All data reported were for food and beverages only, supplements were not included.

Nutrient intakes in pregnant women were compared to nutrient intakes in non-pregnant women. The key nutrients selected for comparison were long-chain omega-3 fatty acids, folate, vitamin $B_6$, vitamin $B_{12}$, calcium, vitamin D and iron. In addition, total energy and macronutrient intake (carbohydrate, protein, and fat) were compared between groups.

## 2.5. Data Entry

Responses to all FFQs were double-entered into a key-punch program utilizing Microsoft Excel® (Excel version 2007) to ensure accuracy.

## 2.6. Statistical Analysis

Assessment for outliers for FFQ data was completed based on unrealistic reported energy intakes of <600 kcal or >3500 kcal per day, as recommended by Csizmadi *et al.* [16]. Independent samples *t*-tests were used to compare differences between groups for continuous demographic variables while chi square analysis and Fisher's exact test were used to examine the differences in categorical demographics between groups. Independent samples *t*-tests were used to compare mean intake between groups of the key nutrients measured by the FFQ.

Analyses were performed using SPSS (version 18.0, SPSS Inc, Chicago, IL, USA) except for demographic variables: parity, education level, household income and BMI classification where STATA (version 10, StataCorp LP, College Station, TX, USA) was used.

## 3. Results

### 3.1. Participant Information

Overall, 98 pregnant women and 103 non-pregnant women completed the study. Nine participants (seven pregnant and two non-pregnant) were excluded from all analyses on the basis of unrealistic energy intake reported on the FFQ [16]. Participant demographic information is described in Table 1. Compared to the non-pregnant women, the women in the pregnant group were more likely to have a higher pre-pregnancy BMI ($p = 0.003$), be married ($p < 0.001$), have more children ($p = 0.005$), be employed ($p = 0.025$), and have a higher household income ($p < 0.001$).

There were no significant differences found between groups for age, ethnicity, chronic illness, or level of education.

## 3.2. FFQ Nutrient Intake Comparison between Groups

Energy, macronutrient, and key micronutrient intakes are shown in Table 2. The pregnant women reported a significantly higher mean intake of saturated fat (SFA) ($p < 0.05$), *trans* fat ($p < 0.01$), and calcium ($p < 0.05$) compared to the non-pregnant group. The non-pregnant women reported a significantly higher mean intake of alcohol ($p < 0.05$). Intakes of energy and all other macronutrients and key micronutrients were similar between groups.

**Table 1.** Participant Demographic Characteristics.

| | Pregnant (*n* = 91) | Non-Pregnant (*n* = 101) | *p* value |
|---|---|---|---|
| | Mean (SD) [a] | | |
| Age (years) | 30.8 ± 5.0 | 29.1 ± 7.7 | 0.072 |
| Weeks Gestation | 31.0 ± 8.2 | N/A | N/A |
| Body Mass Index (BMI) (kg/m²) | 25.1 ± 6.7 | 22.8 ± 3.1 | 0.003 ** |
| | (%) [b] | | |
| **Marital Status** | | | <0.001 ** |
| Married/Common Law | 97% | 51% | |
| Single/Divorced/Other | 3% | 49% | |
| **Parity** | | | 0.005 * |
| 0 | 53% | 68% | |
| 1 | 32% | 13% | |
| 2 or more | 15% | 19% | |
| **Ethnicity** | | | 0.293 |
| Caucasian | 77% | 83% | |
| Other | 23% | 17% | |
| **Chronic Illness** | | | 0.620 |
| No | 80% | 83% | |
| Yes | 20% | 17% | |
| **Education Level** | | | 0.616 |
| High school graduate or less | 7% | 4% | |
| Some college or university | 16% | 20% | |
| College or university degree or above | 77% | 76% | |
| **Employment Status** | | | 0.025 * |
| Employed/Self-Employed | 70% | 55% | |
| Unemployed [c] | 30% | 45% | |
| **Annual Household Income** | | | <0.001 ** |
| <$30,000 | 3% | 35% | |
| $30,000–59,000 | 18% | 23% | |
| >$60,000 | 79% | 42% | |

\* *p*-Value significant at $p < 0.05$ level; \*\* *p*-value significant at $p < 0.01$ level; [a] *t*-test for independent samples; [b] Chi square analysis (marital status, ethnicity, chronic illness, employment status) or Fisher's Exact Test (parity, education, income, BMI) as appropriate; [c] Included students, homemakers, unemployed or other. Abbreviations: BMI (body mass index), kg (kilograms), m (metres), SD (standard deviation).

**Table 2.** Comparison between Groups of Energy and Nutrient Intake Measured by FFQ.

| Nutrient | Pregnant [a] (n = 91) (mean ± SD) | Non-Pregnant [b] (n = 101) (mean ± SD) | p-value |
|---|---|---|---|
| Energy (kcal) | 1927 ± 537 | 1869 ± 529 | 0.456 |
| Carbohydrate (g) | 261.8 ± 82.2 | 246.9 ± 78.9 | 0.204 |
| Fibre (g) | 22.2 ± 9.2 | 24.1 ± 10.2 | 0.169 |
| Protein (g) | 77.6 ± 25.6 | 77.3 ± 26.2 | 0.958 |
| Fat (g) | 67.6 ± 22.1 | 66.1 ± 25.2 | 0.660 |
| Saturated Fat (g) | 22.1 ± 8.6 | 19.6 ± 8.1 | 0.039 * |
| MUFA (g) | 26.6 ± 9.8 | 27.1 ± 12.0 | 0.733 |
| PUFA (g) | 13.1 ± 4.7 | 13.5 ± 5.8 | 0.527 |
| ALA (g) | 1.8 ± 0.8 | 1.7 ± 0.7 | 0.265 |
| EPA/DHA (g) | 0.14 ± 0.13 | 0.17 ± 0.21 | 0.246 |
| *Trans* Fat (g) | 3.5 ± 1.4 | 2.9 ± 1.4 | 0.007 ** |
| Cholesterol (mg) | 200.6 ± 75.6 | 182.7 ± 82.7 | 0.120 |
| Alcohol (g) | 3.7 ± 4.9 | 5.6 ± 7.3 | 0.043 * |
| Folate (µg) | 369 ± 124 | 392 ± 148 | 0.250 |
| Vitamin $B_6$ (mg) | 2.1 ± 0.8 | 2.1 ± 0.8 | 0.856 |
| Vitamin $B_{12}$ (µg) | 5.1 ± 2.3 | 5.0 ± 2.3 | 0.802 |
| Calcium (mg) | 1146 ± 556 | 988 ± 408 | 0.026 * |
| Vitamin D (µg) | 5.8 ± 3.5 | 5.2 ± 3.2 | 0.204 |
| Iron (mg) | 15.3 ± 5.0 | 16.4 ± 6.0 | 0.193 |

* Independent samples *t*-test significant at $p < 0.05$ level; ** Independent samples *t*-test significant at $p < 0.01$ level. [a] Energy and macronutrient intake for the year prior to becoming pregnant; [b] Energy and macronutrient intake for the past year. Abbreviations: FFQ (food frequency questionnaire), kcal (kilocalories), g (grams), mg (milligrams), µg (micrograms), SD (standard deviation), MUFA (monounsaturated fat), PUFA (polyunsaturated fat), ALA (alpha-linolenic acid), EPA/DHA (Eicosapentaenoic acid/Docosahexaenoic acid).

## 4. Discussion

A novel comparison between groups was used in this study to approach the question of whether or not food intake measured by the FFQ was similar between pregnant women reporting intake in the year prior to pregnancy and non-pregnant women reporting intake for the past year. It appeared that there were some differences between groups in dietary intake, however, it is not known whether these differences were due to actual differences in food intake between groups or differences in recall bias between groups. It is not a traditional assessment of the relative validity of a dietary intake tool whereby a tool is compared to a gold standard or secondary method. Assessment of relative validity in this population is difficult. Many studies have examined the relationship between FFQs and alternate methods of diet assessment utilizing a variety of populations, sample sizes, FFQs, reference time periods, and reference diet assessment methods [19]. In general, FFQs are typically believed to overestimate nutrient intake although it may be that some overestimate intake more than others or even underestimate intake [13,20,21].

Overall, the FFQ provided a similar estimate of energy, macronutrients and key micronutrients: folate, vitamin $B_6$, vitamin $B_{12}$, vitamin D and iron between groups. However, saturated fat, *trans* fat, and calcium intakes were reported as significantly higher, and alcohol intake was reported as significantly lower in the pregnant group recalling the year prior to pregnancy compared to the non-pregnant group recalling the past year. Reasons for these differences could be multi-fold but cannot be completely discerned in this study. It is possible that: (1) if planning a pregnancy, some women may have made dietary changes in the year prior to becoming pregnant. For example, a woman planning a pregnancy may decrease or eliminate intake of alcoholic beverages and increase consumption of other beverages, such as milk. The mean difference in calcium intake between groups was 158 mg which is approximately the amount of calcium in half a cup of milk [18]. Saturated and *trans* fats may also be present in milk although in varying amounts depending on the type of milk. Thus even if some of the pregnant women changed their beverage consumption as a result of planning pregnancy, intake of these nutrients may have been higher. (2) There may have been increased recall bias among the pregnant women such that they perceived a "healthier" diet in the year prior to pregnancy. Some research supports the idea that women intending pregnancy make positive behaviour changes including higher levels of physical activity and lower smoking rates compared with non-pregnant women [22], lower alcohol intake [23] and taking a multivitamin [24] and/or folic acid supplement [22,23,25]. In contrast, other pre-conception research indicates that women who are planning a pregnancy do not differ greatly from other non-pregnant women with respect to health behaviours such as alcohol use [22,24,25], smoking [23,25], fruit and vegetable consumption [23,25] and physical activity [25]. There may have been differences between groups in usual intake irrespective of whether the pregnancy was planned or not. In the present study, data on whether the pregnancy was planned was not collected so a definitive statement on this issue cannot be made.

Pre-pregnancy dietary intakes in this study were somewhat similar to pre-pregnancy intake reported by pregnant women in Portugal [26] and the Netherlands [13,20]. Women in the present study were observed to have lower energy intake [20,26], lower fat intake [13], higher vitamin D and lower vitamin $B_{12}$ [26]. However, these studies used different FFQs, examined women who were planning a pregnancy or not [20], and were administered at different time points, such as during the first trimester [26] or after delivery [13], which makes direct comparison difficult.

The primary limitation of this study was that neither FFQs nor any other diet assessment tool is considered a gold standard. A FFQ was chosen because it was the only tool that could retrospectively assess nutrient intake prior to pregnancy. The reality of recruitment procedures for the APrON study as well as the fact that many pregnancies are unplanned [27] limited the method to retrospective assessment. In addition to retrospective assessment, there are other times when FFQs are the appropriate choice for diet assessment. For example, a FFQ may more accurately measure nutrients with sporadic intake as opposed to daily intake. In this case a 24 h recall may miss intake of these nutrients. As such, long-chain omega-3 fatty acid intake may be best measured by FFQ as foods containing high levels of long-chain omega-3 fatty acids (*i.e.*, fatty fish) are typically not eaten on a daily basis in Canada [28].

Another limitation was that the pregnant women were recalling a 12 month period that was approximately seven to eight months prior (*i.e.*, before they were pregnant) as opposed to the non-pregnant women who were simply recalling the past 12 months. In addition, there was variation in the point of gestation of the pregnant women which resulted in some women having to recall a period that was longer than others. The extent to which habitual dietary recall is affected by these differences in time to recall is difficult to quantify. The fact that a FFQ is meant to capture habitual dietary intake may lessen the impact of these differences in recall period.

One of the strengths of the study, was that recruitment took place over approximately 18 months which would minimize the effect of seasonality on reporting food intake. Additionally, in terms of the FFQ, was that every effort was made to update the food list to include new fortified foods as well as an improved variety of foods. However, a weakness of FFQs in general is that they continually need updating to reflect changes in the food supply.

In addition, there were significant differences in the demographic characteristics of the two groups. This may have augmented the differences observed when comparing the FFQ between groups. For example, the significantly lower BMI of non-pregnant women compared to pregnant women may indicate differences in dietary intake patterns between groups.

Future research on this tool should include comparison against a reference tool with multiple days of dietary intake in order to generate stronger conclusions regarding the relative validity of the FFQ. In the future, it would also be important to collect whether the pregnancy was planned or not.

## 5. Conclusions

This is the first time to the researchers' knowledge, that the assessment of a pre-pregnancy dietary assessment tool has been completed. The FFQ has a role in dietary assessment of the pre-pregnancy time period as it is a critical period but is difficult to assess.

The FFQ provided a similar estimate of dietary intake between pre-pregnant and non-pregnant groups for energy, macronutrients, and key micronutrients long-chain omega-3 fatty acids, folate, vitamin $B_6$, vitamin $B_{12}$, vitamin D and iron. With the data collected in the current study, it is not possible to state that the FFQ is relatively valid. However, there is also insufficient evidence to state that the FFQ is invalid. The FFQ is currently being used in the Alberta Pregnancy Outcomes and Nutrition (APrON) cohort study. The APrON study sample size will be very large and it is expected that at the group level, the large sample size will assist with removing some of the variability in intake measured by the FFQ. However, considering the limitations of the tool and the populations recruited in this study, it is essential that data from this questionnaire be interpreted and utilized with caution.

**Acknowledgments:** We are extremely grateful to all the families who took part in this study and the whole APrON team (http://www.apronstudy.ca/), investigators, research assistants, graduate and undergraduate students, volunteers, clerical staff and managers. This cohort was established by an interdisciplinary team grant from the Alberta Heritage Foundation for Medical Research (now Alberta Innovates Health Solutions) and additional funding from the Faculty of Agricultural Life and Environmental Sciences Vitamin Grant at the University of Alberta. Personal funding (for SR) was provided by the Dr. Elizabeth A. Donald MSc Fellowship in Human Nutrition. The individual members of the APrON research team are Nicole Letourneau, Catherine J. Field, Deborah Dewey, Rhonda C. Bell, Francois P. Bernier, Marja Cantell, Linda M. Casey, Misha Eliasziw, Anna Farmer, Lisa Gagnon, Gerald F. Giesbrecht, Laki Goonewardene, David W. Johnston, Bonnie J. Kaplan, Libbe Kooistra, Nicole Letourneau, Donna P. Manca, Jonathan W. Martin, Linda J. McCargar, Maeve O'Beirne, Victor J. Pop, Nalini Singhal.

**Author Contributions:** R.B. and C.B. conceived and designed the experiments; S.R. performed the studies, analyzed the data and wrote the paper; R.B., L.M. and V.H. contributed to data interpretation, and reviewed and edited the manuscript. All authors approved the final version of the manuscript.

**Conflicts of Interest:** The authors declare no conflict of interest.

## References

1. Kind, K.L.; Moore, V.M.; Davies, M.J. Diet around conception and during Pregnancy—Effects on fetal and neonatal outcomes. *Reprod. Biomed. Online* **2006**, *12*, 532–541.

2. Stephenson, J.; Patel, D.; Barrett, G.; Howden, B.; Copas, A.; Ojukwu, O.; Pandya, P.; Shawe, J. How do women prepare for pregnancy? Preconception experiences of women attending antenatal services and views of health professionals. *PLoS ONE* **2014**, *9*, e103085.

3. Guelinckx, I.; Devlieger, R.; Beckers, K.; Vansant, G. Maternal obesity: Pregnancy complications, gestational weight gain and nutrition. *Obes. Rev.* **2008**, *9*, 140–150.

4. Mehta, S. Nutrition and pregnancy. *Clin. Obstet. Gynecol.* **2008**, *51*, 409–418.

5. Melzer, K.; Schutz, Y. Pre-pregnancy and pregnancy predictors of obesity. *Int. J. Obes. (Lond)* **2010**, *34* (Suppl. 2), S44–S52.

6. Montpetit, A.E.; Plourde, H.; Cohen, T.R.; Koski, K.G. Modeling the impact of prepregnancy BMI, physical activity, and energy intake on gestational weight gain, infant birth weight, and postpartum weight retention. *J. Phys. Act. Health* **2012**, *9*, 1020–1029.

7. Institute of Medicine (US); National Research Council (US). *Committee to Reexamine IOM Pregnancy Weight Guidelines*; National Academies Press: Washington, DC, USA, 2009.

8. Gardiner, P.M.; Nelson, L.; Shellhaas, C.S.; Dunlop, A.L.; Long, R.; Andrist, S.; Jack, B.W. The clinical content of preconception care: Nutrition and dietary supplements. *Am. J. Obstet. Gynecol.* **2008**, *199*, S345–S356.

9. Bao, W.; Tobias, D.K.; Olsen, S.F.; Zhang, C. Pre-pregnancy fried food consumption and the risk of gestational diabetes mellitus: A prospective cohort study. *Diabetologia* **2014**, *57*, 2485–2491.

10. Jungheim, E.S.; Schoeller, E.L.; Marquard, K.L.; Louden, E.D.; Schaffer, J.E.; Moley, K.H. Diet-induced obesity model: Abnormal oocytes and persistent growth abnormalities in the offspring. *Endocrinology* **2010**, *151*, 4039–4046.

11. Hori, H.; Umezawa, M.; Uchiyama, M.; Niki, R.; Yanagita, S.; Takeda, K. Effect of high-fat diet prior to pregnancy on hepatic gene expression and histology in mouse offspring. *J. Perinat. Med.* **2014**, *42*, 83–91.

12. De Wals, P.; Tairou, F.; van Allen, M.I.; Uh, S.; Lowry, R.B.; Sibbald, B.; Evans, J.A.; van, D.H.; Zimmer, P.; Crowley, M.; *et al.* Reduction in neural-tube defects after folic acid fortification in Canada. *N. Engl. J. Med.* **2007**, *357*, 135–142.

13. Krapels, I.P.; van Rooij, I.A.; Ocke, M.C.; West, C.E.; van der Horst, C.M.; Steegers-Theunissen, R.P. Maternal nutritional status and the risk for orofacial cleft offspring in humans. *J. Nutr.* **2004**, *134*, 3106–3113.

14. Kaplan, B.J.; Giesbrecht, G.F.; Leung, B.M.; Field, C.J.; Dewey, D.; Bell, R.C.; Manca, D.P.; O'Beirne, M.; Johnston, D.W.; Pop, V.J.; *et al.* The Alberta pregnancy outcomes and nutrition (APrON) cohort study: Rationale and methods. *Matern. Child. Nutr.* **2014**, *10*, 44–60.

15. Serra-Majem, L.; Frost Andersen, L.; Henrique-Sanchez, P.; Doreste-Alonso, J.; Sanchez-Villegas, A.; Ortiz-Andrelluchi, A.; Negri, E.; La Vecchia, C. Evaluating the quality of dietary intake validation studies. *Br. J. Nutr.* **2009**, *102*, S3–S9.

16. Csizmadi, I.; Kahle, L.; Ullman, R.; Dawe, U.; Zimmerman, T.P.; Friedenreich, C.M.; Bryant, H.; Subar, A.F. Adaptation and evaluation of the National Cancer Institute's diet history questionnaire and nutrient database for Canadian populations. *Public Health Nutr.* **2007**, *10*, 88–96.

17. Subar, A.F.; Thompson, F.E.; Kipnis, V.; Midthune, D.; Hurwitz, P.; McNutt, S.; McIntosh, A.; Rosenfeld, S. Comparative validation of the block, willett, and National Cancer Institute food frequency questionnaires: The eating at America's table study. *Am. J. Epidemiol.* **2001**, *154*, 1089–1099.

18. Health Canada. *Canadian Nutrient File, 2007b Version*; Health Canada: Ottawa, Canada, 2007.

19. Molag, M.L.; de Vries, J.H.; Ocke, M.C.; Dagnelie, P.C.; van den Brandt, P.A.; Jansen, M.C.; van Staveren, W.A.; van't Veer, P. Design characteristics of food frequency questionnaires in relation to their validity. *Am. J. Epidemiol.* **2007**, *166*, 1468–1478.

20. De Weerd, S.; Steegers, E.A.; Heinen, M.M.; van den Eertwegh, S.; Vehof, R.M.; Steegers-Theunissen, R.P. Preconception nutritional intake and lifestyle factors: First results of an explorative study. *Eur. J. Obstet. Gynecol. Reprod. Biol.* **2003**, *111*, 167–172.

21. Subar, A.F.; Kipnis, V.; Troiano, R.P.; Midthune, D.; Schoeller, D.A.; Bingham, S.; Sharbaugh, C.O.; Trabulsi, J.; Runswick, S.; Ballard-Barbash, R.; *et al.* Using intake biomarkers to evaluate the extent of dietary misreporting in a large sample of adults: The OPEN study. *Am. J. Epidemiol.* **2003**, *158*, 1–13.

22. Xaverius, P.K.; Tenkku, L.E.; Salas, J.; Morris, D. Exploring health by reproductive status: An epidemiological analysis of preconception health. *J. Womens Health (Larchmt)* **2009**, *18*, 49–56.

23. Inskip, H.M.; Crozier, S.R.; Godfrey, K.M.; Borland, S.E.; Cooper, C.; Robinson, S.M.; Southampton Women's Survey Study Group. Women's compliance with nutrition and lifestyle recommendations before pregnancy: General population cohort study. *BMJ* **2009**, *338*, b481.

24. Green-Raleigh, K.; Lawrence, J.M.; Chen, H.; Devine, O.; Prue, C. Pregnancy planning status and health behaviors among nonpregnant women in a California managed health care organization. *Perspect. Sex. Reprod. Health* **2005**, *37*, 179–183.

25. Chuang, C.H.; Weisman, C.S.; Hillemeier, M.M.; Schwarz, E.B.; Camacho, F.T.; Dyer, A.M. Pregnancy intention and health behaviors: Results from the Central Pennsylvania Women's Health Study Cohort. *Matern. Child Health J.* **2010**, *14*, 501–510.

26. Pinto, E.; Barros, H.; dos Santos Silva, I. Dietary intake and nutritional adequacy prior to conception and during pregnancy: A follow-up study in the north of Portugal. *Public Health Nutr.* **2009**, *12*, 922–931.

27. Wilson, R.D.; Johnson, J.A.; Wyatt, P.; Allen, V.; Gagnon, A.; Langlois, S.; Blight, C.; Audibert, F.; Desilets, V.; Brock, J.A.; *et al.* Pre-conceptional vitamin/folic acid supplementation 2007: The use of folic acid in combination with a multivitamin supplement for the prevention of neural tube defects and other congenital anomalies. *J. Obstet. Gynaecol. Can.* **2007**, *29*, 1003–1026.

28. Innis, S.M.; Elias, S.L. Intakes of essential N-6 and N-3 polyunsaturated fatty acids among pregnant Canadian women. *Am. J. Clin. Nutr.* **2003**, *77*, 473–478.

# Estimated Daily Intake and Seasonal Food Sources of Quercetin in Japan

Haruno Nishimuro, Hirofumi Ohnishi, Midori Sato,
Mayumi Ohnishi-Kameyama, Izumi Matsunaga, Shigehiro Naito,
Katsunari Ippoushi, Hideaki Oike, Tadahiro Nagata, Hiroshi Akasaka,
Shigeyuki Saitoh, Kazuaki Shimamoto and Masuko Kobori

**Abstract:** Quercetin is a promising food component, which can prevent lifestyle related diseases. To understand the dietary intake of quercetin in the subjects of a population-based cohort study and in the Japanese population, we first determined the quercetin content in foods available in the market during June and July in or near a town in Hokkaido, Japan. Red leaf lettuce, asparagus, and onions contained high amounts of quercetin derivatives. We then estimated the daily quercetin intake by 570 residents aged 20–92 years old in the town using a food frequency questionnaire (FFQ). The average and median quercetin intakes were 16.2 and 15.5 mg day$^{-1}$, respectively. The quercetin intakes by men were lower than those by women; the quercetin intakes showed a low correlation with age in both men and women. The estimated quercetin intake was similar during summer and winter. Quercetin was mainly ingested from onions and green tea, both in summer and in winter. Vegetables, such as asparagus, green pepper, tomatoes, and red leaf lettuce, were good sources of quercetin in summer. Our results will help to elucidate the association between quercetin intake and risks of lifestyle-related diseases by further prospective cohort study and establish healthy dietary requirements with the consumption of more physiologically useful components from foods.

Reprinted from *Nutrients*.   Cite as: Nishimuro, H.; Ohnishi, H.; Sato, M.; Ohnishi-Kameyama, M.; Matsunaga, I.; Naito, S.; Ippoushi, K.; Oike, H.; Nagata, T.; Akasaka, H.; Saitoh, S.; Shimamoto, K.; Kobori, M. Estimated Daily Intake and Seasonal Food Sources of Quercetin in Japan. *Nutrients* **2015**, *7*, 2345–2358.

## 1. Introduction

Epidemiological studies have suggested that flavonoids, including quercetin, have a protective effect against cardiovascular diseases, cancers, and other chronic diseases [1–7]. Quercetin is a flavonol that is ubiquitously found in vegetables, fruits, and tea, as the glycosides [6,8]. The antioxidant activity [9–11], the anti-inflammatory effect [12], and/or other molecular mechanisms may prevent lifestyle-related diseases. Our previous study showed that a diet containing quercetin alleviated streptozotocin-induced diabetic symptoms in mice [13]. Quercetin was suggested to recover functions in both the liver and pancreas through oxidative stress reduction and the blockade of cyclin-dependent kinase inhibitor *p21(WAF1/Cip1)* (*Cdkn1a*) expression. Moreover, the consumption of a quercetin-rich diet alleviated obesity, hyperglycemia, hyperinsulinemia, and dyslipidemia in C57BL/6J mice that were fed a Western diet that was rich in fat, cholesterol, and sucrose [14]. Quercetin decreased oxidative stress and reducing peroxisome proliferator-activated receptor α expression that subsequently reduced the expression of genes related to steatosis in the liver. Recently, Dong *et al.* reported that quercetin suggested to suppress obesity-associated macrophage infiltration and inflammation through the adenosine monophosphate-activated protein kinase α1/silent information regulator 1 pathway in mice fed a high-fat diet [15].

Quercetin glycosides are mostly hydrolyzed and absorbed from the small or large intestines [6,8]. The physiological functions utilize the conjugated metabolites of quercetin in the plasma or other tissues, or the deconjugated aglycone in the specific tissues [8,16,17]. The intake of quercetin from dietary sources or supplements increases the plasma quercetin concentration [6]. Cao *et al.* reported that the mean intake over seven days of five flavonoids, including quercetin, was positively correlated to their corresponding plasma concentrations [18]. Ioku *et al.* showed that the quercetin glucoside content in onions did not decrease after frying or microwave heating [19]. Quercetin-4'-glucoside in onions was shown to transfer to the water during boiling without decomposition [19]. Thus, it is likely that the daily intake of food rich in quercetin increases the bioavailability of quercetin and contributes to the prevention of lifestyle-related diseases.

Sapporo Medical University has conducted a longitudinal population-based cohort study in the Tanno and Sobetsu area in Hokkaido. In the Tanno and Sobetsu study, central obesity assessed by waist circumference is shown to be useful for assessing the risk of type 2 diabetes [20]. Moreover, parental hypertension is shown to have an age-independent impact on the elevation of blood pressure, plasma glucose, and triglyceride levels, which may underlie the increase in cardiovascular events due to family history of hypertension [21]. Precise estimation of quercetin intake by subjects in the cohort study will help elucidate the relationship between quercetin intake and health indexes or risks of lifestyle related diseases. Sobetsu town is in an agricultural region and the major industry is fruit growing such as apples and cherries. The quercetin content of plant foods differs depending on the cultivars or cultivation conditions [22,23]. Therefore, in this study, to make a precise estimate of quercetin intake in the local residents, we first determined the quercetin content of the foods available in the markets in the Sobetsu area; we then estimated the daily quercetin intake by the residents in the Sobetsu town using a food frequency questionnaire (FFQ).

## 2. Experimental Section

### 2.1. Materials

One to three bags or bunches (approximately 0.2–1 kg bag$^{-1}$ or bunch) of commonly eaten vegetables and fruits were obtained from three major farmer's markets and the representative supermarket in the Sobetsu area (Sobetsu town, Toya town and Date city) during June, July, and December in 2013. Different bags or bunches of the same food were produced by the different farms. Autumn-planted onions grown on the main island and spring-planted onions grown in Hokkaido were available during summer and winter, respectively. Therefore, we determined the quercetin contents of onions and other vegetables and fruits commonly eaten in winter. The fruits and vegetables, except onions obtained in July, red leaf lettuce obtained in July, asupara-ra, and Chinese cabbage, were grown in the Sobetsu area. The edible parts, which were defined in the "Standard Tables of Food Composition in Japan (Fifth revised and enlarged editions)," in a bag or bunch were combined and reduced by sample division. Approximately 100–200 g of each food sample was frozen with liquid nitrogen, lyophilized, powdered in a grinder, and stored at −30 °C until the analysis. Approximately 150 g and 250 g of asparagus were cooked by boiling before the lyophilization respectively. Onions (200 g × 2) and green peppers (100 g × 2) were cooked by stirring before the lyophilization respectively. Green tea (200 g) and dried buckwheat noodles (400 g) were obtained from the representative supermarket in the Sobetsu area. Four grams of green tea leaves were infused twice with 100 mL of 80 °C water for 1 min. The green tea infusion was lyophilized, powdered, and then stored at −30 °C until the analysis. The dried buckwheat noodles were cooked by boiling before the lyophilization.

### 2.2. Determination of Quercetin Content

The quercetin content of each food sample was quantified by a high-performance liquid chromatography (HPLC) using the validated method of Watanabe et al. [24]. Briefly, quercetin aglycone was extracted from 200 mg of a freeze-dried food sample by hydrolysis with 12 mL of HCl solution (ethanol/water/HCl, 50:20:8, v/v/v) at 90 °C for 60 min, while shaking the sample solutions every 15 min. Five mL of green tea infusion was hydrolyzed with 12.5 mL of ethanol and 2 mL of HCl at 90 °C for 60 min. Each extract of vegetables, fruits, and tea was increased to 25 mL with methanol. Fifteen mL of each sample was filtered through a 0.45 μm polyvinylidene fluoride (PVDF) membrane filter prior to the HPLC analysis.

A Shimadzu HPLC Prominence that contained a degasser (DGU-20A3), binary pump (LC-20AB), auto-sampler (SIL-20AC), column oven (CTO-20A), and photodiode array detector (SPD-M20A) was used as the HPLC system. Ten microliter of each hydrolyzed food sample was applied to the HPLC column (Prodigy ODS (3),

5 µm, 100 A, 4.6 × 250 mm (Phenomenex, Torrance, CA, USA; Part No.00G-4097-E0)) and eluted with methanol/0.85% phosphoric acid (1:1, v/v) at a flow rate of 1.0 mL min$^{-1}$ at 35 °C. The spectra were recorded from 200 nm to 500 nm, and quercetin was measured at 370 nm.

All food samples were determined in triplicate.

Quercetin content of foods are shown in Table 1. The quercetin content of cooked asparagus by boiling was 23.1 mg (100 g)$^{-1}$ fresh weight. The quercetin contents of sautéed onions and green peppers were 7.7 and 7.5 mg per 100g fresh weight, respectively. The quercetin contents were slightly decreased by stir-frying. Among the foods we evaluated, spring-planted onions obtained in winter showed the highest quercetin content. The quercetin contents were less than the detection limit (0.07 mg g$^{-1}$ of dry weight) in green and red shiso (*Perilla frutescens*), eggplants, welsh onions, cabbages, spinach, potatoes, buckwheat noodles, garland chrysanthemum, and Chinese cabbages.

### 2.3. Diet Survey

Sapporo Medical University has been conducting a cohort study called "The Tanno-Sobetsu study" since 1977. In the Tanno-Sobetsu Study, residents of two towns, Tanno and Sobetsu, in Hokkaido, Japan were recruited for annual medical examinations, including standard blood and urine tests. We recruited the study participants in the cohort of Sobetsu town. Sobetsu town is a rural area located in the island of "Hokkaido" in the north of Japan. Most participants in this cohort were middle-aged and elderly people and their life-style, obesity prevalence, blood pressure, blood glucose and lipid levels were similar to those in the results of national survey in Japan. Therefore, this cohort is considered to represent general Japanese population.

Two-day weighed food records (weight, servings, and portion size of food intake) were completed by eight volunteer housewives in July 2013. The FFQ, which asked about the frequency and portion size for 15 food items (onion, spinach, broccoli, potato, green pepper, asparagus, tomato, cherry tomato, cabbage, eggplant, red leaf lettuce, shiso (*Perilla frutescens*), cherry, buckwheat noodles, and green tea) was recorded by 570 residents aged 20–93 years; trained dieticians checked the information through interviews during July–August 2013. A FFQ which asked about the frequency and portion size for 14 food items (onion, spinach, broccoli, potato, green pepper, asparagus, tomato, cherry tomato, Chinese cabbage, garland chrysanthemum, red leaf lettuce, apples, buckwheat noodles, and green tea) was recorded by 60 residents aged 41–91 years; trained dieticians checked the responses through interviews in December 2013 in the same manner. The subjects were informed of the objective of the study and agreed to participate. The study design was approved by the Ethical Committee in Sapporo Medical University.

The intake of quercetin was estimated by the calculations of the food intakes and the quercetin content.

**Table 1.** Quercetin content in commonly-eaten foods in Japan.

| Acquisition period | Food | Quercetin content (mg 100 g$^{-1}$ FW or mg (100 mL)$^{-1}$ *) |
|---|---|---|
| June–July 2013 | Red leaf lettuce (*Lactuca sativa* L. var. *crispa*) | 30.6 |
| | Asparagus (*Asparagus officinalis* L.) | 23.6 |
| | Romaine lettuce (*Lactuca sativa* L. var. *longifolia*) | 12.0 |
| | Onion (*Allium cepa* L.) | 11.0 |
| | Green pepper (*Capsicum annuum* L.) | 9.9 |
| | Asupara-na (Brassica rapa) | 4.3 |
| | Cherry tomato (*Solanum lycopersicum*) | 3.3 |
| | Podded pea (*Pisum sativu* L.) | 1.7 |
| | Tomato (*Solanum lycopersicum*) | 1.6 |
| | Broccoli (*Brassica oleracea* var. *italica*) | 1.6 |
| | Cherry (*Prunus avium* L.) | 1.2 |
| | Green tea infusion | 2.1* |
| | Welsh onion (*Allium fistulosum* L.) | N.D. |
| | Spinach (*Spinacia oleracea* L.) | N.D. |
| | Potato (*Solanum tuberosum* L.) | N.D. |
| | Red shiso[1] (*Perilla frutescent* var. *crispa*) | N.D. |
| | Green shiso[2] (*Perilla frutescent* var. *crispa*) | N.D. |
| | Eggplant (*Solanum melongena* L.) | N.D. |
| | Cabbage (*Brassica oleracea* L. var. *capitata*) | N.D. |
| | Dried buckwheat nudles (boiled) | N.D. |
| December 2013 | Onion (*Allium cepa* L.) | 41.9 |
| | Red leaf lettuce (*Lactuca sativa* L. var. *crispa*) | 10.3 |
| | Apple (Fuji) (*Malus domestica* Borkh.) | 2.3 |
| | Broccoli (*Brassica oleracea* var. *italica*) | 0.5 |
| | Spinach (*Spinacia oleracea* L.) | N.D. |
| | Garland chrysanthemum (*Glebionis coronaria*) | N.D. |
| | Chinese cabbage (*Brassica rapa* var. *pekinensis*) | N.D. |

N.D., not detected; FW, fresh weight. [1] *Perilla frutescens* var. *crispa* f. *crispa*. [2] *Perilla frutescens* var. *crispa* f. *purpurea*. Each food item was purchased 1–3 times and each sample was determined in triplicate. Values are expressed as mean of 1–3 samples.

### 2.4. Statistical Analysis

The statistical analyses were performed using GraphPad Prism 5 for Windows Ver. 5.04 (GraphPad Software, San Diego, CA, USA). The significance of the differences between groups was determined by the Mann–Whitney U test. We applied square root transformation to the daily quercetin intakes, which did not have a normal distribution, before assessing the correlation between quercetin intake and age. The association was established by the Pearson rank correlation test. A $p$ value of <0.05 was considered statistically significant.

# 3. Results

## 3.1. Estimated Dietary Quercetin Intakes by Female Volunteers Using Two-Day Weighted Food Record

Two-day weighed food records were completed by eight volunteer housewives in Sobetsu town in Hokkaido in July 2013. Quercetin intake was estimated using the quercetin contents of foods obtained during June and July 2013. The estimated quercetin and vegetable intakes of each subject are shown in Figure 1a. The estimated daily vegetable intakes and quercetin intakes were 187–573 g day$^{-1}$ and 12.6–49.9 mg day$^{-1}$, respectively. The daily intake of quercetin was higher in subjects who consumed a large amount of vegetables. The average intake of vegetables and quercetin was 381 g day$^{-1}$ and 21.5 mg day$^{-1}$, respectively. The major sources of quercetin were onions, asparagus, green peppers, green tea, and tomatoes (Figure 1b).

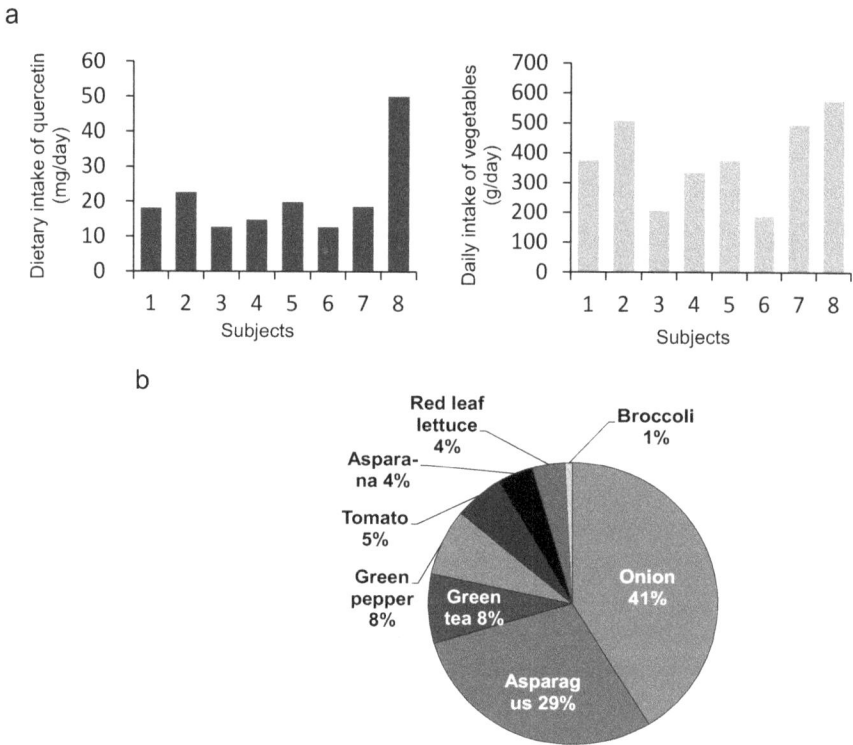

**Figure 1.** (**a**) Estimated intakes of quercetin and vegetables using two-day weighed food records of female volunteers. (**b**) Percentage contribution of foods to daily quercetin intake by the volunteers.

## 3.2. Estimated Daily Quercetin Intakes of Residents by FFQ

The FFQ, which asked about the frequency and portion size of 15 commonly-eaten and quercetin-rich foods, was then completed by 570 residents of Sobetsu during July and August 2013. The subjects were 210 men and 360 women, aged 20–93 years. The average age was 65 years old. Quercetin intake was then estimated using the quercetin content of food obtained in June and July 2013.

Figure 2a shows a frequency distribution chart of quercetin intake by the 570 residents. The estimated quercetin intake ranged from 0.5 to 56.8 mg day$^{-1}$. The average and the median quercetin intakes were 16.2 mg day$^{-1}$ and 15.5 mg day$^{-1}$, respectively. Green tea was the main dietary source of quercetin, followed by onions, asparagus, tomatoes, and green peppers (Figure 3a). The average and median quercetin intakes by men and women were 13.8 and 12.0 mg day$^{-1}$, and 18.3 and 17.2 mg day$^{-1}$, respectively. The daily quercetin intake by women was significantly higher than the intake by men ($p < 0.001$) (Figure 2b).

The coefficients of correlation between quercetin intake and age were 0.242 and 0.292 for men and women, respectively (Figure 2b). Quercetin intake showed low correlations ($p < 0.0001$) with age for both men and women (Figure 2c).

Another FFQ, which asked about the frequency and portion size of 14 commonly-eaten and quercetin-rich foods in winter, was completed by 60 residents of Sobetsu in December 2013. The subjects included 24 men and 36 women, aged 41–91 years. The average age was 66 years old. The quercetin contents of onions, red leaf lettuce, apples, and broccoli in December 2013 were used for estimating the quercetin intake. The estimated quercetin intake ranged from 3.7 to 109.1 mg day$^{-1}$ (Figure 4a). The average and the median quercetin intakes were 18.3 mg day$^{-1}$ and 16.1 mg day$^{-1}$, respectively (Figure 4a). The estimated quercetin intakes in winter were not significantly different from those in summer. The average and median quercetin intakes by men and women were 16.2 and 13.7 mg day$^{-1}$, and 19.6 and 17.3 mg day$^{-1}$, respectively. The daily quercetin intakes of men and women were not significantly different as well (Figure 4b). Quercetin intake during winter did not show a correlation with age for both men and women (Figure 4c). During winter, quercetin was mainly ingested from onions (Figure 3b).

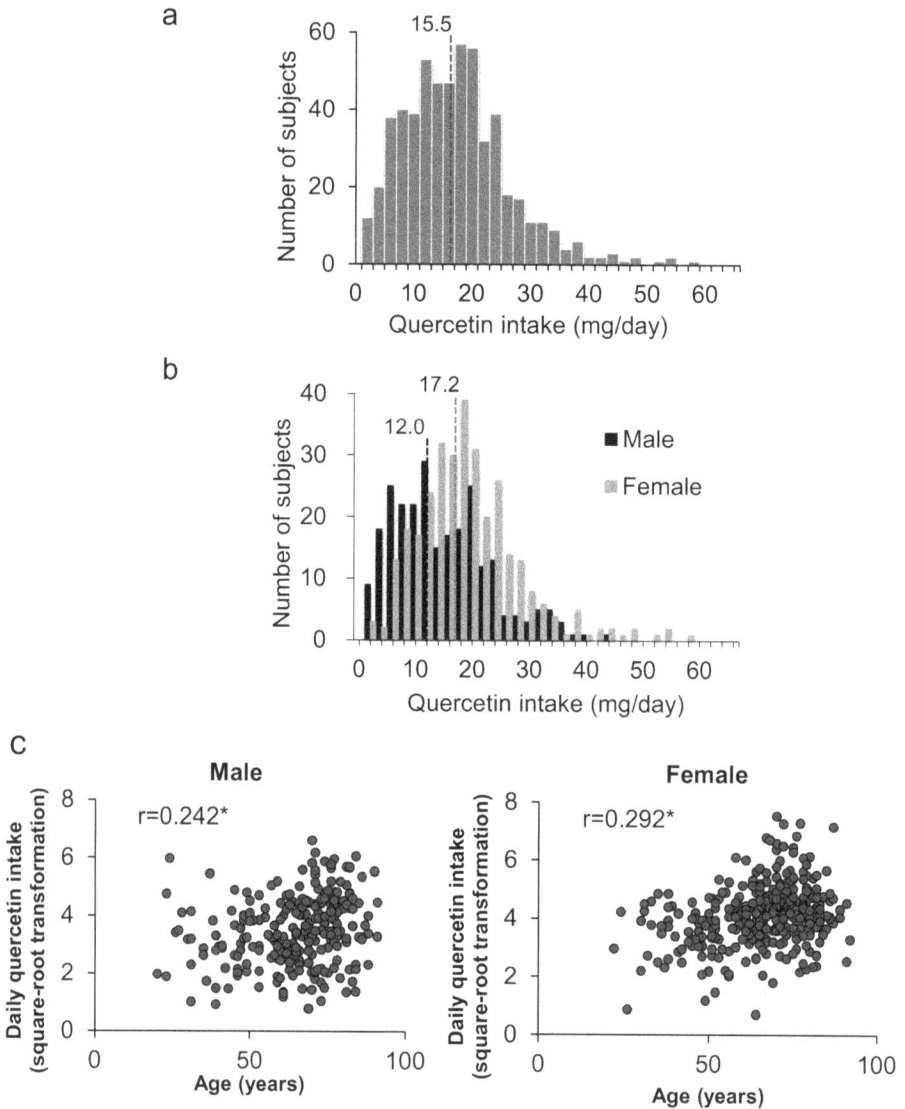

**Figure 2.** (a) Estimated daily quercetin intake by 570 residents of Sobetsu in Hokkaido using the FFQ during summer. (b) Estimated daily quercetin intakes by men and women using the FFQ during summer. Numbers in the figure show the median quercetin intakes by men and women. (c) Correlation between the daily quercetin intakes by men or women and their age. r, correlation coefficient; * $p < 0.0001$; Pearson correlation test.

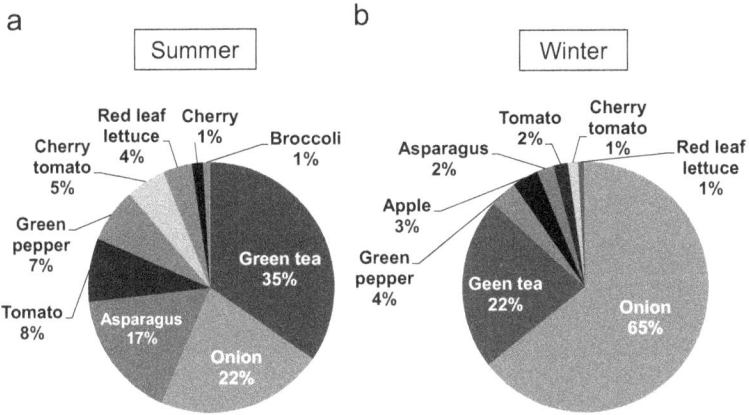

**Figure 3.** Percentage contribution of foods to the daily quercetin intake by residents of Sobetsu in Hokkaido during summer (**a**) and winter (**b**).

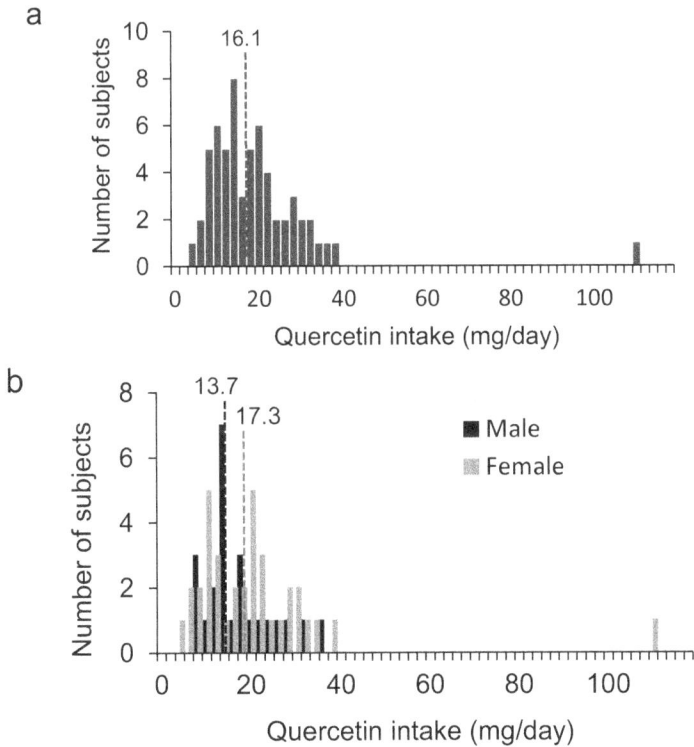

**Figure 4.** *Cont.*

C

**Male**

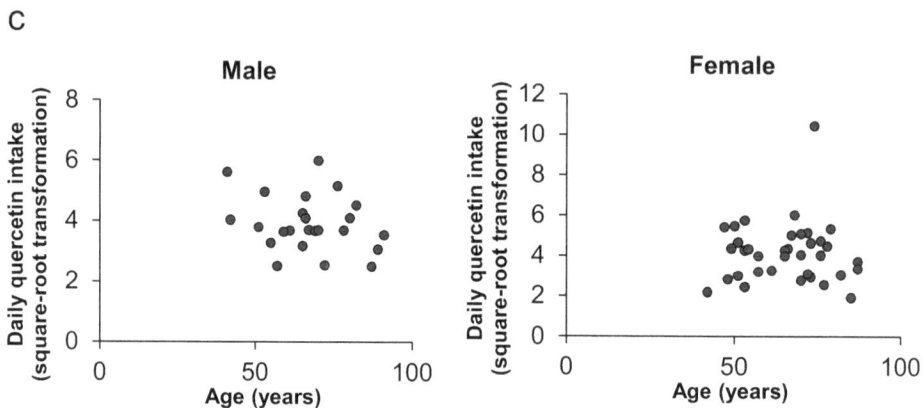

**Female**

Daily quercetin intake (square-root transformation)

Age (years)

**Figure 4.** (**a**) Estimated daily quercetin intake by 60 residents of Sobetsu in Hokkaido using the FFQ during winter. (**b**) Estimated daily quercetin intakes by men and women using the FFQ during winter. Numbers in the figure show the median quercetin intakes by men and women. (**c**) Relationship between quercetin intakes by men or women and their age.

## 4. Discussion

In this study, onions and green tea were shown to be major sources of quercetin intake both in summer and in winter. The quercetin contents of the edible part of onions in Japan were 10–50 mg 100 g$^{-1}$ fresh weight. Onions grown in Hokkaido had been reported to contain 30–50 mg quercetin (100 g)$^{-1}$ fresh weight [25]. The principal cultivar "Kita momiji 2000" contained approximately 40 mg quercetin (100 g)$^{-1}$ [24]. From autumn to spring, the onions grown in the major production area of Hokkaido were eaten throughout Japan. On the other hand, the quercetin content of the green tea infusion was less than that of onions. In our study, the green tea infusion contained 2.1 mg quercetin 100 mL$^{-1}$, whereas it had been previously reported to contain 0.11 mg or 4.23 mg quercetin 100 g$^{-1}$ [26,27]. Because onion and green tea are the most common vegetable and beverage, they appear to be the major food sources of quercetin in Japan.

Epidemiological studies showed that moderate wine consumption reduced the risk of cardiovascular diseases [28]. Consumption of wine rich in polyphenols is expected to have health benefits [29]. Yoo *et al.* reported the positive correlation for quercetin concentration (0.1–1 mg L$^{-1}$) with total phenols and antioxidant activity in red wines [30]. However, the result of our survey on alcohol drinking showed that about 3% and 6% of men and women were habitual wine drinkers, respectively. Wine consumption probably does not contribute to daily quercetin intake in this cohort.

A significant amount of quercetin was consumed from vegetables, such as asparagus, green pepper, tomato, and red leaf lettuce during summer. The results of the two-day weighted food record by eight volunteers also showed that asparagus, green peppers, tomatoes, and red leaf lettuce are also major food sources of quercetin. We showed that cooked asparagus and green pepper maintained a substantial concentration of quercetin. These vegetables, which are in season during summer, contributed more to quercetin intake in summer than that in winter.

Although the contribution percentages for different foods varied, the estimated daily quercetin intake by residents in summer we comparable to that in winter. The results of the FFQ by 570 subjects showed that the estimated quercetin intakes by men were lower than those by women. The daily quercetin intakes by the subjects showed a low correlation with age in both men and women. On the other hand, the quercetin intakes by men and women were not significantly different and the daily quercetin intakes were not correlated with age in winter. This difference may have occurred because there were fewer subjects in the survey during winter.

There have been several reports on the estimated daily quercetin intake by Japanese women but not by men [26,27,31]. The simple FFQ, which asked about the frequency and portion size of 15 commonly-eaten and quercetin-rich food items, enabled estimation of the quercetin intake by men and women, including older people. Although the quercetin content of plant foods differs depending on the cultivars or cultivation conditions, quercetin intakes were estimated using a database established in other country or other period in other epidemiological studies on quercetin and risks of lifestyle-related diseases [1–7]. In this study we precisely estimated the quercetin intake by subjects in a cohort study and found that partial correlation analysis adjusted for age showed that quercetin intake was negatively correlated with diastolic blood pressure (rpar = $-0.145$, $p = 0.008$). Edwards et al. showed that supplementation with 730 mg quercetin day$^{-1}$ for 28 days reduced systolic and diastolic blood pressure in stage 1 hypertensive patients [32]. Egert et al. showed that supplementation of quercetin reduced systolic blood pressure in overweight–obese carriers of the apo $\varepsilon 3/\varepsilon 3$ genotype [33]. Quercetin intake may contribute in decreasing the levels of blood pressure. Arai et al. showed that after adjustment for age, body mass index, and total energy intake, the quercetin intake was inversely correlated with the plasma total cholesterol and LDL cholesterol concentrations in Japanese women [26]. Although the cross-sectional analysis did not show any other significant correlation, further prospective study will be able to elucidate the causal association between quercetin intake and health indexes or risks of lifestyle related diseases.

The antioxidant activity is thought to be a prevention mechanism of lifestyle-related diseases. Although Edward et al. did not find the effect of supplemented quercetin on oxidative stress indices in hypertensive subjects [32], Egert et al. reported that the supplementation of quercetin at a dose of 150 mg day$^{-1}$ for 6 weeks reduced the oxidized LDL concentration in overweight subjects [34]. Terao et al. recently showed that plasma quercetin metabolites detected after combined intake of sautéed onion and tofu were different from those detected after the intake of sautéed onion in healthy volunteers [35]. The antioxidant effect of quercetin depends on the matrix that is it found in the intake of other foods and other factors. Evaluation of the antioxidant effect of the quercetin-rich foods and the foods in diet may help to elucidate the preventive effect of quercetin on lifestyle-related diseases.

The averages of the estimated daily quercetin intake by residents of Sobetsu in Hokkaido were 16.2 mg day$^{-1}$ in summer and 18.3 mg day$^{-1}$ in winter. Arai $et$ $al.$ reported that the average estimated quercetin intake was 9.3 mg day$^{-1}$ using a three-day weighted dietary record by women living in the northern part of Japan [26]. Ioku $et$ $al.$ estimated the average quercetin intake by middle-aged and elderly women living in the Kansai area in Japan as 17.8 mg day$^{-1}$ [27]. Otaki $et$ $al.$ estimated the average intake of quercetin by women in the northern part of Japan as 15.8 mg day$^{-1}$ with a cross-sectional study using a 24 h weighted dietary record [31]. Our results are similar to the results of these previous studies conducted 10–20 years ago.

## 5. Conclusions

In conclusion, we have estimated daily quercetin intake by residents, who are the subjects of the longitudinal cohort study, in a town in Hokkaido. The average and median daily quercetin intake using FFQ was 16.2 and 15.5 mg day$^{-1}$, respectively, during summer. The results were similar to the estimated quercetin intake by Japanese women in the previous studies. The quercetin intake by men was lower than that by women. The quercetin intakes showed a low correlation with age in both men and women. The daily intake of quercetin, which was mainly provided by onions and green tea, was comparable in summer and in winter. Summer vegetables, such as asparagus, green pepper, tomatoes, and red leaf lettuce, were also good sources of quercetin, which is a promising food component for the prevention of lifestyle-related diseases. Further prospective study will probably be able to elucidate the causal association between quercetin intake and health indexes or risks of lifestyle-related diseases.

**Acknowledgments:** This work was financially supported in part by a grant from the Ministry of Agriculture, Forestry and Fisheries (MAFF) research project for the new demand and creation of agricultural products, Japan. The authors would like to thank Enago (Crimson Interactive Japan, Tokyo, Japan) for the English language review.

**Author Contributions:** H.O., M.S., T.N., H.A., S.S., K.S., and M.K. conceived and designed the study. H.N., M.O.K., I.Z., K.I., H.O., and M.K. performed the experiments. H.O., M.S., H.A., S.S., and K.S. performed the diet survey. H.N., H.O., M.O.K., S.N., and M.K. analyzed the data. H.O., M.S., M.O.K., H.A., S.S., K.S., and M.K. contributed reagents/materials/analysis tools. H.N., H.O., M.O.K., and M.K. wrote the paper.

**Conflicts of Interest:** The authors declare no conflict of interest.

# References

1. Formica, J.V.; Regelson, W. Review of the biology of quercetin and related bioflavonoids. *Food Chem. Toxicol.* **1995**, *33*, 1061–1080.

2. Knekt, P.; Jarvinen, R.; Reunanen, A.; Maatela, J. Flavonoid intake and coronary mortality in Finland: A cohort study. *BMJ* **1996**, *312*, 478–481.

3. Arts, I.C.W.; Hollman, P.C.H. Polyphenols and disease risk in epidemiologic studies. *Am. J. Clin. Nutr.* **2005**, *81*, 317s–325s.

4. Hollman, P.C.H.; Katan, M.B. Dietary flavonoids: Intake, health effects and bioavailability. *Food Chem. Toxicol.* **1999**, *37*, 937–942.

5. Hooper, L.; Kroon, P.A.; Rimm, E.B.; Cohn, J.S.; Harvey, I.; Le Cornu, K.A.; Ryder, J.J.; Hall, W.L.; Cassidy, A. Flavonoids, flavonoid-rich foods, and cardiovascular risk: A meta-analysis of randomized controlled trials. *Am. J. Clin. Nutr.* **2008**, *88*, 38–50.

6. Kelly, G.S. Quercetin. Monograph. *Altern. Med. Rev.* **2011**, *16*, 172–194.

7. Peterson, J.J.; Dwyer, J.T.; Jacques, P.F.; McCullough, M.L. Associations between flavonoids and cardiovascular disease incidence or mortality in European and US populations. *Nutr. Rev.* **2012**, *70*, 491–508.

8. Terao, J.; Kawai, Y.; Murota, K. Vegetable flavonoids and cardiovascular disease. *Asia Pac. J. Clin. Nutr.* **2008**, *17*, 291–293.

9. Morales, J.; Gunther, G.; Zanocco, A.L.; Lemp, E. Singlet oxygen reactions with flavonoids. A theoretical-experimental study. *PLoS ONE* **2012**, *7*, e40548.

10. Lagoa, R.; Graziani, I.; Lopez-Sanchez, C.; Garcia-Martinez, V.; Gutierrez-Merino, C. Complex I and cytochrome c are molecular targets of flavonoids that inhibit hydrogen peroxide production by mitochondria. *Biochim. Biophys. Acta* **2011**, *1807*, 1562–1572.

11. Mahesh, T.; Menon, V.P. Quercetin allievates oxidative stress in streptozotocin-induced diabetic rats. *Phytother. Res.* **2004**, *18*, 123–127.

12. Boesch-Saadatmandi, C.; Wagner, A.E.; Wolffram, S.; Rimbach, G. Effect of quercetin on inflammatory gene expression in mice liver *in vivo*—Role of redox factor 1, miRNA-122 and miRNA-125b. *Pharmacol. Res.* **2012**, *65*, 523–530.

13. Kobori, M.; Masumoto, S.; Akimoto, Y.; Takahashi, Y. Dietary quercetin alleviates diabetic symptoms and reduces streptozotocin-induced disturbance of hepatic gene expression in mice. *Mol. Nutr. Food Res.* **2009**, *53*, 859–868.

14. Kobori, M.; Masumoto, S.; Akimoto, Y.; Oike, H. Chronic dietary intake of quercetin alleviates hepatic fat accumulation associated with consumption of a Western-style diet in C57/BL6J mice. *Mol. Nutr. Food Res.* **2011**, *55*, 530–540.

15. Dong, J.; Zhang, X.; Zhang, L.; Bian, H.; Xu, N.; Bao, B.; Liu, J. Quercetin reduces obesity-associated ATM inflammation in mice: A mechanism including AMPKα1/SIRT1. *J. Lipid Res.* **2014**, *55*, 363–374.

16. Murota, K.; Hotta, A.; Ido, H.; Kawai, Y.; Moon, J.H.; Sekido, K.; Hayashi, H.; Inakuma, T.; Terao, J. Antioxidant capacity of albumin-bound quercetin metabolites after onion consumption in humans. *J. Med. Investig.* **2007**, *54*, 370–374.

17. Ishisaka, A.; Kawabata, K.; Miki, S.; Shiba, Y.; Minekawa, S.; Nishikawa, T.; Mukai, R.; Terao, J.; Kawai, Y. Mitochondrial dysfunction leads to deconjugation of quercetin glucuronides in inflammatory macrophages. *PLoS ONE* **2013**, *8*, e80843.

18. Zamora-Ros, R.; Knaze, V.; Lujan-Barroso, L.; Slimani, N.; Romieu, I.; Fedirko, V.; de Magistris, M.S.; Ericson, U.; Amiano, P.; Trichopoulou, A.; *et al.* Estimated dietary intakes of flavonols, flavanones and flavones in the European Prospective Investigation into Cancer and Nutrition (EPIC) 24 hour dietary recall cohort. *Br. J. Nutr.* **2011**, *106*, 1915–1925.

19. Ioku, K.; Aoyama, Y.; Tokuno, A.; Terao, J.; Nakatani, N.; Takei, Y. Various cooking methods and the flavonoid content in onion. *J. Nutr. Sci. Vitaminol.* **2001**, *47*, 78–83.

20. Ohnishi, H.; Saitohi, S.; Takagii, S.; Katohi, N.; Chibai, Y.; Akasakai, H.; Nakamura, Y.; Shimamoto, K. Incidence of type 2 diabetes in individuals with central obesity in a rural Japanese population: The Tanno and Sobetssu study. *Diabetes Care* **2006**, *29*, 1128–1129.

21. Mitsumata, K.; Saitoh, S.; Ohnishi, H.; Akasaka, H.; Miura, T. Effects of parental hypertension on longitudinal trends in blood pressure and plasma metabolic profile: Mixed-effects model analysis. *Hypertension* **2012**, *60*, 1124–1130.

22. Slimestad, R.; Fossen, T.; Vagen, I.M. Onions: A source of unique dietary flavonoids. *J. Agric. Food Chem.* **2007**, *55*, 10067–10080.

23. Jin, J.; Koroleva, O.A.; Gibson, T.; Swanston, J.; Magan, J.; Zhang, Y.; Rowland, I.R.; Wagstaff, C. Analysis of phytochemical composition and chemoprotective capacity of rocket (*Eruca sativa* and *Diplotaxis tenuifolia*) leafy salad following cultivation in different environments. *J. Agric. Food Chem.* **2009**, *57*, 5227–52234.

24. Watanabe, J.; Takebayashi, J.; Takano-Ishikawa, Y.; Yasui, A. Evaluation of a Method to Quantify Quercetin Aglycone in Onion (*Allium cepa*) by Single- and Multi-laboratory Validation Studies. *Anal. Sci.* **2012**, *28*, 1179–1182.

25. Okamoto, D.; Noguchi, Y.; Muro, T.; Morishita, M. Genetic variation of quercetin glucoside content in onion (*Allium cepa* L.). *J. Jpn. Soc. Hortic. Sci.* **2006**, *75*, 100–108.

26. Arai, Y.; Watanabe, S.; Kimira, M.; Shimoi, K.; Mochizuki, R.; Kinae, N. Dietary intakes of flavonols, flavones and isoflavones by Japanese women and the inverse correlation between quercetin intake and plasma LDL cholesterol concentration. *J. Nutr.* **2000**, *130*, 2243–2250.

27. Ioku, K.; Okuda, T.; Higuchi, H.; M., K.; Takei, Y. Investigation of the Flavonoid Intake in a Daily Meal of the Kansai in the Middle-aged women. *Osaka Kyoiku Univ. Repos. II* **2008**, *56*, 1–19.

28. Arranz, S.; Chiva-Blanch, G.; Valderas-Martínez, P.; Medina-Remón, A.; Lamuela-Raventós, R.M.; Estruch, R. Wine, beer, alcohol and polyphenols on cardiovascular disease and cancer. *Nutrients* **2012**, *4*, 750–781.

29. Yoo, Y.J.; Saliba, A.J.; MacDonald, J.B.; Prenzler, P.D.; Ryan, D. A cross-cultural study of wine consumers with respect to health benefits of wine. *Food Qual. Prefer.* **2013**, *28*, 531–538.

30. Yoo, Y.J.; Prenzler, P.D.; Saliba, A.J.; Ryan, D. Assessment of some Australian red wines for price, phenolic content, antioxidant activity, and vintage in relation to functional food prospects. *J. Food Sci.* **2011**, *76*, C1355–C1364.

31. Otaki, N.; Kimira, M.; Katsumata, S.; Uehara, M.; Watanabe, S.; Suzuki, K. Distribution and major sources of flavonoid intakes in the middle-aged Japanese women. *J. Clin. Biochem. Nutr.* **2009**, *44*, 231–238.

32. Edwards, R.L.; Lyon, T.; Litwin, S.E.; Rabovsky, A.; Symons, J.D.; Jalili, T. Quercetin reduces blood pressure in hypertensive subjects. *J. Nutr.* **2007**, *137*, 2405–2411.

33. Egert, S.; Boesch-Saadatmandi, C.; Wolffram, S.; Rimbach, G.; Muller, M.J. Serum lipid and blood pressure responses to quercetin vary in overweight patients by apolipoprotein E genotype. *J. Nutr.* **2010**, *140*, 278–284.

34. Egert, S.; Bosy-Westphal, A.; Seiberl, J.; Kurbitz, C.; Settler, U.; Plachta-Danielzik, S.; Wagner, A.E.; Frank, J.; Schrezenmeir, J.; Rimbach, G.; *et al.* Quercetin reduces systolic blood pressure and plasma oxidised low-density lipoprotein concentrations in overweight subjects with a high-cardiovascular disease risk phenotype: A double-blinded, placebo-controlled cross-over study. *Br. J. Nutr.* **2009**, *102*, 1065–1074.

35. Nakamura, T.; Murota, K.; Kumamoto, S.; Misumi, K.; Bando, N.; Ikushiro, S.; Takahashi, N.; Sekido, K.; Kato, Y.; Terao, J. Plasma metabolites of dietary flavonoids after combination meal consumption with onion and tofu in humans. *Mol. Nutr. Food Res.* **2014**, *58*, 310–307.

# Evaluation of Riboflavin Intakes and Status of 20–64-Year-Old Adults in South Korea

Ji Young Choi, Young-Nam Kim and Youn-OK Cho

**Abstract:** A recent Korea National Health and Nutrition Survey indicated inadequate riboflavin intake in Koreans, but there is limited research regarding riboflavin status in South Korea. The purpose of this study was to determine riboflavin intake and status of Korean adults. Three consecutive 24-h food recalls were collected from 412 (145 men and 267 women) healthy adults, aged 20–64 years, living in South Korea and urine samples were collected from 149 subjects of all subjects. The dietary and total (dietary plus supplemental) riboflavin intake was $1.33 \pm 0.34$ and $2.87 \pm 6.29$ mg/day, respectively. Approximately 28% of the subjects consumed total riboflavin less than the Estimated Average Requirement. Urinary riboflavin excretion was $205.1 \pm 190.1$ µg/g creatinine. Total riboflavin intake was significantly positively correlated to the urinary riboflavin excretion. ($r = 0.17171$, $p = 0.0363$). About 11% of the Korean adults had urinary riboflavin <27 µg/g creatinine indicating a riboflavin deficiency and 21% had low status of riboflavin (27 µg/g creatinine $\leq$ urinary riboflavin < 80 µg/g creatinine). Thus, one-third of Korean adults in this study had inadequate riboflavin status. In some adults in Korea, consumption of riboflavin-rich food sources should be encouraged.

Reprinted from *Nutrients*. Cite as: Choi, J.Y.; Kim, Y.-N.; Cho, Y.-O. Evaluation of Riboflavin Intakes and Status of 20–64-Year-Old Adults in South Korea. *Nutrients* **2015**, *7*, 253–264.

## 1. Introduction

Assessment of dietary intake is essential to investigate the relationships between diet and health in epidemiological studies and to design nutrient intervention studies. Particularly, determination of usual intake is critical to estimate the prevalence of inadequate intakes. The Korea Centers for Disease Control and Prevention have indicated that riboflavin is one of nutrients consumed inadequately by Koreans in the Korea National Health and Nutrition Survey (KNHANES) [1–3]. The KNHANES 2012 reported that a half of the Koreans consumed riboflavin less than the Estimated Average Requirement (EAR) for Koreans [3]. The KNHANES is a complex, stratified, multistage, probability-cluster survey of a representative sample of the non-institutionalized civilian Korean population. In the Nutrition Survey of KNHANES, one day of 24-h recall from participants is collected and dietary nutrient intakes calculated, which may not be captured as usual intake for some individuals with highly variable intakes. In addition, the results of nutrient intakes in KNHANES did not count the intake from dietary supplements, causing errors in the calculated nutrient intakes [4]. Thus, the prevalence of inadequate riboflavin intake in KNHANES might be overestimated.

Riboflavin—Vitamin $B_2$ is a water-soluble vitamin that is involved for a number of oxidative enzyme systems in electron transport [4]. Riboflavin coenzymes, flavin mononucleotide and flavin adenine dinucleotide, are involved in diverse redox reactions to human metabolism as electron carriers [5], which play in the metabolism of energy, other B vitamins, drugs, and lipids [6,7]. A high prevalence of inadequate riboflavin intake and status has been reported in various population groups in many countries including USA, UK, France, Poland, and Japan [8–11]. Also, the recent studies have indicated that riboflavin deficiency increases risk of cancer at certain sites; lung, distal stomach, esophagus, and rectum [12–16]. Some epidemiological studies have identified relationships between cardiovascular diseases and diets low in riboflavin [17,18]. In South Korea, several studies reported dietary riboflavin intakes of Koreans [19,20], however, there is no study regarding current riboflavin status for Koreans including both intakes and biochemical measurements.

Therefore, the objectives of this study were to estimate total riboflavin intakes (dietary plus supplemental) and urinary riboflavin excretion as a biochemical measurement for riboflavin status and to evaluate current riboflavin status for Korean adults aged 20–64 years.

## 2. Experimental Section

### 2.1. Subjects

Four hundred and twelve healthy adults participated as subjects (145 men and 267 women), aged 20–64 years, living in the Seoul metropolitan area and the cities of Kwangju and Gumi, South Korea, during January 2010 to January 2012. Urine samples were collected from 149 adults (70 men and 79 women) who voluntarily provided the samples among 412 subjects. The subjects were recruited by advertisement in a convenience sampling of universities, gyms, and welfare centers. Adults who were not in good health, had known illnesses, or took medications were not included in the study. The Institutional Review Board of Duksung Women's University approved the study (2010-1 & 2011-04-0001). Informed consent was obtained from each subject. The subjects were interviewed to obtain information regarding age, gender, current illness, medications taken, intake of vitamin and mineral supplements within 30 days of the interview, and appetite. All interviews were conducted by trained interviewers. Interviewers measured weights and heights of the subjects in light clothing and barefoot. Body mass index (BMI) was calculated as weight divided by squared height ($kg/m^2$).

## 2.2. Calculation of Intakes of Selected Nutrients and Riboflavin

Three consecutive 24-h recalls (2 weekdays and 1 weekend day) were obtained from each subject by a trained interviewer. Intakes of macronutrients and vitamins were estimated using a computer-aided nutritional analysis program (CAN-Pro 4.0) developed by the Korean Nutrition Society [21]. The nutrient database of Can-pro 4.0 is based on the Korean Food Composition Table (Korean Rural Development Administration, 2006) and the Food Values (Korean Nutrition Society, 2009). The subjects consuming such supplements were asked to offer information on the names of the supplements and the amount, frequency, and duration of the use. Among 129 subjects taking any types of dietary supplements in this study, 80 subjects (19.4%, 31 men and 49 women) of all subjects took supplements containing riboflavin. In the subjects providing urine samples, 23% took riboflavin supplements. Thus, the amounts of riboflavin consumed by the subjects were reported as dietary riboflavin (from foods only) and total riboflavin intakes (dietary plus supplemental riboflavin). The EAR for riboflavin is 1.3 mg/day for men aged 19–64 years and 1.0 mg/day for women aged 19–64 years, respectively. The dietary and total intakes of riboflavin were compared with EARs for Koreans [22]. The top 10 major food sources of riboflavin consumed by the subjects were also determined.

## 2.3. Measurement of Urinary Riboflavin Excretion

First urine samples in the morning of an interview were collected from the 149 subjects in this study. Urine was protected from light and was kept in crushed ice. The samples were distributed in vials and can be stored at $-70\,^{\circ}C$ until analysis. Urinary riboflavin was analyzed using the high-performance liquid chromatography (HPLC) method by Gatautis and Natio [23]. The standard of riboflavin was purchased from Sigma-Aldrich (St. Louis, MO, USA). All reagents were the HPLC grade in this study. The HPLC system consisted of UltiMate 3000 pump, UltiMate Injector and autosampler, FLD-3000 fluorescence detector (Thermo Scientific, Waltham, MA, USA), and C18 reversed-phase HPLC column (Waters, Ireland, $3.9 \times 300$ mm, 10 µm particle size). Riboflavin standard and urine were detected with $\lambda_{excitation}$ of 450 nm and $\lambda_{emission}$ 530 nm. Minimum detectable level was 0.0042 ng riboflavin. The coefficient of variance between assays was <5% for urine riboflavin. Urine creatinine was analyzed using an assay kit (Cayman Chemical Company, Ann Arbon, MI, USA). Interpretive criteria for the urinary excretion of riboflavin are <27 µg/g creatinine for deficient and 27–79 µg/g creatinine for low status [4].

## 2.4. Statistical Analysis

Data were analyzed by gender and by riboflavin supplementation using SAS version 9.1.3 software (SAS Institute, INC., Cary, NC, US). Values are reported as means $\pm$ standard deviations, and the differences by gender and by riboflavin supplementation (nonusers *vs.* users of riboflavin supplements) were analyzed using Student's *t*-test. Histogram and Q-Q plots were used to determine whether the variables were normally distributed. Percentile values of riboflavin intakes were also reported by gender and by urinary riboflavin excretion. Pearson's correlation coefficients were calculated to determine the correlations between riboflavin intake and urinary riboflavin excretion. Differences were considered significant $p < 0.05$.

## 3. Results

### 3.1. Subject Characteristics and Selected Nutrient Intakes

Table 1 shows general characteristics and selected nutrient intakes of 412 Korean adults aged 20–64 years. The mean age of all subjects was $38.8 \pm 12.6$ years and BMI was $22.9 \pm 3.0$ kg/m$^2$. Energy intake of the subjects was $1866.9 \pm 376.7$ kcal/day. Energy intake of men was significantly higher than that of women ($p < 0.001$). Significantly higher mean intakes of macronutrients and selected vitamins were observed for men compared with women, except vitamin A and vitamin C ($p < 0.001$).

**Table 1.** General characteristics and selected nutrient intakes of 412 Korean adults by gender.

| Variable | Men ($n$ = 145) | Women ($n$ = 267) | Total ($n$ = 412) |
|---|---|---|---|
| Age (year) [**] | 36.6 $\pm$ 12.7 | 40.1 $\pm$ 12.4 | 38.8 $\pm$ 12.6 |
| Weight (kg) [***] | 72.3 $\pm$ 9.8 | 56.8 $\pm$ 8.1 | 62.3 $\pm$ 11.4 |
| Height (cm) [***] | 173.3 $\pm$ 6.0 | 159.9 $\pm$ 4.6 | 164.6 $\pm$ 8.2 |
| BMI (kg/m$^2$) [***] | 24.0 $\pm$ 2.7 | 22.2 $\pm$ 3.0 | 22.9 $\pm$ 3.0 |
| *Macronutrients* | | | |
| Energy (kcal/day) [***] | 2119.5 $\pm$ 389.3 | 1729.7 $\pm$ 289.1 | 1866.9 $\pm$ 376.7 |
| Carbohydrate (g/day) [***] | 275.3 $\pm$ 50.8 | 251.5 $\pm$ 54.0 | 259.9 $\pm$ 54.1 |
| Protein (g/day) [***] | 89.7 $\pm$ 23.8 | 69.9 $\pm$ 15.7 | 76.9 $\pm$ 21.2 |
| Total fat (g/day) [***] | 60.6 $\pm$ 18.6 | 48.7 $\pm$ 15.2 | 52.9 $\pm$ 17.5 |
| *Vitamins* | | | |
| Vitamin A ($\mu$g RE [1]/day) | 803.9 $\pm$ 302.1 | 813.7 $\pm$ 329.2 | 810.3 $\pm$ 319.6 |
| Vitamin E (mg $\alpha$-TE [2]/day) [***] | 19.4 $\pm$ 12.4 | 16.0 $\pm$ 5.1 | 17.2 $\pm$ 8.6 |
| Thiamin (mg/day) [***] | 1.4 $\pm$ 0.4 | 1.2 $\pm$ 0.3 | 1.2 $\pm$ 0.3 |
| Niacin (mg NE [3]/day) [***] | 19.8 $\pm$ 5.5 | 15.9 $\pm$ 4.0 | 17.3 $\pm$ 4.9 |
| Vitamin B$_6$ (mg/day) [***] | 1.9 $\pm$ 0.6 | 1.8 $\pm$ 0.6 | 1.8 $\pm$ 0.5 |
| Vitamin C (mg/day) [***] | 96.5 $\pm$ 45.8 | 119.9 $\pm$ 63.0 | 111.6 $\pm$ 58.5 |

Values are means $\pm$ standard deviations; [**] $p < 0.01$, [***] $p < 0.001$ by *t*-test; [1] Retinol Equivalent; [2] $\alpha$-Tocopherol Equivalent; [3] Niacin Equivalent.

## 3.2. Riboflavin Intakes

The dietary and total riboflavin intake of the subjects was $1.33 \pm 0.34$ mg/day and $2.87 \pm 6.29$ mg/day, respectively (Table 2) and there were no significant differences in the intakes by gender ($p \geq 0.05$). The ratio of dietary riboflavin intake to energy intake of women was significantly higher than that of men ($p < 0.001$). Users of riboflavin supplements consumed more total riboflavin than nonusers ($p < 0.001$). Approximately 42.8% of men and 29.2% of women had dietary riboflavin intakes less than EAR, but the prevalence of inadequate riboflavin intake was reduced by counting riboflavin supplements to 33.8% in men and 24.7% in women. Only two subjects taking riboflavin supplements had total riboflavin intakes less than EAR. The top 10 major dietary sources of riboflavin consumed by the subjects were whole egg, citrus fruit, whole milk, Ra Myeon (Korean instant noodle), Kimchi, pork (loin), mackerel, spinach, chicken, and pork (belly). There were no riboflavin fortified foods that the subjects consumed except cereals. Cereal was the 27th largest source of riboflavin in this study and approximately 2.7% of the subjects consumed cereals.

## 3.3. Urinary Riboflavin Excretion and Riboflavin Status

Urinary riboflavin excretion was $205.1 \pm 190.1$ µg/g creatinine (Table 3). No significant difference in riboflavin excretion was observed by gender ($p \geq 0.05$), but the excretion of users of riboflavin supplements was significantly higher than that of nonusers ($p < 0.001$). Approximately 11% of the Korean adults had a riboflavin concentration <27 µg/g creatinine indicating a biochemical deficiency of riboflavin. The subjects having low status (27 µg/g creatinine $\leq$ urinary riboflavin < 80 µg/g creatinine) were 20.8% of all subjects and 8.8% of the users.

## 3.4. Percentile Values of Riboflavin Intake

Percentile values of dietary and total riboflavin intakes by gender and by urinary riboflavin excretion are shown in Table 4. Median dietary and total riboflavin intakes of men were 1.37 and 1.46 mg/day, respectively. Women had median dietary and total riboflavin intakes of 1.18 and 1.24 mg/day, respectively. Median dietary and total riboflavin intakes of men with urinary riboflavin $\geq$27 µg/g creatinine were 1.37 and 1.44 mg/day, respectively. Median dietary and total riboflavin intakes of women with urinary riboflavin $\geq$27 µg/g creatinine were 1.33 and 1.43 mg/day, respectively.

## 3.5. Associations among Riboflavin Intakes and Urinary Riboflavin Excretion

There was no significant correlation between urinary riboflavin and dietary riboflavin intakes including the ratio of dietary riboflavin to energy intake ($p \geq 0.05$) (Table 5). However, urinary riboflavin excretion was significantly positively correlated with total riboflavin intake ($r = 0.17171$, $p = 0.0363$).

**Table 2.** Riboflavin intakes of 412 Korean adults by gender and by riboflavin supplementation.

| Variable | Gender | | Riboflavin Supplementation | | Total ($n = 412$) |
|---|---|---|---|---|---|
| | Men ($n = 145$) | Women ($n = 267$) | Nonusers of Riboflavin Supplements ($n = 332$) | Users of Riboflavin Supplements ($n = 80$) | |
| Dietary riboflavin intake (mg/day) | $1.35 \pm 0.34$ | $1.31 \pm 0.33$ | $1.25 \pm 0.35$ | $1.27 \pm 0.32$ | $1.33 \pm 0.34$ |
| Dietary riboflavin/energy (mg/1000 kcal) | $0.65 \pm 0.14$ [***] | $0.74 \pm 0.16$ | $0.68 \pm 0.16$ | $0.67 \pm 0.15$ | $0.69 \pm 0.16$ |
| Total riboflavin intake (diet + supplements) (mg/day) | $2.62 \pm 5.51$ | $3.08 \pm 6.94$ | $1.25 \pm 0.35$ [***] | $5.72 \pm 9.31$ | $2.87 \pm 6.29$ |
| Using supplements with riboflavin (% ($n$)) | 21.4 (31) | 18.4 (49) | 0 (0) | 100 (80) | 19.4 (80) |
| Not meeting the Estimated Average Requirement with dietary riboflavin (% ($n$)) | 42.8 (62) | 29.2 (78) | 33.7 (112) | 35.0 (28) | 33.9 (140) |
| Not meeting the Estimated Average Requirement with total riboflavin (% ($n$)) | 33.8 (49) | 24.7 (66) | 33.7 (112) | 2.5 (2) | 27.6 (114) |

Values are means $\pm$ standard deviations; The Estimated Average Requirement for riboflavin is 1.3 mg/day for men aged 19–64 years and 1.0 mg/day for women aged 19–64 years; [***] $p < 0.001$ by $t$-test.

**Table 3.** Urinary riboflavin excretion of 149 Korean adults by gender and by riboflavin supplementation.

| Variable | Gender | | Riboflavin Supplementation | | Total ($n = 149$) |
|---|---|---|---|---|---|
| | Men ($n = 70$) | Women ($n = 79$) | Nonusers of Riboflavin Supplements ($n = 115$) | Users of Riboflavin Supplements ($n = 34$) | |
| Urinary riboflavin (µg/g creatinine) | $193.8 \pm 183.3$ | $215.1 \pm 196.4$ | $175.8 \pm 164.2$ [***] | $304.3 \pm 236.2$ | $205.1 \pm 190.1$ |
| 27 µg/g creatinine $\leq$ Urinary riboflavin < 80 µg/g creatinine (%($n$)) | 21.4 (15) | 20.3 (16) | 24.3 (28) | 8.8 (3) | 20.8 (31) |
| Urinary riboflavin < 27 µg/g creatinine (%($n$)) | 12.9 (9) | 10.1 (8) | 11.3 (13) | 11.8 (4) | 11.4 (17) |

Values are means $\pm$ standard deviations. [***] $p < 0.001$ by $t$-test.

**Table 4.** Percentile values of dietary and total riboflavin intakes of Korean adults.

| Subject | n | Dietary Riboflavin (mg/day) | | | | | Total Riboflavin [1] (mg/day) | | | | |
|---|---|---|---|---|---|---|---|---|---|---|---|
| | | 5th | 25th | 50th | 75th | 95th | 5th | 25th | 50th | 75th | 95th |
| *Total subjects (n = 412)* | | | | | | | | | | | |
| Men | 145 | 0.76 | 1.11 | 1.37 | 1.58 | 1.96 | 0.77 | 1.16 | 1.46 | 1.83 | 3.76 |
| Women | 267 | 0.71 | 0.95 | 1.18 | 1.39 | 1.78 | 0.72 | 1.00 | 1.24 | 1.63 | 2.94 |
| *Selected subjects (n=149)* [2] | | | | | | | | | | | |
| Total men | 70 | 0.73 | 1.08 | 1.38 | 1.60 | 1.96 | 0.76 | 1.29 | 1.47 | 1.77 | 6.33 |
| Men with urinary riboflavin ≥ 27 μg/g creatinine | 61 | 0.73 | 1.08 | 1.37 | 1.54 | 1.93 | 0.76 | 1.19 | 1.44 | 1.66 | 6.33 |
| Total women | 79 | 0.71 | 1.09 | 1.30 | 1.51 | 1.97 | 0.81 | 1.11 | 1.39 | 1.78 | 21.31 |
| Women with urinary riboflavin ≥ 27 μg/g creatinine | 71 | 0.81 | 1.11 | 1.33 | 1.53 | 1.97 | 0.93 | 1.17 | 1.43 | 1.78 | 5.20 |

[1] Dietary + supplemental riboflavin; [2] Subjects providing urine sample for urine riboflavin analysis.

**Table 5.** Correlations between riboflavin intakes and urinary riboflavin excretion.

| Riboflavin Intake | Urinary Riboflavin |
|---|---|
| Dietary riboflavin | 0.082 (0.318) [1] |
| Dietary riboflavin per energy | 0.129 (0.116) |
| Total riboflavin (diet + supplements) | 0.171 (0.036) * |

[1] *p*-value; * significant at $p < 0.05$.

## 4. Discussion

Recent studies have reported the relationships between riboflavin status and some diseases such as certain types of cancers [12–16] and cardiovascular disease [18]. Riboflavin is involved in the folate-mediated one-carbon. Thus, poor riboflavin status may lead to an elevated rate of DNA damage and altered methylation of DNA, both of which are important risk factors for cancer [24]. Inadequate riboflavin intake has been indicated by a national dietary survey of several countries [25–27] including South Korea [1–3]. However, in Korea, a study regarding riboflavin status for Korean adults is very limited. Therefore, this study estimated intakes and urinary excretion of riboflavin and evaluated riboflavin status of 20–64-year-old adults living in the Seoul metropolitan area and the cities of Kwangju and Gumi, South Korea.

In this study, the mean dietary riboflavin intake (1.33 mg/day) is similar to recently reported dietary riboflavin intake of 20–64-year-old adults reported in KNHANES 2010–2012 [3]. However, dietary riboflavin intakes of Koreans were lower than those of Chinese adults (1.6 mg/day) [25], American adults (2.19 mg/day) [28], and British adults (1.97 mg/day for men and 1.50 mg/day for women) [26]. In the current study, dietary supplements providing riboflavin increased mean intake from food sources alone by 21% for men, from 1.35–2.62 mg, and by 25% for women, from 1.31–3.08 mg. Approximately 19% of the subjects took riboflavin supplements and their mean total riboflavin intake was 5.72 mg/day, much lower than that of American adults taking riboflavin supplements (11.23–11.61 mg/day) [28]. In this study, a 24-h recall method was used for calculation of riboflavin intake. However, food frequency questionnaire or food diary methods were used for estimation of riboflavin intake in other countries [26–28].

The Korean Dietary Reference Intakes (KDRIs) for riboflavin are set as EAR and Recommended Nutrient Intake in all age groups older than one year old. EAR is the daily nutrient intake estimated to meet the requirement of half of healthy individuals in a life-stage group, thus are set at the median of the distribution or requirements. EAR is used to estimate the prevalence of inadequate intake within a group of individuals. EAR of e KDRIs for riboflavin is set at 1.3 mg/day for men and 1.0 mg/day for women aged 19–64 years, based on reports that the riboflavin requirement is at least more than 1 mg/day in Koreans to maintain normal urinary riboflavin excretion and based on median intake of Korean adults in KNHANES 2007 [22]. In this study, median (50th percentile) dietary riboflavin intake of men and women was 1.37 and 1.18 mg/day, respectively. Median dietary intake of men and women with urinary riboflavin $\geq 27$ µg/g creatinine, a cut-off point of riboflavin deficiency, was 1.37 and 1.33 mg/day, respectively. Thus, current riboflavin EAR for men of KDRIs may be appropriate, but EAR for women might be underestimated. KNHANES 2010–2012 [3] reported that about 45% of men ($n = 3127$) and 46% of women ($n = 4081$) consumed the dietary riboflavin less than EAR. In the current study, a low proportion of participants (33.9%) had dietary riboflavin intakes below EAR and the proportion for total (dietary + supplemental) riboflavin intake was much lowered (27.6%). In the US, the prevalence of American adults consuming dietary riboflavin less than Recommended Dietary Allowance was 3% [28]. In British adults, 8% had total riboflavin intake less than the Reference Nutrient Intakes, a nutrient requirement to meet the needs of 97%–98% of healthy individuals [22,26]. Therefore, the prevalence of inadequate riboflavin intake with riboflavin supplementation in this study was much lower than that of KNHANES. However, the prevalence of inadequate intake in Korean adults was still high compared to the prevalence of other countries.

Balance studies in human subjects show clearly that as riboflavin intake increases there is a progressive rise in urinary excretion of riboflavin [29]. Urinary excretion of riboflavin reflects an excess of current intake over tissue requirement and the measurement of urinary excretion provides useful information regarding tissue saturation [18,29,30] under the circumstance of optimum nutritional status for riboflavin. Thus, urinary riboflavin excretion could be used as a potential biomarker to assess its mean estimated intakes in a group. [30–33]. Urinary losses decrease when riboflavin stores decrease. Besides the urinary excretion, the determination of erythrocyte glutathione reductase activity coefficient (EGRAC) is also used. EGRAC is sensitive to changes in riboflavin intake up to levels of intake approaching tissue saturation of riboflavin. However, differences in the relationship between intake and EGRAC values among different population groups have indicated [33] that re-evaluation of EGRAC threshold for riboflavin deficiency should be considered [34]. In this study, urinary excretion was used for evaluation of riboflavin status. The study conducted by Lim and Yoon [20] in 1997 reported that 8.8% and 14.2% of Korean women ($n$ = 38) had riboflavin deficient and low status, respectively, based on urinary excretion, which is in line with the prevalence of riboflavin deficiency and low status in Korean adults of this study. The national survey of UK in 2014 indicated the rate of riboflavin deficiency was 69% of British adults [26]. Whitfield *et al.* [35] reported that 67% of Canadian women ($n$ = 51) had a suboptimal (low) status in 2014. The difference in rates of inadequate riboflavin status between the current study and the studies of UK and Canada may be due to a use of different biochemical index, EGRAC, in UK and Canadian studies. In this study, seven subjects (20%) of users of riboflavin supplements had inadequate riboflavin status. The mean riboflavin intake only from supplements of users with normal status was 6.80 mg/day (0.36–40 mg/day), but those of users with deficiency and low status was 0.94 mg/day (0.51–1.6 mg/day). Additional riboflavin intakes from supplements were low in users with inadequate status; therefore, it seems that the intake from supplements did not affect riboflavin status of them.

A positive relationship has been observed between riboflavin intake and urinary excretion [31,36]. In this study, no significant correlation was observed between dietary riboflavin intake and urinary riboflavin. However, urinary riboflavin excretion showed a positive correlation with total riboflavin intake ($r = 0.1717$, $p < 0.0363$). Because the subjects supplementing riboflavin additionally consumed 0.36–40 mg/day of riboflavin, total riboflavin intake showed significant correlation with urinary riboflavin rather than dietary intake. These findings show that the urinary riboflavin level reflects riboflavin intake and the intake in population affects their riboflavin status as well. The nutrient database in this study is based on raw foods. In raw foods, nutrient contents are changed by food preparation, cooking conditions (e.g., time and temperature), and the addition of different ingredients depending on household preferences. Therefore, riboflavin cooked foods consumed by the subjects might be underestimated [37]. Three consecutive 24-h recalls were obtained from each subject, which may not be captured as usual intake. Thus, the correlation between urinary riboflavin excretion and total riboflavin intake might not be strong.

## 5. Conclusions

In Korean adults of this study, the prevalence of inadequate riboflavin intake including riboflavin supplementation was much lower than that of KNHANES of South Korea, but the prevalence of inadequacy in Korean adults was still high compared to other countries. One-third of Korean adults in the current study had inadequate riboflavin status, thus consumption of good sources of riboflavin should be encouraged in Koreans such as milk and milk products, whole egg, pork, and mandarins.

**Acknowledgments:** This research was supported by the 2013 research fund from the National Research Foundation of Korea (NRF-2011-0021273).

**Author Contributions:** Young-Nam Kim and Youn-Ok Cho contributed to the design of the study. Ji Young Choi performed experiments and wrote the manuscript, and Young-Nam Kim and Youn-Ok Cho read and corrected the final version of the manuscript. All authors read and approved.

**Conflicts of Interest:** The authors declare no conflict of interest.

## References

1.  Ministry of Health and Welfare; Korea Centers for Disease Control and Prevention. *Korea Health Statistics 2008: Korea National Health and Nutrition Examination Survey (KNHANES IV-2)*; Korea Centers for Disease Control and Prevention: Osong, Korea, 2009.

2.    Ministry of Health and Welfare; Korea Centers for Disease Control and Prevention. *Korea Health Statistics 2007–2009: Korea National Health and Nutrition Examination Survey (KNHANES IV-3)*; Korea Centers for Disease Control and Prevention: Osong, Korea, 2010.

3.    Ministry of Health and Welfare; Korea Centers for Disease Control and Prevention. *Korea Health Statistics 2010–2012: Korea National Health and Nutrition Examination Survey (KNHANES V-3)*; Korea Centers for Disease Control and Prevention: Osong, Korea, 2013.

4.    Gibson, R.S. *Principles of Nutritional Assessment*, 2nd ed.; Oxford University Press, Inc.: New York, NY, USA, 2005; pp. 554–562.

5.    Akimoto, M.; Sato, Y.; Okubo, T.; Todo, H.; Hasegawa, T.; Sugibayashi, K. Conversion of FAD to FMN and riboflavin in plasma: Effects of measuring method. *Pharm. Soc. Jpn.* **2006**, *29*, 1779–1782.

6.    Hustad, S.; Ueland, P.M.; Schneede, J. Quantification of riboflavin, flavin mononucleotide, flavin adenine dinucleotide in human plasma by capillary electrophoresis and laser-induced fluorescence detection. *Clin. Chem.* **1999**, *45*, 862–868.

7.    Shaw, N.S. Prevalence of thiamin and riboflavin deficiency among the elderly in Taiwan. *Asia Pac. J. Clin. Nutr.* **2005**, *14*, 238–243.

8.    Anderson, J.J.; Suchindran, C.M.; Roggenkamp, K.J. Micronutrient intakes in two US populations of older adults: Lipid research clinics program prevalence study findings. *J. Nutr. Health Aging* **2009**, *13*, 595–600.

9.    Preziosi, P.; Galan, P.; Deheeger, M.; Yacoup, N.; Drewnowski, A.; Hercberg, S. Breakfast type, daily nutrient intakes and vitamin and mineral status of French children, adolescents, and adults. *J. Am. Coll. Nutr.* **1999**, *18*, 171–178.

10.   Matrix, J.; Aranda, P.; Sanchez, C.; Montellano, M.A.; Planells, E.; Liopis, J. Assessment of thiamin (vitamin $B_1$) and riboflavin (vitamin $B_2$) status in an adult Mediterranean population. *Br. J. Nutr.* **2003**, *90*, 661–666.

11.   Szczuko, M.; Seidler, T.; Mierzwa, M.; Stachowska, E.; Chlubek, D. Effect of riboflavin supply on student body's provision in north-western Poland with riboflavin measured by activity of glutathione reductase considering daily intake of other nutrients. *Int. J. Food Sci. Nutr.* **2011**, *62*, 431–438.

12.   Kweon, S.S.; Shu, X.O.; Xiang, Y.; Yang, G.; Ji, B.T.; Li, H.; Gao, Y.T.; Zheng, W.; Shrubsole, M.J. One-carbon metabolism dietary factors and distal gastric cancer risk in Chinese woman. *Cancer Epidemiol. Biomark. Prev.* **2014**, *23*, 1–20.

13.   Powers, H.J.; Hill, M.H.; Welfare, M.; Spiers, A.; Bal, W.; Russell, J.; Dukworth, T.; Gibney, E.; Williams, E.A.; Mathers, J.C. Responses of biomarkers of folate and riboflavin status to folate and riboflavin supplementation in healthy and colorectal polyp patients (The FAB2 study). *Cancer Epidemiol. Biomark. Prev.* **2007**, *16*, 2128–2134.

14.   Vogel, S.; Dindore, V.; Engeland, M.; Goldbohm, R.A.; Brandt, P.A.; Weijenberg, M.P. Dietary folate, methionine, riboflavin, and vitamin $B_6$ and risk of sporadic colorectal cancer. *J. Nutr.* **2008**, *138*, 2372–2378.

15.   Bassett, J.K.; Hodgem, A.M.; English, D.R.; Baglietto, L.; Hopper, J.L.; Giles, G.G.; Severi, G. Dietary intake of B vitamins and methionine and risk of lung cancer. *Eur. J. Clin. Nutr.* **2012**, *66*, 182–187.

16. He, Y.; Ye, L.; Shan, B.; Song, G.; Meng, F.; Wang, S. Effect of riboflavin-fortified salt nutrition intervention on esophageal squamous cell carcinoma in a high incidence area, China. *Asian Pac. J. Cancer Prev.* **2009**, *10*, 619–622.

17. Azizi-Namini, P.; Ahmed, M.; Yan, A.T.; Keith, M. The role of B vitamins in the Management of heart Failure. *Nutr. Clin. Prat.* **2012**, *27*, 363–374.

18. Powers, H.J. Riboflavin and health. *Am. J. Clin. Nutr.* **2003**, *77*, 1352–1360.

19. Yoon, J.S.; Lim, W.J.; Kim, S.Y. A human metabolic study for determination of daily requirement of riboflavin. *Korean J. Nutr.* **1989**, *22*, 507–515.

20. Lim, W.J.; Yoon, J.S. A longitudinal study on seasonal variation of riboflavin status of rural women: Dietary intake, erythrocyte glutathione reductase activity coefficient, and urinary riboflavin excretion. *Korean J. Nutr.* **1997**, *29*, 507–516.

21. The Korean Nutrition Society. *Computer Aided Nutritional Analysis Program for Professionals*; The Korean Nutrition Society: Seoul, Korea, 2011.

22. The Korean Nutrition Society. *Dietary Reference Intakes for Koreans*; The Korean Nutrition Society: Seoul, Korea, 2010.

23. Gatautis, V.J.; Naito, H.K. Liquid-chromatographic determination of urinary riboflavin. *Clin. Chem.* **1981**, *27*, 1672–1675.

24. Huang, J.; Vieira, A. DNA methylation, riboswitches, and transcription factor activity: Fucdamental mechanisms of gene-nutrient interactions involving vitamins. *Mol. Biol. Rep.* **2006**, *381*, 1029–1036.

25. Bian, S.; Gao, Y.; Zhang, M.; Wang, X.; Liu, W.; Zhang, D.; Huang, G. Dietary nutrient intake and metabolic syndrome risk in Chinese adults: A case-control study. *Nutr. J.* **2013**, *12*, 106–112.

26. Beverley, B.; Alison, L.; Ann, P.; Chris, B.; Polly, P.; Sonja, N.; Gillian, S. *National Diet and Nutrition Survey: Results from Years 1, 2, 3 and 4 (Combined) of the Rolling Programme (2008/2009–2011/2012)*; Public Health England and the Food Standards Agency: London, UK, 2014; pp. 88–111.

27. Shi, Z.; Zhen, S.; Wittert, G.A.; Yuan, B.; Zuo, H.; Taylor, A.W. Inadequate riboflavin intake and anemia risk in a Chinese population: Five-year follow up of the Jiangsu Nutrition Survey. *PLoS One* **2014**, *9*.

28. What We Eat in America, NHANES 2009–2010, Individuals 2 Years and over (Excluding Pregnant and/or Lactating Females and Breast-Fed Children), Day 1 Food and Supplement Intake Data, Weighted. Available online: http://www.ars.usda.gov/ba/bhnrc/fsrg (accessed on 29 September 2014).

29. Horwitt, M.K. Interpretations of requirements for thiamin, riboflavin, niacin-tryptophan, and vitamin E plus comments on balance studies and vitamin $B_6$. *Am. J. Clin. Nutr.* **1986**, *44*, 973–985.

30. Zempleni, J.; Galloway, J.R.; McCormick, D.B. Pharmacokinetics of orally and intravenously administered riboflavin in healthy humans. *Am. J. Clin. Nutr.* **1996**, *63*, 54–66.

31. Tsuji, T.; Fukuwatari, T.; Shihata, K. Twenty-four-hour urinary water-soluble vitamin levels correlate with their intakes in free-living Japanese schoolchildren. *Public Health Nutr.* **2010**, *14*, 327–333.

32. Tasevska, N.; Runswick, S.A.; McTaggart, A.; Bingham, S.A. Twenty-four hour urinary thiamine as a biomarker for the assessment of thiamin intake. *Eur. J. Clin. Nutr.* **2007**, *62*, 1139–1147.

33. Fukuwatari, T.; Shibata, K. Urinary water-soluble vitamins and their metabolite contents as nutritional marker for evaluating vitamin intakes in young Japanese women. *J. Nutr. Sci. Vitaminol.* **2008**, *54*, 223–229.

34. Hill, M.H.E.; Bradley, A.; Mushtaq, S.; Williams, E.A.; Powers, H.J. Effects of methodological variation on assessment of riboflavin status using the erythrocyte glutathione reductase activation coefficient assay. *Br. J. Nutr.* **2009**, *102*, 273–278.

35. Whitfield, K.; McCann, A.; Karakochuk, C.; Talukder, A.; Ward, M.; McNulty, H.; McLean, J.; Green, T. High rates of riboflavin deficiency in women of childbearing age in Cambodia and Canada. *FASEB J.* **2014**, *28* (Suppl. 1).

36. Fukuwatari, T. Urinary water-soluble vitamins as potential nutritional biomarkers to assess their intakes. *J. Nutr. Food Sci.* **2011**, *6*, 1–9.

37. Kim, Y.N.; Cho, Y.O. Evaluation of vitamin $B_6$ intake and status of 20- to 64-year-old Koreans. *Nutr. Res. Pract.* **2014**, *8*, 688–694.

# Suboptimal Micronutrient Intake among Children in Europe

Boris Kaganov, Margherita Caroli, Artur Mazur, Atul Singhal and Andrea Vania

**Abstract:** Adequate dietary intake of micronutrients is not necessarily achieved even in resource-rich areas of the world wherein overeating is a public health concern. In Europe, population-based data suggests substantial variability in micronutrient intake among children. Two independent surveys of micronutrient consumption among European children were evaluated. Stratified by age, the data regarding micronutrient intake were evaluated in the context of daily requirements, which are typically estimated in the absence of reliable absolute values derived from prospective studies. The proportion of children living in Europe whose intake of at least some vitamins and trace elements are at or below the estimated average requirements is substantial. The most common deficiencies across age groups included vitamin D, vitamin E, and iodine. Specific deficiencies were not uniform across countries or by age or gender. Micronutrient intake appears to be more strongly influenced by factors other than access to food. Substantial portions of European children may be at risk of reversible health risks from inadequate intake of micronutrients. Despite the growing health threat posed by excess intake of calories, adequate exposure to vitamins, trace elements, and other micronutrients may deserve attention in public health initiatives to optimize growth and development in the European pediatric population.

Reprinted from *Nutrients*. Cite as: Kaganov, B.; Caroli, M.; Mazur, A.; Singhal, A.; Vania, A. Suboptimal Micronutrient Intake among Children in Europe. *Nutrients* **2015**, *7*, 3524–3535.

## 1. Introduction

While recognizing that comprehensive data regarding diet and nutrition among children in Europe remain limited, well-documented nutritional deficiencies do exist across the European pediatric population. The aim of this review article is to raise awareness of the importance of ensuring children who have ready access to food are maintaining adequate levels of micronutrients through proper food choices and appropriate use of nutritional supplements.

Based on the clear relationship between adequate intake of vitamins as well as other micronutrients and health, authorities in most countries of Europe publish recommendations for appropriate population-based daily nutrient intake [1]. In 2006 the European Food Safety Authority (EFSA) published its first consensus document regarding appropriate consumption within the European Union [2]. In that document, appropriate levels were defined as dietary reference values (DRVs). These and other terms, like dietary reference intakes (DRIs), recommended dietary allowances (RDAs) and estimated daily requirements (EDRs), express best estimates of nutrient intakes that will reduce the risk of adverse health consequences associated with a specific nutrient. Table 1.

**Table 1.** Common Terms for Describing Nutritional Values.

---

- **DRV** (*Dietary Reference Value*) or EAR (*Estimated Average Requirment*): how much of a nutrient meets the needs of 50% of the healthy subjects of a specific population's group

---

- **DRI** or **RDA** (*Dietary Reference Intake* or *Recommended Dietary Allowance*): how much of a nutrient meets the needs of 97.5% (mean + 2SD) of healthy subjects of a specific population group

---

- **EDR** (*Estimated Daily Requirement*): estimate of nutrient intakes that will reduce risk of adverse health consequences

---

- **AI** (*Adequate Intake*): how much of a nutrient is adequate for a population's group, according to the average intakes of apparently healthy people

---

- **UL** (tolerable *Upper* intake *Levels*): maximum intake of a nutrient not bound to any adverse effect

---

- **LTI** (*Lowest Threshold Intake*): lowest acceptable intake, under which nearly all individuals in a population's group will not maintain metabolic integrity and efficiency

---

In the absence of reliable information of an absolute threshold at which a nutrient deficit leads to complications, DRVs are often derived from average intakes in a healthy population. Values are typically set at two standard deviations above the average to accommodate variability in physiologic demands [3]. Discrepancies between DRVs from different guidelines can arise from several causes including differences in the sampled populations and in the methods with which studies were conducted. Nevertheless, comparisons of population-based nutritional recommendations, such as those included on food labels, typically reveal relatively modest differences across Europe and countries outside of Europe [4].

In children, the disparity among available nutritional guidelines has been modest within Europe where many countries continue to issue independent recommendations for the pediatric population. The differences stem from methodology regarding how data is collected and interpreted across age ranges that are not necessarily stratified identically. For example, in Italy recommendations are made for five age groups in post-breastfed children (ages 1–3, 4–6, 7–10, 11–14, 15–17 years), whereas a recently published Nordic (Denmark, Finland, Norway, and Sweden) consensus document divided infants aged younger than 2 years into three groups and older children into four groups (ages 2–5, 6–9, 10–13, 14–17 years) [5] Recently published EFSA guidelines were limited to infants and children of 36 months of age or younger with multiple stratifications within this age range [6].

Specific stratifications are relevant to nutritional analyses. In general, children require higher levels of many nutrients proportional to body weight than adults [7] but their specific needs evolve rapidly at different points in growth. Metabolically active organs, such as the brain, liver, and heart, represent a far greater proportion of body weight in infants than adults and have reached 50% of adult size by 2 years of age [8]. In deriving data about health nutrient intake from a sample population, the specific age stratifications could therefore influence normative data. Moreover, the methodologies for evaluating food consumption, such as 7-day dietary recall or standardized questionnaire, as well as the statistical methods for data analysis have the potential for producing differences that complicate comparisons.

Finally, the presentation of data from different nutritional guidelines may vary. In the EFSA guidelines, tables outlining nutrients represent a synthesis of available data in a format intended to be simple to consult. In contrast, tables in the Italian guidelines include information on the quality of data, drawing attention to values for which average intake (AI) has been substituted for average requirements (AR) when reliable data to calculate ARs are absent. This increased detail may be of use when considering nutrition in special populations, such as those with gastrointestinal (GI) dysfunction, even if it renders the tables more complex.

Due to potentially irreversible physical or cognitive deficits, the consequences of micronutrient deficiency are potentially greater in children than adults. Many of these deficiencies and complications, such as inadequate vitamin D intake leading to abnormal bone formation [9], are well known and readily recognizable. Others, such as the impact of micronutrient deficiency on cognition, may be both complex and subtle [10]. Micronutrients implicated in cognitive development include iodine [11], for which deficiencies have correlated with lower intelligence quotient (IQ) scores [12], iron, which is important for oxygen transport to the brain [13], as well as zinc [14] and thiamine [15].

In Europe, deficiencies in micronutrients are mostly related to the quality of the diet but not to the quantity of food consumed. For this reason, the risks of micronutrient deficiency have the potential to persist in otherwise resource-rich areas of the world. Due to the importance of these micronutrients for growth and development, risks posed by deficiencies may be greater in children, who may also have lower stores of micronutrients than adults to bridge periods of deficiency. In both, nutritional assessments have the potential to avoid preventable disease.

## 2. Methods

Two studies, employing different methodologies, have evaluated micronutrient consumption among children living in Europe. In a report from the Directorate General of the European Commission, Health and Consumers, nutritional data was compared across regions of Europe [16]. In this study, data was collected utilizing the EU-supported Data Food Networking (DAFNE) methodology over a one year period in order to capture seasonal variations in food intake. In the other study, representative dietary survey data were collected and compared from Belgium, Denmark, France, Germany, The Netherlands, Poland, Spain, and the United Kingdom (UK) [17]. In this study, a number of different design and dietary assessment methods were used in the surveys, including single or repeated 24 h recalls; 2, 3, 4 or 7 day prospective food records; estimated or weighed amounts consumed; and modified dietary histories with a reference period of 4 weeks. All the surveys, except for those from Belgium and Poland, covered all seasons of the year.

In both studies, data were stratified by types of micronutrients within predefined age groups. Although the methods of data collection and analysis varied, including definitions of adequate and inadequate micronutrient consumption, these two sets of data provide a basis for considering potential trends. They provide a context for evaluating the variability in diet and its potential impact on endpoints relevant to pediatric health.

No human subjects nor their data were prospectively collected in the execution of this work. All of the data used herein were extracted from published sources.

## 3. Results

In the European survey, nutritional information from 16 countries was collected for analysis in four geographical regions. The north region included countries from Scandinavia. The east region included Germany, Austria, and countries of Eastern Europe. The south region included Greece, Italy, and the Iberian countries. The west region included Belgium, France, Ireland, The Netherlands, and the UK. Reference values for adequate nutrient intake were drawn from 2003 World Health Organization (WHO) guidelines [18].

The data were not collected concurrently but in country-specific surveys conducted between the years 2000 and 2008. There were also differences in the methodology of collection, such as 3-day *vs.* 7-day dietary recall. Despite efforts to homogenize the data, the authors emphasized its limitations. The findings were considered suitable to an overview of nutrition in Europe, which was the objective of this evaluation, but of limited reliability for rigorous conclusions about relative nutritional intake for cross-country comparisons.

Across the four age groups evaluated (4 to 6 years, 7 to 9 years, 10 to 14 years, and 15 to 18 years) the most commonly observed deficiencies involved vitamin D, folate, iron, calcium, iodine, and phosphate. For most of the remaining micronutrients, such as the trace minerals selenium and magnesium, and the vitamins B6 and vitamin C, deficiencies were rare or not observed. However, there was substantial regional variability in reported deficiencies by individual nutrient within age groups and gender (Figure 1).

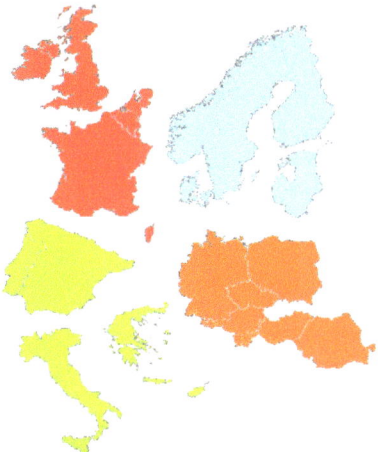

| Age (years) | Region | Sex | Folate (Ref 300 mcg) | Vitamin D (Ref: 5 mcg) | Vitamin B6 (Ref: 0.7 mg) |
|---|---|---|---|---|---|
| 4–6 | North | Male | 135–256 | 2.3–6.8 | 1.1–1.6 |
| 4–6 | North | Female | 132–235 | 2.0–6.5 | 1.0–1.5 |
| 7–9 | North | Male | 204–290 | 2.5–6.4 | 1.3–2.5 |
| 7–9 | North | Female | 187–264 | 2.2–5.1 | 1.2–1.6 |
| 4–6 | South | Male | 198 | 2.3 | 1.6 |
| 4–6 | South | Female | 199 | 2.2 | 1.6 |
| 7–9 | South | Male | 242 | 2.8 | 1.8 |
| 7–9 | South | Female | 211 | 2.1 | 1.7 |
| 4–6 | Central-East | Male | 190–214 | 1.8–2.3 | 1.5–1.8 |
| 4–6 | Central-East | Female | 164–190 | 1.5–2.3 | 1.2–1.9 |
| 7–9 | Central-East | Male | 154–229 | 1.5–2.8 | 1.2–1.8 |
| 7–9 | Central-East | Female | 145–212 | 1.5–2.7 | 1.1–1.8 |
| 4–6 | West | Male | 120–225 | 2.2–2.4 | 1.3–1.8 |
| 4–6 | West | Female | 109–196 | 1.9 | 1.2–1.7 |
| 7–9 | West | Male | 144–256 | 2.2–2.9 | 1.3–2.2 |
| 7–9 | West | Female | 133–226 | 2.4–2.8 | 1.2–1.9 |

**Figure 1.** Folate and Vitamin D levels that fell below recommended reference values compared to normal ranges of Vitamin B6 levels in children in different regions of Europe.

The most consistent finding across all age groups was deficiency in vitamin D and folate. Both the minimum and maximum average intake of vitamin D and folate fell below reference standards in most age groups in all four geographic regions. Although both the minimum and maximum average intake are relevant to epidemiologic studies of nutrition, the terms differ for their relevance to the definition of malnutrition. An intake below the minimum average, unlike the maximum intake, indicates the potential for inadequacy, or malnutrition as it applies to that nutrient.

No deficiencies other than vitamin D and folate were observed as consistently (Figure 2), but other types of deficiencies were observed frequently. For example, the maximum average intake of iron was below recommended levels among females aged 4–6 years in the north and west and in all older females from any region. The maximum average intake of iodine was below recommended levels in the central region for both sexes at all age groups and for older females in the west region.

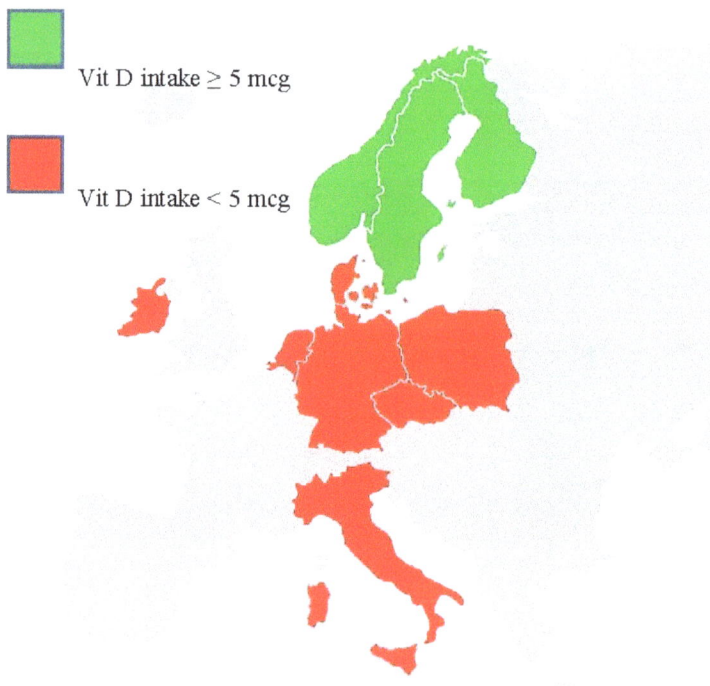

Figure 2. Vitamin D intake in European children aged 4–18 years old.

Among children aged 7–9 years, both the minimum and maximum average intake of iron also fell below the reference standard among females in the north, south, and west as did iodine for females in the east. Minimum averages, but not maximum averages, were below reference standards for calcium among both males and females in the north and east, and, for iron, among males and females in the north and west. For all other nutrients, both minimum and maximum average intakes exceeded reference standards.

Relative to younger children, the frequency with which both the minimum and maximum average intake for any given nutrient fell below the reference standard was greater in both those aged 10 to 14 years and in adolescents. In those aged 10–14 years, this included calcium among males and females in all four regions and iron among males and females in the north, south, and west. Both minimum and maximum average intake of iron was also below reference standards among both girls and boys in all regions with the exception of males in the east. Maximum and minimum average iodine intake was below the reference standard for both genders in the east and west. In the oldest age group, both the minimum and maximum average intake of calcium fell below the reference standard in both genders in most regions and average minimum intake were commonly deficient for iron, zinc, and iodine.

In the second study, which included both adults and children, nutritional experts from European countries were invited to submit data that met predefined quality criteria. Data from eight countries were included. The nutrients selected for analysis included those for which there were reference values and for which there were known or suspected deficiencies. These were calcium, copper, iodine, iron, magnesium, potassium, selenium, zinc, and the vitamins A, B1, B2, B6, B12, C, D, E, and folate. The reference values were taken from values originally established in the UK in 1991 [19], or for those missing, from the 2004 Nordic Nutrient recommendations [20]. The age of these reference values in the context of dietary changes is a potential weakness of this study but more recent UK values were unavailable. Results were expressed in several ways, including the proportion of the population with an estimated daily intake below the lower reference nutrient intake (LRNI) and estimated average requirement (EAR).

For the majority of nutrients evaluated, the proportion of children with daily intakes below the EAR, suggesting a potential for a health risk was measurable in at least some countries in one or more of the five pediatric age ranges evaluated (ages 1–3 years, 4–6 years, 7–10 years, 11–14 years, 15–17 years) (Table 2). Iodine is one example. For this nutrient, 61% of girls and 55% of boys aged 4–10 years in Germany had intakes below the EAR. Iron is another example. In this case, 94% of girls in Germany aged 4–10 years had average intakes below the EAR. The average intakes of vitamin D, a third example, were below the EAR in essentially all children in every age group and country.

Even when deficiencies were uncommon across most countries, there were exceptions. For example, the proportion of patients with an average intake of vitamin E below the EAR was consistently low across all countries with the exception of boys aged 4–10 in Belgium, where more than 20% were deficient by the reference standard. In addition, it is reasonable to consider whether low prevalence rates in relative terms are still clinically meaningful. In children who face complications for readily reversible nutrient deficiencies, small but measurable prevalence rates may signal a need for simple screening so that dietary modification or supplementation can be implemented.

**Table 2.** Percent of children with intakes of select micronutrients intake estimated average requirement (EAR) as reported in various surveys in several European countries.

| Country | Iodine | | | Iron | | Magnesium | Selenium | Zinc | |
|---|---|---|---|---|---|---|---|---|---|
| | C♂ (75–82.5 µg/day) | C♀ (75–82.5 µg/day) | T♂♀ (5.3 mg/day) | C♀ (4.7–6.7 mg/day) | A♀ (8.7 mg/day) | A♀ (230–250 mg/day) | A♀ (33.8–45 mg/day) | C♀ (5.0–5.4 mg/day) | A♀ (5.5–7.0 mg/day) |
| BE | - | - | 23.4 | 10.2 | - | 0.4 | - | 7.6 | - |
| DK | 0.0 | 0.0 | | 18.8 | 93.9 | 0.5 | 79.6 | 4.9 | 23.0 |
| FR | 11.8 | 25.3 | | 3.5 | 73.6 | 4.7 | 54.1 | 4.6 | 18.4 |
| DE * | 55.1 | 60.8 | | 5.5 | 24.8 | 1.6 | - | 13.8 | 6.0 |
| PL | 41.9 | 45.5 | 55.1 | 28.3 | 67.5 | 11.2 | - | 27.0 | 19.2 |
| ES | - | - | | 0.3 | 23.8 | 0.3 | - | - | - |
| NL | - | - | 32.0 | 12.0 | 85.1 | 0.2 †; 5.6 ‡ | 67.9 | 39.0; 13.0 | 21.0 |
| UK | 9.2 | 16.3 | 32.3 | 25.9 | 67.0 | 8.6 | 60.8 | 27.1 | 47.5 |

Reference values for respective nutrient in (parenthesis); * Age range for a child in Germany is 6–10 years old; T = Toddler (<3 years old); C = Child (ranges between 4–10 years old depending on country); A = Adolescent (11–17 years old); † Children 4–6 years old; ‡ Children 7–10 years old.

## 4. Discussion

The obstacles to determine adequate micronutrient intake are complex. In regions where fruits, fresh vegetables, and proteins are readily available and well represented in the average diet, nutritional deficiencies are likely to be uncommon. Yet, dietary decisions made by individuals within such regions may still lead to nutritional deficiencies, including nutritional deficiencies concurrent with excess body weight. Despite modern food distribution, which has improved consistent access to diverse food groups in countries with short growing seasons, food choices by parents for young children and older children for themselves are not necessarily influenced the goal of healthy eating.

Public health initiatives in Europe to address common nutritional deficiencies vary by country. For example, iodine fortification of salt is mandatory in some countries such as Denmark but voluntary in others, such as Finland and Italy. Fortification of milk with vitamin D is required or strongly encouraged in most countries but fortification of milk products or margarine with vitamin A or E is less common. Fortification of fruit juices with vitamin C is not mandatory and may vary by country according to consumer demand.

Differences in fortification policies are likely to explain some portion of the disparity in the prevalence of some nutrient deficiencies among children living in Europe but the diet of any individual child may deviate grossly from those of peers. Parents who avoid individual food groups due to preference or belief, or children who refuse specific food categories, are vulnerable to deficiencies even when consuming an otherwise quantitatively well balanced diet. Indeed, the "picky eater" child is a well-recognized phenomenon with prevalence rates estimated as high as 50% in children 24-months-of age [21] A greater relative risk of nutritional deficiencies is likely in children on exclusion diets, such as those on a vegetarian (especially vegan), gluten-free, or lactose-free diet.

Due to the evidence of persistent deficiencies among children, a systematic approach to ensuring adequate access to vital vitamins, trace elements, and other nutrients essential to healthy growth, such as calcium, is reasonable in routine pediatric care. In otherwise healthy children, a formal dietary assessment, although potentially valuable for increasing the rate of detection, may not be justified by time and expense, but general questions about diet may identify potential inadequacies. Several relatively simple tools, such as the Child and Diet Evaluation Tool (CADET) [22], have been validated for identifying children with low intake of fruits and vegetable. Clinical inquiries about diet have the potential to reveal inadequacies at the same time that they serve to convey the message that a healthy diet plays a role in disease prevention.

When informal dietary surveys suggest potential problems in nutrient acquisition, further evaluation, including a referral to a nutritionist or dietician, may be appropriate. It is important not to underestimate the complexity of adequate nutrition. The interplay and heterogeneity of variables that affect how micronutrients are metabolized and stored remains a focus of study. In experimental studies, for example, metabolism of iron is affected by dietary exposure to both zinc and nicotinic acid [23] Clinical studies in resource-poor areas of the world have suggested that coexisting micronutrient deficiencies can impair the response to single micronutrient replacement therapy [24].

In children suspected or at risk of micronutrient deficiencies, nutritional supplementation may be a valuable approach for ensuring adequate intakes. Supplementation of specific nutrients is helpful in those with chronic diseases affecting liver or gut function, such as Crohn's disease, or in those on exclusion diets liable to limit intake of specific vitamins. There is also a strong rationale for supplements in preventing deficiencies in otherwise healthy children at risk for micronutrient deficiencies. This may be particularly important in specific stages of development, such as vitamin D in infants or vitamin D and iron in toddlers and other young children in whom there is evidence of adverse health consequences when these nutrients are deficient. Published studies have associated supplementation of vitamin D, which appears to enhance metabolism in several organs other than bone, such as immune function [25], with improved nutrient adequacy in both children and adults. [26,27] This finding has lead public health agencies in some countries (e.g., the U.K.) to recommend supplementation, particularly for children younger than age 5 years.

Due to the evidence that there may be interactions within a healthy diet important to the metabolism of nutrients, supplementation should not be considered a substitute for a well-balanced healthy diet. Although suitable for adjunctive use when nutrient deficiencies are known or suspected, nutritional supplementation does not provide any additional benefit in individuals who are already obtaining adequate nutrients by diet alone. Specific supplements should be recommended on the basis of the nutrients relevant to the risk of deficiency at recommended dosages. Whether or not supplements are being considered, parents and older children should receive explicit information on the essential role of a healthy diet to maximize growth and development while minimizing health risks.

In Europe, the persistence of nutritional deficiencies in the midst of an obesity epidemic should not be misunderstood as a paradox. Ready access to food does not ensure healthy food choices required to achieve adequate nutrition. In young children, food choices may be dictated by adults responding to well marketed prepared products high in fat and low in nutritional value. Modern food distribution has largely eliminated seasonal gaps in adequate access to fruits and vegetables but individual choice can thwart efforts to promote healthy eating. The data from two large surveys suggest that prevalence rates of selected nutritional deficiencies among European children are clinically meaningful. The rates for specific nutrient deficiencies vary by country but several, including vitamin D, folate, and iron, are common. Due to the threat these deficiencies pose for impaired growth and other adverse health consequences, the data should encourage public health initiatives designed to improve nutrition on a population basis and to consider routine inquiries about diet in the care of healthy children. In children with normal metabolism, the risks posed by nutritional deficiencies may be circumvented if detected and reversed in early stages of development.

**Acknowledgments:** We would like to acknowledge Janice Harland, a nutritional consultant in Cirencester, UK, who made valuable contributions to the pediatric nutrition roundtable held in Rome, Italy on 3 September 2013. Kevin Taylor of Procter & Gamble was instrumental in organizing the Rome pediatric nutrition roundtable and stimulating the gathering of data critical to this manuscript. We would like to thank Theodore Bosworth, a medical writer based in New York who provided medical writing services on behalf of P & G Health Care and PGT Healthcare.

**Author Contributions:** The premise for this article was developed from data presented and analyzed in a pediatric nutrition roundtable convened in Rome, Italy on 3 September 2013 and at the 3rd Global Congress for Consensus in Pediatrics and Child Health (CIP) in Bangkok, 15 February 2014. In Rome, data were presented and included in this manuscript from

Kaganov and Singhal. In Bangkok, data were presented and included in this manuscript from Kaganov, Caroli, Vania, and Mazur. All of the authors equally contributed to the writing of this manuscript.

**Conflicts of Interest:** Funding for the Rome Roundtable, CIP Symposium, and manuscript submission fee was provided by Procter & Gamble Health Care (Cincinnati, OH, USA) and PGT Healthcare (Geneva, Swithzerland). The authors declare that have no other competing interests.

## References

1.  Doets, E.L.; de Wit, L.S.; Dhonukshe-Rutten, R.A.; Cavelaars, A.E.J.M.; Raats, M.M.; Timotijevic, L.; Brzozowska, A.; Wijnhoven, T.M.A.; Pavlovic, M.; Totland, T.H.; *et al.* Current micronutrient recommendations in Europe: Towards understanding their differences and similarities. *Eur. J. Nutr.* **2008**, *47*, 17–40.

2.  European Food Safety Authority (EFSA). Tolerable Upper Intake Levels for Vitamins and Minerals, 2006. Available online: Http://www.efsa.europa.eu/it/ndatopics/docs/ndatolerableuil.pdf (accessed on 18 September 2014).

3.  Leaf, A.A. Vitamins for babies and young children. *Arch. Dis. Child.* **2007**, *92*, 160–164.

4.  Dwyer, J.T. *Present Knowledge in Nutrition*, 10th ed.; Erdman, J.S., MacDonald, I.A., Zeisel, S.H., Eds.; Wiley-Blackwell: New York, NY, USA, 2012.

5.  Nordic Council of Ministers. *Nordic Nutrition Recommendations 2012. Integrating Nutrition and Physical Activity*, 4th ed.; Nordic Council of Ministers: Copenhagen, Denmark, 2014.

6.  EFSA NDA Panel. Scientific opinion on nutrient requirements and dietary intakes of infants and young children in the European Union. *EFSA J.* **2013**.

7.  Lucas, B.L.; Feucht, S.A. *Krause's Food & Nutrition Therapy*, 12th ed.; Mahan, L.K., Escott-Stump, S., Eds.; Saunders Elsevier: St. Louis, MS, USA, 2008.

8.  Prentice, A.M.; Ward, K.A.; Goldberg, G.R.; Jarjou, L.M.; Moore, S.E.; Fulford, A.J.; Prentice, A. Critical windows for nutritional interventions against stunting. *Am. J. Clin. Nutr.* **2013**, *97*, 911–918.

9.  Holick, M.F. Resurrection of vitamin D deficiency and rickets. *J. Clin. Investig.* **2006**, *116*, 2062–2072.

10. Antonow-Schlorke, I.; Schwab, M.; Cox, L.A.; Li, C.; Stuchlik, K.; Witte, O.W.; Nathanielsz, P.W.; McDonald, T.J. Vulnerability of the fetal primate brain to moderate reduction in maternal global nutrient availability. *Proc. Natl. Acad. Sci. USA* **2011**, *108*, 3011–3016.

11. Pharoah, P.O.; Buttfield, I.H.; Hetzel, B.S. Neurological damage to the fetus resulting from severe iodine deficiency during pregnancy. *Lancet* **1971**, *1*, 308–310.

12. Qian, M.; Wang, D.; Watkins, W.E.; Gebski, V.; Yan, Y.Q.; Li, M.; Chen, Z.P. The effects of iodine on intelligence in children: A meta-analysis of studies conducted in China. *Asia. Pac. J. Clin. Nutr.* **2005**, *14*, 32–42.

13. Walker, S.P.; Wachs, T.D.; Meeks-Gardner, J.M.; Lozoff, B.; Wasserman, G.A.; Pollitt, E.; Carter, J.A. Child development: Risk factors for adverse outcomes in developing countries. *Lancet* **2007**, *369*, 145–157.

14. Black, M.M.; Baqui, A.H.; Zaman, K.; el Arifeen, S.E.; Le, K.; McNary, S.W.; Parveen, M.; Hamadani, J.D.; Black, R.E. Iron and zinc supplementation promote motor development and exploratory behavior among Bangladeshi infants. *Am. J. Clin. Nutr.* **2004**, *80*, 903–910.

15. Fattal, I.; Friedmann, N.; Fattal-Valevski, A. The crucial role of thiamine in the development of syntax and lexical retrieval: a study of infantile thiamine deficiency. *Brain* **2011**, *134*, 1720–1739.

16. Elmadfa, I. *European Nutrition and Health Report*; Forum of Nutrition, Elmadfa, I., Eds.; Karger: Vienna, Austria, 2009; Volume 62.

17. Mensink, G.B.; Fletcher, R.; Gurinovic, M.; Huybrechts, I.; Lafay, L.; Serra-Majem, L.; Szponar, L.; Tetens, I.; Verkaik-Kloosterman, J.; Baka, A.; Stephen, A.M. Mapping low intake of micronutrients across Europe. *Br. J. Nutr.* **2013**, *110*, 755–773.

18. World Health Organization (WHO). *Diet, Nutrition, and the Prevention of Chronic Diseases, Joint WHO/FAO Technical Report Series*; WHO: Geneva, Switzerland, 2003; No. 916.

19. Department of Health. *Dietary Reference Values for Food, Energy and Nutrients in the United Kingdom*; HSMO: London, UK, 1992.

20. Nordic Council of Ministers. *Nordic Nutrition Recommendations 2004. Integrating Nutrition and Physical Activity*, 4th ed.; Nordic Council of Ministers: Copenhagen, Denmark, 2005.

21. Carruth, B.R.; Ziegler, P.J.; Gordon, A.; Barr, S.I. Prevalence of picky eaters among infants and toddlers and their caregivers' decisions about offering a new food. *J. Am. Diet. Assoc.* **2004**, *104*, s57–s64.

22. Cade, J.E.; Frear, L.; Greenwood, D.C. Assessment of diet in young children with an emphasis on fruit and vegetable intake: Using CADET—Child and Diet Evaluation Tool. *Public Health Nutr.* **2006**, *9*, 501–508.

23. Agte, V.V.; Paknikar, K.M.; Chiplonkar, S.A. Effect of nicotinic acid on zinc and iron metabolism. *Biometals* **1997**, *10*, 271–276.

24. Thurlow, R.A.; Winichagoon, P.; Pongcharoen, T.; Gowachirapant, S.; Boonpraderm, A.; Manger, M.S.; Bailey, K.B.; Wasantwisut, E.; Gibson, R.S. Risk of zinc, iodine and other micronutrient deficiencies among school children in North East Thailand. *Eur. J. Clin. Nutr.* **2006**, *60*, 623–632.

25. Aranow, C. Vitamin D and the immune system. *J. Investig. Med.* **2011**, *59*, 881–886.

26. Briefel, R.; Hanson, C.; Fox, M.K.; Novak, T.; Ziegler, P. Feeding Infants and Toddlers Study: Do vitamin and mineral supplements contribute to nutrient adequacy or excess among US infants and toddlers? *J. Am. Diet. Assoc.* **2006**, *106*, S52–S65.

27. Weeden, A.; Remig, V.; Holcomb, C.A.; Herald, T.J.; Baybutt, R.C. Vitamin and mineral supplements have a nutritionally significant impact on micronutrient intakes of older adults attending senior centers. *J. Nutr. Elder.* **2010**, *29*, 241–254.

# Cod Liver Oil Supplement Consumption and Health: Cross-sectional Results from the EPIC-Norfolk Cohort Study

Marleen A.H. Lentjes, Ailsa A. Welch, Angela A. Mulligan, Robert N. Luben, Nicholas J. Wareham and Kay-Tee Khaw

**Abstract:** Supplement users (SU) make healthy lifestyle choices; on the other hand, SU report more medical conditions. We hypothesised that cod liver oil (CLO) consumers are similar to non-supplement users, since CLO use might originate from historical motives, *i.e.*, rickets prevention, and not health consciousness. CLO consumers were studied in order to identify possible confounders, such as confounding by indication. The European Prospective Investigation into Cancer (EPIC) investigates causes of chronic disease. The participants were 25,639 men and women, aged 40–79 years, recruited from general practices in Norfolk, East-Anglia (UK). Participants completed questionnaires and a health examination between 1993 and 1998. Supplement use was measured using 7-day diet diaries. CLO was the most common supplement used, more prevalent among women and associated with not smoking, higher physical activity level and more favourable eating habits. SU had a higher occurrence of benign growths and bone-related diseases, but CLO was negatively associated with cardiovascular-related conditions. Although the results of SU characteristics in EPIC-Norfolk are comparable with studies worldwide, the CLO group is different from SU in general. Confounding by indication takes place and will need to be taken into account when analysing prospective associations of CLO use with fracture risk and cardiovascular diseases.

Reprinted from *Nutrients*. Cite as: Lentjes, M.A.H.; Welch, A.A.; Mulligan, A.A.; Luben, R.N.; Wareham, N.J.; Khaw, K.-T. Cod Liver Oil Supplement Consumption and Health: Cross-sectional Results from the EPIC-Norfolk Cohort Study. *Nutrients* **2014**, *6*, 4320–4337.

## 1. Introduction

Since the 19th century, cod liver (CLO), for its source of vitamin D, has been used as one of the remedies to cure rickets [1]. It has been the most commonly used supplement in the UK for decades [2–6]. In EPIC-Norfolk, 32% of men and 45% of women used dietary supplements between 1993 and 1998 [7] with nearly 25% of all participants consuming CLO [8]. Special interest in CLO supplement use is warranted for several reasons. Firstly, for its nutrients, CLO contains eicosapentaenoic acid and docosahexaenoic acid, which in observational studies have been negatively associated with several cancer sites [9,10]; on the other hand, meta-analyses of trial and/or cohort data have shown no effect of these omega-3 fatty acids in supplement form on cardiovascular disease [11,12]. CLO also provides vitamins A, D and E of which vitamin D prevents osteomalacia and has been associated with osteoporosis [13]; while chronic intake above 1500 µg/day of vitamin A might increase the risk of fractures [14]. Secondly, methodological reasons: there is no such person as "a supplement user" [5,15], supplement users (SU) are heterogeneous and ignoring these differences can lead to bias [16]. These differences are not only due to lifestyle [17], but also to what is referred to as "confounding by indication" [5,18,19]. Meaning that certain co-morbidities make the use of certain dietary supplements more likely, which, if not taken into account, could lead to the conclusion that there is an association between the exposure, *i.e.*, dietary supplements, and outcome (e.g., fracture) when in fact the co-morbidity (e.g., osteoporosis) is merely an indication for, or increases, supplement use.

Before public health messages can be formulated to encourage or discourage CLO use, also in the light of possible harmful effects when overdosed [20], a careful analysis of eating habits and other possible confounders in CLO consumers will have to precede this [16]. Supplement use in general in the United Kingdom [3–5,21], Europe [22], the United States [23] and Australia [24,25] has been associated with socio-demographic factors such as being a woman, being older, having a higher socio-economic status; behaviour-wise, SU exercise more, smoke less, eat more healthily and have a lower body mass index (BMI). Whether CLO consumers share the same characteristics as SU in general, and as a result would confound the association found between CLO consumption and health, requires further study. The high proportion of CLO consumers, as well as the detailed information collected in this aging cohort, puts EPIC-Norfolk in a position to study such associations.

This paper describes the socio-demographics, eating habits, anthropometry and self-reported health of NSU and SU in EPIC-Norfolk, with a special focus on the most commonly consumed supplement: CLO.

## 2. Methods

### 2.1. Study Design and Participant Selection

This study was conducted according to the guidelines laid down in the Declaration of Helsinki and all procedures were approved by the Norfolk District Health Authority Ethics Committee. Written informed consent was obtained from all participants. The study started in 1993 with participants aged between 40 and 79 years. Participants lived in the Norfolk area of East Anglia and were recruited from general practitioners' (GP) age-sex registers [26]. Of the 77,630 invited participants, 30,447 gave their informed consent and received a Health and Lifestyle Questionnaire.

Of this group, 25,639 attended a health examination at their GP-clinic and were given a 7-day Diet Diary (7dDD).

## 2.2. Data Collection

The Health and lifestyle Questionnaire was sent to the participants in advance of their GP clinic appointment. Participants were asked about the following: smoking habits (never, former or current smoker); final level of education obtained (no qualifications, O-level, A-level, Degree or equivalent); current profession, from which socio-economic class was derived (unskilled, semi-skilled, skilled manual, skilled non-manual, managerial or professional); marital status (married, single, widowed, divorced or separated); a validated physical activity score combining occupational and recreational physical activity (active, moderately active, moderately inactive, inactive) [27]; and self-reported illnesses, such as cardiovascular diseases, diabetes, cancer and osteoporosis, measured by the question: "Has the doctor ever told you that you have any of the following". The participant's postcode was linked to the Townsend residential area deprivation score. This score identifies material deprivation by using four components: unemployment, non-car ownership, non-house ownership and overcrowding, *i.e.*, the number of people who live per room in a house [28].

Participants were taken through the research protocol by a trained nurse [26]. During the health examination, weight (kg) and height (cm) were measured from which Body Mass Index (BMI) was calculated (kg/m$^2$).

A 7dDD was handed out at the health examination [29,30]. This diary was a 45-page, A5 booklet, with detailed instructions regarding how food and drink should be recorded, as well as seventeen series of colour photos, depicting portions of food items on plates in increasing quantities. The nurse completed a 24-h diet recall as a means of instruction ($n$ = 25,507; 99%). The remainder of the 7dDD was completed at the participant's home, 23,638 (92%) of the participants completed more than one day.

The 7dDD ended with general questions, referred to as the "Back Of Diary (BOD)", and was completed by 23,309 (91%) participants [8]. The BOD included the question relating to supplement use ("Please name any vitamins, minerals or other food supplements taken on each day of last week"). If this question was left open, crossed out or answered with "no/none", then participants were categorised as NSU; however, if participants had recorded any supplements taken, they were categorised as SU. Kappa-statistics with instruments recalling supplement use over the past year in EPIC-Norfolk ranged from 0.72–0.78 [7]. Supplements were coded according to the Vitamin and Minerals Supplement (ViMiS) system described in detail elsewhere [8]. Summarised, supplements were grouped into 45 distinct groups of which CLO was one. This group included CLO or any other type of fish oil, and CLO supplements combined with multivitamins or with, for example, evening primrose oil in the *same* capsule. For the purpose of this analysis, participants who reported medication containing vitamins and/or minerals without further supplement use were classified as NSU.

The 7dDD were entered by trained data-entry clerks using a program called DINER, Data Into Nutrients for Epidemiological Research [30] and checked and calculated by nutritionists using DINERMO [31]. Alcohol intake in grams was divided by 8 to obtain the number of units in alcoholic beverages. Food group data were calculated by summing the weight of each food item consumed, belonging to either fruit, vegetables, red, white or processed meat or white and fatty fish, as well as the percentage contribution to these food groups from composite food items (e.g., Beef stew including vegetables) [31]. These food groups were chosen because of established associations with cancer and cardiovascular risk factors [32].

*2.3. Statistical Analysis*

The characteristics of participants were compared using two different groupings. First, NSU *vs.* SU, followed by two SU subgroups in order to elucidate possible confounding factors for CLO users: SU+CLO, participants who used CLO *or* supplements where cod liver oil/fish oil was an ingredient, also when used in combination with non-CLO supplements (*i.e.*, multiple supplement users of which at least one contained CLO); SU-CLO, participants who consumed one or more supplements that did not contain CLO.

Both comparisons were firstly carried out without adjustment, stratified by sex, using the Chi-squared statistic, followed by multivariable binary (SU *vs.* NSU) and multinomial (SU+CLO *vs.* NSU and SU-CLO *vs.* NSU) logistic regression to compare these groups adjusted for all presented socio-demographic variables.

Differences in food consumption between NSU and SU groups were tested using the Mann-Whitney U and Kruskal-Wallis statistic. Associations between self-reported illnesses and supplement use were adjusted for age using multinomial logistic regression, with supplement use as the dependent variable (NSU/SU+CLO/SU-CLO). Analyses were performed using SPSS v19 (IBM Corp., Armonk, NY, USA). *p*-values below 0.05 were considered significant.

# 3. Results

*3.1. Supplement Consumption*

Out of 23,039 participants who answered the BOD, 3253 (31.7%) of men ($n$ = 10,247) and 5736 (44.8%) of women ($n$ = 12,792) used a supplement ($\chi^2$ (1) = 410.01, $p$ < 0.001). A total of 5262 and 10,732 supplements were consumed by men and women respectively. For both men and women, CLO was the most commonly consumed supplement (43% and 32% respectively), followed by garlic

(12%) and multivitamins (11%) for men and multivitamins (11%) and evening primrose oil (10%) for women. For CLO supplements, 94% of men and 96% of women used these on a daily basis compared to 89% and 90% respectively for non-CLO supplements. CLO supplements were consumed by 22% of men and 26% of women. Only 10% of men consumed supplements that did not contain CLO, compared to 19% of women.

### 3.2. Socio-Demographic Characteristics of Supplement Users

Supplement use in general was associated with sex-dependent characteristics (see columns NSU and SU in Table 1 for men and Table 2 for women). Male SU were older than NSU, whereas female SU completed higher levels of education than female NSU. Marital status was not, and Townsend score only weakly, associated with supplement use. All other characteristics had, in general, stronger associations among women compared to men. In summary, supplement use indicated a healthier lifestyle and higher socio-economic class.

The characteristics of the participants who consumed a supplement that contained CLO (SU+CLO) vs. NSU and participants who consumed other types of supplements (SU-CLO) vs. NSU (see Tables 1 and 2), resulted in stronger associations with socio-demographic characteristics with supplement use, especially among women. Notably, younger age in women was strongly associated with the SU-CLO category, similarly for higher education level; however, such associations among SU+CLO were not present. In men, not being married as well as a higher education level, though not associated with supplement use in general, was associated with SU-CLO.

Results of the fully adjusted analysis (NSU vs. SU) are to be found in Tables 1 and 2 (see column SU vs. NSU). 3.6% of the participants were lost due to missing values for one or more variables ($n$ = 22,205). For supplement use in general, results remained the same as in the unadjusted analysis, except for the area deprivation score in both sexes. Smoking had the strongest association with supplement use, decreasing the odds of supplement use with 41% in men and 29% in women; followed by physical inactivity in men and winter season and lower social class in women. The analysis was repeated with sex in the model (data not shown) and showed a significant independent effect of sex on supplement use in general (OR = 0.54; 95% CI: 0.51–0.58).

Multinomial logistic regression compared NSU with the two SU subgroups (SU+CLO and SU-CLO, see last two columns in Tables 1 and 2). Results were similar compared to the unadjusted analysis, with exception of education level among men and area deprivation score in both sexes, which lost their significance. Strongest associations were again seen for current smoking; other variables, particularly social class and education, were more strongly associated with the SU-CLO group and not with the SU+CLO group when compared to supplement use in general.

335

**Table 1.** Characteristics of European Prospective Investigation into Cancer (EPIC)-Norfolk participants (men only) according to supplement status (Non-supplement User (NSU)/Supplement User (SU)) and supplement subgroup (NSU/SU/SU+cod liver oil (CLO)/SU-CLO). Analyses are shown unadjusted (Chi-squared test). Logistic regression (NSU/SU) and multinomial logistic regression (NSU/SU+CLO/SU-CLO) were adjusted for all variables in this table (n = 9943). Boldly printed OR were statistically significant findings.

| MEN | NSU N | % | SU N | % | SU+CLO N | % | SU-CLO N | % | SU vs. NSU OR | 95% CI | SU+CLO vs. NSU OR | 95% CI | SU-CLO vs. NSU OR | 95% CI |
|---|---|---|---|---|---|---|---|---|---|---|---|---|---|---|
| **Age** | 6994 | | 3253 | | 2215 | | 1038 | | | | | | | |
| <=50 years | 1696 | 24.2 | 528 | 16.2 | 285 | 12.9 | 243 | 23.4 | **1.15** | 1.12–1.18 | **1.21** | 1.17–1.24 | **1.05** | 1.01–1.09 |
| >50–60 years | 2199 | 31.4 | 950 | 29.2 | 649 | 29.3 | 301 | 29.0 | | | OR represents the % change in odds of being | | | |
| >60–70 years | 2120 | 30.3 | 1218 | 37.4 | 876 | 39.5 | 342 | 32.9 | | | a SU for every 5 year increment in age | | | |
| >70 years | 979 | 14.0 | 557 | 17.1 | 405 | 18.3 | 152 | 14.6 | | | | | | |
| | $\chi^2 (3) = 118.51, p < 0.001$ | | | | $\chi^2 (6) = 170.43, p < 0.001$ | | | | | | | | | |
| **Marital status** | 6967 | | 3227 | | 2198 | | 1029 | | | | | | | |
| Married | 6110 | 87.7 | 2839 | 88.0 | 1956 | 89.0 | 883 | 85.8 | Ref | | Ref | | Ref | |
| Not married [a] | 857 | 12.3 | 388 | 12.0 | 242 | 11.0 | 146 | 14.2 | 1.01 | 0.88–1.15 | 0.88 | 0.75–1.03 | **1.30** | 1.07–1.58 |
| | $\chi^2 (1) = 0.16, p < 0.001$ n.s. | | | | $\chi^2 (2) = 6.76, p < 0.05$ | | | | | | | | | |
| **Social class** | 6881 | | 3197 | | 2174 | | 1023 | | | | | | | |
| Non-Manual [b] | 3935 | 57.2 | 1961 | 61.3 | 1265 | 58.2 | 696 | 68.0 | Ref | | Ref | | Ref | |
| Manual [c] | 2946 | 42.8 | 1236 | 38.7 | 909 | 41.8 | 327 | 32.0 | **0.87** | 0.79–0.95 | 1.00 | 0.90–1.11 | **0.63** | 0.55–0.74 |
| | $\chi^2 (1) = 15.50, p < 0.001$ | | | | $\chi^2 (2) = 43.29, p < 0.001$ | | | | | | | | | |
| **Education level** | 6991 | | 3249 | | 2211 | | 1038 | | | | | | | |
| Any qualification [d] | 4829 | 69.1 | 2276 | 70.1 | 1508 | 68.2 | 768 | 74.0 | Ref | | Ref | | Ref | |
| No qualifications | 2162 | 30.9 | 973 | 29.9 | 703 | 31.8 | 270 | 26.0 | 0.93 | 0.84–1.03 | 0.95 | 0.84–1.06 | 0.89 | 0.76–1.05 |
| | $\chi^2 (1) = 1.00,$ n.s. | | | | $\chi^2 (2) = 12.12, p < 0.01$ | | | | | | | | | |
| **Townsend index [e]** | 6968 | | 3245 | | 2211 | | 1034 | | | | | | | |
| Score < 0 | 5859 | 84.1 | 2786 | 85.9 | 1910 | 86.4 | 876 | 84.7 | Ref | | Ref | | Ref | |
| Score > 0 | 1109 | 15.9 | 459 | 14.1 | 301 | 13.6 | 158 | 15.3 | 0.93 | 0.82–1.05 | 0.88 | 0.76–1.02 | 1.04 | 0.86–1.26 |
| | $\chi^2 (1) = 5.34, p < 0.05$ | | | | $\chi^2 (2) = 6.85, p < 0.05$ | | | | | | | | | |
| **Smoking** | 6951 | | 3226 | | 2197 | | 1029 | | | | | | | |
| Never | 2295 | 33.0 | 1111 | 34.4 | 730 | 33.2 | 381 | 37.0 | Ref | | Ref | | Ref | |
| Former | 3756 | 54.0 | 1872 | 58.0 | 1309 | 59.6 | 563 | 54.7 | 0.95 | 0.87–1.05 | 0.97 | 0.87–1.08 | 0.91 | 0.79–1.05 |

**Table 1.** *Cont.*

| MEN | NSU N | % | SU N | % | SU+CLO N | % | SU-CLO N | % | SU vs. NSU OR | 95% CI | SU+CLO vs. NSU OR | 95% CI | SU-CLO vs. NSU OR | 95% CI |
|---|---|---|---|---|---|---|---|---|---|---|---|---|---|---|
| Current | 900 | 12.9 | 243 | 7.5 | 158 | 7.2 | 85 | 8.3 | **0.59** | 0.50–0.69 | **0.58** | 0.48–0.70 | **0.61** | 0.47–0.79 |
| | | $\chi^2(2) = 65.22$, $p < 0.001$ | | | | $\chi^2(4) = 71.95$, $p < 0.001$ | | | | | | | | | |
| Physical activity [f] | 6991 | | 3249 | | 2211 | | 1038 | | | | | | | |
| (Moderately) active | 3060 | 43.8 | 1475 | 45.4 | 1000 | 45.2 | 475 | 45.8 | Ref | | Ref | | Ref | |
| (Moderately) inactive | 3931 | 56.2 | 1774 | 54.6 | 1211 | 54.8 | 563 | 54.2 | **0.82** | 0.75–0.90 | **0.82** | 0.74–0.91 | **0.81** | 0.71–0.93 |
| | | $\chi^2(1) = 2.38$, n.s. | | | | $\chi^2(2) = 2.46$, n.s. | | | | | | | | | |
| Start 7dDD [g] | 6994 | | 3252 | | 2215 | | 1037 | | | | | | | |
| Spring/Summer | 3507 | 50.1 | 1541 | 47.4 | 1066 | 48.1 | 475 | 45.8 | Ref | | Ref | | Ref | |
| Autumn/Winter | 3487 | 49.9 | 1711 | 52.6 | 1149 | 51.9 | 562 | 54.2 | **1.12** | 1.03–1.22 | 1.09 | 0.98–1.20 | **1.20** | 1.05–1.37 |
| | | $\chi^2(1) = 6.75$, $p < 0.01$ | | | | $\chi^2(2) = 8.27$, $p < 0.05$ | | | | | | | | | |

NSU, Non-supplement User; SU, Supplement User; CLO, cod liver oil; $\chi^2$, Chi-squared test; OR, odds ratio; CI, confidence interval; Ref, Reference category. [a] Not married included the categories (NSU/SU): single ($n = 290/128$), widowed ($n = 213/106$), separated ($n = 69/19$) and divorced ($n = 286/135$); [b] Non-manual included the categories (NSU/SU): professional ($n = 544/222$), managerial ($n = 2531/1315$), skilled non-manual ($n = 860/424$); [c] Manual included the categories (NSU/SU): skilled manual ($n = 1787/760$), semi-skilled ($n = 934/397$) and non-skilled ($n = 225/79$); [d] Any qualification included (NSU/SU): O-level ($n = 587/291$), A-level ($n = 3177/1518$), Degree or equivalent ($n = 1065/467$); [e] Townsend index score $< 0$ means district in which the participant lives is more affluent than the mean in England; score $> 0$ means a district in which the participant lives is more deprived than the mean in England; [f] Included the categories (NSU/SU): active (1467/705), moderately active (1593/770), moderately inactive (1685/837), inactive (2246/937); [g] Created from first date in the diary; Spring: March–May, Summer: June–August, Autumn: September–November, Winter: December–February.

**Table 2.** Characteristics of EPIC-Norfolk participants (women only) according to supplement status (NSU/SU) and supplement subgroup (NSU/SU+CLO/SU-CLO). Analysis are shown unadjusted (Chi-squared test). Logistic regression (NSU/SU) and multinomial logistic regression (NSU/SU+CLO/SU-CLO) were adjusted for all variables in this table ($n = 12,262$). Boldly printed OR were statistically significant findings.

| WOMEN | NSU N | % | SU N | % | SU+CLO N | % | SU-CLO N | % | SU vs. NSU OR | 95% CI | SU+CLO vs. NSU OR | 95% CI | SU-CLO vs. NSU OR | 95% CI |
|---|---|---|---|---|---|---|---|---|---|---|---|---|---|---|
| Age | 7056 | | 5736 | | 3389 | | 2347 | | | | | | | |
| <=50 years | 1833 | 26.0 | 1356 | 23.6 | 611 | 18.0 | 745 | 31.7 | 1.02 | 1.00–1.04 | **1.09** | 1.06–1.12 | **0.93** | 0.90–0.95 |
| >50–60 years | 2185 | 31.0 | 1862 | 32.5 | 1107 | 32.7 | 755 | 32.2 | | | | | | |
| >60–70 years | 2100 | 29.8 | 1792 | 31.2 | 1170 | 34.5 | 622 | 26.5 | | | | | | |
| >70 years | 938 | 13.3 | 726 | 12.7 | 501 | 14.8 | 225 | 9.6 | | | | | | |
| | $\chi^2(3) = 12.43\ p < 0.01$ | | | | $\chi^2(6) = 175.26\ p < 0.001$ | | | | | OR represents the % change in odds of being a SU for every 5 year increment in age | | | | | |
| Marital status | 7025 | | 5691 | | 3363 | | 2328 | | | | | | | |
| Married | 5400 | 76.9 | 4315 | 75.8 | 2519 | 74.9 | 1796 | 77.1 | Ref | | Ref | | Ref | |
| Not married [a] | 1625 | 23.1 | 1376 | 24.2 | 844 | 25.1 | 532 | 22.9 | 1.06 | 0.98–1.16 | 1.06 | 0.96–1.17 | 1.06 | 0.94–1.20 |
| | $\chi^2(1) = 1.91$ n.s. | | | | $\chi^2(2) = 5.75$ n.s. | | | | | | | | | |
| Social class | 6865 | | 5612 | | 3299 | | 2313 | | | | | | | |
| Non-Manual [b] | 4063 | 59.2 | 3610 | 64.3 | 2049 | 62.1 | 1561 | 67.5 | Ref | | Ref | | Ref | |
| Manual [c] | 2802 | 40.8 | 2002 | 35.7 | 1250 | 37.9 | 752 | 32.5 | **0.84** | 0.78–0.91 | **0.90** | 0.82–0.99 | **0.76** | 0.69–0.85 |
| | $\chi^2(1) = 34.48\ p < 0.001$ | | | | $\chi^2(2) = 51.09\ p < 0.001$ | | | | | | | | | |
| Education level | 7052 | | 5732 | | 3386 | | 2346 | | | | | | | |
| Any qualification [d] | 3942 | 55.9 | 3423 | 59.7 | 1869 | 55.2 | 1554 | 66.2 | Ref | | Ref | | Ref | |
| No qualifications | 3110 | 44.1 | 2309 | 40.3 | 1517 | 44.8 | 792 | 33.8 | **0.91** | 0.84–0.99 | 1.02 | 0.93–1.11 | **0.77** | 0.69–0.86 |
| | $\chi^2(1) = 18.88\ p < 0.001$ | | | | $\chi^2(2) = 88.08\ p < 0.001$ | | | | | | | | | |
| Townsend index [e] | 7030 | | 5710 | | 3375 | | 2335 | | | | | | | |
| Score <0 | 5845 | 83.1 | 4845 | 84.9 | 2851 | 84.5 | 1994 | 85.4 | Ref | | Ref | | Ref | |
| Score >0 | 1185 | 16.9 | 865 | 15.1 | 524 | 15.5 | 341 | 14.6 | 0.91 | 0.82–1.01 | 0.91 | 0.81–1.02 | 0.91 | 0.80–1.05 |
| | $\chi^2(1) = 6.80\ p < 0.01$ | | | | $\chi^2(2) = 7.67\ p < 0.05$ | | | | | | | | | |
| Smoking | 6992 | | 5680 | | 3350 | | 2330 | | | | | | | |
| Never | 3,949 | 56.5 | 3260 | 57.4 | 1939 | 57.9 | 1321 | 56.7 | Ref | | Ref | | Ref | |
| Former | 2179 | 31.2 | 1930 | 34.0 | 1162 | 34.7 | 768 | 33.0 | 1.08 | 1.00–1.17 | 1.07 | 0.98–1.17 | 1.09 | 0.98–1.21 |
| Current | 864 | 12.4 | 490 | 8.6 | 249 | 7.4 | 240 | 10.3 | **0.71** | 0.63–0.80 | **0.61** | 0.53–0.72 | **0.85** | 0.72–0.99 |

**Table 2.** *Cont.*

| WOMEN | NSU N | % | SU N | % | SU+CLO N | % | SU-CLO N | % | SU vs. NSU OR | 95% CI | SU+CLO vs. NSU OR | 95% CI | SU-CLO vs. NSU OR | 95% CI |
|---|---|---|---|---|---|---|---|---|---|---|---|---|---|---|
| Physical activity [f] | 7052 | | 5732 | | 3386 | | 2346 | | | | | | | |
| | $\chi^2 (2) = 48.93\ p < 0.001$ | | $\chi^2 (1) = 12.89\ p < 0.001$ | | $\chi^2 (4) = 61.43\ p < 0.001$ | | $\chi^2 (2) = 21.34\ p < 0.001$ | | | | | | | |
| (Moderately) active | 2561 | 36.3 | 2259 | 39.4 | 1282 | 37.9 | 977 | 41.6 | Ref | | Ref | | Ref | |
| (Moderately) inactive | 4491 | 63.7 | 3473 | 60.6 | 2104 | 62.1 | 1369 | 58.4 | 0.87 | 0.80–0.94 | 0.87 | 0.80–0.96 | 0.86 | 0.77–0.95 |
| Start 7dDD [g] | 7056 | | 5736 | | 3389 | | 2347 | | | | | | | |
| | $\chi^2 (1) = 17.28\ p < 0.001$ | | $\chi^2 (1) = 17.28\ p < 0.001$ | | $\chi^2 (2) = 17.39\ p < 0.001$ | | | | | | | | | |
| Spring/Summer | 3662 | 51.9 | 2765 | 48.2 | 1640 | 48.4 | 1125 | 47.9 | Ref | | Ref | | Ref | |
| Autumn/Winter | 3394 | 48.1 | 2971 | 51.8 | 1749 | 51.6 | 1222 | 52.1 | 1.16 | 1.08–1.25 | 1.15 | 1.06–1.26 | 1.17 | 1.07–1.29 |

NSU, Non-supplement User; SU, Supplement User; CLO, cod liver oil; $\chi^2$, Chi-squared test; CI, confidence interval; Ref, Reference category. [a] Not married includes the categories (NSU/SU): single ($n = 281/230$), widowed ($n = 806/670$), separated ($n = 67/65$) and divorced ($n = 471/411$); [b] Non-manual includes the categories (NSU/SU): professional ($n = 421/372$), managerial ($n = 2343/2026$), skilled non-manual ($n = 1299/1212$); [c] Manual includes the categories (NSU/SU): skilled manual ($n = 1511/1115$), semi-skilled ($n = 971/702$) and non-skilled ($n = 320/185$); [d] Any qualification included (NSU/SU): O-level ($n = 830/640$), A-level ($n = 2363/2163$), Degree or equivalent ($n = 749/620$); [e] Townsend index score < 0 means district in which the participant lives is more affluent than the mean in England; score > 0 means a district in which the participant lives is more deprived than the mean in England; [f] Included the categories (NSU/SU): active ($1012/954$), moderately active ($1549/1305$), moderately inactive ($2186/1924$), inactive ($2305/1549$); [g] Created from first date in the diary: Spring: March-May, Summer: June-August, Autumn: September-November, Winter: December-February.

339

### 3.3. Food Choices of Supplement Users

SU in general consumed significantly more fruit, vegetables and fatty fish and less red and processed meat than NSU (Table 3). In both men and women, the lower intake of red and processed meats amongst SU in general appeared to be mainly driven by the SU-CLO group, which had a significantly lower intake compared to the SU+CLO group ($p < 0.025$). Although there were no associations between alcohol consumption and supplement use in men, we observed a higher proportion of alcohol consumers among women using supplements, particularly the SU-CLO group, as well as an increment in their median weekly intake ($p < 0.025$).

### 3.4. Health and Supplement Use

BMI was associated with both age and supplement use. The mean (95% CI), age-adjusted BMI for male NSU was 26.6 (26.5–26.7) kg/m$^2$, for SU+CLO 26.3 (26.2–26.4) kg/m$^2$ and for SU-CLO 26.1 (25.9–26.2) kg/m$^2$ (F = 15.6 [2;10217], $p < 0.001$). Among women, the association between supplement use and BMI was stronger; the mean BMI for female NSU was 26.4 (26.3–26.5) kg/m$^2$, for SU+CLO 25.9 (25.7–26.0) kg/m$^2$ and for SU-CLO 25.6 (25.4–25.8) kg/m$^2$ (F = 42.4 [2;12750], $p < 0.001$).

In this *cross-sectional* study, the use of different types of dietary supplements was associated with self-reported illnesses (Table 4). For participants who reported having had benign growths, the odds of being a SU-CLO increased by 36% in men and 35% in women compared to NSU. Diseases affecting the heart and circulation were *negatively* associated with CLO supplement use and not associated with non-CLO supplement use. Men who reported having had a heart attack had a 42% lower odds of using CLO compared to men free of a prevalent heart attack; women who reported having been diagnosed with diabetes had a 50% reduced odds of being a SU+CLO. Participants who reported diseases that affect bone health were reporting more supplement use. Women who reported arthritis had a 60% increased odds of using CLO and 15% increased use of other types of supplements; similar results for CLO use were found for men. Women who reported osteoporosis had a 58% increased odds of using a non-CLO supplement.

**Table 3.** Comparison of food group intake distributions between Non-Supplement Users and Supplement Users (NSU/SU) and between SU subgroups (NSU/SU+CLO/SU-CLO) in the EPIC-Norfolk study.

| Food groups | NSU Median | IQR | SU Median | IQR | SU+CLO Median | IQR | SU-CLO Median | IQR | p-value [a] NSU vs. SU | p-value [b] NSU vs. SU+CLO vs. SU-CLO |
|---|---|---|---|---|---|---|---|---|---|---|
| MEN (n) | 6994 | | 3252 | | 2215 | | 1037 | | | |
| Fruit (g/day) | 127 | 60–212 | 161 | 86–253 | 161 | 89–257 | 158 | 79–244 | p < 0.001 | p < 0.001 |
| Vegetables (g/day) | 139 | 99–188 | 145 | 106–198 | 146 | 108–197 | 145 | 102–202 | p < 0.001 | p < 0.001 |
| Meat | | | | | | | | | | |
| Red (g/day) | 38 | 20–59 | 33 | 16–54 | *34 | 16–55 | 31 | 14–52 | p < 0.001 | p < 0.001 |
| White (g/day) | 22 | 7–40 | 22 | 7–40 | 22 | 8–40 | 21 | 6–40 | n.s. | n.s. |
| Processed (g/day) | 25 | 13–40 | 22 | 11–37 | *23 | 12–38 | 21 | 9–35 | p < 0.001 | p < 0.001 |
| Fish | | | | | | | | | | |
| White(g/day) | 16 | 0–25 | 16 | 0–27 | 16 | 0–27 | 15 | 0–27 | p < 0.01 | p < 0.01 |
| Fatty (g/day) | 1 | 0–19 | 8 | 0–24 | 7 | 0–24 | 8 | 0–24 | p < 0.001 | p < 0.001 |
| Alcoholic beverages (units/diary) | 8.1 | 1.2–21.0 | 8.2 | 1.2–21.1 | 8.1 | 1.3–20.9 | 8.4 | 0.9–21.8 | n.s. | n.s. |
| Alcohol consumers only (units/diary) [c] | 13.0 | 5.3–25.5 | 13.0 | 5.4–25.5 | 12.8 | 5.1–25.1 | 13.9 | 6.0–26.8 | n.s. | n.s. |
| WOMEN (n) | 7056 | | 5736 | | 3389 | | 2347 | | | |
| Fruit (g/day) | 151 | 83–238 | 180 | 107–267 | *183 | 110–269 | 174 | 104–263 | p < 0.001 | p < 0.001 |
| Vegetables (g/day) | 136 | 97–183 | 145 | 107–194 | 145 | 108–192 | 146 | 105–197 | p < 0.001 | p < 0.001 |
| Meat | | | | | | | | | | |
| Red (g/day) | 27 | 12–45 | 24 | 9–41 | *25 | 10–42 | 23 | 7–40 | p < 0.001 | p < 0.001 |
| White (g/day) | 18 | 5–34 | 19 | 6–35 | 19 | 5–36 | 19 | 6–35 | p < 0.05 | n.s. |
| Processed (g/day) | 16 | 7–27 | 14 | 6–25 | *15 | 6–25 | 14 | 4–24 | p < 0.001 | p < 0.001 |
| Fish | | | | | | | | | | |
| White (g/day) | 12 | 0–21 | 12 | 0–22 | *13 | 0–23 | 11 | 0–21 | n.s. | p < 0.001 |
| Fatty (g/day) | 3 | 0–16 | 6 | 0–20 | 6 | 0–21 | 6 | 0–19 | p < 0.001 | p < 0.001 |
| Alcoholic beverages (units/diary) | 2.1 | 0.0–9.2 | 3.3 | 0–10.3 | *3.1 | 0.0–9.8 | 3.9 | 0.0–11.2 | p < 0.001 | p < 0.001 |
| Alcohol consumers only (units/diary) [d] | 6.9 | 3.0–14.6 | 7.3 | 3.3–14.7 | *7.0 | 3.2–14.1 | 7.7 | 3.5–15.2 | n.s. | p < 0.05 |

NSU, Non-supplement User; SU, Supplement User; CLO, cod liver oil; IQR, Inter Quartile Range. [a] Differences between groups tested using Mann-Whitney U test; [b] Differences between groups tested using Kruskal-Wallis test and if significant, followed by Mann-Whitney U test to test for differences in SU subgroups. p-values < 0.025 were considered significant (Bonferroni correction applied: 0.05/2, marked with an * in the SU+CLO column); [c] Men: NSU n = 5411 (77%), SU+CLO n = 1748 (79%), SU-CLO n = 799 (77%); [d] Women: NSU n = 4352 (62%), SU+CLO n = 2233 (66%), SU-CLO n = 1611 (69%); * p-value < 0.025 (see also footnote b).

**Table 4.** Differences in self-reported health between non-supplement users (NSU) and supplement user subgroups (SU+CLO, SU-CLO) in EPIC-Norfolk.

| Health condition | Answer category | N | % | NSU N | % | SU+CLO N | % | SU-CLO N | % | SU+CLO vs NSU OR[a] | 95% C.I. | SU-CLO vs. NSU OR[a] | 95% C.I. |
|---|---|---|---|---|---|---|---|---|---|---|---|---|---|
| MEN | | 10,247 | | 6994 | 68.3 | 2215 | 21.6 | 1038 | 10.1 | | | | |
| Mean age (SD) | | 58.9 | | 58.9 | | 61.8 | | 59.4 | | **1.19** | 1.16–1.22 | 1.03 | 0.99–1.07 |
| Benign growth | Yes | 993 | 9.7 | 634 | 9.1 | 234 | 10.6 | 125 | 12.1 | 1.12 | 0.96–1.32 | **1.36** | 1.11–1.67 |
| | No | 9235 | 90.3 | 6348 | 90.9 | 1975 | 89.4 | 912 | 87.9 | Ref | | Ref | |
| Cancer | Yes | 405 | 4.0 | 259 | 3.7 | 94 | 4.3 | 52 | 5.0 | 0.98 | 0.76–1.24 | 1.33 | 0.98–1.89 |
| | No | 9830 | 96.0 | 6727 | 96.3 | 2117 | 95.7 | 986 | 95.0 | Ref | | Ref | |
| Heart attack | Yes | 560 | 5.5 | 409 | 5.9 | 94 | 4.3 | 57 | 5.5 | **0.58** | 0.46–0.74 | 0.90 | 0.68–1.20 |
| | No | 9668 | 94.5 | 6573 | 94.1 | 2116 | 95.7 | 979 | 94.5 | Ref | | Ref | |
| Stroke | Yes | 189 | 1.8 | 139 | 2.0 | 36 | 1.6 | 14 | 1.4 | **0.65** | 0.45–0.94 | 0.64 | 0.37–1.12 |
| | No | 10,041 | 98.2 | 6846 | 98.0 | 2173 | 98.4 | 1022 | 98.6 | Ref | | Ref | |
| High blood pressure | Yes | 1469 | 14.4 | 979 | 14.0 | 328 | 14.9 | 162 | 15.6 | 0.92 | 0.80–1.05 | 1.11 | 0.92–1.33 |
| | No | 8753 | 85.6 | 5999 | 86.0 | 1879 | 85.1 | 875 | 84.4 | Ref | | Ref | |
| Diabetes | Yes | 333 | 3.3 | 236 | 3.4 | 69 | 3.1 | 28 | 2.7 | 0.78 | 0.59–1.03 | 0.77 | 0.52–1.14 |
| | No | 9898 | 96.7 | 6747 | 96.6 | 2141 | 96.9 | 1010 | 97.3 | Ref | | Ref | |
| Arthritis | Yes | 1932 | 18.9 | 1137 | 16.3 | 604 | 27.4 | 191 | 18.5 | **1.72** | 1.53–1.93 | 1.14 | 0.96–1.35 |
| | No | 8282 | 81.1 | 5837 | 83.7 | 1602 | 72.6 | 843 | 81.5 | Ref | | Ref | |
| Osteoporosis | Yes | 60 | 0.6 | 42 | 0.6 | 12 | 0.5 | 6 | 0.6 | 0.75 | 0.39–1.43 | 0.93 | 0.39–2.19 |
| | No | 10,166 | 99.4 | 6940 | 99.4 | 2194 | 99.5 | 1032 | 99.4 | Ref | | Ref | |
| WOMEN | | 12792 | | 7056 | 55.2 | 3389 | 26.5 | 2347 | 18.3 | | | | |
| Mean age (SD) | | 56.9 | | 56.9 | | 60.0 | | 56.9 | | **1.09** | 1.07–1.12 | **0.91** | 0.88–0.93 |
| Benign growth | Yes | 2448 | 19.2 | 1227 | 17.4 | 703 | 20.8 | 518 | 22.1 | **1.25** | 1.12–1.38 | **1.35** | 1.21–1.52 |
| | No | 10,304 | 80.8 | 5812 | 82.6 | 2671 | 79.2 | 1821 | 77.9 | Ref | | Ref | |
| Cancer | Yes | 883 | 6.9 | 468 | 6.6 | 258 | 7.6 | 157 | 6.7 | 1.11 | 0.94–1.30 | 1.07 | 0.89–1.30 |
| | No | 11,898 | 93.1 | 6582 | 93.4 | 3127 | 92.4 | 2189 | 93.3 | Ref | | Ref | |
| Heart attack | Yes | 168 | 1.3 | 105 | 1.5 | 39 | 1.2 | 24 | 1.0 | **0.66** | 0.46–0.96 | 0.82 | 0.52–1.28 |
| | No | 12,608 | 98.7 | 6941 | 98.5 | 3345 | 98.8 | 2322 | 99.0 | Ref | | Ref | |
| Stroke | Yes | 127 | 1.0 | 86 | 1.2 | 26 | 0.8 | 15 | 0.6 | **0.55** | 0.35–0.86 | 0.61 | 0.35–1.06 |
| | No | 12,651 | 99.0 | 6962 | 98.8 | 3358 | 99.2 | 2331 | 99.4 | Ref | | Ref | |
| High blood pressure | Yes | 1840 | 14.4 | 1067 | 15.1 | 483 | 14.3 | 290 | 12.4 | **0.84** | 0.74–0.94 | 0.89 | 0.77–1.03 |
| | No | 10,926 | 85.6 | 5977 | 84.9 | 2899 | 85.7 | 2050 | 87.6 | Ref | | Ref | |
| Diabetes | Yes | 205 | 1.6 | 139 | 2.0 | 37 | 1.1 | 29 | 1.2 | **0.50** | 0.35–0.73 | 0.69 | 0.46–1.03 |
| | No | 12,571 | 98.4 | 6908 | 98.0 | 3347 | 98.9 | 2316 | 98.8 | Ref | | Ref | |
| Arthritis | Yes | 3495 | 27.4 | 1717 | 24.4 | 1195 | 35.4 | 583 | 25.0 | **1.60** | 1.46–1.76 | **1.15** | 1.03–1.28 |
| | No | 9247 | 72.6 | 5316 | 75.6 | 2180 | 65.6 | 1751 | 75.0 | Ref | | Ref | |
| Osteoporosis | Yes | 340 | 2.7 | 164 | 2.3 | 100 | 3.0 | 76 | 3.2 | 1.17 | 0.91–1.51 | **1.58** | 1.20–2.09 |
| | No | 12,418 | 97.3 | 6877 | 97.7 | 3276 | 97.0 | 2265 | 96.8 | Ref | | Ref | |

NSU, Non-supplement user; SU, Supplement User; CLO, cod liver oil; OR, odds ratio; CI, confidence interval. [a] Age-adjusted OR (per 5 year) using multinomial logistic regression. Boldly printed OR were statistically significant findings.

## 4. Discussion

Supplement use in EPIC-Norfolk is more prevalent among women and is associated with not smoking, a higher social class, higher physical activity levels and more favourable eating habits. These SU characteristics were found to be stronger for subgroups of SU, than for SU in general. Moreover, a participant's self-report of medical conditions at baseline was associated with subgroups of supplements, with CLO supplements being strongly positively associated with arthritis and negatively associated with cardiovascular conditions.

The associations found between supplement use in general and socio-demographic variables are in line with previous findings from a UK survey and cohort studies [4,5,21]. Our finding of more and stronger associations in women compared to men, has also been observed in the MRC National Survey of Health and Development [4]. However, important socio-demographic differences exist within SU. For example, in our study social class appeared to be mainly associated with SU-CLO use in men and women's education was only associated with SU-CLO use and not SU+CLO use. Also, while most "unhealthy behaviours" were less prevalent among SU, exceptions were smoking and alcohol consumption among women in the SU-CLO group. The Norwegian Women and Cancer (NoWAC) study grouped participants into categories by frequency of consumption of CLO use [33]. Their average age of 45 years was 15 years lower than in EPIC-Norfolk; even so, participants' age was positively associated with daily CLO consumption, as well as being an ex-smoker and being more physically active. Again, this stresses the different possible confounders within subgroups of SU.

In EPIC-Norfolk, SU, particularly the SU+CLO group, were found to have a higher consumption of fruit, vegetables and fatty fish and especially the SU-CLO group had a lower consumption of red and processed meat compared to NSU. These associations are comparable with other studies [4,5,21,33] and are indicative that SU are a group of people who are least likely to need supplements. Although SU have in general been characterised as "healthy eating" consumers, this might not necessarily be so [15,34]. A longitudinal study in Switzerland found that 21% of daily/weekly vitamin and mineral SU were clustered around a "healthy" food pattern (16% among NSU); whereas 31% of daily/weekly vitamin and mineral SU consumed an "unhealthy" food pattern (compared to 39% in NSU); the SU were also found to have the most positive attitude towards fortification and could have used supplements as a means of compensation. In the current analysis, only a limited set of foods were compared between NSU and SU in order to avoid multiple testing, but future analyses could compare clusters of a greater variety of foods.

In this cross-sectional analysis, participants who reported having had benign growths were more likely to report non-CLO supplement use. Cancer was not associated with supplement use in the EPIC-Norfolk study, contrary to what has been found in the UK Women's Cohort Study [35]. Also the VITAL cohort [18] reports significant associations between high dose vitamin E and cancer in women as well as a study among cancer survivors [36], where only vitamin use, but not mineral, herbal or other types of supplement use, was associated with cancer. In the VITAL cohort, the number of supplements consumed among women with a medical condition was higher than in men; however, the associations between supplement use and medical conditions were stronger in *men* [18]. It was suggested that women might use supplements to prevent illness, whereas men might start to take supplements after diagnosis. In EPIC-Norfolk, the associations between supplement use and medical conditions were of similar strength for men and women, but data collected at later health examinations will be able to answer important questions related to the onset of illness and the starting or stopping of supplement use. Although the time between diagnosis and the start of the use of dietary supplements is also of importance since participants might make a change in their habits shortly after diagnosis, but return to their former habits after some time has passed [36], the surveys in EPIC-Norfolk might not be frequent enough to capture these changes.

A limitation of our analysis is the stratification of results into SU+CLO and SU-CLO groups, since this is likely to have underestimated the heterogeneity among the SU-CLO subgroup. A recent analysis of the Hertfordshire Cohort Study (HCS) used cluster analysis to describe five groups of SU; however, plant and fish oils were grouped together [15]. The aim of our analysis was to study possible confounding variables of participants consuming fish and CLO supplements. SU+CLO reported more illnesses such as arthritis and less (symptoms of) cardiovascular disease and stroke, contrary to what is reported in the HCS [15]. A UK survey [5] and a survey among 65-98 year old Australians [24,25] however found similar associations to EPIC-Norfolk. The data collected at later health examinations, will have to be taken into account before causal inferences between CLO and cardiovascular diseases can be made, especially since meta-analyses have not shown benefits [11,12]. The fact that CLO is positively associated with age, and that it is more likely to be taken on a daily basis, makes the SU+CLO subgroup of particular interest to investigate further since exposure to CLO is likely to have been for an extended period of time and follow-up time in this prospective cohort is by now two decades, contrary to trials. The nutrients of these supplements are quantified in the ViMiS database where missing values for omega-3 fatty acids were completed, and units of measure were made compatible for food and supplement sources enabling the calculation of a "total nutrient exposure" in a detailed way [8,37]. The wide range of endpoints collected will enable us to look at potential positive as well as harmful effects of CLO.

## 5. Conclusions

Significant socio-demographic associations were found in this study with weaker and fewer associations in SU+CLO than in SU-CLO group, especially among men. Associations between supplement use and age, smoking, social class and education were strong, but not uniform across all SU or between sexes. Participants, who had prevalent heart attack or stroke, were less likely to report CLO supplements; however, self-reported arthritis was associated with increased CLO use. The differences we found between subgroups of SU provide important information that will be necessary for later endpoint analysis of this and other studies, since confounding by indication as well as lifestyle confounders will need to be taken into account depending on the type of supplement consumed.

**Acknowledgments:** The authors wish to thank the EPIC-Norfolk participants and research and administrative staff, particularly Amit Bhaniani for his input in the revision of the supplement database. The EPIC-Norfolk study received grants from the Medical Research Council (G9502233) and Cancer Research UK (SP2024-0201 and SP2024-0204).

**Author Contributions:** The study was designed by K.-T. Khaw, N.J. Wareham. The data collection was organised by A.A. Welch, R.N. Luben. A.A. Welch, A.A. Mulligan and R.N. Luben commenced work on the supplement database; M.A.H. Lentjes revised the supplement database, supervised by A.A. Welch. M.A.H. Lentjes and A.A. Mulligan obtained data from 7-day diet diaries. The research question was formulated by M.A.H. Lentjes, who also analysed the data and wrote the manuscript. All authors read and contributed to the manuscript.

**Conflicts of Interest:** The authors declare no conflict of interest.

## References

1. Rajakumar, K. Vitamin D, cod-liver oil, sunlight, and rickets: A historical perspective. *Pediatrics* **2003**, *112*, e132–e135.
2. Bates, C.J.; Prentice, A.; van der Pols, J.C.; Walmsley, C.; Pentieva, K.D.; Finch, S.; Smithers, G.; Clarke, P.C. Estimation of the use of dietary supplements in the National Diet and Nutrition Survey: People aged 65 years and Over. An observed paradox and a recommendation. *Eur. J. Clin. Nutr.* **1998**, *52*, 917–923.
3. Henderson, L.; Gregory, J.; Swan, G. *The National Diet & Nutrition Survey: Adults Aged 19 to 64 Years. Types and Quantities of Foods Consumed*; Her Majesty's Stationary Office (HMSO): London, UK, 2002; Volume 1.
4. McNaughton, S.A.; Mishra, G.D.; Paul, A.A.; Prynne, C.J.; Wadsworth, M.E.J. Supplement use is associated with health status and health-related behaviors in the 1946 British birth cohort. *J. Nutr.* **2005**, *135*, 1782–1789.
5. Harrison, R.A.; Holt, D.; Pattison, D.J.; Elton, P.J. Are those in need taking dietary supplements? A survey of 21 923 adults. *Br. J. Nutr.* **2004**, *91*, 617–623.
6. Bates, B.; Lennox, A.; Bates, C.; Swan, G. *National Diet and Nutrition Survey. Headline Results from Years 1 and 2 (Combined) of the Rolling Programme (2008/2009–2009/10)*; Department of Health, Food Standards Agency: London, UK, 2011.

7. Lentjes, M.A.H.; Welch, A.A.; Luben, R.N.; Khaw, K.-T. Differences in dietary supplement use and secular and seasonal trends assessed using three different instruments in the EPIC-Norfolk population study. *J. Diet. Suppl.* **2013**, *10*, 142–151.

8. Lentjes, M.A.H.; Bhaniani, A.; Mulligan, A.A.; Khaw, K.-T.; Welch, A.A. Developing a database of vitamin and mineral supplements (ViMiS) for the Norfolk arm of the European Prospective Investigation into Cancer (EPIC-Norfolk). *Public Health Nutr.* **2011**, *14*, 459–471.

9. Brasky, T.M.; Lampe, J.W.; Potter, J.D.; Patterson, R.E.; White, E. Specialty supplements and breast cancer risk in the VITamins And Lifestyle (VITAL) Cohort. *Cancer Epidemiol. Biomark. Prev.* **2010**, *19*, 1696–1708.

10. Skeie, G.; Braaten, T.; Hjartåker, A.; Brustad, M.; Lund, E. Cod liver oil, other dietary supplements and survival among cancer patients with solid tumours. *Int. J. Cancer* **2009**, *125*, 1155–1160.

11. Chowdhury, R.; Stevens, S.; Gorman, D.; Pan, A.; Warnakula, S.; Chowdhury, S.; Ward, H.; Johnson, L.; Crowe, F.; Hu, F.B.; *et al.* Association between fish consumption, long chain omega 3 fatty acids, and risk of cerebrovascular disease: Systematic review and meta-analysis. *BMJ* **2012**, *345*, e6698.

12. Rizos, E.C.; Ntzani, E.E.; Bika, E.; Kostapanos, M.S.; Elisaf, M.S. Association between omega-3 fatty acid supplementation and risk of major cardiovascular disease events: A systematic review and meta-analysis. *JAMA* **2012**, *308*, 1024–1033.

13. Scientific Advisory Committee on Nutrition (SACN). *Update on Vitamin D*; The Stationary Office (TSO): London, UK, 2007.

14. Mulholland, C.A.; Benford, D.J. What is known about the safety of multivitamin-multimineral supplements for the generally healthy population? Theoretical basis for harm. *Am. J. Clin. Nutr.* **2007**, *85*, 318S–322S.

15. Denison, H.J.; Jameson, K.A.; Syddall, H.E.; Dennison, E.M.; Cooper, C.; Sayer, A.A.; Robinson, S.M. Patterns of dietary supplement use among older men and women in the UK: Findings from the Hertfordshire Cohort Study. *J. Nutr. Health Aging* **2012**, *16*, 307–311.

16. White, E.; Patterson, R.E.; Kristal, A.R.; Thornquist, M.; King, I.; Shattuck, A.L.; Evans, I.; Satia-Abouta, J.; Littman, A.J.; Potter, J.D. VITamins And Lifestyle cohort study: Study design and characteristics of supplement users. *Am. J. Epidemiol.* **2004**, *159*, 83–93.

17. Hoggatt, K.J. Commentary: Vitamin supplement use and confounding by lifestyle. *Int. J. Epidemiol.* **2003**, *32*, 553–555.

18. Satia-Abouta, J.; Kristal, A.R.; Patterson, R.E.; Littman, A.J.; Stratton, K.L.; White, E. Dietary supplement use and medical conditions: The VITAL study. *Am. J. Prev. Med.* **2003**, *24*, 43–51.

19. Gunther, S.; Patterson, R.E.; Kristal, A.R.; Stratton, K.L.; White, E. Demographic and health-related correlates of herbal and specialty supplement use. *J. Am. Diet. Assoc.* **2004**, *104*, 27–34.

20. Expert group on vitamins and minerals. *Safe Upper Levels for Vitamins and Minerals*; Food Standards Agency: London, UK, 2003.

21. Kirk, S.F.; Cade, J.E.; Barrett, J.H.; Conner, M. Diet and lifestyle characteristics associated with dietary supplement use in women. *Public Health Nutr.* **1999**, *2*, 69–73.

22. Skeie, G.; Braaten, T.; Hjartåker, A.; Lentjes, M.; Amiano, P.; Jakszyn, P.; Pala, V.; Palanca, A.; Niekerk, E.M.; Verhagen, H.; *et al.* Use of dietary supplements in the European Prospective Investigation into Cancer and Nutrition calibration study. *Eur. J. Clin. Nutr.* **2009**, *63*, S226–S238.

23. Patterson, R.E.; White, E.; Kristal, A.R.; Neuhouser, M.L.; Potter, J.D. Vitamin supplements and cancer risk: The epidemiologic evidence. *Cancer Causes Control* **1997**, *8*, 786–802.

24. Brownie, S.; Rolfe, M. Health characteristics of older Australian dietary supplement users compared to non-supplement users. *Asia Pac. J. Clin. Nutr.* **2004**, *13*, 365–371.

25. Brownie, S. Predictors of dietary and health supplement use in older Australians. *Aust. J. Adv. Nurs.* **2006**, *23*, 26–32.

26. Day, N.; Oakes, S.; Luben, R.; Khaw, K.T.; Bingham, S.; Welch, A.; Wareham, N. EPIC-Norfolk: Study design and characteristics of the cohort. European Prospective Investigation of Cancer. *Br. J. Cancer* **1999**, *80* (Suppl. S1), 95–103.

27. Wareham, N.J.; Jakes, R.W.; Rennie, K.L.; Schuit, J.; Mitchell, J.; Hennings, S.; Day, N.E. Validity and repeatability of a simple index derived from the short physical activity questionnaire used in the European Prospective Investigation into Cancer and Nutrition (EPIC) study. *Public Health Nutr.* **2003**, *6*, 407–413.

28. Shohaimi, S.; Luben, R.; Wareham, N.; Day, N.; Bingham, S.; Welch, A.; Oakes, S.; Khaw, K.-T. Residential area deprivation predicts smoking habit independently of individual educational level and occupational social class. A cross sectional study in the Norfolk cohort of the European Investigation into Cancer (EPIC-Norfolk). *J. Epidemiol. Commun. Health* **2003**, *57*, 270–276.

29. Bingham, S.A.; Welch, A.A.; McTaggart, A.; Mulligan, A.A.; Runswick, S.A.; Luben, R.; Oakes, S.; Khaw, K.T.; Wareham, N.; Day, N.E. Nutritional methods in the European Prospective Investigation of Cancer in Norfolk. *Public Health Nutr.* **2001**, *4*, 847–858.

30. Welch, A.A.; McTaggart, A.; Mulligan, A.A.; Luben, R.; Walker, N.; Khaw, K.T.; Day, N.E.; Bingham, S.A. DINER (Data Into Nutrients for Epidemiological Research)—A new data-entry program for nutritional analysis in the EPIC-Norfolk cohort and the 7-day diary method. *Public Health Nutr.* **2001**, *4*, 1253–1265.

31. Lentjes, M.A.H.; McTaggart, A.; Mulligan, A.A.; Powell, N.A.; Parry-Smith, D.; Luben, R.N.; Bhaniani, A.; Welch, A.A.; Khaw, K.-T. Dietary intake measurement using 7 d diet diaries in British men and women in the European Prospective Investigation into Cancer-Norfolk study: A focus on methodological issues. *Br. J. Nutr.* **2014**, *111*, 516–526.

32. World Cancer Research Fund/American Institute for Cancer Research. *Food, Nutrition, Physical Activity, and the Prevention of Cancer: A Global Perspective*; AICR: Washington, DC, USA, 2007.

33. Brustad, M.; Braaten, T.; Lund, E. Predictors for cod-liver oil supplement use–the Norwegian Women and Cancer Study. *Eur. J. Clin. Nutr.* **2004**, *58*, 128–136.

34. Van der Horst, K.; Siegrist, M. Vitamin and mineral supplement users. Do they have healthy or unhealthy dietary behaviours? *Appetite* **2011**, *57*, 758–764.

35. Hutchinson, J.; Burley, V.J.; Greenwood, D.C.; Thomas, J.D.; Cade, J.E. High-dose vitamin C supplement use is associated with self-reported histories of breast cancer and other illnesses in the UK Women's Cohort Study. *Public Health Nutr.* **2011**, *14*, 768–777.

36. Miller, M.F.; Bellizzi, K.M.; Sufian, M.; Ambs, A.H.; Goldstein, M.S.; Ballard-Barbash, R. Dietary supplement use in individuals living with cancer and other chronic conditions: A population-based study. *J. Am. Diet. Assoc.* **2008**, *108*, 483–494.

37. Lentjes, M.A.H.; Mulligan, A.A.; Welch, A.A.; Bhaniani, A.; Luben, R.N.; Khaw, K.-T. Contribution of cod liver oil-related nutrients (vitamins A, D, E and eicosapentaenoic acid and docosahexaenoic acid) to daily nutrient intake and their associations with plasma concentrations in the EPIC-Norfolk cohort. *J. Hum. Nutr. Diet.* **2014**.

# Nutritional Adequacy of Dietary Intake in Women with Anorexia Nervosa

Susan K. Raatz, Lisa Jahns, LuAnn K. Johnson, Ross Crosby, James E. Mitchell, Scott Crow, Carol Peterson, Daniel Le Grange and Stephen A. Wonderlich

**Abstract:** Understanding nutrient intake of anorexia nervosa (AN) patients is essential for the treatment. Therefore, estimates of total energy and nutrient consumption were made in a group of young women (19 to 30 years) with restricting and binge purge subtypes of AN participating in an ecological momentary assessment study. Participants completed three nonconsecutive 24-hour diet recalls. Mean nutrient intakes were stratified by subtype and by quartiles of energy intake and compared to the age specific Dietary Reference Intake (DRI) levels, as well as to the reported intakes from the What We Eat In America (WWEIA) dietary survey 2011–2012. Reported intake was determined for energy, macronutrients, and micronutrients. The mean body mass index (BMI) for all participants was $17.2 \pm 0.1$ kg/m$^2$. Reported nutrient intake was insufficient for participants in quartiles 1–3 of both AN subtypes when compared to the DRIs. Intake reported by participants in quartile 4 of both subgroups met requirements for most nutrients and even met or exceeded estimated energy needs. Counseling of AN patients should be directed to total food consumption to improve energy intake and to reduce individual nutritional gaps.

Reprinted from *Nutrients*. Cite as: Raatz, S.K.; Jahns, L.; Johnson, L.K.; Crosby, R.; Mitchell, J.E.; Crow, S.; Peterson, C.; Le Grange, D.; Wonderlich, S.A. Nutritional Adequacy of Dietary Intake in Women with Anorexia Nervosa. *Nutrients* **2015**, 7, 3652–3665.

## 1. Introduction

Anorexia nervosa (AN) is a psychiatric disorder that results in considerable morbidity and mortality. The estimated prevalence is between 0.3% and 0.6% in adolescents and young adult women [1]. Prolonged dietary restriction in this disorder results in overt malnutrition, leading to significant decline in health status. In addition to the obvious wasting and loss of lean and fat mass, patients experience bone loss and often amenorrhea [2]. Onset of AN at an early age leads to reduced growth and an inability to attain genetic height potential despite accelerated growth following nutritional therapy [3]. Long-term mortality associated with the disease is ~10% per decade mainly due to cachexia and suicide [1,4].

AN is characterized by two subtypes-those with primarily food restricting behavior and those with associated binge eating and purging behavior [5]. Although definitions of the subtypes are quite distinct, frequent crossover can occur, with up to 62% of restricting patients developing binge purge behavior [6]. Knowledge of the AN subtype is important for selection of therapeutic approaches to treatment, and may play an important role in the nutritional and medical status of the individual [7].

Understanding the nutrient intake of AN patients is essential for nutritional counseling and treatment. Assessment of dietary intake in this population is fraught with error [8]. Studies of dietary consumption with retrospective recall of intake have obvious shortcomings as individuals with AN are often less than candid about their eating behavior; however, their knowledge of what was consumed may be greater than that of the general population [9]. Obtaining dietary intake information by observation in a hospital or clinic setting is not representative of usual intake; therefore, dietary recall is the best available technique to assess consumption and has high agreement between reported total energy intake and predicted energy expenditure [10].

Recently the Academy of Nutrition and Dietetics published its Position Paper on *Nutrition Intervention in the Treatment of Eating Disorders* [11]. This statement contends that "nutrition intervention, including nutrition counseling by a registered dietitian, is an essential component of the team treatment of patients with anorexia nervosa, bulimia nervosa, and other eating disorders during assessment and treatment across the continuum of care" [11]. Information on adequacy of nutrient intake in this group will direct clinically relevant medical nutrition therapy emphasizing common key nutritional deficiencies in the context of a treatment plan for a healthy and nutritionally complete diet.

In evaluation of dietary intake of individuals with AN, emphasis has been primarily given to the reduced intake of energy and macronutrients. Little work has been done to describe the effect of diet restriction on the total micronutrient intake levels in AN [10,12,13]. Our objective was to quantify nutrient intake in a group of participants with AN who were taking part in an ecological momentary assessment study (EMA). Therefore, we assessed total reported energy and nutrient intake in a sample of young women, aged 19 to 30 years, with both restricting and binge purge subtypes of AN and compared them to the Dietary Reference Intakes (DRIs) [14] for women aged 19–30 years. We also compared this group to the reported intake of a representative group of women who participated in What We Eat in America (WWEIA) the dietary intake segment of the of the National Health and Nutrition Examination Survey (NHANES) 2011–2012 [15,16]. We discuss the relevance of our results to RDs and other practitioners working with AN patients.

## 2. Experimental Section

### 2.1. Experimental Protocol

This study is an analysis of dietary recall data that was part of an EMA study in which participants with AN provided information on eating behavior, emotions, stress and coping on hand held computers over 14 days [17]. Participants also completed three non-consecutive 24-hours dietary recalls (DR) during the two weeks. The study was conducted between 2006 and 2010. The main outcome, adequacy of energy and nutrient intakes, is compared to the DRI and intake of participants in WWEIA/NHANES 2011–2012. Studies were carried out at the Neuropsychiatric Institute, Fargo, ND; The University of Minnesota, Minneapolis, MN and The University of Chicago, Chicago, IL. Approval for this protocol was obtained from Institutional Review Boards of all facilities involved in this research: The University of North Dakota, Grand Forks, ND; Sanford Health, Fargo, ND; the University of Minnesota; and the University of Chicago. All participants provided written informed consent prior to enrollment in the study.

### 2.2. Participants

Participants in the trial included women aged 17 to 58 years ($n = 118$) with a diagnosis of AN. volunteers were recruited to meet the criteria for AN, either restricting or binge purge type, as defined in the Diagnostic and Statistical Manual of Mental Disorders [5] or subclinical AN as previously described [17].

A subset of all recruited participants was included in this analysis, who were between the ages of 19 and 30 years, and had three complete days of random DR ($n = 75$; 64% of sample). This age group was used for this assessment as it corresponds to the life stage and sex grouping of the DRI for the purpose of comparison of nutritional adequacy. There were not enough women in the other age groups (14–18, 31–50, or 51–70 years) to provide appropriate aggregate intake data for comparison to the DRIs.

### 2.3. Diagnostic Assessment

Participants were assessed with structured interviews at baseline to evaluate the status of their disorder and to classify their subtype of AN, including the Structured Clinical Interview for DSM IV, Axis I [18] and the Eating Disorders Examination [19]. Body Mass Index (BMI) ($kg/m^2$) of participants was determined by measurement of height in cm and weight in kg by trained clinic staff.

### 2.4. Dietary Assessment

Participants were called three times to obtain detailed 24-hours dietary recall information. The recalls were performed by trained interviewers and detailed diet

351

information was directly entered during the interview and analyzed utilizing the 2005 version of the Nutrition Data System for Research (NDS-R) [20,21] from the Nutrition Coordinating Center at the University of Minnesota. The multiple-pass methodology used by trained interviewers during recalls is similar to the methodology used to collect 24-hours DR data in the WWEIA/NHANES survey [22].

## 2.5. Comparison to Dietary Reference Intakes

Use of DRIs as part of the nutrition care process was discussed in detail in a recent practice dietetics paper [23]. Given the restrictive eating habits of individuals with AN, many nutrient shortfalls in the diet are expected. Individual nutrition assessments include many indicators of nutritional status and often include dietary intake measured by 24-hours DR or food records. If dietary intake has been assessed for $\geq 3$ days, nutrient intake can be compared to the DRIs and included in the treatment process [23]. Current dietary intake data can be used to identify nutrient intakes that are relevant for planning treatment and follow-up goals [24].

The Estimated Average Requirement (EAR) is the median usual intake estimated to meet the physiological needs of half of the individuals in a life stage and sex group. The recommended dietary allowance (RDA) is sufficient to meet or exceed the estimated needs of 98% of the population of interest and is set at two standard deviations above the EAR. An Adequate Intake (AI) is set when there is insufficient scientific evidence to set an EAR and RDA and is the estimated intake of an apparently healthy population.

The Practice Paper of the American Dietetic Association: *Using the Dietary Reference Intakes* provides guidelines for the application of the DRIs to patient assessment: (1) if the reported intake of a specific nutrient exceeds the RDA or AI, intake may be considered adequate; (2) if intake is less than the AI, it cannot be considered inadequate, but the dietitian may choose to encourage increased consumption to meet the AI; (3) if intake is below the RDA but exceeds the EAR, there is a 50% chance that intake does not meet the individual requirement and increased consumption should be encouraged; (4) if intake is below the EAR there is a greater chance that intake is not sufficient to meet requirements [23].

Estimated Energy Requirement (EER) is defined as "the average dietary intake that is predicted to maintain energy balance in a healthy adult of a defined age, gender, weight, height, and level of physical activity consistent with good health" [25]. The EER does not address energy needs of AN patients, as additional energy requirements to restore healthy weight depends upon factors such as initial deficit, desired rate of recovery, and catch-up growth. Therefore, the EER may underestimate the energy requirements of patients with AN, despite their low body weight. On the other hand, AN patients are hypometabolic and the EER may overestimate their maintenance energy needs if they are not physically active [2]. Due to the uncertainty of AN patients energy needs, the description of EER was calculated and presented at moderate physical activity levels [25].

$$EER = 354 - 6.91 \times age\ [y] + PA \times (9.36 \times weight\ [kg] + 726 \times height\ [m]) \quad (1)$$

where PA is 1.27 if moderately active.

*2.6. Comparison to NHANES*

For comparison to an apparently healthy population, the nutrient intake of non-pregnant women aged 19–30 years was derived from the 2011–2012 WWEIA/NHANES survey [16]. WWEIA/NHANES is a nationally representative, cross-sectional survey of the non-institutionalized, civilian U.S. population. The survey uses a complex, stratified, multistage probability cluster sampling design. WWEIA/HANES participants were asked to complete a single in-person 24-hours DR. A second 24-hours DR was collected via telephone within 10 days of the first; however, only the day 1 recalls are used in our analysis ($n$ = 403 women) [26–28].

*2.7. Statistical Analysis*

Nutrient values computed from the three DR were averaged for each subject and divided into quartiles based on reported energy intake within restricting and binge purge subtypes of AN. Means and 95% confidence intervals (CI) were calculated for each nutrient within each quartile. The percentage of women whose reported intakes were less than the EAR or AI, as appropriate, were calculated for each nutrient. Mean and 95% CI of nutrient intakes of women ages 19–30 who participated in WWEIA/NHANES 2011–2012 were calculated using the Survey means procedure in SAS (SAS Institute, Cary, NC). Analyses included the sampling strata and primary sampling units and were weighted using the appropriate NHANES sample weights. Consonance of the AN subjects intakes with those of the nationally representative sample of women aged 19–30 was estimated by calculating the percentage consumed by an AN subject relative to the mean intakes reported by the WWEIA/NHANES respondents.

Age and BMI values for all women and for AN subgroup by quartile were calculated and presented as mean ± standard error of the mean (SEM). Mean ± SEM of the EER was calculated for each quartile for each AN subgroup. The percentage of subject consuming at least 100% of the EER was calculated for each of the 3 activity levels. All analyses were performed with SAS V9.3 (SAS Institute, Inc., Cary, NC, USA).

## 3. Results

The overall mean age of participants was $22.5 \pm 0.4$ years and the average BMI was $17.2 \pm 0.1$ kg/m$^2$. There were no significant differences in age and BMI between the diagnostic subtypes across the quartiles. Age in years (mean $\pm$ SEM) and BMI (mean $\pm$ SEM) for participants by AN subtype of restricting and binge purge were, respectively Quartile 1: age: $23 \pm 1$, $20 \pm 1$, BMI: $17.3 \pm 0.3$; $17.3 \pm 0.3$; Quartile 2: age: $22 \pm 1$, $25 \pm 1$, BMI: $17.8 \pm 0.2$; $17.2 \pm 0.6$, Quartile 3: age: $22 \pm 1$, $25 \pm 1$. BMI: $17.0 \pm 0.3$, $17.3 \pm 0.3$; Quartile 4: age: $21 \pm 1$, $24 \pm 1.3$, BMI: $17.0 \pm 0.3$; $17.0 \pm 0.5$.

Table 1 presents mean and 95% CI for reported dietary intake of participants by AN subtype (quartiles) in reference to the DRI. For all nutrients under consideration the percentage of individuals reporting intakes lower than the EAR are shown. Participants of both subtypes in quartiles 1 and 2 reported low energy intake and consequently were below the DRI EAR for those nutrients evaluated. As reported energy intake increased in both AN subtype groups in quartiles 3 and 4, the number of participants not reporting intakes below the EAR is reduced the only macronutrient with an EAR is carbohydrate. The DRIs also suggest evaluating diets based upon the Acceptable Macronutrient Distribution Range (AMDR). These ranges are based upon energy intake. The AMDR for fat, protein and carbohydrate is 20%–25% en, 10%–35% en and 45%–65% en, respectively. However, with the wide variability in reported energy intake in this population it may be more clinically relevant to use the AMDRs to plan diets based upon on estimated energy needs, not reported intake.

Table 2 provides mean reported dietary intake by AN subtype (quartiles) compared to mean reported intake by WWEIA/NHANES for women of the same age range. Reported intakes are substantially lower for all subjects except those in the 4th quartile of both the restrictor and binge purge subtype of AN. Estimated energy requirements for participants at a moderate activity level are $2242 \pm 27$ kcal, $2292 \pm 32$ kcal, $2281 \pm 28$ kcal, $2313 \pm 32$ kcal, for quartiles 1 through 4, respectively, of the AN restrictor subtype and $2253 \pm 25$ kcal, $2248 \pm 48$ kcal, $2355 \pm 31$ kcal, $2304 \pm 37$ kcal for quartiles 1–4, respectively, for the AN binge-purge subtype participants. Participants in quartiles 1–3 of both subtypes of AN have very low concordance with energy needs at moderate activity levels with none of the participants reporting intake equivalent to EER. Sixty four percent (64%) of participants in quartile 4 of the AN restrictor subtype and 86% of those in quartile 4 of the AN binge purge subtype meet the EER.

**Table 1.** Reported dietary intake of individuals with anorexia nervosa (by subtype and quartile) and percent not meeting the Dietary Reference Intakes.

| | DRI[1] *EAR **AI | Quartile 1 Restrictor (n = 12) Mean (95% CI) | % Below EAR | Quartile 1 Binge/Purge (n = 8) Mean (95% CI) | % Below EAR | Quartile 2 Restrictor (n = 11) Mean (95% CI) | % Below EAR | Quartile 2 Binge/Purge (n = 7) Mean (95% CI) | % Below EAR | Quartile 3 Restrictor (n = 12) Mean (95% CI) | % Below EAR | Quartile 3 Binge/Purge (n = 7) Mean (95% CI) | % Below EAR | Quartile 4 Restrictor (n = 11) Mean (95% CI) | % Below EAR | Quartile 4 Binge/Purge (n = 7) Mean (95% CI) | % Below EAR |
|---|---|---|---|---|---|---|---|---|---|---|---|---|---|---|---|---|---|
| Energy (kcal) | | 736 (567–904) | | 671 (571–771) | | 1308 (1194–1421) | | 1082 (965–1200) | | 1799 (1706–1892) | | 1662 (1445–1880) | | 2639 (2130–3147) | | 4102 (2301–5904) | |
| *Carbohydrate (g) | 100 | 110 (81–138) | 50 | 128 (104–151) | 25 | 203 (175–230) | 0 | 161 (122–200) | 0 | 252 (233–270) | 0 | 238 (208–267) | 0 | 382 (316–448) | 0 | 533 (278–788) | 0 |
| Protein (g) | | 33 (22–44) | | 22 (15–29) | | 54 (45–63) | | 41 (25–56) | | 78 (67–88) | | 59 (39–80) | | 93 (76–110) | | 143 (65–221) | |
| Fat (g) | | 17 (13–23) | | 17 (7.6–16) | | 35 (30–40) | | 33 (23–43) | | 54 (46–63) | | 57 (46–68) | | 84 (58–110) | | 159 (78–240) | |
| **Dietary Fiber (g) | 25 | 12 (6.4–17) | | 12 (7–18) | | 19 (14–23) | | 12 (0.2–24) | | 21 (14–28) | | 17 (10–24) | | 27 (21–33) | | 31 (19–43) | |
| *Calcium (mg) | 800 | 545 (291–799) | 75 | 451 (281–621) | 88 | 761 (578–944) | 55 | 676 (306–1046) | 57 | 1073 (829–1317) | 25 | 926 (413–1440) | 57 | 1514 (1191–1838) | 9 | 2271 (769–3772) | 0 |
| *Iron (mg) | 8.1 | 7.9 (4.1–12) | 67 | 9 (2.9–16) | 63 | 15 (10–19) | 9 | 10 (6–13) | 43 | 18 (13–22) | 0 | 15 (8–23) | 29 | 24 (17–31) | 0 | 28 (15–40) | 0 |
| *Phosphorus (mg) | 580 | 607 (403–811) | 42 | 453 (308–597) | 63 | 962 (814–1109) | 0.0 | 812.7 (470–1156) | 29 | 1355.6 (1156–1556) | 0 | 1063 (714–1413) | 0 | 1745 (1453–2037) | 0 | 2815 (1052–4578) | 0 |
| *Thiamin (mg) | 0.9 | 0.7 (0.4–0.9) | 67 | 1 (0.4–1.7) | 75 | 1 (1.1–1.6) | 0.0 | 1.0 (0.7–1.3) | 43 | 1.7 (1.5–2.0) | 0 | 1.5 (1.1–1.9) | 14 | 2.6 (1.9–3.4) | 0 | 3.43 (1.7–5.2) | 0 |
| *Riboflavin (mg) | 0.9 | 1.1 (0.8–1.5) | 25 | 2 (0.9–2.0) | 0.0 | 2 (1.4–2.0) | 0.0 | 2.6 (0.4–4.7) | 14 | 2.4 (2.1–2.8) | 0 | 2.1 (1.3–2.8) | 0 | 3.8 (2.7–4.9) | 0 | 5.3 (1.9–8.8) | 0 |
| *Niacin | 11 | 8.6 (5.5–12) | 67 | 13 (4.8–21) | 75 | 19 (14–23) | 9 | 11.6 (8.3–15) | 29 | 23.3 (19–28) | 0 | 18.5 (13–24) | 0 | 35.0 (25–45) | 0 | 43.9 (22–665) | 0 |
| *Folate (µg) | 320 | 234 (145–324) | 75 | 291 (158–423) | 63 | 458 (316–601) | 18 | 235 (115–355) | 71 | 497 (341–654) | 25 | 434 (228–640) | 43 | 690 (499–882) | 9 | 764 (343–1185) | 14 |
| *Vitamin B6 (mg) | 1.1 | 0.9 (0.6–1.3) | 67 | 1 (0.2–1.8) | 88 | 2 (1.2–1.8) | 27 | 1.0 (0.5–1.4) | 71 | 2.1 (1.3–2.9) | 8 | 1.6 (0.8–2.4) | 43 | 3.1 (2.3–4.0) | 0 | 3.6 (1.4–5.8) | 0 |

Table 1. Cont.

| | | Quartile 1 | | | | Quartile 2 | | | | Quartile 3 | | | | Quartile 4 | | | |
|---|---|---|---|---|---|---|---|---|---|---|---|---|---|---|---|---|---|
| | | Restrictor (n = 12) | | Binge/Purge (n = 8) | | Restrictor (n = 11) | | Binge / Purge (n = 7) | | Restrictor (n = 12) | | Binge / Purge (n = 7) | | Restrictor (n = 11) | | Binge / Purge (n = 7) | |
| | DRI[1] *EAR **AI | Mean (95% CI) | % Below EAR | Mean (95% CI) | % Below EAR | Mean (95% CI) | % Below EAR | Mean (95% CI) | % Below EAR | Mean (95% CI) | % Below EAR | Mean (95% CI) | % Below EAR | Mean (95% CI) | % Below EAR | Mean (95% CI) | % Below EAR |
| *Vitamin B12 (µg) | 2 | 2.2 (1.0-3.4) | 58 | 2 (0.3-4.3) | 63 | 3 (2.0-3.9) | 18 | 3.2 (1.3-5.0) | 43 | 5.8 (3.9-8.0) | 0 | 4.8 (2.0-7.6) | 29 | 8.4 (5.8-11.0) | 0 | 11.7 (1.6-22) | 0 |
| *Vitamin C (mg) | 60 | 70 (38-102) | 50 | 85 (25-146) | 50 | 77 (37-117) | 55 | 44 (2-87) | 71 | 116 (76-157) | 17 | 96 (39-153) | 14 | 129 (85-174) | 27 | 107 (54-160) | 29 |
| *Vitamin A (µg RE) | 500 | 503 (286-720) | 50 | 536 (110-962) | 50 | 850 (580-1120) | 18 | 567 (229-905) | 57 | 811 (543-1078) | 33 | 916 (374-1457) | 29 | 1235 (887-1584) | 9 | 2421 (449-4394) | 0 |
| *Vitamin D (µg) | 10 | 1.7 (0.5-2.9) | 100 | 2 (0.6-2.4) | 100 | 3 (2.4-4.5) | 100 | 2.5 (0.5-4.6) | 100 | 6.0 (3.2-8.9) | 92 | 4.3 (1.6-7.0) | 100 | 6.7 (4.6-8.8) | 91 | 14.7 (3.9-26) | 43 |
| *Vitamin E (mg) | 12 | 2.7 (1.5-3.9) | 100 | 5 (0.3-9.9) | 88 | 6 (4.0-7.0) | 100 | 4.4 (2.2-6.5) | 100 | 8.7 (5.0-12) | 67 | 6.2 (4.2-8.2) | 100 | 16.2 (9.6-23) | 64 | 12.2 (8.8-16) | 57 |
| **Vitamin K (µg) | 90 | 88 (34-142) | | 112 (7-217) | | 112 (47-178) | | 68 (19-117) | | 90 (49-131) | | 107 (35-247) | | 139 (69-208) | | 143 (75-211) | |
| *Selenium (µg) | 45 | 39 (27-52) | 67 | 37 (17-56) | 88 | 76 (65-88) | 9 | 59 (37-80) | 43 | 107 (88-126) | 0 | 83 (47-119) | 14 | 125 (104-146) | 0 | 202 (89-314) | 0 |
| *Zinc (mg) | 6.8 | 5.4 (3.4-7.3) | 67 | 7 (2.6-5.7) | 88 | 9 (6.4-12) | 27 | 5.6 (3.0-8.2) | 86 | 10.6 (9.6-12) | 0 | 9.6 (5.3-14) | 29 | 16.3 (12-21) | 0 | 19.9 (7.2-33) | 0 |

[1] DRI, Dietary Reference Intakes; * EAR, Estimated Average Requirement; ** AI, Adequate Intake.

356

**Table 2.** Reported dietary intake of individuals with anorexia nervosa (by subtype and quartile) and comparison (%) to a representative group from NHANES 2011–2012

| | NHANES | Quartile 1 Restrictor (n = 12) | | Quartile 1 Binge/Purge (n = 8) | | Quartile 2 Restrictor (n = 11) | | Quartile 2 Binge/Purge (n = 7) | | Quartile 3 Restrictor (n = 12) | | Quartile 3 Binge/Purge (n = 7) | | Quartile 4 Restrictor (n = 11) | | Quartile 4 Binge/Purge (n = 7) | |
|---|---|---|---|---|---|---|---|---|---|---|---|---|---|---|---|---|---|
| | Mean (95% CI) | Mean (95% CI) | % | Mean (95% CI) | % | Mean (95% CI) | % | Mean (95% CI) | % | Mean (95% CI) | % | Mean (95% CI) | % | Mean (95% CI) | % | Mean (95% CI) | % |
| Energy (kcal) | 2003 (1913–2094) | 736 (567–904) | 37 | 671 (571–771) | 34 | 1308 (1194–1421) | 65 | 1082 (965–1200) | 54 | 1799 (1706–1892) | 90 | 1662 (1445–1880) | 83 | 2639 (2130–3147) | 132 | 4102 (2301–5904) | 205 |
| Carbohydrate (g) | 252 (239–264) | 110 (81–138) | 44 | 128 (104–151) | 51 | 203 (175–230) | 80 | 161 (122–200) | 64 | 252 (233–270) | 100 | 238 (208–267) | 95 | 382 (316–448) | 152 | 533 (278–788) | 212 |
| Protein (g) | 72 (68–75) | 33 (22–44) | 46 | 22 (15–29) | 31 | 54 (45–63) | 75 | 41 (25–56) | 57 | 78 (67–88) | 108 | 59 (39–80) | 83 | 93 (76–110) | 129 | 143 (65–221) | 199 |
| Fat (g) | 75 (71–79) | 17 (13–23) | 23 | 17 (7.6–16) | 15 | 35 (30–40) | 47 | 33 (23–43) | 44 | 54 (46–63) | 73 | 57 (46–68) | 76 | 84 (58–110) | 112 | 159 (78–240) | 213 |
| *Dietary Fiber (g) | 16 (14–17) | 12 (6.4–17) | 73 | 12 (7–18) | 78 | 19 (14–23) | 118 | 12 (0.2–24) | 76 | 21 (14–28) | 134 | 17 (10–24) | 108 | 27 (21–33) | 171 | 31 (19–43) | 199 |
| Calcium (mg) | 909 (835–983) | 545 (291–799) | 60 | 451 (281–621) | 50 | 761 (578–944) | 84 | 676 (306–1046) | 74 | 1073 (829–1317) | 118 | 926 (413–1440) | 102 | 1514 (1191–1838) | 167 | 2271 (769–3772) | 250 |
| Iron (mg) | 14 (13–15) | 7.9 (4.1–12) | 57 | 9 (2.9–16) | 68 | 15 (10–19) | 106 | 10 (6–13) | 68 | 18 (13–22) | 127 | 15 (8–23) | 110 | 24 (17–31) | 171 | 28 (15–40) | 197 |
| Phosphorus (mg) | 1229 (1168–1290) | 607 (403–811) | 49 | 453 (308–597) | 37 | 962 (814–1109) | 78 | 812.7 (470–1156) | 66 | 1355.6 (1156–1556) | 110 | 1063 (714–1413) | 87 | 1745 (1453–2037) | 142 | 2815 (1052–4578) | 229 |
| Thiamin (mg) | 1.6 (1.4–1.7) | 0.7 (0.4–0.9) | 44 | 1 (0.4–1.7) | 66 | 1 (1.1–1.6) | 89 | 1.0 (0.7–1.3) | 63 | 1.7 (1.5–2.0) | 109 | 1.5 (1.1–1.9) | 97 | 2.6 (1.9–3.4) | 166 | 3.43 (1.7–5.2) | 219 |
| Riboflavin (mg) | 1.8 (1.7–2.0) | 1.1 (0.8–1.5) | 61 | 2 (0.9–2.0) | 79 | 2 (1.4–2.0) | 93 | 2.6 (0.4–4.7) | 138 | 2.4 (2.1–2.8) | 131 | 2.1 (1.3–2.8) | 112 | 3.8 (2.7–4.9) | 206 | 5.3 (1.9–8.8) | 287 |
| Niacin | 23 (22–25) | 8.6 (5.5–12) | 37 | 13 (4.8–21) | 56 | 19 (14–23) | 80 | 11.6 (8.3–15) | 50 | 23.3 (19–28) | 101 | 18.5 (13–24) | 80 | 35.0 (25–45) | 152 | 43.9 (22–665) | 190 |
| Folate (µg) | 390 (349–430) | 234 (145–324) | 60 | 291 (158–423) | 75 | 458 (316–601) | 118 | 235 (115–355) | 60 | 497 (341–654) | 128 | 434 (228–640) | 111 | 690 (499–882) | 177 | 764 (343–1185) | 196 |
| Vitamin B6 (mg) | 1.9 (1.8–2.1) | 0.9 (0.6–1.3) | 47 | 1 (0.2–1.8) | 51 | 2 (1.2–1.8) | 77 | 1.0 (0.5–1.4) | 50 | 2.1 (1.3–2.9) | 107 | 1.6 (0.8–2.4) | 84 | 3.1 (2.3–4.0) | 163 | 3.6 (1.4–5.8) | 186 |
| Vitamin B12 (µg) | 4.5 (4.0–4.9) | 2.2 (1–3.4) | 48 | 2 (0.3–4.3) | 52 | 3 (2.0–3.9) | 66 | 3.2 (1.3–5.0) | 71 | 5.8 (3.9–8.0) | 130 | 4.8 (2.0–7.6) | 107 | 8.4 (5.8–11.0) | 188 | 11.7 (1.6–22) | 261 |

Table 2. Cont.

| | NHANES | Quartile 1 Restrictor (n = 12) | | Binge/Purge (n = 8) | | Quartile 2 Restrictor (n = 11) | | Binge/Purge (n = 7) | | Quartile 3 Restrictor (n = 12) | | Binge/Purge (n = 7) | | Quartile 4 Restrictor (n = 11) | | Binge/Purge (n = 7) | |
|---|---|---|---|---|---|---|---|---|---|---|---|---|---|---|---|---|---|
| | Mean (95% CI) | Mean (95% CI) | % | Mean (95% CI) | % | Mean (95% CI) | % | Mean (95% CI) | % | Mean (95% CI) | % | Mean (95% CI) | % | Mean (95% CI) | % | Mean (95% CI) | % |
| Vitamin C (mg) | 83 (69–96) | 70 (38–102) | 85 | 85 (25–146) | 103 | 77 (37–117) | 93 | 44 (2–87) | 54 | 116 (76–157) | 141 | 96 (39–153) | 117 | 129 (85–174) | 156 | 107 (54–160) | 130 |
| Vitamin A (µg RE) | 595 (511–679) | 503 (286–720) | 85 | 536 (110–962) | 90 | 850 (580–1120) | 143 | 567 (229–905) | 95 | 811 (543–1078) | 136 | 916 (374–1457) | 154 | 1235 (887–1584) | 208 | 2421 (449–4394) | 407 |
| Vitamin D (µg) | 3.7 (3.1–4.3) | 1.7 (0.5–2.9) | 47 | 2 (0.6–2.4) | 40 | 3 (2.4–4.5) | 92 | 2.5 (0.5–4.6) | 68 | 6.0 (3.2–8.9) | 163 | 4.3 (1.6–7.0) | 116 | 6.7 (4.6–8.8) | 181 | 14.7 (3.9–26) | 398 |
| Vitamin E (mg) | 7.9 (7.1–8.7) | 2.7 (1.5–3.9) | 34 | 5 (0.3–9.9) | 65 | 6 (4.0–7.0) | 70 | 4.4 (2.2–6.5) | 55 | 8.7 (5.0–12) | 110 | 6.2 (4.2–8.2) | 78 | 16.2 (9.6–23) | 205 | 12.2 (8.8–16) | 153 |
| *Vitamin K (µg) | 118 (94–142) | 88 (34–142) | 75 | 112 (7–217) | 95 | 112 (47–178) | 95 | 68 (19–117) | 57 | 90 (49–131) | 76 | 107 (35–247) | 90 | 139 (69–208) | 117 | 143 (75–211) | 121 |
| Selenium (µg) | 101 (96–106) | 39 (27–52) | 39 | 37 (17–56) | 36 | 76 (65–88) | 75 | 59 (37–80) | 58 | 107 (88–126) | 106 | 83 (47–119) | 82 | 125 (104–146) | 124 | 202 (89–314) | 200 |
| Zinc (mg) | 9.8 (9.2–10.4) | 5.4 (3.4–7.3) | 55 | 7 (2.6–5.7) | 42 | 9 (6.4–12) | 91 | 5.6 (3.0–8.2) | 57 | 10.6 (9.6–12) | 108 | 9.6 (5.3–14) | 98 | 16.3 (12–21) | 167 | 19.9 (7.2–33) | 203 |

# 4. Discussion

The mean BMI for all participants ($17.2 \pm 0.1$ kg/m$^2$) was, as expected, below the lower limit of normal for healthy individuals. Reported nutrient intake was insufficient for participants in quartiles 1–3 of both AN subtypes when compared with DRIs. Intake reported by quartile 4 of both subgroups met or exceeded the requirements for most nutrients. Reported energy intake ranges from extremely low (~25%–40% of estimated needs) in quartile 1 of both AN subgroups to very high (158%–220% of estimated needs) for participants in quartile 4 of the binge purge AN subtype. Interestingly, when compared to the national sample, participants of both subtypes falling in quartiles 3 and 4 reported similar or higher energy and nutrient intakes. The higher reported intakes may in part be due to over-reporting by the AN population, or reflective of the increased food intake found among individuals engaging in binge-purge behaviors.

Difference in reported energy and nutrient intake by AN subtype did not present as much separation as anticipated. Eddy *et al.* [6] suggest that crossover from restricting to binge purge behavior in AN is suggestive of phases in the course of the disease. This notion is supported by Peat *et al.* [7] who suggest there is generally progression from restrictor to binge purge AN to bulimia nervosa in a sizeable number of patients, although other cross-over patterns are seen as well. Furthermore, a recent study from this dataset comparing restricting *versus* binge purge AN revealed that the binge purge type tended to engage in more episodes of virtually all eating disorder behaviors, including restriction, suggesting that subtype distinction may reflect a dimension of severity as opposed to a true qualitative subtype differentiation [29].

Participants reporting high energy intakes in quartile 4 of each AN subtype have a substantial discrepancy between body weight and energy intake as their body weights do not reflect adequate or excessive calorie consumption. It is possible that they over-reported their intake. Schebendach *et al.* [8] suggest that weight restored AN patients tend to significantly over-report intake and that this bias is increased at higher intake levels. It is possible that some women with AN, particularly the binge purge subtype, engaged in various forms of purging behavior to compensate for eating or binge eating episodes. Similarly, physical activity may be elevated in AN, and may account for the discrepancies observed in quartile 4. Indeed, two studies using doubly labeled water to assess total energy expenditure in young women with AN and bulimia nervosa show that because of high levels of physical activity, they expend as much energy as their healthy weight counterparts despite decreased basal metabolic rate [30,31]. These data support the notion that AN participants have a failure to consume enough energy to maintain a healthy body weight no matter what their reported intake is, which may be an important element in the diagnosis of AN.

A primary limitation of our study is the use of three 24-hours DRs as representative of actual dietary intake. Although this is generally considered acceptable for healthy individuals, it may not be adequate to represent usual nutrient intake in patients with eating disorders. By comparing reported intake of the present group to the DRIs, we may be substantially overestimating adequacy of these women's diets as these standards represent usual rather than optimal intake. In this study, we report nutrients from foods, not supplements, and may therefore not be reporting total intake. Additionally, the number of subjects in each cell is small and may, therefore, affect our outcomes.

Reported nutrient intake may not reflect the quantity of absorbed nutrients due to purging behaviors. The timing of and type of purging behaviors will affect the actual nutrients absorbed. We have no way to assess the bioavailability of consumed nutrients but can make the assumption that food and nutrient utilization is lower in this group than in healthy populations.

Analysis of nutrient intake of reported diets does not provide any information on eating patterns or eating behaviors. The present analysis did not assess if there are differences in the patterns of food intake, such as meal timing, volume consumed per eating episode, or specific food avoidance behaviors of participants with restricting *versus* binge purge types of AN. Recent EMA studies have examined the relationship of several eating disorder behaviors and their precipitating factors [9,17].

## 5. Conclusions

Our data demonstrate that intake is below adequate for most nutrients in participants reporting reduced energy intake and approaching adequate in those reporting high intake. However, reported intake of participants in quartile 4 exceeds estimated energy needs, yet they maintain very low body weights. Recognizing that AN patients diagnosed with either subtype may display characteristics of both types (*i.e.*, restriction and binge purge behaviors) will allow for more individualized nutrition care plans. The goal of nutritional intervention in patients with AN is the attainment of healthy body weight and improved nutrient intake.

Although nutrient intake assessment is subject to error of both over- and under-reporting, our results provide insight into the dietary intake of malnourished AN patients. Counseling of these patients should be directed to dietary improvements in total food consumption to increase energy intake with additional focus on nutritional gaps presented by evaluation of individual food intake. Although these data provide some insight into possible nutrient inadequacies, thorough assessment of dietary intake and physical activity patterns of patients with AN is required to design appropriate individualized medical nutrition therapy.

**Acknowledgments:** This work was funded by National Institutes of Health RO1-MH059674 and the United States Department of Agriculture 3062-51000-051-00D and 3062-51000-053-00D.

**Author Contributions:** SKR, LJ, SW and JEM conceived and designed this nutrient analysis project. The ecological momentary assessment study was conducted by SW, JM, RC, SC, DL CP and RC. LKJ and RC analyzed the data. SKR, LJ and SW wrote the paper. All authors read and approved the final manuscript.

**Conflicts of Interest:** The authors declare no conflict of interest.

## References

1.  Hoek, H.W. Incidence, prevalence and mortality of anorexia nervosa and other eating disorders. *Curr. Opin. Psychiatry* **2006**, *19*, 389–394.

2.  Mitchell, J.E.; Crow, S. Medical complications of anorexia nervosa and bulimia nervosa. *Curr. Opin. Psychiatry* **2006**, *19*, 438–443.

3.  Lantzouni, E.; Frank, G.R.; Golden, N.H.; Shenker, R.I. Reversibility of growth stunting in early onset anorexia nervosa: A prospective study. *J. Adolesc. Health* **2002**, *31*, 162–165.

4.  Harris, E.C.; Barraclough, B.M.; Winslow, F. Suicide as an outcome for medical disorders. *Medicine* **1994**, *73*, 281–296.

5.  American Psychiatric Association. *Diagnostic and Statistical Manual for Mental Disorders*, 4th ed.; American Psychiatric Association: Washington, DC, USA, 1994.

6.  Eddy, K.T.; Keel, P.K.; Dorer, D.J.; Delinsky, S.S.; Franko, D.L.; Herzog, D.B. Longitudinal comparison of anorexia nervosa subtypes. *Int. J. Eat. Disord.* **2002**, *31*, 191–201.

7.  Peat, C.; Mitchell, J.E.; Hoek, H.W.; Wonderlich, S.A. Validity and utility of subtyping anorexia nervosa. *Int. J. Eat. Disord.* **2009**, *42*, 590–594.

8.  Schebendach, J.E.; Porter, K.J.; Wolper, C.; Walsh, B.T.; Mayer, L.E. Accuracy of self-reported energy intake in weight-restored patients with anorexia nervosa compared with obese and normal weight individuals. *Int. J. Eat. Disord.* **2012**, *45*, 570–574.

9.  Smyth, J.; Wonderlich, S.A.; Heron, K.; Sliwinski, M.; Crosby, R.D.; Mitchell, J.E.; Engel, S.G. Daily and momentary mood and stress predict binge eating and vomiting in bulimia nervosa patients in the natural environment. *J. Consult. Clin. Psychol.* **2007**, *75*, 629–638.

10. Hadigan, C.M.; Anderson, E.J.; Miller, K.K.; Hubbard, J.L.; Herzog, D.B.; Klibanski, A.; Grinspoon, S.K. Assessment of macronutrient and micronutrient intake in women with anorexia nervosa. *Int. J. Eat. Disord.* **2000**, *28*, 284–292.

11. Ozier, A.D.; Henry, B.W. Position of the American Dietetic Association: Nutrition intervention in the treatment of eating disorders. *J. Am. Diet. Assoc.* **2011**, *111*, 1236–1241.

12. Beumont, P.; Chambers, T.L.; Rouse, L.; Abraham, S.F. The diet composition and nutritional knowledge of patients with anorexia nervosa. *Int. J. Food. Sci. Nutr.* **1981**, *35*, 265–273.

13. Misra, M.; Tsai, P.; Anderson, E.J.; Hubbard, J.L.; Gallagher, K.; Soyka, L.A.; Miller, K.K.; Herzog, D.B.; Klibanski, A. Nutrient intake in community-dwelling adolescent girls with anorexia nervosa and in healthy adolescents. *Am. J. Clin. Nutr.* **2006**, *84*, 698–706.

14. Institute of Medicine. *Dietary Reference Intakes: Applications in Dietary Assessment*; National Academy Press: Washington, DC, USA, 2000.

15. U.S. Department of Agriculture, A.R.S.; Beltsville Human Nutrition Research Center; Food Surveys Research Group (Beltsville, MD); U.S. Department of Health and Human Services; Centers for Disease Control and Prevention; National Center for Health Statistics (Hyattsville, MD). What We Eat in America, NHANES 2011–2012 Fact Sheet: Dietary Intake Data. 2014. Available online: http://www.ars.usda.gov/News/docs.htm?docid=13793 (accessed on 11 May 2015).

16. USDA. *Nutrient Intakes from Food: Mean Amounts Consumed per Individual, by Race/Ethnicity and Age, What We Eat in America, NHANES 2011–2012*. Available online: http://www.ars.usda.gov/Services/docs.htm?docid=18349 (accessed on 11 May 2015).

17. Engel, S.G.; Wonderlich, S.A.; Crosby, R.D.; Mitchell, J.E.; Crow, S.; Peterson, C.B.; Le Grange, D.; Simonich, H.K.; Cao, L.; Lavender, J.M.; *et al.* The role of affect in the maintenance of anorexia nervosa: Evidence from a naturalistic assessment of momentary behaviors and emotion. *J. Abnorm. Psychol.* **2013**, *122*, 709–719.

18. First, M.B.; Gibbon, M. *User's guide for the structured clinical interview for DSM-IV Axis I Sisorders: SCID-1 Clinician Version*; American Psychiatric Pub: Arlington, VA, USA, 1997.

19. Cooper, Z.; Fairburn, C. The eating disorder examination: A semi-structured interview for the assessment of the specific psychopathology of eating disorders. *Int. J. Eat. Disord.* **1987**, *6*, 1–8.

20. Schakel, S.; Sievert, Y.; Buzzard, I. Sources of data for developing and maintaining a nutrient database. *J. Am. Diet. Assoc.* **1988**, *88*, 1268.

21. Feskanich, D.; Sielaff, B.H.; Chong, K.; Buzzard, I.M. Computerized collection and analysis of dietary intake information. *Comput. Methods Programs Biomed.* **1989**, *30*, 47–57.

22. Centers for Disease Control and Prevention; National Center for Health Statistics. National Health and Nutrition Examination Survey Phone Follow-Up Dietary Interviewer Procedure Manual. Available online: http://www.cdc.gov/nchs/data/nhanes/nhanes_07_08/manual_dietarypfu.pdf (accessed on 11 May 2015).

23. Murphy, S.P.B. Susan I Practice paper of the American Dietetic Association: Using the dietary reference intakes. *J. Am. Diet. Assoc.* **2011**, *111*, 762.

24. Institute of Medicine. *Dietary Reference Intakes: Applications in Dietary Planning*; National Academy Press: Washington, DC, USA, 2003.

25. Institute of Medicine. *Standing Committee on the Scientific Evaluation of Dietary Reference Intakes; Dietary Reference Intakes for Energy, Carbohydrate, Fiber, Fat, Fatty Acids, Cholesterol, Protein, and Amino Acids (Macronutrients)*; Natl Academy Press: Washington, DC, USA, 2005; Volume 1.

26. Department of Agriculture, A.R.S.; Beltsville Human Nutrition Research Center; Food Surveys Research Group (Beltsville, MD); U.S. Department of Health and Human Services; Centers for Disease Control and Prevention. What We Eat in America, NHANES 2007–2008 Data: Dietary Interview-Total Nutrients Intakes-First Day. Available online: http://wwwn.cdc.gov/nchs/nhanes/2007-2008/DR1TOT_E.htm (accessed on 11 May 2015).

27. Agricultural Research Service; Food Survey Research Group. *USDA Food and Nutrient Database for Dietary Studies*, version 4.1; Agricultural Research Service, Food Survey Research Group: Beltsville, MD, USA, 2011.

28. U.S. Department of Agriculture, Agricultural Research Service. USDA National Nutrient Database for Standard Reference, Release 22. Available online: https://catalog.data.gov/dataset/usda-national-nutrient-database-for-standard-reference-release-22 (accessed on 11 May 2015).

29. De Young, K.P.; Lavender, J.M.; Steffen, K.; Wonderlich, S.A.; Engel, S.G.; Mitchell, J.E.; Crow, S.J.; Peterson, C.B.; Le Grange, D.; Wonderlich, J.; *et al.* Restrictive eating behaviors are a non-weight-based marker of severity in anorexia nervosa. *Int. J. Eat. Disord.* **2013**, *46*, 849–854.

30. Casper, R.C.; Schoeller, D.A.; Kushner, R.; Hnilicka, J.; Gold, S.T. Total daily energy expenditure and activity level in anorexia nervosa. *Am. J. Clin. Nutr.* **1991**, *53*, 1143–1150.

31. Pirke, K.M.; Trimborn, P.; Platte, P.; Fichter, M. Average total energy expenditure in anorexia nervosa, bulimia nervosa, and healthy young women. *Biol. Psychiatry* **1991**, *30*, 711–718.

# The Contribution of Fortified Ready-to-Eat Cereal to Vitamin and Mineral Intake in the U.S. Population, NHANES 2007–2010

Victor L. Fulgoni III and Rita B. Buckley

**Abstract:** Micronutrients play a pivotal role in achieving and maintaining optimum health across all life stages. Much of the U.S. population fails to meet Estimated Average Requirements (EARs) for key nutrients. This analysis aims to assess the contribution of fortified ready-to-eat cereals (RTEC) to micronutrient intake for U.S. residents aged 2–18, 19–99, and 2–99 years of age according to National Health and Nutrition Examination Survey (NHANES) 2007–2010 data. We used the National Cancer Institute (NCI) method to assess usual intake of 21 micronutrients and the percentage of the population under EARs and above Tolerable Upper Intake Levels (UL). Without fortification of RTECs, the percentage of those aged 2–18 years that were below EARs increased by 155%, 163%, 113%, and 35% for niacin, iron, thiamin, and vitamin A, respectively. For vitamins B6 and zinc, the respective numbers were 118% and 60%. Adults aged 19–99 and 2–99 had lower percentages but similar outcomes. RTECs are associated with improved nutrient adequacy and do not widely affect prevalence above the UL. The data indicate that large proportions of the population fail to achieve micronutrient sufficiency without fortification, and that its use can help Americans reach national nutrient intake goals.

Reprinted from *Nutrients*. Cite as: Fulgoni, V.L., III; Buckley, R.B. The Contribution of Fortified Ready-to-Eat Cereal to Vitamin and Mineral Intake in the U.S. Population, NHANES 2007–2010. *Nutrients* **2015**, 7, 3949–3958.

## 1. Introduction

Micronutrients play a pivotal role in achieving and maintaining optimal health across all life stages [1]. Vitamins are essential nutrients for many body functions, and are particularly important during growth as well as for certain vulnerable groups, such as pregnant women, young children, and the elderly. In addition to increasing nutrient intakes within the population, fortification has an impact on consumer purchasing decisions that can ultimately affect health and well-being [2].

Despite the availability of diverse foods, large-scale population-based dietary intake surveys, such as NHANES, indicate a gap between vitamin intakes and estimated average requirements for a significant proportion of the population; for example, more than 75% of the U.S. population does not get enough vitamin E [3]. A high percentage of all children/adolescents have inadequate intakes of numerous micronutrients, with the greatest inadequacy among older girls [4]. Many Americans would not achieve recommended micronutrient intakes without fortification of the food supply [2].

According to the Dietary Guidelines for Americans 2010 [5], consumption of vegetables, fruits, whole grains, milk and milk products, and seafood is lower than recommended. This makes some micronutrients—potassium, dietary fiber, calcium, and vitamin D—low enough to be a public health issue. Other vitamins of concern include iron, folate, and vitamin B12 [5].

Shortfalls in nutrition intakes could result from changing lifestyles, with increased food choices that have low micronutrient densities. These products have an impact on the quality of an individual's daily diet, and thus, nutrition status [3].

Diet and physical inactivity are the most important contributors to the epidemic of overweight and obesity among men, women, and children in all segments of our society [5]. Fortified ready-to-eat cereals (RTEC) with lower calories appear to be an effective tool for addressing nutritional deficiencies among populations [6]; for instance, encouraging RTEC consumption by pregnant women is a simple, safe, and inexpensive intervention that could help optimize nutrient intake for successful placental and fetal development [7].

Fortified RTECs remain a major contributor of micronutrients within the U.S. diet. Enriched and/or fortified foods provide a large proportion of the intakes of vitamins A, C and D, as well as thiamin, iron, and folate, although some of these nutrients are still below the EARs for a significant portion of the population [8]. Trends observed in the types of fortification in RTECs demonstrate positive changes in nutrient composition that may have an important impact on public health [9].

It is also important to consider fortification in the context of potential micronutrient overexposure. For example, excessive niacin intake can lead to potential skin reactions; too much vitamin A can lead to liver damage; and high levels of zinc can inhibit immune function [10]. Whether intake of some nutrients in fortified foods will result in total consumption above the UL depends, in part, on how the upper intake thresholds are estimated and how the target population is assessed [2].

The aim of this study was to determine the impact of RTEC fortification on micronutrient sufficiency in U.S. youths aged 2–18 and adults 19–99 and 2–99 years of age.

## 2. Subjects and Methods

### 2.1. Study Design

We performed a secondary analysis of data from the National Health and Nutrition Examination Survey (NHANES) 2007–2010. NHANES is a continuous cross-sectional survey on the health and nutrition status of a nationally representative sample of the civilian, non-institutionalized population of the United States [11]. The database is a publicly available resource for use by researchers throughout the world. No permission or IRB approval is needed to access NHANES data.

NHANES uses a complex, stratified, multistage probability cluster sampling design to collect demographic, socioeconomic, dietary, and general health data. Survey participants undergo a comprehensive health examination in a mobile examination center (MEC). Trained interviewers collect dietary data via in-person 24 h dietary recalls using USDA automated multi-pass methods during the MEC examination [12]. A second 24 h dietary recall is conducted by telephone 3–10 days after the first. Survey participants 12 years and older complete the dietary interview on their own. Proxy respondents report for children less than 11 years of age.

For this analysis, we used the 2007–2010 NHANES data set for ages 2–18 ($n = 6090$), 19–99 ($n = 11,297$), and 2–99 years ($n = 17,387$), with exclusions for unreliable data and pregnant or lactating females. We only included dietary records deemed reliable and complete by the USDA Foods Surveys Research Group.

The analysis included 21 different micronutrients—vitamin A, thiamin, riboflavin, niacin, total choline, vitamin B6, vitamin B12, folate (DFE), vitamin C, vitamin D, vitamin E (as alpha-tocopherol), vitamin K, calcium, phosphorus, magnesium, iron, zinc, copper, selenium, sodium, and potassium. We estimated amounts consumed from RTECs with fortification, and then used modeling that removed all 21 nutrients from RTECs to estimate intakes without fortification. Given that there is no way to estimate inherent nutrients in all RTEC, we assumed that all nutrients added were from fortification. Dietary supplements and medicines were excluded. All micronutrients are shown in Tables 1–4; only statistically significant ($p < 0.05$) results are included in the Results and Discussion sections.

Cereal consumers were defined as individuals who had eaten some RTEC on the first NHANES 24 h dietary recall sample day. Dietary Reference Intakes (DRIs) for populations came from the U.S. Food and Nutrition Board, Institute of Medicine, and the National Academies of Science.

## 2.2. Statistical Analyses

Intake was determined on daily and usual bases with and without fortification calculated using the National Cancer Institute (NCI) method [13], as were percentiles of intakes, and when applicable, percent of the population below the EAR, AI, and above the UL for the 21 nutrients used in the analysis. The NCI-supplied SAS programs Mixtran v1.1 and Distrib v1.1 were respectively used to generate parameter effects after covariate adjustment and estimate the distribution of usual intake via the Monte Carlo method [14]. The covariates used in the NCI usual intake estimation were sequence coded by day (weekend, Friday through Sunday) or (weekday, Monday through Thursday) and DRI age groups (2–18, 19–99 and 2–99 years).

We used the balanced repeated replication (BRR) method with a non-response adjustment for variance estimates, standard errors, and confidence intervals for usual intake means and percentiles. SAS software (version 9.3, SAS Institute, Cary, NC, USA) was used to perform all analyses. We used dietary sample weights to account for differential non-response, adjust for oversampling of some groups, and account for the complex sample design of NHANES [15]. We used a Z-statistic to determine differences in population groups, and conducted food source analyses and sources of nutrients in the diets of children and adults, respectively. The level of significance was set at $p < 0.05$.

RTECs are major dietary sources of micronutrients. Thus, we created separate categories for 21 nutrients in the analyses using data from the first NHANES 24 h recall. We determined the mean and standard error (SE) of nutrient intakes contributed from the total diets and from each food group with PROC DESCRIPT of SUDAAN (version 11.0; RTI International, Research Triangle Park, NC, USA).

## 3. Results

### 3.1. Estimated Average Requirements (EAR) and Contribution of RTEC Fortification

Among those 2–18 years of age with intake below EAR, significant ($p < 0.05$) nutrient increases resulting from RTEC fortification ranged from 3.3% for vitamin D (D2 + D3) to 161.5% for folate, DFE. Beside folate and vitamin D, there were significant increases in iron; thiamin (vitamin B1); riboflavin (vitamin B2); vitamin A, RAE; vitamin B6; vitamin E (alpha-tocopherol); niacin ($p = 0.01$); and zinc (Table 1).

In the 19–99 year old age group, significant percentage increases for nutrients below EAR ranged from 8.3% for magnesium to 84.8% for folate. Other micronutrient intakes that increased as a result of RTEC fortification were iron; riboflavin (vitamin B2); thiamin (vitamin B1); vitamin A, RAE; vitamin B12; vitamin B6; zinc; niacin; and vitamin E (Table 2).

Significant percentage increases toward EAR in the population aged 2–99 years ranged from 2.7% for vitamin E to 91.9% for folate, DFE. Other nutrients that showed higher intakes with fortification of RTECs were iron; magnesium; riboflavin (vitamin B2); thiamin; vitamin A, RAE; vitamin B6; zinc, calcium; niacin; vitamin B12; vitamin C; and vitamin D (Table 3).

Table 4 shows the contribution of RTEC fortification to micronutrient intake (% increase compared to when fortification was removed) across all age groups.

**Table 1.** Percentage of the U.S. population below EAR or AI [a] with and without micronutrient fortification, ages 2–18 ($n$ = 6090).

| Micronutrient | With Fortification | No Fortification | % Increase * |
|---|---|---|---|
| Calcium (mg) | 45.32 ± 1.05 | 47.58 ± 1.03 | 5.0 |
| Copper | 3.96 ± 0.48 | 4.68 ± 1.03 | 18.1 |
| Folate, DFE (mcg) [c] | 4.42 ± 0.46 | 11.56 ± 1.03 | 161.5 * |
| Iron (mg) [c] | 2.43 ± 0.25 | 6.40 ± 0.47 | 16.3 * |
| Magnesium (mg) | 35.35 ± 0.96 | 37.60 ± 0.96 | 6.3 |
| Niacin (mg) [c] | 0.60 ± 0.16 | 1.53 ± 0.34 | 155.0 * |
| Phosphorus (mg) | 16.29 ± 0.95 | 17.67 ± 0.94 | 8.4 |
| Potassium | 98.22 ± 0.20 | 98.4 7± 0.16 | 0.2 |
| Vitamin B2 (mg) [c] | 1.38 ± 0.20 | 2.31 ± 0.31 | 67.3 * |
| Selenium (mcg) | 0.19 ± 0.07 | 0.23 ± 0.09 | 21.0 |
| Sodium (mg) [a] | 0.53 ± 0.14 | 0.72 ± 0.18 | 35.8 |
| Thiamin (vitamin B1, mg) [c] | 2.15 ± 0.38 | 4.58 ± 0.64 | 113.0 * |
| Total choline (mg) [a] | 77.99 ± 0.83 | 78.65 ± 0.81 | 0.85 |
| Vitamin A, RAE (mcg) [c] | 24.90 ± 0.98 | 33.70 ± 0.88 | 35.3 * |
| Vitamin B12 (mcg) [c] | 1.51 ± 0.98 | 2.48 ± 0.49 | 64.2 |
| Vitamin B6 (mg) [c] | 3.29 ± 0.42 | 7.18 ± 0.80 | 118.2 * |
| Vitamin C (mg) | 21.34 ± 0.82 | 23.77 ± 0.97 | 11.3 |
| Vitamin D (D2 + D3, mcg) | 88.21 ± 0.69 | 91.14 ± 0.55 | 3.3 * |
| Vitamin E [b] (mg) | 77.77 ± 0.79 | 80.83 ± 0.77 | 3.9 * |
| Vitamin K (mcg) [a] | 58.84 ± 1.27 | 59.37 ± 0.77 | 0.9 |
| Zinc (mg) [c] | 8.55 ± 0.89 | 13.75 ± 1.15 | 60.8 * |

[a] Percentages below adequate intake (AI) levels where EAR was not available; [b] alpha-tocopherol; * $p < 0.05$; [c] RTEC contributes 10% or more of the mean usual micronutrient intake.

### 3.2. Percentage of Population with Micronutrient Intake above the UL

Sodium was above the UL in 89.26% ± 0.93% of those in the 2–18 year age group and 89.27% ± 0.79% of those aged 19–99 years. Removing fortification reduced these levels by 2.3% and 1.4%, respectively. Among those aged 2–18 years, the prevalence of potential risk from excessive micronutrient intake (>UL) was <1% for calcium and iron. Risk of overconsumption was 14.73% ± 0.73% for zinc, with a 41.9% decline without fortification, and 2.37% ± 0.22% for selenium, with a 12.6% decline. Among those aged 19–99 years, <1% of the population was above the ULs for calcium and iron. In those aged 2–99 years, 3.58% ± 0.18% of the population was above the UL for zinc, with a 42.1% decline without fortification.

**Table 2.** Percentage of the U.S. population below EAR or AI [a] with and without micronutrient fortification, ages 19–99 ($n = 11,297$).

| Micronutrient | With Fortification | No Fortification | % Increase * |
|---|---|---|---|
| Calcium (mg) | 42.07 ± 0.70 | 44.00 ± 0.68 | 4.5 * |
| Copper | 4.12 ± 0.55 | 4.93 ± 0.63 | 19.6 |
| Folate, DFE (mcg) [c] | 10.77 ± 0.61 | 19.91 ± 0.94 | 84.7 * |
| Iron (mg) [c] | 4.58 ± 0.32 | 6.99 ± 0.36 | 52.2 * |
| Magnesium (mg) | 55.85 ± 0.78 | 60.50 ± 0.73 | 8.3 * |
| Niacin (mg) [c] | 1.30 ± 0.28 | 2.34 ± 0.39 | 80.0 * |
| Phosphorus (mg) | 0.74 ± 0.17 | 0.85 ± 0.18 | 14.8 |
| Potassium | 97.73 ± 0.29 | 98.06 ± 0.27 | 0.3 |
| Riboflavin (vitamin B2, mg) | 2.23 ± 0.20 | 3.04 ± 0.25 | 36.3 * |
| Selenium (mcg) | 0.39 ± 0.13 | 0.50 ± 0.16 | 28.2 |
| Sodium (mg) [a] | 0.25 ± 0.10 | 0.31 ± 0.12 | 24.0 |
| Thiamin (vitamin B1, mg) [c] | 5.28 ± 0.63 | 8.90 ± 0.91 | 68.5 * |
| Total choline (mg) [a] | 94.12 ± 0.53 | 94.32 ± 0.50 | 0.21 |
| Vitamin A, RAE (mcg) [c] | 46.84 ± 1.15 | 54.84 ± 1.11 | 17.0 * |
| Vitamin B12 (mcg) [c] | 2.75 ± 0.33 | 4.27 ± 0.61 | 55.2 * |
| Vitamin B6 (mg) [c] | 11.18 ± 0.79 | 18.07 ± 0.99 | 61.6 * |
| Vitamin C (mg) | 42.02 ± 0.85 | 44.83 ± 0.86 | 4.2 |
| Vitamin D (D2 + D3, mcg) | 95.71 ± 0.45 | 96.75 ± 0.37 | 4.2 |
| Vitamin E [b] (mg) | 91.18 ± 0.61 | 93.37 ± 0.60 | 2.4 * |
| Vitamin K (mcg) [a] | 68.37 ± 0.99 | 68.39 ± 0.98 | 0.03 |
| Zinc (mg) [c] | 12.32 ± 0.72 | 17.09 ± 0.88 | 38.7 * |

[a] Percentages below adequate intake (AI) levels where EAR was not available; [b] alpha-tocopherol; * $p < 0.05$; [c] RTEC contributes 10% or more of the mean usual micronutrient intake.

### 3.3. Percentage of Individuals below the AI with Fortified RTEC Micronutrients

Analysis of NHANES 2007–2010 data indicates that even with fortification of RTECs, certain nutrients (*i.e.*, potassium, total choline, and vitamin K) are below AI across all age groups. Inadequate intakes of potassium affected approximately 98% of all individuals. The respective figures for total choline below AI for those aged 2–18, 19–99, and 2–99 years were 77.99% ± 0.83%, 94.12% ± 0.53%, and 90.19% ± 0.49%; for vitamin K, they were 58.84% ± 1.27%, 94.12% ± 0.53% and 66.03% ± 0.84%, respectively.

**Table 3.** Percentage of the U.S. population below EAR or AI [a] with and without micronutrient fortification, ages 2–99 ($n$ = 17,387).

| Micronutrient | With Fortification | No Fortification | % Increase * |
|---|---|---|---|
| Calcium (mg) | 42.87 ± 0.62 | 44.87 ± 0.62 | 4.6 * |
| Copper | 4.12 ± 0.49 | 4.79 ± 0.54 | 16.2 |
| Folate, DFE (mcg) [c] | 9.33 ± 0.53 | 17.91 ± 0.81 | 91.9 * |
| Iron (mg) [c] | 4.06 ± 0.28 | 6.85 ± 0.33 | 687 * |
| Magnesium (mg) | 50.82 ± 0.57 | 55.05 ± 0.60 | 8.3 * |
| Niacin (mg) [c] | 1.12 ± 0.23 | 2.18 ± 0.36 | 94.6 * |
| Phosphorus (mg) | 4.51 ± 0.30 | 4.96 ± 0.32 | 9.9 |
| Potassium | 97.81 ± 0.27 | 98.16 ± 0.23 | 0.36 |
| Riboflavin (vitamin B2, mg) | 2.00 ± 0.19 | 2.88 ± 0.25 | 44.0 * |
| Selenium (mcg) | 0.34 ± 0.11 | 0.44 ± 0.13 | 29.4 |
| Sodium (mg) [a] | 0.30 ± 0.11 | 0.41 ± 0.13 | 36.6 * |
| Thiamin (vitamin B1, mg) [c] | 4.48 ± 0.53 | 7.83 ± 0.78 | 74.7 * |
| Total choline (mg) [a] | 90.19 ± 0.49 | 90.56 ± 0.46 | 0.4 |
| Vitamin A, RAE (mcg) [c] | 41.53 ± 0.97 | 49.74 ± 0.93 | 19.7 * |
| Vitamin B12 (mcg) [c] | 2.47 ± 0.29 | 3.84 ± 0.55 | 55.4 * |
| Vitamin B6 (mg) [c] | 9.27 ± 0.68 | 15.46 ± 0.84 | 66.7 * |
| Vitamin C (mg) | 37.73 ± 0.66 | 39.65 ± 0.62 | 5.0 * |
| Vitamin D (D2 + D3, mcg) | 93.91 ± 0.46 | 95.42 ± 0.38 | 1.6 * |
| Vitamin E [b] (mg) | 87.90 ± 0.56 | 90.35 ± 0.53 | 2.7 * |
| Vitamin K (mcg) [a] | 66.03 ± 0.84 | 66.22 ± 0.83 | 0.2 |
| Zinc (mg) [c] | 11.47 ± 0.69 | 16.33 ± 0.82 | 42.3 * |

[a] Percentages below adequate intake (AI) levels where EAR was not available; [b] alpha-tocopherol; * $p$ < 0.05; [c] RTEC contributes 10% or more of the mean usual micronutrient intake.

**Table 4.** Contribution of RTEC fortification to micronutrient intake (% increase) across all age groups.

| Micronutrient | Ages 2–18 % Increase | p-Values [a] | Ages 19–99 % Increase | p-Values [a] | Ages 2–99 % Increase | p-Values * |
|---|---|---|---|---|---|---|
| Calcium | 5.0 | 0.12 | 4.5 | 0.04 * | 4.6 | 0.02 * |
| Copper | 18.1 | 0.31 | 19.6 | 0.33 | 16.2 | 0.35 |
| Folate, DFE | 161.5 | 0.00 * | 84.8 | 0.00 * | 91.9 | 0.00 * |
| Iron | 163.3 | 0.00 * | 52.6 | 0.00 * | 68.7 | 0.00 * |
| Magnesium | 6.3 | 0.09 | 8.3 | 0.00 * | 8.3 | 0.00 * |
| Niacin | 155.0 | 0.01 * | 80.0 | 0.02 * | 94.6 | 0.01 * |
| Phosphorous | 8.4 | 0.30 | 14.8 | 0.63 | 9.9 | 0.30 |
| Potassium | 0.25 | 0.32 | 0.34 | 0.39 | 0.36 | 0.33 |
| Riboflavin (vitamin B2) | 67.3 | 0.01 * | 36.3 | 0.01 * | 44.0 | 0.00 * |
| Selenium | 21.0 | 0.66 | 28.2 | 0.60 | 29.4 | 0.57 |
| Sodium | 33.8 | 0.40 | 24.0 | 0.69 | 36.6 | 0.02 * |
| Thiamin (vitamin B1) | 113.0 | 0.00 * | 68.5 | 0.00 * | 74.7 | 0.00 * |
| Total choline | 0.85 | 0.56 | 0.21 | 0.77 | 0.41 | 0.57 |
| Vitamin A, RAE | 35.3 | 0.00 * | 17.0 | 0.00 * | 19.7 | 0.00 * |
| Vitamin B12 | 64.2 | 0.09 | 55.2 | 0.02 * | 55.4 | 0.02 * |
| Vitamin B6 | 118.2 | 0.00 * | 61.6 | 0.00 * | 66.7 | 0.00 * |
| Vitamin C | 11.3 | 0.05 | 4.2 | 0.13 | 5.0 | 0.03 |
| Vitamin D | 3.3 | 0.00 * | 1.0 | 0.07 | 1.6 | 0.01 * |
| Vitamin E | 3.9 | 0.00 * | 2.4 | 0.01 * | 2.7 | 0.00 * |
| Vitamin K | 0.90 | 0.77 | 0.03 | 0.99 | 0.29 | 0.87 |
| Zinc | 60.8 | 0.00 * | 38.7 | 0.00 * | 42.3 | 0.00 * |

* Statistically significant ($p$ < 0.05).

## 4. Discussion

To our knowledge, our observations are the first to model the potential impact of a lack of fortification on overall dietary intake among a nationally representative sample of U.S. youths and adults who consume fortified and nonfortified RTECs. The prevalence of dietary inadequacy (assessed as the proportion of the population with intakes below the EAR) was significantly lower for consumers of fortified RTECs compared with nonfortified RTECs.

The results of this study confirm prior reports of higher mean nutrient intakes from food sources among breakfast consumers and/or those who ate RTECs for breakfast in nationally representative samples of American children and young adults [16,17] as well as Australian boys [18] and adults [19]. Galvin *et al.* [20] found that in Irish adults, fortified RTECs were associated with a more nutrient-dense diet and a reduced risk of dietary inadequacy for calcium, iron, riboflavin, and folate. These outcomes did not increase the risk of excessive intakes of micronutrients [20].

Barr *et al.* [21] demonstrated that among Canadian children and adolescents, the prevalence of nutrition inadequacy for vitamin D, calcium, iron, and magnesium was lowest in consumers of RTEC breakfasts compared with those who skipped breakfast or ate other types of breakfasts. In all groups, the potential risk of excessive nutrient intakes was low.

Food fortification is a proven and effective tool for tackling nutritional deficiencies among populations, especially among 'emergent deficiencies' that were not previously considered a problem [6].

In the U.S., current micronutrients of public health concern include potassium, calcium, and vitamin D. For specific population groups (e.g., those 50 years and older and women of childbearing age), intakes of iron, folate, and vitamin B12 are also of concern [5]. Several of the nutrients enhanced by RTEC consumption iron, folate, vitamin B12, and vitamin D. RTEC fortification increased the consumption of these nutrients across all age groups, particularly among those aged 2–18 years (Table 4). However, it fell short of AI for potassium, total choline, and vitamin K.

Overall, fortification improved nutrient adequacy and had scant impact on the prevalence of intakes with slightly higher proportions above the ULs. Intakes in excess of the UL were not associated with the addition of these micronutrients to RTECs. In addition, the proportion of individuals with intakes exceeding the UL remained largely unchanged when the added micronutrients were excluded from the intake estimate [20]. This indicates that consumption above the ULs was not driven by fortification.

Although the potential for nutrient overconsumption cannot be disregarded, particularly in the case of zinc in the 2–18 year and 2–99 year age groups, the benefits of fortified RTECs on reducing nutrient inadequacy appear to outweigh the potential risks for adverse effects of excess intake [22]. This study found that fortified

371

RTEC was associated with better nutrient adequacy and did not meaningfully affect prevalence above UL for all micronutrients other than zinc.

*Strengths and Limitations*

The strengths of this report include a large, nationally representative sample with validated data collection, and the use of sophisticated, readily available software to estimate intake distributions (*i.e.*, the NCI method). Another includes the use of advanced modeling techniques to estimate consumption of RTECs without fortification among the various age groups.

Limitations include the assessment of dietary nutrient adequacy and excess based on food sources alone, without the potential contribution of supplements. NHANES data are also cross-sectional (points in time) and rely on different subjects each year. In addition, we assumed that all nutrients examined in RTEC were from fortification, but there may have been small amounts of some nutrients still in RTEC after processing; thus, we may have slightly overestimated the impact of fortification removal.

## 5. Conclusions

This study supports previous reports that demonstrate the positive impact of fortified cereals on micronutrient intakes in the diets of adults [22] and children [23], with relatively small risk for adverse effects from excessive intake [1,22]. It shows that RTEC fortification is a cost-effective way to improve vitamin and mineral intake and ensure a healthy and productive life for many at-risk individuals in the U.S. [3].

**Acknowledgments:** This manuscript was prepared using NHANES 2007–2010 data obtained by the Centers for Disease Control and Prevention (CDC). It was funded by an unrestricted research grant from Kellogg's. The funder had no role in study design, data collection and analysis, decision to publish, or preparation of the manuscript. The content is solely the responsibility of the authors and does not necessarily represent the views of the funder.

**Author Contributions:** Victor L. Fulgoni collected, modeled, and provided all data, reviewed the manuscript, and added vital intellectual content. Rita B. Buckley analyzed the data, drafted the manuscript, and provided vital intellectual content.

**Conflicts of Interest:** Rita B. Buckley has no conflicts of interest to declare. Victor L. Fulgoni consults with the members of the food industry and conducts analyses of NHANES for numerous food and beverage companies and associated organizations.

## References

1.  Hennessy, A.; Walton, J.; Flynn, A. The impact of voluntary food fortification on micronutrient intakes and status in European countries: A review. *Proc. Nutr. Soc.* **2013**, *72*, 433–440.

2.    Dwyer, J.T.; Woteki, C.; Bailey, R.; Britten, P.; Carriquiry, A.; Gaine, P.C.; Miller, D.; Moshfegh, A.; Murphy, M.M.; Smith Edge, M. Fortification: New findings and implications. *Nutr. Rev.* **2014**, *72*, 127–141.

3.    Hoeft, B.; Weber, P.; Eggersdorfer, M. Micronutrients—A global perspective on intake, health benefits and economics. *Int. J. Vitam. Nutr. Res.* **2012**, *82*, 316–320.

4.    Berner, L.A.; Keast, D.R.; Bailey, R.L.; Dwyer, J.T. Fortified foods are major contributors to nutrient intakes in diets of US children and adolescents. *J. Acad. Nutr. Diet.* **2014**, *114*, 1009–1022.

5.    U.S. Department of Agriculture; U.S. Department of Health and Human Services. *Dietary Guidelines for Americans*, 7th ed.U.S. Government Printing Office: Washington, DC, USA, 2010.

6.    De Lourdes Samaniego-Vaesken, M.; Alonso-Aperte, E.; Varela-Moreiras, G. Vitamin food fortification today. *Food Nutr. Res.* **2012**, *56*, 5459–5467.

7.    Snook Parrott, M.; Bodnar, L.M.; Simhan, H.N.; Harger, G.; Markovic, N.; Roberts, J.M. Maternal cereal consumption and adequacy of micronutrient intake in the periconceptional period. *Public Health Nutr.* **2009**, *12*, 1276–1283.

8.    Fulgoni, V.L., III; Keast, D.R.; Bailey, R.L.; Dwyer, J. Foods, fortificants, and supplements: Where do Americans get their nutrients? *J. Nutr.* **2011**, *141*, 1847–1854.

9.    Thomas, R.G.; Pehrsson, P.R.; Ahuja, J.K.C.; Smieja, E.; Miller, K.B. Recent trends in ready-to-eat breakfast cereals in the US. *Procedia Food Sci.* **2013**, *2*, 20–26.

10.   Environmental Working Group. *How Much is Too Much? Excess Vitamins and Minerals in Food Can Harm Kids' Health.*; Environmental Working Group: Washington, DC, USA, 2014.

11.   Centers for Disease Control and Prevention; National Center for Health Statistics. Overview: NHANES Sample Design. Available online: http://www.cdc.gov/nchs/tutorials/Nhanes/SurveyDesign/SampleDesign/intro.htm (accessed on 25 November 2014).

12.   Blanton, C.A.; Moshfegh, A.J.; Baer, D.J.; Kretsch, M.J. The USDA Automated Multiple-Pass Method accurately estimates group total energy and nutrient intake. *J. Nutr.* **2006**, *136*, 2594–2599.

13.   National Cancer Institute. Usual Dietary Intakes: The NCI Method. Available online: http://riskfactor.cancer.gov/diet/usualintakes/method.html (accessed on 25 November 2014).

14.   National Cancer Institute. Usual Dietary Intakes: SAS Macros for Analysis of a Single Dietary Component. Available online: http://www.riskfactor.cancer.gov/diet/usualintakes/macros_single.html (accessed on 25 November 2014).

15.   The National Center for Health Statistics. Analytic and Reporting Guidelines The National Health and Nutrition Examination Survey (NHANES). Available online: http://www.cdc.gov/nchs/data/nhanes/nhanes_03_04/nhanes_analytic_guidelines_dec_2005.pdf (accessed on 25 November 2014).

16.   Deshmukh-Taskar, P.R.; Radcliffe, J.D.; Liu, Y.; Nicklas, T.A. Do breakfast skipping and breakfast type affect energy intake, nutrient intake, nutrient adequacy, and diet quality in young adults? NHANES 1999–2002. *J. Am. Coll. Nutr.* **2010**, *29*, 407–418.

17. Deshmukh-Taskar, P.R.; Nicklas, T.A.; O'Neil, C.E.; Keast, D.R.; Radcliffe, J.D.; Cho, S. The relationship of breakfast skipping and type of breakfast consumption with nutrient intake and weight status in children and adolescents: The National Health and Nutrition Examination Survey 1999–2006. *J. Am. Diet. Assoc.* **2010**, *110*, 869–878.

18. Grieger, J.A.; Cobiac, L. Comparison of dietary intakes according to breakfast choice in Australian boys. *Eur. J. Clin. Nutr.* **2012**, *66*, 667–672.

19. Williams, P. Breakfast and the diets of Australian adults: An analysis of data from the 1995 National Nutrition Survey. *Int J Food Sci Nutr* **2005**, *56*, 65–79.

20. Galvin, M.A.; Kiely, M.; Flynn, A. Impact of ready-to-eat breakfast cereal (RTEBC) consumption on adequacy of micronutrient intakes and compliance with dietary recommendations in Irish adults. *Public Health Nutr.* **2003**, *6*, 351–363.

21. Barr, S.I.; DiFrancesco, L.; Fulgoni, V.L., III. Breakfast consumption is positively associated with nutrient adequacy in Canadian children and adolescents. *Br. J. Nutr.* **2014**, *112*, 1373–1383.

22. Barr, S.I.; DiFrancesco, L.; Fulgoni, V.L., III. Consumption of breakfast and the type of breakfast consumed are positively associated with nutrient intakes and adequacy of Canadian adults. *J. Nutr.* **2013**, *143*, 86–92.

23. Serra-Majem, L. Vitamin and mineral intakes in European children. Is food fortification needed? *Public Health Nutr.* **2001**, *4*, 101–107.

# Section 5:
# Assessment of Dietary Patterns and Dietary Quality

# Role of Dietary Pattern Analysis in Determining Cognitive Status in Elderly Australian Adults

Kimberly Ashby-Mitchell, Anna Peeters and Kaarin J. Anstey

**Abstract:** Principal Component Analysis (PCA) was used to determine the association between dietary patterns and cognitive function and to examine how classification systems based on food groups and food items affect levels of association between diet and cognitive function. The present study focuses on the older segment of the Australian Diabetes, Obesity and Lifestyle Study (AusDiab) sample (age 60+) that completed the food frequency questionnaire at Wave 1 (1999/2000) and the mini-mental state examination and tests of memory, verbal ability and processing speed at Wave 3 (2012). Three methods were used in order to classify these foods before applying PCA. In the first instance, the 101 individual food items asked about in the questionnaire were used (no categorisation). In the second and third instances, foods were combined and reduced to 32 and 20 food groups, respectively, based on nutrient content and culinary usage—a method employed in several other published studies for PCA. Logistic regression analysis and generalized linear modelling was used to analyse the relationship between PCA-derived dietary patterns and cognitive outcome. Broader food group classifications resulted in a greater proportion of food use variance in the sample being explained (use of 101 individual foods explained 23.22% of total food use, while use of 32 and 20 food groups explained 29.74% and 30.74% of total variance in food use in the sample, respectively). Three dietary patterns were found to be associated with decreased odds of cognitive impairment (CI). Dietary patterns derived from 101 individual food items showed that for every one unit increase in ((Fruit and Vegetable Pattern: $p = 0.030$, OR 1.061, confidence interval: 1.006–1.118); (Fish, Legumes and Vegetable Pattern: $p = 0.040$, OR 1.032, confidence interval: 1.001–1.064); (Dairy, Cereal and Eggs Pattern: $p = 0.003$, OR 1.020, confidence interval: 1.007–1.033)), the odds of cognitive impairment decreased. Different results were observed when the effect of dietary patterns on memory, processing speed and vocabulary were examined. Complex patterns of associations between dietary factors and cognition were evident, with the most consistent finding being the protective effects of high vegetable and plant-based food item consumption and negative effects of 'Western' patterns on cognition. Further long-term studies and investigation of the best methods for dietary measurement are needed to better understand diet-disease relationships in this age group.

Reprinted from *Nutrients*. Cite as: Ashby-Mitchell, K.; Peeters, A.; Anstey, K.J. Role of Dietary Pattern Analysis in Determining Cognitive Status in Elderly Australian Adults. *Nutrients* **2015**, *7*, 1052–1067.

## 1. Introduction

Cognitive impairment is a condition in which a person has difficulty with memory, learning, concentrating or making decisions that affect their daily life [1]. Diet is among several modifiable factors found to influence cognitive function [2–4]. Age is presently the strongest known predictor for cognitive decline, and cognitive impairment (CI) has been shown to adversely affect quality of life and functional ability [5,6]. Risk reduction is especially important because there is still no effective treatment for dementia [7].

Studies aimed at elucidating the association between diet and cognitive function have utilised both the single nutrient and dietary pattern approaches [8,9]. While the single-nutrient approach has addressed various public health problems, many researchers theorise that due to high correlations between individual food constituents, there should be a shift toward analysis using a dietary pattern approach [10,11]. Evidence on the effect of dietary lipids, B-vitamins, antioxidants, fish, alcohol, vegetables and legumes have all produced varying results, and further research is needed into biomarkers for particular nutrients and cognitive endpoints in order for any definitive population-based conclusions to be reached [2,12–15]. Diets low in saturated fat, high in legumes, fruits and vegetables, moderate in ethanol intake and low in meat and dairy have also been highlighted as being beneficial to neurological function. One of the most studied dietary patterns is the Mediterranean diet, a diet rich in cereals, olive oil, fish, fruits and vegetables and low in dairy and meat, with a moderate consumption of red wine. This diet has been linked to increased survival, reduced risk of cancers, cardiovascular disease, longevity and cognitive impairment [16]. However, it is important to consider that there may be other dietary patterns, yet to be identified, that may have similar benefits and that can be applied to various sociocultural and demographic settings.

Few studies have examined the effect of dietary patterns on cognitive function using a data-driven method and even fewer of these studies have utilised Australian data. We identified only two studies utilising a data-driven approach to dietary analysis that have examined links with cognition in an Australian sample. The first used data from the Melbourne Collaborative Cohort Study in conducting factor analysis to determine the effect of dietary intake on psychological distress in older Australians [17] and the second utilised data from the Personality and Total Health (PATH) Through Life Study to examine the diet-depression relationship in three cohorts [18].

PCA is a data-driven approach that reduces a large number of food variables into a smaller set that captures the major dietary traits in the population [19]. In nutritional epidemiology, PCA can be used to investigate exposure-disease associations. As it relates to older age groups, such information can serve to develop age-specific guidelines and policies. One of the major criticisms of PCA, however, is that results can differ based on the methods employed during variable reduction and classification [20,21] and there is presently no accepted gold standard for dietary analysis to guide researchers.

The present study therefore has two aims. First, it addresses the question of how classification systems used to reduce food variables before the application of PCA affect the observed association between diet and cognitive function. Second, it evaluates the association between dietary patterns and cognitive function in a population-based cohort of Australian adults. In addition, it aims to determine the variance in food use explained by the different variable reduction methods employed, *i.e.* using 101 individual food items, 32 food groups and 20 food groups.

## 2. Experimental Section

### 2.1. Study Design and Sample

The study utilised secondary data derived from the AusDiab study, a population-based national survey of the general (non-institutionalised) Australian population aged 25 years and older [22]. The baseline examination was undertaken in 1999–2000 ($n$ = 11,247), with follow-ups conducted in 2004–2005 ($n$ = 8798) and 2011–2012 ($n$ = 6186) [22]. Dietary data were obtained from a sub-group of the sample using a questionnaire (Wave 1: $n$ = 3298) [22]. Measurement of cognitive function was conducted on those who attended survey sites in the third Wave of data collection ($n$ = 4764) [23]. The present study focuses on the older segment of the sample (age 60+ at baseline) that completed the food frequency questionnaire at Wave 1 and the mini-mental state examination and tests of memory, verbal ability and processing speed at Wave 3 ($n$ = 577).

We excluded 2721 participants from the current analysis since these participants had no dietary and/or cognitive data recorded.

### 2.2. Cognitive Outcome Measurement

The mini-mental state examination (MMSE) was used for data collection in 2011–2012 (AusDiab Wave 3) to determine CI status. Participants were classified based on their MMSE score as either cognitively impaired (score of 0–23) or not cognitively impaired (score of 24–30) [24].

The California Verbal Learning Test (CVLT) was used to assess memory using a 16-point scoring system. For this test, participants were asked to recall and repeat a list of 16 common shopping items that had been read to them by an interviewer. During a short delay of 20 min, during which participants were given other tasks to perform, the interviewer then asked the participant to recall the 16 common shopping list items again (delayed recall). The Spot-the-Word test (STW) was used in this study to test participants' vocabulary and verbal knowledge with scores ranging from 0 to 60. STW testing involved presenting participants with pairs of items, one of which was a real word and the other a non-word, and then requiring participants to identify the word. Performance on the STW has not been shown to decline with age and is highly correlated with verbal acumen [25]. Finally, processing speed was tested using the Symbol-Digit Modalities Test (SDMT). Participants were provided with a reference key and asked to pair geometric figures with specific numbers. Using the SDMT, participants were scored from 0–60 on the number of correct answers provided in 90 s.

## 2.3. Food Consumption Data and Classification

The AusDiab semi-quantitative food frequency questionnaire consisted of 121 items that asked participants about their consumption of 101 food items [26]. This questionnaire assessed usual intake and recorded the amount and types of specific food items consumed by participants. In some cases, for example casseroles and potatoes, pictures of serving sizes were provided so that persons could indicate whether they had more or less of a given food item each day and each week, using the past 12 months as a reference. Participants were asked to specify the number of times they had specific food items in the past year by checking 1 of 10 frequency categories ranging from 'never' to 'three or more times per day'. The average daily intake of food weight in grams was subsequently computed and used in the present analysis.

Three methods were used in order to classify these foods before applying PCA. In the first instance, the 101 individual food items asked about in the questionnaire were used (no categorisation). In the second and third instances, foods were combined and reduced to 32 and 20 food groups, respectively, based on nutrient content and culinary usage—a method employed in several other published studies for PCA [21,27] (see Table 1). Some foods were not categorised and were kept separate since they did not comfortably fit into any of the categories, e.g. pizza and meat pies [21,28]. More specifically, for the reduction of 101 items to 32 food groups, individual items were classed into groups, e.g., the item 'Processed Meats' was a tally of a participant's bacon, ham, salami and sausage consumption in grams/day, while the item 'Red Meats' was a tally of beef, pork, lamb, veal and hamburger in grams/day. In the final classification system, the 32 food groups were further categorised into broader groups, which resulted in 20 food groups, e.g. the item

'Meats' was a tally of a participant's 'Processed Meats' and 'Red Meats' consumption in grams/day.

**Table 1.** Food groupings used in the dietary pattern analysis.

| *Method 1* | *Method 2* | *Method 3* |
|---|---|---|
| **Food Item** | **Food Category** | **Food Category** |
| Bacon, ham, salami, sausages | Processed Meats | Meat |
| Beef, pork, lamb, veal, hamburger | Red Meats | Meat |
| Fish, fried fish, tinned fish | Fish | Fish |
| Chicken | Poultry | Poultry |
| Eggs | Eggs | Eggs |
| Butter | Butter | Fats and Oils |
| Margarine, poly/mono-unsaturated margarine | Margarine | Fats and Oils |
| Butter and margarine blends | Butter and Margarine Blends | Fats and Oils |
| Reduced-fat/skim milk, low-fat cheese, yoghurt | Low-fat Dairy Products | Dairy |
| Full-cream milk, hard/firm/soft/ricotta/cottage/cream cheese, ice-cream, flavoured-milk drink | High-fat Dairy Products | Dairy |
| Red/white/fortified wine | Wine | Alcohol |
| Light/heavy beer | Beer | Alcohol |
| Other spirits | Other Spirits | Alcohol |
| Tinned fruit, oranges, apples, pears, bananas, melon, pineapple, strawberries, apricots, peaches, mango | Fruit | Fruit |
| Fruit juice | Fruit Juice | Fruit Juice |
| Cabbage, cauliflower, broccoli | Cruciferous Vegetables | Vegetables |
| Carrot, pumpkin | Dark-yellow Vegetables | Vegetables |
| Tomatoes, tomato sauce | Tomatoes | Vegetables |
| Lettuce, spinach | Green, leafy Vegetables | Vegetables |
| Peas, green beans, bean sprouts, baked beans, tofu, other beans, soya milk | Legumes | Vegetables |
| Cucumber, celery, beetroot, mushrooms, zucchini, capsicum, avocado | Other Vegetables | Vegetables |
| Onion, garlic | Garlic and Onions | Vegetables |
| Potatoes | Potatoes | Vegetables |
| Chips | Chips/French fries | Chips/French Fries |
| All-bran, bran flakes, Weet-Bix, cornflakes, porridge, muesli, wholemeal/rye/multi-grain bread | Whole Grains | Whole Grains |

Table 1. *Cont.*

| *Method 1* | *Method 2* | *Method 3* |
|---|---|---|
| **Food Item** | **Food Category** | **Food Category** |
| High-fibre white/white bread, rice, pasta, crackers | Refined Grains | Refined Grains |
| Pizza | Pizza | Pizza |
| Sweet biscuits, cakes, crisps, chocolate | Snacks | Snacks |
| Nuts, peanut butter | Nuts | Nuts |
| Jam, vegemite | Condiments | Condiments |
| Sugar | Sugar | Sugar |
| Meat pies | Meat Pies | Meat Pies |

## 2.4. Statistical Analysis

PCA using SPSS version 22 was conducted to identify underlying dietary patterns. In determining the number of components to retain for further analysis, we considered component eigenvalues greater than 1 along with examination of scree plots. Components were rotated by an orthogonal (varimax) rotation to improve interpretability. Overall though, the comprehensibility and interpretability of the rotated factors were considered along with the aforementioned criteria. Similar to other studies, derived components were labelled based on our description of the observed patterns [29].

Dietary pattern scores were calculated for each individual at Wave 1 using all three classification methods (individual food items, 32 food groups and 20 food groups). Scores for an observed pattern were computed using the following equation: $i = \sum_j \left[ (b_{ij}/\lambda_i) X_j \right]$ [29]. Variables with factor loadings of $\geq 0.30$ were included in the weighted average [30,31].

Logistic regression analysis was performed to determine the association between dietary pattern scores at Wave 1 and cognitive status at Wave 3 using all three food item categorisation methods, *i.e.* PCA based on 101 individual food items, 32 food groups or 20 food groups. The interaction between dietary pattern score and exercise time was also examined to determine whether there was any association with cognitive status using all three food categorisation methods.

Generalized linear models (GLM) were used to estimate the associations between dietary pattern scores at Wave 1 and memory, verbal ability and processing speed using all three food variable reduction methods.

## 3. Results

Descriptive statistics for the sample are presented in Table 2. A total of 577 participants (49.22% female) had both diet and cognitive data recorded at Wave 1.

**Table 2.** Descriptive statistics at Wave 1 for the AusDiab sample included in the study ($n$ = 577).

| Variables | Wave 1 |
|---|---|
| Age Range | 60–83 |
| Mean Age (SD) | 66.07 (4.85) |
| Female (%) | 284 (49.22) |
| BMI (SD) | 26.89 (4.09) |
| Secondary School (%) | 242 (24.4) |
| Tertiary Level (%) | 229 (40.1) |
| Other - Trade, Technician, Primary Only (%) | 100 (17.4) |
| Current Smoker (%) | 29 (5.1) |
| Ex-Smoker (%) | 182 (32.0) |
| Non-Smoker | 357 (62.9) |
| Exercise Mean (SD), mins./week | 292.45 (324.21) |
| MMSE Score | 27.41 (2.44) |
| CVLT Score | 5.17 (2.30) |
| STW Score | 50.30 (6.84) |
| SDMT Score | 38.63 (10.74) |
| Impaired (%) | 44 (7.63) |

## 3.1. Dietary Pattern Analysis

Classification method affected the number and components of the patterns identified. Variable reduction using 20 food groups explained a greater proportion of variance in the sample than variable reduction using 32 food groups and 101 individual food items. Use of 20 food groups explained 30.74% of total variance in food use in the sample. Comparatively, use of 101 individual foods explained 23.22% and use of 32 food groups explained 29.74% of total variance in food use.

### 3.1.1. Wave 1 Dietary Patterns Using 101 Individual Food Items

Seven dietary patterns were extracted using PCA with varimax rotation. The rotated component matrix with factor loadings is shown in Supplementary Table 1.

The first dietary pattern identified was labelled 'Fruit and Vegetable' because of the high loadings of unprocessed fruit and vegetables observed. The second dietary pattern identified was labelled 'Snack and Processed Food' due to the high factor loadings observed for foods that could be qualified as such, e.g., cakes, jam, ice cream, sausages, and salami. Dietary pattern labels for the other observed dietary structures can be viewed in Supplementary Table 1. Together, the dietary patterns identified accounted for 23% of total variance in the sample.

**Table 3.** Results of logistic regression analyses showing associations between CI at Wave 3 and dietary patterns obtained using 101 food items, 32 food groups and 20 food groups at Wave 1 (odds ratios with 95% confidence intervals shown in brackets).

| | Dietary Pattern 1 | Dietary Pattern 2 | Dietary Pattern 3 | Dietary Pattern 4 | Dietary Pattern 5 | Dietary Pattern 6 | Dietary Pattern 7 |
|---|---|---|---|---|---|---|---|
| 101 Food Items | Fruit & Vegetable | Snack & Processed Foods | Vegetable | Meat | Fish, Legumes & Vegetable | Vegetable, Pasta & Alcohol | Dairy, Cereal & Eggs |
| OR (95% CI) | 1.061 (1.006–1.118) $p = 0.030$ * | 1.051 (0.967–1.143) $p = 0.239$ | 0.986 (0.916–1.061) $p = 0.701$ | 1.005 (0.964–1.048) $p = 0.806$ | 1.032 (1.001–1.064) $p = 0.040$ * | 1.000 (0.965–1.037) $p = 0.994$ | 1.020 (1.007–1.033) $p = 0.003$ ** |
| 32 Food Groups | Western | Prudent | Vegetable, Grains & Wine | High-Fat | | | |
| OR (95% CI) | 1.005 (0.994–1.016) $p = 0.409$ | 0.997 (0.984–1.010) $p = 0.643$ | 1.008 (0.995–1.020) $p = 0.229$ | 0.999 (0.992–1.007) | | | |
| 20 Food Groups | Variety | Western | Dairy, Grains & Alcohol | | | | |
| OR (95% CI) | 1.006 (0.994–1.018) $p = 0.333$ | 1.008 (0.986–1.031) $p = 0.497$ | 1.001 (0.998–1.005) $p = 0.383$ | | | | |

Model adjusted for age, sex, energy, education, BMI, smoking status, STW and exercise time; * $p < 0.05$; ** $p < 0.01$.

### 3.1.2. Wave 1 Dietary Patterns Using 32 Food Groups

After applying PCA, four dietary patterns were extracted. The rotated component matrix with factor loadings is shown in Supplementary Table 2.

The first pattern identified was labelled 'Western' because of the predominantly high loadings of processed meats, refined grains and convenience foods. The second dietary pattern identified was labelled 'Prudent' and had characteristically high factor loadings of fish, vegetables and fruit. Dietary pattern labels for the other observed dietary structures can be viewed in Supplementary Table 4. Together, the dietary patterns identified accounted for 30% of total variance in the sample.

### 3.1.3. Wave 1 Dietary Patterns Using 20 Food Groups

Three dietary patterns were extracted using PCA with varimax rotation. The rotated component matrix with factor loadings is shown in Supplementary Table 3.

The first pattern identified was labelled 'Variety' because of the high loadings of a wide variety of foods—vegetables, fruit, fish, meat and nuts. The second dietary pattern was labelled 'Western' because of the high factor loadings of high-fat and high-sugar foods. The final dietary pattern was labelled 'Dairy, Grains and Alcohol' due to the high factor loadings of these foods recorded. Together, these dietary patterns identified accounted for 31% of total variance in the sample.

### 3.2. Dietary Pattern as a Predictor of CI Using the MMSE

Logistic regression analysis using dietary pattern scores obtained from all three variable reduction techniques (*i.e.*, 101 individual food items, 32 food groups and 20 food groups) was conducted to examine the relationship between dietary pattern and CI. Covariates included the independent variables age, sex, energy, education, BMI, smoking status, exercise time and Spot-the-Word (as a control for premorbid intelligence) [32].

The only significant dietary predictors of CI were obtained using 101 individual food items. Three of the seven dietary patterns identified were observed to be significant predictors of CI. For every one unit increase in these pattern scores, the odds of CI decreased ((Fruit and Vegetable Pattern: $p = 0.030$, OR 1.061, confidence interval: 1.006–1.118); (Fish, Legumes and Vegetable Pattern: $p = 0.040$, OR 1.032, confidence interval: 1.001–1.064); (Dairy, Cereal and Eggs Pattern: $p = 0.003$, OR 1.020, confidence interval: 1.007–1.033)).

**Table 4.** Results of GLM showing associations between cognitive function at Wave 3 and dietary patterns obtained using 101 individual food items, 32 food groups and 20 food groups at Waves 1, 2 and 3 ($\beta$ values with Standard Errors shown in brackets).

| | Dietary Pattern 1 | Dietary Pattern 2 | Dietary Pattern 3 | Dietary Pattern 4 | Dietary Pattern 5 | Dietary Pattern 6 | Dietary Pattern 7 |
|---|---|---|---|---|---|---|---|
| 101 Food Items | Fruit & Vegetable | Snack & Processed Foods | Vegetable | Meat | Fish, Legumes & Vegetable | Vegetable, Pasta & Alcohol | Dairy, Cereal & Eggs |
| CVLT | 0.012 (0.013) $p = 0.336$ | 0.020 (0.015) $p = 0.186$ | −0.001 (0.012) $p = 0.930$ | 0.000 (0.005) $p = 0.984$ | −0.002 (0.007) $p = 0.793$ | 0.004 (0.006) $p = 0.551$ | −4.474 (0.002) $p = 0.986$ |
| SDMT | 0.097 (0.057) $p = 0.091$ | 0.060 (0.067) $p = 0.365$ | 0.013 (0.054) $p = 0.801$ | 0.014 (0.023) $p = 0.536$ | −0.062 (0.032) $p = 0.054$ | −0.003 (0.028) $p = 0.916$ | −0.016 (0.011) $p = 0.149$ |
| STW | 0.077 (0.039) $p = 0.051$ | 0.080 (0.046) $p = 0.086$ | 0.046 (0.037) $p = 0.224$ | 0.007 (0.020) $p = 0.722$ | 0.000 (0.022) $p = 0.994$ | 0.000 (0.021) $p = 0.982$ | 0.002 (0.008) $p = 0.799$ |
| 32 Food Groups | Western | Prudent | Vegetable, Grains & Wine | High-Fat | | | |
| CVLT | −0.008 (0.003) $p = 0.001$ ** | −0.005 (0.003) $p = 0.067$ | 0.001 (0.003) $p = 0.764$ | −0.001 (0.001) $p = 0.711$ | | | |
| SDMT | −0.024 (0.011) $p = 0.035$ * | −0.035 (0.011) $p = 0.002$ ** | 0.024 (0.012) $p = 0.034$ * | 0.005 (0.006) $p = 0.403$ | | | |
| STW | −0.006 (0.008) $p = 0.467$ | −0.006 (0.008) $p = 0.425$ | 0.013 (0.008) $p = 0.119$ | 0.001 (0.005) $p = 0.774$ | | | |
| 20 Food Groups | Variety | Western | Dairy, Grains & Alcohol | | | | |

Table 4. *Cont.*

|  | Dietary Pattern 1 | Dietary Pattern 2 | Dietary Pattern 3 | Dietary Pattern 4 | Dietary Pattern 5 | Dietary Pattern 6 | Dietary Pattern 7 |
|---|---|---|---|---|---|---|---|
| CVLT | −0.003 (0.003) $p = 0.272$ | −0.004 (0.005) $p = 0.376$ | −0.002 (0.001) $p = 0.005**$ | | | | |
| SDMT | −0.026 (0.011) $p = 0.018*$ | −0.007 (0.021) $p = 0.740$ | −0.005 (0.003) $P = 0.149$ | | | | |
| STW | −0.008 (0.008) $p = 0.291$ | 0.002 (0.015) $p = 0.901$ | −0.001 (0.002) $p = 0.618$ | | | | |

Model adjusted for age, sex, energy, education, BMI, smoking status, STW and exercise time; * $p < 0.05$, ** $p < 0.01$.

When the interaction term 'dietary pattern score × exercise time' was included in the model, no significant results were obtained.

### 3.3. Dietary Pattern as a Predictor of Memory, Vocabulary and Verbal Knowledge and Processing Speed

Using dietary pattern scores calculated from 101 individual food items, there were no dietary patterns observed to be significantly predictive of memory, processing speed or verbal knowledge.

Using 32 food groups, however, the 'Western' dietary pattern was a predictor of poorer memory and processing speed ($\beta = -0.008$, SE = 0.003, $p = 0.001$ and $\beta = -0.024$, SE = 0.011, $p = 0.035$). In addition, the 'Prudent' dietary pattern was also a predictor of poorer processing speed ($\beta = -0.035$, SE = 0.011, $p = 0.002$).

When 20 food groups were used to calculate dietary pattern scores, the 'Dairy, grains and alcohol' dietary pattern was predictive of poorer memory while the 'Variety' dietary pattern was associated with poorer processing speed ( = -0.002, SE = 0.001, $p = 0.005$ and When 20 food groups were used to calculate dietary pattern scores, the 'Dairy, grains and alcohol' dietary pattern was predictive of poorer memory while the 'Variety' dietary pattern was associated with poorer processing speed ($\beta = -0.002$, SE = 0.001, $p = 0.005$ and $\beta = -0.026$, SE = 0.011, $p = 0.018$ respectively).

## 4. Discussion

The present study is one of the few that use a data-driven method of dietary analysis to assess the relationship between diet and cognitive function in older Australian adults. A number of findings from this study are noteworthy. First, the broader the categories used in grouping foods, the greater the variability in food use that was explained. It was observed, however, that the results of logistic regression were more sensitive when dietary analysis was based on individual food items than food groups. From these data we observed that for every one unit increase in 'Fruit and Vegetable', 'Fish, Legumes and Vegetable' and 'Dairy, Cereal and Eggs' dietary pattern scores, the odds of CI decreased.

When looking at the relationship between dietary pattern and memory, processing speed and vocabulary, no significant results were observed using 101 individual food items. Using 32 food groups, the 'Western' dietary pattern was found to be predictive of poorer memory and processing speed, the 'Vegetable, Grains and Wine' pattern was a predictor of better processing speed while the 'Prudent' pattern was predictive of poorer processing speed. Using 20 food groups we observed that the 'Variety' dietary pattern was a predictor of poorer processing speed and the 'Dairy, Grains and Alcohol' pattern predictive of poorer memory.

We found that the method of reducing food variables affected the amount of variance in food use that was explained. Similarly to other published findings, the broader the categories used, the greater the variability in food use explained [21]. We suggest this may be due to the inclusion of foods that are both weakly and strongly correlated with a specific pattern in the broader categorisations which leads to an increase in the information captured [21]. Interestingly, for logistic regression analyses, it was only when the level of detail in the items included in PCA-derived dietary patterns increased that significant associations between diet and cognitive impairment were observed, *i.e.*, it was variable reduction that utilised dietary pattern scores from individual foods that produced the only significant results. This may be because analysis using individual foods captures more meaningful results as it is able to show whether consumption or non-consumption of specific food items is associated with disease.

Our results are consistent with previous studies in showing that diets with high loadings of vegetables and other plant-based food items (fruit, grains and legumes) resulted in reduced odds of disease and improved cognitive function [21,27]. In a study of 6911 Chinese subjects aged 65 and older who formed part of the Chinese Longitudinal Health Longevity Study, lower intakes of vegetables and legumes were associated with cognitive decline when using MMSE as a measure of cognitive function [33]. Multivariate logistic regression showed that always eating vegetables and always consuming legumes were inversely associated with cognitive decline [33]. Additionally, in a study of 2,148 community-based elderly subjects without dementia in New York, higher intakes of cruciferous and dark and green leafy vegetables were found to be associated with a decreased risk of developing AD [34]. The benefits of diets high in vegetables extend beyond the cognitive domain. In a European study aimed to investigate the effect of the Mediterranean diet (MeDi) on mortality, greater adherence was associated with a more than 50% lower rate of all-causes and cause-specific mortality [35]. McCann *et al.* [21], in a study examining the effect of dietary patterns on estimation of endometrial cancer risk, found that dietary patterns high in fruit, vegetables and whole-grains resulted in reduced endometrial cancer risks. Similarly, dietary patterns high in vegetables, grain and fruit have been found to be associated with a modestly lower risk for type 2 diabetes [27]. This seemingly protective association between plant-based foods and disease may be the result of the high concentration of antioxidant nutrients present in vegetables and fruits and their role in suppressing inflammation. There is evidence that oxidative stress and inflammation can lead to impaired cognitive function because of an increase in free radicals and the damage they cause to neuronal cells [14].

The Mediterranean diet (MeDi), one of the most studied dietary patterns, describes a diet rich in cereals, olive oil, fish, fruits and vegetables and low in dairy and meat with a moderate consumption of red wine. This diet has been linked to increased survival, reduced risk of cancers, cardiovascular disease, longevity and CI [11,16,36–38]. In the present study, diets rich in vegetables, grain and wine were found to be predictive of better processing speed and diets high in vegetables and plant-based food items were generally associated with better cognitive outcomes.

Worth noting is the finding that the 'Prudent' dietary pattern was predictive of poorer processing speed. This dietary pattern was so labelled because of its high loadings of fish, fruit and vegetables, nuts and whole-grains. Perhaps an explanation of this lies in the method in which food items are prepared or in analysing whether there is actually a protective effect of foods contained in this pattern. For instance, while many studies have examined the effect of fish consumption on cognition, some clarification is still needed on the purported link between the two. In a study of 6150 Chicago residents aged 65 and older to examine whether intake of fish and omega-3 fatty acids protects against age-related cognitive decline, it was reported that fish consumption may be associated with slower cognitive decline with age [39]. Similar findings were also reported by Kalmijn *et al.* in 1997, who found statistically significant decreased risks of AD with higher fish consumption [40]. In two more recent Australian studies, one reported that higher fish consumption was associated with an increased risk of cognitive disorder [15] while the other found no evidence to support the hypothesis that higher proportions of fish intake benefits cognitive performance in normal older adults [41].

The 'Variety' dietary pattern was also found to be predictive of poorer processing speed. This pattern, so named because of high factor loadings in a variety of foods, is of interest because dietary guidelines for Australia and the rest of the world highlight the benefits of consuming a wide variety of foods. Therefore, in food and nutrition policy, there is a need to ensure that messages about the method of food preparation, processing and portion sizes of consumables are equally stressed.

In the present study, the 'Western' dietary pattern was predictive of poorer memory and processing speed. This is supported by other research which has reported that the 'Western' dietary pattern is associated with cognitive decline and reduced executive function [42].

One of the limitations of this study lies in its inability to report disease incidence as cognitive data were only collected at one time point (Wave 3). Additionally, no data were collected on executive function, and dietary intake is self-reported. There is also some subjectivity in determining food groups before application of PCA, but the method of food variable reduction we employed has been widely used in other studies [21,27]. It is also possible that the results observed may represent a selection bias, as only older adults with dietary and cognitive data were included in the study ($n = 577$). This has the effect of limiting the generalizability of the study's findings. Finally, while we focused on the methodology of grouping foods in this paper, we were still unable to clearly identify guidelines for future researchers to follow.

This is a major issue for diet-cognition research and suggests the need for further investigation and development of more robust and consensus-led methodologies in the field.

Despite its limitations, this study adds to the sparse body of literature examining the relationship between dietary patterns and CI among older adults, both in Australia and internationally. Furthermore, the study's focus on older age groups whose dietary patterns have not been widely studied and reported is noteworthy. Finally, the study's ability to answer a methodological question that has been one of the main critiques of PCA makes it noteworthy—how do variable reduction methods before the application of PCA affect the results obtained? This question is significant when examining the relationship between dietary patterns and cognition since there is a level of subjectivity involved in reducing food variables, and these can affect the observed associations with cognitive function [27].

Future studies examining the association between dietary intake and cognitive status will be useful to identify other patterns associated with CI and to examine more nuanced issues as they relate to diet and cognitive function.

## 5. Conclusions

Our findings showed that diets with high factor loadings of fruit, vegetables and plant-based food items conferred cognitive benefits, while those with high factor loadings of high-fat and convenience foods are linked to poorer cognitive outcomes. These results are similar to those of other studies which show that diets with high loadings of vegetables, fruit and grain reduce the odds of a myriad of diseases [21,27,43]. In addition, we demonstrated that the method of variable reduction in dietary studies may influence results, and suggest that further work is required to establish robust and replicable methods of dietary analysis for use in research into cognitive ageing. Additional studies that focus on the dietary habits of those over age 60 would be useful in order to further elucidate more specific details between dietary patterns, types and amount of fat, protein and carbohydrates, number of calories, and micro and macronutrients that are linked with optimal cognitive function and reduced risk of CI in older adults. Such information is required to provide support for the development of policies that promote optimal cognitive health in ageing.

**Acknowledgments:** This research was supported by the Australian Research Council Centre of Excellence in Population Ageing Research (project number CE110001029). AP is supported by a National Health and Medical Research Council Career Development Award (1045456). KJA is funded by NHMRC Fellowship #1002560. We acknowledge support from the NHMRC Dementia Collaborative Research Centres. The AusDiab study co-coordinated by the Baker IDI Heart and Diabetes Institute, gratefully acknowledges the support and assistance given by: K Anstey, B Atkins, B Balkau, E Barr, A Cameron, S Chadban, M de Courten, D Dunstan, A Kavanagh, D Magliano, S Murray, N Owen, K Polkinghorne, J Shaw, T Welborn, P Zimmet and all the study participants. Also, for funding or logistical support, we are grateful to: National Health and Medical Research Council (NHMRC grants 233200 and 1007544),

Australian Government Department of Health and Ageing, Abbott Australasia Pty Ltd., Alphapharm Pty Ltd., Amgen Australia, AstraZeneca, Bristol-Myers Squibb, City Health Centre-Diabetes Service-Canberra, Department of Health and Community Services —Northern Territory, Department of Health and Human Services—Tasmania, Department of Health—New South Wales, Department of Health—Western Australia, Department of Health—South Australia, Department of Human Services—Victoria, Diabetes Australia, Diabetes Australia Northern Territory, Eli Lilly Australia, Estate of the Late Edward Wilson, GlaxoSmithKline, Jack Brockhoff Foundation, Janssen-Cilag, Kidney Health Australia, Marian & FH Flack Trust, Menzies Research Institute, Merck Sharp & Dohme, Novartis Pharmaceuticals, Novo Nordisk Pharmaceuticals, Pfizer Pty Ltd., Pratt Foundation, Queensland Health, Roche Diagnostics Australia, Royal Prince Alfred Hospital, Sydney, Sanofi Aventis, Sanofi-Synthelabo, and the Victorian Government's OIS Program.

**Author Contributions:** Kimberly Ashby-Mitchell was responsible for designing the study, conducting analyses, interpreting the output of analyses and preparing the manuscript for submission. Anna Peeters interpreted data and revised the manuscript for intellectual content. Kaarin J. Anstey interpreted data and revised the manuscript for intellectual content.

**Conflicts of Interest:** The authors have reported no conflicts of interest.

## References

1. U.S. Department of Health and Human Services Centers for Disease Control and Prevention. *Cognitive Impairment: A Call for Action Now*; U.S. Department of Health and Human Services Centers for Disease Control and Prevention: Atlanta, GA, USA, 2011.

2. Gillette-Guyonnet, S.; Secher, M.; Vellas, B. Nutrition and neurodegeneration: Epidemiological evidence and challenges for future research. *Br. J. Clin. Pharmacol.* **2013**, *75*, 738–755.

3. McNeill, G.; Winter, J.; Jia, X. Diet and cognitive function in later life: A challenge for nutrition epidemiology. *Eur. J. Clin. Nutr.* **2009**, *63*, S33–S37.

4. Shatenstein, B.; Ferland, G.; Belleville, S.; Gray-Donald, K.; Kergoat, M.-J.; Morais, J.; Gaudreau, P.; Payette, H.; Greenwood, C. Diet quality and cognition among older adults from the NuAge study. *Exp. Gerontol.* **2012**, *47*, 353–360.

5. Barnes, D.E.; Yaffe, K. Predicting dementia: Role of dementia risk indices. *Future Neurol.* **2009**, *4*, 555–560.

6. Matthews, F.E.; Jagger, C.; Miller, L.L.; Brayne, C. Education differences in life expectancy with cognitive impairment. *J. Gerontol. Ser. A: Biol. Sci. Med. Sci.* **2009**, *64*, 125–131.

7. Andrade, C.; Radhakrishnan, R. The prevention and treatment of cognitive decline and dementia: An overview of recent research on experimental treatments. *Indian J. Psychiatry* **2009**, *51*, 12.

8. Jacobs, D.R.; Steffen, L.M. Nutrients, foods, and dietary patterns as exposures in research: A framework for food synergy. *Am. J. Clin. Nutr.* **2003**, *78*, 508–513.

9. Waijers, P.M.; Feskens, E.J.; Ocké, M.C. A critical review of predefined diet quality scores. *Br. J. Nutr.* **2007**, *97*, 219–231.

10. Jacobs, D.R.; Tapsell, L.C. Food, not nutrients, is the fundamental unit in nutrition. *Nutr. Rev.* **2007**, *65*, 439–450.

11. Scarmeas, N.; Stern, Y.; Mayeux, R.; Manly, J.J.; Schupf, N.; Luchsinger, J.A. Mediterranean diet and mild cognitive impairment. *Arch. Neurol.* **2009**, *66*, 216–225.

12. Morris, M.; Evans, D.A.; Bienias, J.L.; Tangney, C.C.; Bennett, D.A.; Wilson, R.S.; Aggarwal, N.; Schneider, J. Consumption of fish and *n*-3 fatty acids and risk of incident Alzheimer disease. *Arch. Neurol.* **2003**, *60*, 940–946.

13. Nelson, C.; Wengreen, H.J.; Munger, R.G.; Corcoran, C.D. Dietary folate, vitamin B-12, vitamin B-6 and incident Alzheimer's disease: The Cache County memory, health, and aging study. *J. Nutr. Health Aging* **2009**, *13*, 899–905.

14. Wärnberg, J.; Gomez-Martinez, S.; Romeo, J.; Díaz, L.-E.; Marcos, A. Nutrition, inflammation, and cognitive function. *Ann. N. Y. Acad. Sci.* **2009**, *1153*, 164–175.

15. Cherbuin, N.; Anstey, K.J. The Mediterranean diet is not related to cognitive change in a large prospective investigation: The PATH through life study. *Am. J. Geriatr. Psychiatry* **2012**, *20*, 635–639.

16. Scarmeas, N.; Stern, Y.; Tang, M.-X.; Mayeux, R.; Luchsinger, J.A. Mediterranean diet and risk for Alzheimer's disease. *Ann. Neurol.* **2006**, *59*, 912–921.

17. Hodge, A.; Almeida, O.P.; English, D.R.; Giles, G.G.; Flicker, L. Patterns of dietary intake and psychological distress in older Australians: Benefits not just from a Mediterranean diet. *Int. Psychogeriatr.* **2013**, *25*, 456–466.

18. Jacka, F.N.; Cherbuin, N.; Anstey, K.J.; Butterworth, P. Dietary patterns and depressive symptoms over time: Examining the relationships with socioeconomic position, health behaviours and cardiovascular risk. *PLoS One* **2014**, *9*, e87657.

19. Reedy, J.; Wirfält, E.; Flood, A.; Mitrou, P.N.; Krebs-Smith, S.M.; Kipnis, V.; Midthune, D.; Leitzmann, M.; Hollenbeck, A.; Schatzkin, A. Comparing 3 dietary pattern methods—Cluster analysis, factor analysis, and index analysis—With colorectal cancer risk the NIH–AARP diet and health study. *Am. J. Epidemiol.* **2010**, *171*, 479–487.

20. Fabrigar, L.R.; Wegener, D.T.; MacCallum, R.C.; Strahan, E.J. Evaluating the use of exploratory factor analysis in psychological research. *Psychol. Methods* **1999**, *4*, 272.

21. McCann, S.E.; Marshall, J.R.; Brasure, J.R.; Graham, S.; Freudenheim, J.L. Analysis of patterns of food intake in nutritional epidemiology: Food classification in principal components analysis and the subsequent impact on estimates for endometrial cancer. *Public Health Nutr.* **2001**, *4*, 989–997.

22. Dunstan, D. *Diabesity and Associated Disorders in Australia,2000: The Accelerating Epidemic: The Australian Diabetes, Obesity and Lifestyle Study (AusDiab)*; International Diabetes Institute: Melbourne, Australia, 2001.

23. Tanamas, S.K. *The Australian Diabetes, Obesity and Lifestyle Study*; Baker IDI Heart and Diabetes Institute: Melbourne, Australia, 2013.

24. Anstey, K.J.; von Sanden, C.; Luszcz, M.A. An 8-year prospective study of the relationship between cognitive performance and falling in very old adults. *J. Am. Geriatr. Soc.* **2006**, *54*, 1169–1176.

25. Baddeley, A.; Emslie, H.; Nimmo-Smith, I. The Spot-the-Word test: A robust estimate of verbal intelligence based on lexical decision. *Br. J. Clin. Psychol./Br. Psychol. Soc.* **1993**, *32*, 55–65.

26. Grantham, N.M.; Magliano, D.J.; Hodge, A.; Jowett, J.; Meikle, P.; Shaw, J.E. The association between dairy food intake and the incidence of diabetes in Australia: The Australian diabetes obesity and lifestyle study (AusDiab). *Public Health Nutr.* **2013**, *16*, 339–345.

27. Van Dam, R.M.; Rimm, E.B.; Willett, W.C.; Stampfer, M.J.; Hu, F.B. Dietary patterns and risk for type 2 diabetes Mellitus in U.S. men. *Ann. Intern. Med.* **2002**, *136*, 201–209.

28. Khani, B.R.; Ye, W.; Terry, P.; Wolk, A. Reproducibility and validity of major dietary patterns among Swedish women assessed with a food-frequency questionnaire. *J. Nutr.* **2004**, *134*, 1541–1545.

29. Hu, F.B.; Rimm, E.; Smith-Warner, S.A.; Feskanich, D.; Stampfer, M.J.; Ascherio, A.; Sampson, L.; Willett, W.C. Reproducibility and validity of dietary patterns assessed with a food-frequency questionnaire. *Am. J. Clin. Nutr.* **1999**, *69*, 243–249.

30. Hosking, D.; Danthiir, V. Retrospective lifetime dietary patterns are associated with demographic and cardiovascular health variables in an older community-dwelling Australian population. *Br. J. Nutr.* **2013**, *110*, 2069–2083.

31. Northstone, K.; Ness, A.; Emmett, P.; Rogers, I. Adjusting for energy intake in dietary pattern investigations using principal components analysis. *Eur. J. Clin. Nutr.* **2007**, *62*, 931–938.

32. Crowell, T.A.; Vanderploeg, R.D.; Small, B.J.; Graves, A.B.; Mortimer, J.A. Elderly norms for the Spot-the-Word test. *Arch. Clin. Neuropsychol.* **2002**, *17*, 123–130.

33. Chen, X.; Huang, Y.; Cheng, H.G. Lower intake of vegetables and legumes associated with cognitive decline among illiterate elderly Chinese: A 3-year cohort study. *J. Nutr. Health Aging* **2012**, *16*, 549–552.

34. Gu, Y.; Nieves, J.W.; Stern, Y.; Luchsinger, J.A.; Scarmeas, N. Food combination and Alzheimer disease risk: A protective diet. *Arch. Neurol.* **2010**, *67*.

35. Knoops, K.B.; de Groot, L.M.; Kromhout, D.; Perrin, A.E.; Moreiras-Varela, O.; Menotti, A.; van Staveren, W.A. Mediterranean diet, lifestyle factors, and 10-year mortality in elderly european men and women: The hale project. *JAMA* **2004**, *292*, 1433–1439.

36. Sofi, F.; Abbate, R.; Gensini, G.F.; Casini, A. Accruing evidence on benefits of adherence to the Mediterranean diet on health: An updated systematic review and meta-analysis. *Am. J. Clin. Nutr.* **2010**, *92*, 1189–1196.

37. Solfrizzi, V.; Panza, F.; Frisardi, V.; Seripa, D.; Logroscino, G.; Imbimbo, B.P.; Pilotto, A. Diet and Alzheimer's disease risk factors or prevention: The current evidence. *Expert Rev. Neurother.* **2011**, *11*, 677–708.

38. Trichopoulou, A.; Costacou, T.; Bamia, C.; Trichopoulos, D. Adherence to a Mediterranean diet and survival in a Greek population. *N. Engl. J. Med.* **2003**, *348*, 2599–2608.

39. Morris, M.C. The role of nutrition in Alzheimer's disease: Epidemiological evidence. *Eur. J. Neurol.: Off. J. Eur. Fed. Neurol. Soc.* **2009**, *16* (Suppl. 1), 1–7.

40. Kalmijn, S.; Launer, L.J.; Ott, A.; Witteman, J.C.; Hofman, A.; Breteler, M.M. Dietary fat intake and the risk of incident dementia in the Rotterdam Study. *Ann. Neurol.* **1997**, *42*, 776–782.

41. Danthiir, V.; Hosking, D.; Burns, N.R.; Wilson, C.; Nettelbeck, T.; Calvaresi, E.; Clifton, P.; Wittert, G.A. Cognitive performance in older adults is inversely associated with fish consumption but not erythrocyte membrane *n*-3 fatty acids. *J. Nutr.* **2014**, *144*, 311–320.

42. Gardener, S.L.; Rainey-Smith, S.R.; Barnes, M.B.; Sohrabi, H.R.; Weinborn, M.; Lim, Y.Y.; Harrington, K.; Taddei, K.; Gu, Y.; Rembach, A. Dietary patterns and cognitive decline in an Australian study of ageing. *Mol. Psychiatry* **2014**, *29*.

43. Chan, R.; Chan, D.; Woo, J. A cross sectional study to examine the association between dietary patterns and cognitive impairment in older Chinese people in Hong Kong. *J. Nutr. Health Aging* **2013**, *17*, 757–765.

# The Comparative Validity and Reproducibility of a Diet Quality Index for Adults: The Australian Recommended Food Score

Clare E. Collins, Tracy L. Burrows, Megan E. Rollo, May M. Boggess, Jane F. Watson, Maya Guest, Kerith Duncanson, Kristine Pezdirc and Melinda J. Hutchesson

**Abstract:** Adult diet quality indices are shown to predict nutritional adequacy of dietary intake as well as all-cause morbidity and mortality. This study describes the reproducibility and validity of a food-based diet quality index, the Australian Recommended Food Score (ARFS). ARFS was developed to reflect alignment with the Australian Dietary Guidelines and is modelled on the US Recommended Food Score. Dietary intakes of 96 adult participants (31 male, 65 female) age 30 to 75 years were assessed in two rounds, five months apart. Diet was assessed using a 120-question semi-quantitative food frequency questionnaire (FFQ). The ARFS diet quality index was derived using a subset of 70 items from the full FFQ. Reproducibility of the ARFS between round one and round two was confirmed by the overall intraclass correlation coefficient of 0.87 (95% CI 0.83, 0.90), which compared favourably to that for the FFQ at 0.85 (95% CI 0.80, 0.89). ARFS was correlated with FFQ nutrient intakes, particularly fiber, vitamin A, beta-carotene and vitamin C (0.53, 95% CI 0.37–0.67), and with mineral intakes, particularly calcium, magnesium and potassium (0.32, 95% CI 0.23–0.40). ARFS is a suitable brief tool to evaluate diet quality in adults and reliably estimates a range of nutrient intakes.

Reprinted from *Nutrients*. Cite as: Collins, C.E.; Burrows, T.L.; Rollo, M.E.; Boggess, M.M.; Watson, J.F.; Guest, M.; Duncanson, K.; Pezdirc, K.; Hutchesson, M.J. The Comparative Validity and Reproducibility of a Diet Quality Index for Adults: The Australian Recommended Food Score. *Nutrients* **2015**, *7*, 785–798.

## 1. Introduction

The evaluation of relationships between health and intakes of single nutrients does not address the complexities of food and nutrient interactions in the human diet [1]. A focus solely on nutrients does not allow for assessment of the cumulative impact of nutrient interactions from a range of foods on health outcomes over time. Individuals do not usually consume single foods, but combinations of several foods and beverages that contain both nutritive and non-nutritive substances [2]. Given the complexity of assessing individual intakes, measurement of overall diet quality and variety by brief indices allows evaluation of several related aspects of dietary intake concurrently [3], and may provide a better measure of usual dietary intake patterns [4]. Diet quality refers to the nutritional adequacy of an individual's dietary pattern and how closely this aligns with national dietary guidelines [3,5]. Scores or indexes of diet quality are being increasingly used in research as proxies for nutrient intakes, due to their lower researcher and respondent burden. The relationship between diet quality indices and nutritional adequacy, morbidity and mortality in adults has been reviewed [3,6]. This highlights that across these indices the risk for some health outcomes, including biomarkers of disease, incidence and risk of cardiovascular disease, some cancers and both cancer mortality and all-cause mortality can be quantified.

Diet quality indices have been derived by applying a scoring system to dietary intakes assessed by a variety of measures, including food frequency questionnaires (FFQ) and 24 h recalls. Indices are constructed by assigning higher scores within sub-scales based on more frequent or higher intakes of foods, nutrients, or both [3]. Generally there are two types of diet quality scores. These are either food-based or nutrient-based. A food-based diet quality index considers the number of foods or food groups consumed in a given period and assigns points based on diversity and/or frequency of intake [3,5], however no consideration is usually given to the sources or intakes of nutrients. Food-based scores rely on food consumption data only, meaning they can be scored quickly, but they typically have a limited food list and so may not fully reflect overall variety of foods consumed. This may be particularly for some population sub-groups, such as specific ethnic groups where food items may not have been included in the original FFQ food list. In comparison, nutrient-based scores require the dietary intake record to be analysed first in order to derive nutrient intakes, form which the diet quality scores can be calculated. For this reason food-based scores may be preferable for clinical settings and education purposes as they are more easily adapted to this purpose [3,6]. Given differences in food supply, consumption patterns and nutrition recommendations, diet quality indices should be country-specific.

The aim of this study was to evaluate the reproducibility of the Australian Recommended Food Score (ARFS) and its validity against a food frequency questionnaire from which it is derived.

## 2. Experimental Section

### 2.1. Subjects

Data from the Family Diet Quality Study was used in the current analysis. The methods have been published previously elsewhere [7]. Briefly, the population was healthy adults living full-time with at least one child aged 8 to 10 years, in New South

Wales, Australia. Participants were recruited through a range of avenues, such as newspapers and school newsletters. Demographic and anthropometric data, together with the AES FFQ data scanned by an optical reader, were collected at baseline (September 2010–July 2011) and repeated at follow-up (January 2011–February 2012) 5 months later.

*2.2. Australian Eating Survey Food Frequency Questionnaire (AES FFQ)*

The AES FFQ was previously validated in adults [7] using standard adult portion sizes derived from unpublished data, purchased from the Australian Bureau of Statistics, from the National Nutrition Survey [8] and the "natural" serving size from standard items such as a slice of bread. The FFQ is a self-administered 120 item semi-quantitative FFQ that asks respondents to report usual dietary intake over the previous 6 months and takes approximately 30 min to complete [9–16]. It contains 15 supplementary questions (vitamin supplements, food behaviour, and sedentary behaviours). The FFQ has 24 questions on vegetables, 11 on fruit, nine on breads/cereals, nine on dairy foods, 32 on lunch/main meal food items, nine on beverages, 20 on snack foods/dessert and six on sandwich spreads/dressings and sauces. The response for each question is a frequency with options ranging from "never" to "≥7 times per day". Nutrient intakes from the FFQ were computed from the AusNut 1999 database (All Foods) Revision 17 and AusFoods (Brands) Revision 5 [17] by summing over all food items, the product of the number of serves, the portion size in grams and the amount of the nutrient in a gram of that food.

*2.3. Australian Recommended Food Score (ARFS)*

The ARFS was modelled on the Recommended Food Score by Kant and Thompson [18] and the Australian Child and Adolescent Recommended Food Score (ACARFS) [19] as a brief food based diet quality index. The ARFS focuses on dietary variety within food groups recommended in the Australian Dietary Guidelines [20] for example the meat and alternatives food group encapsulates a range of differing foods each with unique nutrient profiles *i.e.*, red meat, fish, eggs, nuts and legumes. It takes approximately 10 min to complete and uses a sub-set of 70 AES FFQ questions. The ARFS has eight sub-scales with 20 questions related to vegetables, 12 to fruit, 7 to meat/flesh foods, six to non-meat/flesh protein foods, 12 to breads and cereals, 10 to dairy foods, one to water and two to spreads/sauces. Most foods are awarded one point for a consumption frequency of ≥once per week, which varies based on national dietary guidelines [20,21]. The ARFS score was calculated by summing the points for each item. The total score ranges from zero to 73 (Supplementary Table 1).

## 2.4. Statistical Methods

Food data were initially screened for implausible energy intakes however none were removed for this reason. Medians and interquartile ranges (IQR) were calculated for all nutrients. Univariate relationships were assessed using Fisher Exact tests to compare categorical variables by gender within data collection round, and exact symmetry tests [22] to compare categorical variables by gender on paired data. Continuous variables were similarly assessed using Wilcoxon rank-sum tests and Wilcoxon signed-rank tests for paired data.

*Reproducibility*: This was conducted separately for both the ARFS and the FFQ and evaluated by comparing the administration of the FFQ twice, five months apart using correlations and intra-class correlation coefficients (ICC) [23]. The ICC, the total variance, and its component parts, the within and the between person variance, are estimated using a linear regression model with a person-level random effect [24]. This model was bootstrapped [25] to obtain standard errors that accounted for the probable correlation between members of the same family.

*Validation:* The relationships between ARFS and FFQ nutrients and the percent energy (% E) from food groups were assessed using correlations, which were estimated by fitting a linear regression models to standardized variables, with standard errors clustered on family [26]. For the validation both rounds of measures were included which was possible due to aa random effects model being used. Total FFQ energy was included as an explanatory variable since both scores increase as the amount of foods increases.

Statistical significance is determined at the 5% level. Normality was visually checked where necessary using probability plots and box plots. Square root transforms were applied as necessary to improve the normality of the residuals of linear regression models. All nutrient calculations, data manipulation and statistical analysis was performed using Stata MP version 12.1 [27].

## 2.5. Ethics

This study was conducted according to the guidelines laid down in the Declaration of Helsinki and all procedures involving human subjects/patients were approved by the University of Newcastle Human Research Ethics Committee (Approval No. H-2010-1170). Written informed consent was obtained from all study participants.

## 3. Results

A total of 96 participants, from 68 separate families, completed FFQs at baseline and 68 at follow-up. Of these 67 completed the survey in both administration rounds. Thirty one participants were male and 65 were female in the initial administration round and of these 20 males and 48 females remained for round 2. Table 1 reports demographic and anthropometric variables for the two FFQ administration rounds and, by sex for $n = 67$ participants, Supplementary Table 2 provides details of all observations $n = 151$. There were no significant differences by sex or by administration round in education, smoking habits and general health. While there were some significant differences in weight, height, BMI and waist by sex, there were no significant differences in these variables between the two administrations rounds.

**Table 1.** Demographic and anthropometric data (151 observations on $N = 67$ participants (31 male) in 64 families). * Fisher's exact test of homogeneity; † Wilcoxon rank-sum test for equality of populations; § No significant difference by gender in Round 1, Round 2 or in total according to the exact symmetry test of homogeneity for paired data; ** No significant difference by gender in Round 1, Round 2 or in total according to the Wilcoxon signed-rank test for equality of distributions on paired data.

| | Round 1 | | | Round 2 | | |
|---|---|---|---|---|---|---|
| | Male $N = 20$ | Female $N = 47$ | $p$ * | Male $N = 20$ | Female $N = 47$ | $p$ * |
| | N (%) | N (%) | | N (%) | N (%) | |
| Education § | | | | | | |
| Year 10 | 1 (5%) | 3 (6%) | | 1 (5%) | 3 (6%) | |
| Year 12 | 1 (5%) | 7 (15%) | | 1 (5%) | 7 (15%) | |
| Trade | 3 (15%) | 1 (2%) | | 5 (25%) | 1 (2%) | |
| Certificate | 4 (20%) | 11 (23%) | | 2 (10%) | 11 (23%) | |
| Degree | 5 (25%) | 13 (28%) | | 3 (15%) | 14 (30%) | |
| Postgrad | 6 (30%) | 12 (26%) | | 8 (40%) | 11 (23%) | |
| Total | 20 | 47 | 0.44 | 20 | 47 | 0.03 |
| Smoked within 10yrs § | | | | | | |
| Yes | 2 (10%) | 2 (4%) | | 3 (15%) | 3 (6%) | |
| No | 18 (90%) | 45 (96%) | | 17 (85%) | 44 (94%) | |
| Total | 20 | 47 | 0.58 | 20 | 47 | 0.35 |
| Current Smoker § | | | | | | |
| Yes | 1 (5%) | 0 (0%) | | 1 (5%) | 0 (0%) | |
| No | 19 (95%) | 47 (100%) | | 19 (95%) | 47 (100%) | |
| Total | 20 | 47 | 0.30 | 20 | 47 | 0.30 |
| General Health § | | | | | | |
| Excellent | 3 (33%) | 6 (29%) | | 1 (14%) | 8 (35%) | |
| Very Good | 2 (22%) | 11 (52%) | | 5 (71%) | 11 (48%) | |
| Good | 4 (44%) | 4 (19%) | | 1 (14%) | 4 (17%) | |
| Fair/Poor | 0 (0%) | 0 (0%) | | 0 (0%) | 0 (0%) | |
| Total | 9 | 21 | 0.25 | 7 | 23 | 0.62 |
| | Median (IQR) | Median (IQR) | $p$ † | Median (IQR) | Median (IQR) | $p$ † |
| Age (years) | 43.6 (41–47) | 41.3 (38–45) | 0.03 | 44.2 (41–47) | 41.9 (39–46) | 0.07 |
| Height (cm) ** | 179 (174–182) | 165 (162–170) | <0.01 | 179 (172–183) | 164 (162–169) | <0.01 |
| Weight (kg) ** | 81.7 (74–89) | 64.9 (60–72) | <0.01 | 81.6 (74–91) | 65.0 (60–73) | <0.01 |
| BMI (kg/m²) ** | 25.7 (24–28) | 23.5 (22–26) | 0.06 | 26.8 (23–28) | 23.5 (22–26) | 0.12 |
| Waist (cm) ** | 90.3 (84–98) | 80.8 (74–86) | <0.01 | 91.4 (85–99) | 80.4 (75–87) | <0.01 |

Table 2 reports the median FFQ nutrient intakes and the proportion of the sample by sex who met the Recommended Dietary Intake (RDI) targets. These results confirm that the sample is representative of the Australian adult population, having similar nutrient profiles as the last Australian National Nutrition Survey [28].

**Table 2.** Comparison of adult nutrient intakes, as assessed by the Australian Eating Survey (AES) food frequency questionnaire (FFQ), to Australian Recommended Dietary Intakes (RDI), Adequate Intake (AI) and upper limit, by gender.

| Intake per day | Male (N = 31) | | | Female (N = 65) | | |
|---|---|---|---|---|---|---|
| Meeting | RDI/AI | Median | Meeting RDI | RDI/AI | Median | Meeting RDI |
| Protein (g) | 64 | 124.54 | 96% | 46 | 92.25 | 95% |
| Fiber (g) AI | 30 | 37.95 | 73% | 25 | 28.41 | 70% |
| Vitamin A (µg) | 900 | 1323.77 | 88% | 700 | 1198.36 | 87% |
| Thiamine (mg) | 1.2 | 2.27 | 90% | 1.1 | 1.6 | 84% |
| Riboflavin (mg) | 1.3 | 3.24 | 100% | 1.1 | 2.42 | 97% |
| Niacin equiv. (mg) | 16 | 56.95 | 100% | 14 | 43.28 | 100% |
| Folate (µg) | 420 | 468.17 | 65% | 420 | 341.22 | 31% |
| Vitamin C (mg) | 45 | 198.1 | 100% | 45 | 174.38 | 98% |
| Calcium (mg) | 1000 | 1375.59 | 71% | 1000 | 1172.81 | 70% |
| Iron (mg) | 8 | 19.09 | 100% | 18 | 13.95 | 37% |
| Magnesium (mg) | 420 | 540.95 | 75% | 320 | 411.14 | 80% |
| Phosphorus(mg) | 1000 | 2132.67 | 100% | 1000 | 1642.88 | 95% |
| Potassium(mg) AI | 3800 | 4447.83 | 73% | 2800 | 3681.6 | 79% |
| Zinc (mg) | 14 | 16.44 | 67% | 8 | 13.14 | 82% |
| Exceeding | Upper Limit | Median | Exceeding Upper limit | Upper Limit | Median | Exceeding Upper limit |
| Sodium(mg) | 920 | 2768.22 | 100% | 920 | 2161.33 | 97% |
| % E Saturated fat | 10 | 11 | 71% | 10 | 13 | 79% |

## 3.1. FFQ Reproducibility

Table 3 lists medians, correlations and intraclass correlation coefficients (ICC) for FFQ food group and nutrient intakes. Since observations for both administration rounds need to be present to estimate correlation between then, the number of observations available for use was only 67. When calculating the ICC however, all observations from both rounds can be utilized, thus the sample size was 163. The median correlation for nutrients was 0.72 (95% CI 0.51–0.92), which was attained by both thiamin and riboflavin. The least correlated was the percent energy (%E) from protein 0.49 (95% CI 0.19–0.78), and the most highly correlated was carbohydrate 0.83, (95% CI 0.68–0.98). We can expect tighter confidence intervals when using this approach. The median ICC was thiamin 0.73 (95% CI 0.55–0.80). The lowest ICC was the percent energy (% E) from protein 0.50 (95% CI 0.33–0.58), and the highest ICC was vitamin C, 0.88 (95% CI 0.92–0.93).

Data summarising the ARFS component subscales, the medians percentage energy from FFQ food groups are presented in Table 4. The median correlation was

0.66 (95% CI 0.48–0.84), which was attained by meat. The lowest correlation was for packaged snacks 0.52 (95% CI 0.32–0.72), and the most strongly correlated was for breakfast cereal 0.83, (95% CI 0.57–1.0). The median ICC was grains 0.62 (95% CI 0.53–0.70), with the lowest for condiments 0.44 (95% CI 0.28–0.61), and the highest for vegetables, 0.84% (95% CI 0.79–0.89).

**Table 3.** Reproducibility of Food Frequency Questionnaire (FFQ) nutrients: Median, interquartile range (IQR) and correlation, with 95% confidence interval, between round 1 and round 2.

| | Round 1 N = 96 | | Round 2 N = 67 | | Correlation N = 67 | | ICC N = 163 | |
|---|---|---|---|---|---|---|---|---|
| Nutrients/day Energy | Median | IQR | Median | IQR | ρ | 95% CI | ICC | 95% CI |
| Energy (kJ) | 9601 | (8024–11501) | 8938 | (7298–11085) | 0.81 | (0.67, 0.96) | 0.85 | (0.80, 0.89) |
| Protein (g) | 101 | (82–125) | 96.5 | (77.3–124.8) | 0.65 | (0.46, 0.84) | 0.70 | (0.62, 0.77) |
| Total fat (g) | 75.5 | (62.6–85.2) | 73.6 | (53.5–89.8) | 0.71 | (0.49, 0.93) | 0.69 | (0.61, 0.78) |
| Saturated fat (g) | 30.1 | (25.0–35.9) | 30.6 | (20.7–34.8) | 0.67 | (0.43, 0.90) | 0.65 | (0.55, 0.76) |
| Polyunsat. Fat (g) | 9.7 | (7.52–10.98) | 9.15 | (7.26–11.91) | 0.76 | (0.58, 0.94) | 0.69 | (0.63, 0.76) |
| Monounsat. Fat (g) | 27.8 | (22.9–31.7) | 27.3 | (19.6–35.5) | 0.73 | (0.52, 0.93) | 0.72 | (0.65, 0.79) |
| Cholesterol (mg) | 283 | (224–360) | 252 | (211–329) | 0.66 | (0.45, 0.87) | 0.70 | (0.60, 0.80) |
| Carbohydrate (g) | 262 | (217–341) | 243 | (192–337) | 0.83 | (0.68, 0.98) | 0.85 | (0.81, 0.89) |
| Sugars (g) | 141 | (100–182) | 119 | (97–168) | 0.82 | (0.68, 0.95) | 0.83 | (0.77, 0.90) |
| Alcohol (g) | 12 | (1.6–20.3) | 8.14 | (1.58–14.29) | 0.79 | (0.64, 0.95) | 0.82 | (0.75, 0.90) |
| Nutrients | | | | | | | | |
| Fiber (g) | 30.5 | (23.8–37.4) | 29.7 | (23.9–35.6) | 0.76 | (0.65, 0.87) | 0.79 | (0.70, 0.87) |
| Vitamin A (µg) | 1228 | (1004–1511) | 1225 | (970–1667) | 0.62 | (0.36, 0.87) | 0.69 | (0.55, 0.83) |
| Retinol (µg) | 297 | (227–410) | 317 | (214–480) | 0.69 | (0.42, 0.97) | 0.67 | (0.57, 0.76) |
| Beta-carotene(µg) | 5316 | (3997–6581) | 5122 | (3824–6959) | 0.61 | (0.35, 0.88) | 0.72 | (0.54, 0.89) |
| Thiamin (mg) | 1.77 | (1.41–2.21) | 1.74 | (1.38–2.16) | 0.72 | (0.52, 0.92) | 0.73 | (0.66, 0.80) |
| Riboflavin (mg) | 2.59 | (2.10–3.19) | 2.54 | (2.06–3.34) | 0.72 | (0.51, 0.92) | 0.72 | (0.66, 0.78) |
| Niacin (mg) | 45.3 | (38.8–55.7) | 43.8 | (36.4–54.7) | 0.70 | (0.51, 0.88) | 0.74 | (0.67, 0.81) |
| Vitamin C (mg) | 184 | (140–235) | 167 | (133–213) | 0.81 | (0.61, 0.101) | 0.88 | (0.82, 0.93) |
| Folate (µg) | 372 | (288–455) | 357 | (279–459) | 0.78 | (0.62, 0.93) | 0.80 | (0.74, 0.85) |
| Calcium (mg) | 1200 | (949–1413) | 1205 | (903–1603) | 0.72 | (0.55, 0.89) | 0.71 | (0.63, 0.79) |
| Iron (mg) | 15.1 | (11.5–18.1) | 14.3 | (11.2–17.7) | 0.75 | (0.60, 0.91) | 0.76 | (0.70, 0.83) |

Table 3. *Cont.*

| | Round 1 N = 96 | | Round 2 N = 67 | | Correlation N = 67 | | ICC N = 163 | |
|---|---|---|---|---|---|---|---|---|
| Magnesium (mg) | 450 | (371–531) | 430 | (344–541) | 0.83 | (0.70, 0.95) | 0.85 | (0.80, 0.90) |
| Phosphorus(mg) | 1743 | (1421–2148) | 1704 | (1273–2256) | 0.73 | (0.57, 0.89) | 0.75 | (0.68, 0.82) |
| Potassium(mg) | 3881 | (3247–4610) | 3730 | (3093–4580) | 0.73 | (0.58, 0.88) | 0.78 | (0.72, 0.83) |
| Sodium(mg) | 2272 | (1783–2846) | 2313 | (1765–2865) | 0.76 | (0.58, 0.93) | 0.80 | (0.75, 0.85) |
| Zinc (mg) | 13.9 | (11.3–17.2) | 13.5 | (11.1–16.4) | 0.71 | (0.54, 0.87) | 0.75 | (0.68, 0.81) |
| Water (mL) | 3469 | (2977–4024) | 3388 | (2987–3837) | 0.80 | (0.64, 0.96) | 0.87 | (0.83, 0.91) |
| Percent Energy | | | | | | | | |
| Protein | 18 | (16.0–20.0) | 18 | (16.0–20.0) | 0.49 | (0.19, 0.78) | 0.50 | (0.33, 0.68) |
| Carbohydrate | 47.5 | (44.0–52.5) | 48 | (43.0–52.0) | 0.68 | (0.50, 0.87) | 0.66 | (0.58, 0.74) |
| Total Fats | 30 | (27.0–33.0) | 30 | (28.0–34.0) | 0.64 | (0.47, 0.81) | 0.60 | (0.50, 0.69) |
| Saturated Fat | 12 | (11.0–14.0) | 12 | (11.0–14.0) | 0.64 | (0.42, 0.85) | 0.63 | (0.55, 0.72) |
| Alcohol | 4 | (0.50–6.00) | 2 | (1.00–5.00) | 0.77 | (0.63, 0.91) | 0.78 | (0.71, 0.85) |
| Percent Fat | | | | | | | | |
| Saturated | 45 | (42.0–49.0) | 45 | (42.0–48.0) | 0.72 | (0.56, 0.89) | 0.73 | (0.64, 0.81) |
| Polyunsaturated | 14 | (12.0–15.5) | 15 | (13.0–16.0) | 0.80 | (0.59, 0.102) | 0.76 | (0.68, 0.84) |
| Monounsaturated | 41 | (39.0–43.0) | 41 | (39.0–42.0) | 0.57 | (0.36, 0.79) | 0.64 | (0.51, 0.76) |

## 3.2. ARFS Reproducibility

The median correlation between the two rounds for ARFS food groups was 0.66 (95% CI 0.48–0. 84), which was attained by meat (Table 4). The lowest correlation was for was vegetables, 0.59 (95% CI 0.34–0.83), and the strongest for ARFS total score, 0.83 (95% CI 0.68–0.98). Similarly, the median ICC was thiamin 0.69 (95% CI 0.55–0.80). The lowest ICC was for meat, 0.62 (95% CI 0.51–0.73), and the highest ICC was for ARFS total score, 0.87 (95% CI 0.83–0.90).

## 3.3. Validity between ARFS and FFQ

Table 5 summarises the correlations between the ARFS sub-scale components and FFQ nutrients adjusted for total FFQ energy, significant at the 5% level. Negative correlations were found for % energy from saturated fat and ARFS total score and ARFS components of fruit, vegetables and grains, this is likely as foods high in SFA are not accounted for in ARFS so as the total ARFS increases intake of SFA decreases. ARFS was highly correlated with FFQ nutrient intakes, particularly for fiber, 0.38 (95% CI 0.27–0.49); vitamin A, 0.45 (95% CI 0.23–0.61); beta-carotene, 0.51 (95% CI

0.34–0.69); and vitamin C, 0.53 (95% CI 0.37–0.67). There were also strong correlations with mineral intakes, particularly calcium, 0.23 (95% CI 0.10–0.46); magnesium, 0.30 (95% CI 0.21–0.40); and potassium, 0.32 (95% CI 0.23–0.40) (See Supplementary Figure 1).

**Table 4.** Reproducibility of The Australian Recommended Food Score (ARFS) components and the AES FFQ percentage of energy (%E) from core and non-core food groups: Median, interquartile range (IQR) and correlation between rounds.

| Scores | Round 1 N = 96 | | Round 2 N = 67 | | Correlation N = 67 | | ICC N = 163 | |
|---|---|---|---|---|---|---|---|---|
| ARFS (max avail. score) | Median | IQR | Median | IQR | ρ | 95% CI | ICC | 95% CI |
| ARFS total(73) | 36 | (32.0–42.5) | 35 | (31.0–41.0) | 0.83 | (0.68, 0.98) | 0.87 | (0.83, 0.90) |
| Vegetables(21) | 14 | (12.0–16.0) | 13 | (11.0–15.0) | 0.59 | (0.34, 0.83) | 0.69 | (0.58, 0.80) |
| Fruit(12) | 7 | (4.0–8.0) | 6 | (4.0–8.0) | 0.64 | (0.47, 0.81) | 0.68 | (0.61, 0.75) |
| Meat(7) | 2 | (2.0–3.0) | 2 | (1.0–3.0) | 0.66 | (0.48, 0.84) | 0.62 | (0.51, 0.73) |
| Meat alternatives(6) | 2 | (1.0–3.0) | 2 | (1.0–3.0) | 0.78 | (0.62,0. 93) | 0.79 | (0.72, 0.86) |
| Grains(13) | 6 | (4.0–7.0) | 6 | (5.0–7.0) | 0.64 | (0.48, 0.80) | 0.68 | (0.59, 0.77) |
| Dairy(11) | 5 | (3.0–6.0) | 5 | (4.0–6.0) | 0.77 | (0.63, 0.91) | 0.79 | (0.73, 0.84) |
| Extras(2) | 1 | (0.0–1.0) | 1 | (0.0–1.0) | 0.65 | (0.44, 0.85) | 0.66 | (0.56, 0.76) |
| %E from food groups | | | | | | | | |
| FFQ CORE | 67.5 | (58.0–76.0) | 69 | (60.0–75.0) | 0.71 | (0.51, 0.91) | 0.76 | (0.68, 0.85) |
| Vegetables | 8 | (6.0–11.0) | 8 | (6.0–10.0) | 0.79 | (0.66, 0.93) | 0.84 | (0.79, 0.89) |
| Fruit | 8 | (5.0–11.5) | 8 | (5.0–11.0) | 0.60 | (0.46, 0.74) | 0.57 | (0.39, 0.74) |
| Meat | 11.5 | (8.0–15.0) | 11 | (7.0–14.0) | 0.53 | (0.15, 0.91) | 0.52 | (0.31, 0.74) |
| Meat alternatives | 4 | (2.0–7.0) | 5 | (2.0–7.0) | 0.53 | (0.26, 0.80) | 0.57 | (0.42, 0.71) |
| Grains | 22 | (15.0–27.0) | 22 | (18.0–25.0) | 0.60 | (0.45, 0.76) | 0.62 | (0.53, 0.70) |
| Dairy | 9 | (7.0–14.0) | 11 | (7.0–16.0) | 0.54 | (0.32, 0.76) | 0.52 | (0.39, 0.64) |
| FFQ NON-CORE | 32.5 | (24.0–42.0) | 31 | (25.0–40.0) | 0.71 | (0.51, 0.91) | 0.77 | (0.69, 0.84) |
| Sweet drinks, fruit juice | 1 | (0.0–4.0) | 1 | (0.0–4.0) | 0.78 | (0.59, 0.97) | 0.78 | (0.70, 0.87) |
| Packaged snacks | 1 | (0.5–3.5) | 1 | (0.0–3.0) | 0.52 | (0.32, 0.72) | 0.56 | (0.38, 0.74) |
| Confectionary | 4 | (2.0–7.0) | 3 | (1.0–6.0) | 0.63 | (0.47, 0.78) | 0.54 | (0.41, 0.67) |
| Baked sweet products | 4 | (2.0–7.0) | 3 | (2.0–7.0) | 0.76 | (0.62, 0.90) | 0.72 | (0.58, 0.85) |
| Take-away | 6 | (4.0–8.0) | 6 | (4.0–8.0) | 0.77 | (0.53, 0.100) | 0.76 | (0.69, 0.84) |
| Condiments | 2 | (1.0–3.5) | 2 | (1.0–5.0) | 0.60 | (0.38, 0.82) | 0.44 | (0.28, 0.61) |
| Processed fatty meats | 2 | (1.0–3.0) | 2 | (1.0–3.0) | 0.69 | (0.50, 0.88) | 0.57 | (0.39, 0.76) |
| Breakfast cereal | 7 | (4.0–10.0) | 8 | (5.0–11.0) | 0.83 | (0.57, 0.100) | 0.70 | (0.58, 0.82) |
| Meat meals with veg. | 7 | (4.5–10.0) | 6 | (4.0–9.0) | 0.52 | (0.19, 0.85) | 0.54 | (0.36, 0.71) |
| Meat meals no veg. | 1 | (0.0–2.0) | 1 | (0.0–1.0) | 0.53 | (0.26, 0.79) | 0.54 | (0.43, 0.65) |

Table 6 displays the correlations between the ARFS components and FFQ nutrients, adjusted for total FFQ energy, significant at the 5% level. There were significant, strong correlations between the corresponding ARFS and FFQ food groups vegetables, fruit, meat, meat alternatives, grains and dairy (0.50, 0.68, 0.42, 0.56, 0.28, 0.46, respectively) (See Supplementary Figure 2).

ARFS was strongly positively correlated with FFQ %E food group intakes, particularly for fruit, 0.38 (95% CI 0.27–0.49); vegetable, 0.45 (95% CI 0.23–0.61), meat alternatives, 0.51 (95% CI 0.34–0.69); and dairy, 0.53 (95% CI 0.37–0.67). There were also strong correlations with mineral intakes, particularly calcium, 0.23 (95% CI 0.10–0.46); magnesium, 0.30 (95% CI 0.21–0.40); and potassium, 0.32 (95% CI 0.23–0.40).

Table 5. Correlations between the Australian Recommended Food Score (ARFS) and the Australian Eating Survey (AES) FFQ components, adjusted for total FFQ energy, significant at the 5% level. Shaded cells are negative correlations.

| | ARFS Total | ARFS Veg | ARFS Fruit | ARFS Meat | ARFS Meat Alt | ARFS Grains | ARFS Dairy | ARFS Extra |
|---|---|---|---|---|---|---|---|---|
| Protein (g) | | | | 0.19 | | 0.10 | 0.22 | |
| Saturated fat (g) | | −0.09 | −0.13 | | | | 0.14 | |
| Cholesterol (mg) | | | | 0.26 | | | 0.21 | |
| Carbohydrate (g) | | | | −0.09 | −0.09 | | −0.07 | |
| Sugars (g) | | | 0.15 | | −0.14 | | | |
| Fiber (g) | 0.38 | 0.31 | 0.37 | | 0.25 | 0.16 | | |
| Vitamin A (µg) | 0.45 | 0.38 | 0.37 | | 0.29 | | | |
| Retinol (µg) | | | | | | | | |
| Beta-carotene(µg) | 0.51 | 0.43 | 0.47 | | 0.30 | | | |
| Thiamine (mg) | | | | | | | | 0.17 |
| Riboflavin (mg) | 0.16 | | | | | 0.14 | 0.24 | |
| Niacin equiv. (mg) | 0.12 | | | 0.20 | | 0.09 | 0.12 | |
| Folate (µg) | 0.27 | 0.20 | 0.19 | | 0.15 | 0.17 | | |
| Vitamin C (mg) | 0.53 | 0.49 | 0.51 | 0.16 | 0.22 | | | |
| Calcium (mg) | 0.23 | | | | | 0.15 | 0.40 | |
| Iron (mg) | 0.12 | | | | | 0.13 | | |
| Magnesium (mg) | 0.30 | 0.20 | 0.22 | | 0.19 | 0.18 | 0.15 | −0.10 |
| Phosphorus (mg) | 0.32 | 0.24 | 0.28 | 0.15 | 0.13 | 0.12 | 0.20 | −0.13 |
| Potassium(mg) | 0.32 | | | 0.09 | | 0.14 | 0.27 | −0.07 |
| Sodium(mg) | | | −0.12 | | | | | 0.13 |
| Zinc (mg) | | | | 0.13 | | | 0.17 | |
| % E Saturated Fat | −0.23 | −0.22 | −0.29 | | | −0.20 | | 0.18 |

Table 6. Correlations between the Australian Recommended Food Score (ARFS) and the Australian Eating Survey (AES) FFQ food groups, adjusted for total FFQ energy, significant at the 5% level. Light grey shaded cells are those with the same group in row and column where positive correlation would be anticipated. Dark grey shaded cells are negative correlations.

| Percentage of Energy From | ARFS Total | ARFS Veg | ARFS Fruit | ARFS Meat | ARFS Meat Alt | ARFS Grains | ARFS Dairy | ARFS Extra |
|---|---|---|---|---|---|---|---|---|
| CORE | 0.31 | 0.30 | 0.32 | | 0.25 | | | −0.26 |
| Vegetables | 0.22 | 0.50 | 0.20 | | | | | |
| Fruit | 0.37 | 0.33 | 0.68 | | | | | |
| Meat | | | | 0.42 | −0.30 | | | |
| Meat alternatives | 0.31 | 0.28 | 0.23 | | 0.56 | | | |
| Grains | | | | | | 0.28 | | |
| Dairy | 0.23 | | | | | 0.21 | 0.46 | |
| NON-CORE | −0.31 | | −0.32 | | −0.25 | | | 0.26 |
| Sweet drinks, fruit juice | −0.25 | −0.27 | −0.18 | | −0.19 | | | |
| Packaged snacks | | −0.20 | | | −0.17 | | | |
| Confectionary | | −0.25 | | | −0.23 | | | |
| Baked sweet products | | | −0.24 | −0.26 | | | | 0.19 |
| Take-away | −0.29 | −0.26 | −0.25 | | | −0.26 | | |
| Condiments | | | | | | 0.21 | | 0.40 |
| Processed fatty meats | | | −0.26 | | −0.27 | | | |
| Breakfast cereal | | | | | | 0.23 | | −0.21 |
| Meat meals with vegetables | | | | 0.32 | −0.26 | | | |
| Meat meals without vegetables | | | | | | | | 0.15 |

## 4. Discussion

The reproducibility and comparative validity of the ARFS in Australian adults was assessed in the current study by comparing food and nutrient intake data from the AES FFQ over two administration rounds five months apart, to estimate intra-class correlation coefficients (ICC). The reproducibility of the ARFS was confirmed as shown by ICCs for each nutrient assessed as being similar to those for the AES FFQ. The median ICC for ARFS nutrients was 0.66 (0.48–0.84) was similar when compared with the median ICC for FFQ nutrients 0.72 (0.51–0.92). These results confirm that the ARFS can be used when a brief evaluation of overall diet quality is required and with the advantages of considerably lower participant and researcher burden compared to other methods of dietary intake assessment.

ARFS was found to be highly correlated with FFQ nutrient intakes, particularly fiber, vitamin A, beta-carotene, and vitamin C. There were also strong positive correlations with mineral intakes for calcium, magnesium and potassium. These results indicate that the ARFS reflects the intake of a variety of nutrients which are known to be associated with health outcomes. These results are similar to a larger validation study in 6542 adults by Toft *et al.* [29], that used an FFQ to validate a food based diet quality score for fiber and vitamin C. However correlations in our study were higher for calcium (0.23), magnesium (0.30) and vitamin A (0.45) [29]. In the present study there were significant and positive correlations between the corresponding ARFS sub-scale score and the corresponding FFQ food groups of vegetables, fruit, meat and vegetarian alternatives, grains and dairy. This was not completely expected as although the ARFS score is based on sub-set of FFQ questions, only nutrient dense foods and drink are included. The approach to scoring is also different with the ARFS being a simple count based on foods usually consumed at least weekly, while the FFQ incorporates the total number of daily serves, portion size and nutrient content. Similar correlations have been previously found between fruits and vegetables assessed by FFQ and diet quality scores [29]. Toft *et al.* [29] found correlations with grams of fruit ($r$ 0.55) and vegetables ($r$ 0.48) and in the current study, $r = 0.68$ and 0.50 respectively. These results suggest that the ARFS does reflect intakes across a variety of nutrients. In addition to food groups and that the foods included in the ARFS are representative of the AES.

The correlation coefficients from the current study are comparable to those found in the validation study conducted in children and adolescents [9]. This was anticipated given that adult AES FFQ was modified from the child and adolescent version [9] and both studies had a similar design. When the results of the current analysis are compared to those in children and adolescents, which reported a median energy adjusted correlation between FFQ and food records of 0.32, the median correlation of all nutrients in the current study are stronger at 0.72, suggesting that frequency based on weekly consumption of a range of nutrient-dense foods is a stronger predictor of nutrient intakes in adults compared to children.

For dietary instruments to be used to examine associations between diet and disease outcomes, it is suggested that correlations between the instrument and the reference method need to be in the range of at least 0.3 or 0.4 [30]. The current study found correlations significantly greater than 0.3 for all nutrients indicating that the ARFS is an appropriate tool to assess dietary patterns and that it has the potential to be used to evaluate relationships between diet and health status.

The ARFS food based diet quality score accounts for diet variety, particularly fruits and vegetables and assesses the healthiness of diet in relation to National Dietary guidelines however does not account for non-core foods. The ARFS has application as a brief tool to assess overall diet quality and provide a cross-sectional snapshot of dietary intake in relation to dietary guidelines and dietary compliance however may not be sensitive to detect change over time.

A general limitation of validation studies is that the results are not necessarily transferable to other populations. This is generally due to the dietary assessment method such as an FFQ being based on the local food supply and portion size data from national-level surveys [31]. A sample size of at least 50 is desirable for each demographic group [32], and ideally between 100 and 200 participants [33]. Although the sample size in the present study was adequate at the group level it was inadequate to confirm validity and reproducibility for subsets based on age, ethnicity or BMI category. The current sample included 65 female (68%) and therefore results likely to represent females as sub-category, but not males, however all participants are parents of primary school aged children so more likely to reflect a younger age group of adults. Performance of the AES FFQ also needs to be evaluated in populations of varying socioeconomic status and ethnicity. Strengths of the current study include that data were screened for implausible intakes. The reporting period of the FFQ was the previous six months so is likely to reflect differing intake due to seasonality. Lastly, by using statistical methods appropriate for repeated measures and correlated data, that is bootstrapped ICC, strong correlations were revealed.

## 5. Conclusions

This study demonstrated that the Australian Recommended Food Score diet quality index is acceptable in classifying participants into quintiles of nutrient and food intakes. The ARFS was found to be reproducible over a five month period and provides an important contribution to the diet quality indices available for assessing usual intakes in adults. Further research is required to evaluate it use in clinical practice, epidemiologic research and public health interventions in terms of evaluating dietary change and predicting disease risk and evaluating in more diverse populations such as older Australians.

**Acknowledgments:** This research project was funded by a Meat and Livestock Australia Human Nutrition Research Program grant. The funding body had no role in the research study and the views expressed in this manuscript are those of the authors. Melinda J. Hutchesson is funded by a National Heart Foundation Postdoctoral Research Fellowship. The authors acknowledge the families who participated in the study as well as the student support for data collection and data entry.

**Author Contributions:** C.E.C., J.W., T.B. and M.G. designed the study. K.D. and K.P. collected the data. K.P. entered the data. J.W., T.B., M.H. and M.R. drafted the manuscript. M.M.B. and M.G. undertook the statistical analysis. All authors read and approved the final manuscript.

**Conflicts of Interest:** The authors declare no conflict of interest.

## References

1. Nicklas, T. Assessing diet quality in children and adolescents. *J. Am. Diet. Assoc.* **2004**, *104*, 1383–1384.

2. Mertz, W. Foods and nutrients. *J. Am. Diet. Assoc.* **1984**, *84*, 769–770.

3. Kant, A. Indexes of overall diet quality: A review. *J. Am. Diet. Assoc.* **1996**, *96*, 785–791.

4. McNaughton, S. Foods and nutrients provide important insights into optimal eating patterns. *Nutr. Diet.* **2006**, *63*, 66.

5. Ruel, M. Operationalizing diet diversity: A review of measurement issues and research priorities. *J. Nutr.* **2003**, *133*, S3911–S3926.

6. Waijers, P.; Feskens, E.; Ocke, M. A critical review of predefined diet quality scores. *Brit. J. Nutr.* **2007**, *97*, 219–231.

7. Collins, C.E.; Boggess, M.M.; Watson, J.F.; Guest, M.; Duncanson, K.; Pezdirc, K.; Rollo, M.; Hutchesson, M.J.; Burrows, T.L. Reproducibility and comparative validity of a food frequency questionnaire for adults. *Clin. Nutr.* **2014**, *33*, 906–914.

8. ABS. *National Nutrition Survey: Nutrient Intakes and Physical Measurements*; Australian Bureau of Statistics: Canberra, Australia, 1998.

9. Watson, J.F.; Collins, C.E.; Sibbritt, D.W.; Dibley, M.J.; Garg, M.L. Reproducibility and comparative validity of a food frequency questionnaire for Australian children and adolescents. *Int. J. Behav. Nutr. Phys. Act.* **2009**, *6*, 62.

10. Burrows, T.L.; Warren, J.M.; Baur, L.A.; Collins, C.E. Impact of a child obesity intervention on dietary intake and behaviors. *Int. J. Obes.* **2008**, *32*, 1481–1488.

11. Jones, R.A.; Okley, A.D.; Collins, C.E.; Morgan, P.J.; Steele, J.R.; Warren, J.M.; Baur, L.A.; Cliff, D.P.; Burrows, T.L.; Cleary, J. The HIKCUPs trial: A multi-site randomized controlled trial of a combined physical activity skill-development and dietary modification program in overweight and obese children. *BMC Pub. Health* **2007**, *7*, 1–9.

12. Lubans, D.R.; Morgan, P.J.; Dewar, D.; Collins, C.E.; Plotnikoff, R.C.; Okley, A.D.; Batterham, M.J.; Finn, T.; Callister, R. The nutrition and enjoyable activity for teen girls (neat girls) randomized controlled trial for adolescent girls from disadvantaged secondary schools: Rationale, study protocol and baseline results. *BMC Pub. Health* **2010**, *10*.

13. Hall, L.; Collins, C.E.; Morgan, P.J.; Burrows, T.L.; Lubans, D.R.; Callister, R. Children's intake of fruit and selected energy-dense nutrient-poor foods is associated with father's intake. *J. Acad. Nutr. Diet.* **2013**, *111*, 1039–1044.

14. Morgan, P.J.; Lubans, D.R.; Callister, R.; Okley, A.D.; Burrows, T.L.; Fletcher, R.; Collins, C.E. The "healthy dads, healthy kids" randomized controlled trial: Efficacy of a healthy lifestyle program for overweight fathers and their children. *Int. J. Obes.* **2011**, *35*, 436–447.

15. Burrows, T.; Truby, H.; Morgan, P.J.; Callister, R.; Davies, P.S.W.; Collins, C.E. A comparison and validation of child versus parent reporting of children's energy intake using food frequency questionnaires versus food records: Who's an accurate reporter? *Clin. Nutr.* **2013**, *32*, 613–618.

16. Burrows, T.; Berthton, B.; Garg, M.; Collins, C. Validation of food frequency questionnaire using red blood cell membrane fatty acids. *Eur. J. Clin. Nutr.* **2012**, *66*, 825–829.

17. *AUSNUT Australian Food and Nutrient Database*; Australian New Zealand Food Authority, Australian Government Publishing Service: Canberra, Australia, 1999.

18. Kant, A.; Thompson, F. Measures of overall diet quality from a food frequency questionnaire: National health interview survey 1992. *Nutr. Rev.* **1997**, *17*, 1443–1456.

19. Marshall, S.; Watson, J.; Burrows, T.; Guest, M.; Collins, C.E. The development and evaluation of the australian child and adolescent recommended food score: A cross-sectional study. *Nutr. J.* **2012**, *11*, 96.

20. National Health and Medical Research Council. *Australian Dietary Guidelines (2013)*; NHMRC: Canberra, Australia, 2013.

21. *The Australian Guide to Healthy Eating*; Commonwealth Department of Health and Family Services under the National Food and Nutrition Policy Program: Canberra, Australia, 1998.

22. Good, P.I. *Permutation, Parametric and Bootstrap Tests of Hypotheses*; Springer: New York, NY, USA, 2005.

23. Weir, J.P. Quantifying test-retest reliability using the intraclass correlation coefficient and the sem. *J. Strength Cond. Res.* **2005**, *19*, 231–240.

24. Lee, J.; Koh, D.; Ong, C.N. Statistical evaluation of agreement between two methods for measuring a quantitative variable. *Comput. Biol. Med.* **1989**, *19*, 61–70.

25. Efron, B.; Tibshirani, R. *An Introduction to the Bootstrap*; Chapman & Hall/CRC: New York, NY, USA, 1993.

26. Williams, R.L. A note on robust variance estimation for cluster-correlated data. *Biometrics* **2000**, *56*, 645–646.

27. *Stata*, version 12; Stata Press: College Station, TX, USA, 2012.

28. ABS. *National Nutrition Survey: Selected Highlights, Australia, 1995*. Available online: http://www.abs.gov.au/ausstats/abs@.nsf/Lookup/1173B761B1662AE9CA 2568A900139371 (accessed on 20 January 2015).

29. Toft, U.; Kristoffersen, L.; Lau, C.; Borch-Johnsen, K.; Jørgensen, T. The dietary quality score: Validation and association with cardiovascular risk factors: The inter99 study. *Eur. J. Clin. Nutr.* **2007**, *61*, 270–278.

30. Cade, J.; Thompson, R.; Burley, V.; Warm, D. Development, validation and utilisation of food-frequency questionnaires—A review. *Pub. Health Nutr.* **2002**, *5*, 567–587.

31. Plummer, M.; Kaaks, R. Commentary: An open assessment of dietary measurement errors. *Int. J. Epidemiol.* **2003**, *32*, 1062–1063.

32. Cade, J.E.; Burley, V.J.; Warm, D.L.; Thompson, R.L.; Margetts, B.M. Food-frequency questionnaires: A review of their design, validation and utilisation. *Nutr. Res. Rev.* **2004**, *17*, 5–22.

33. Willett, W.; Lenart, E. Reproducibility and validity of food-frequency questionnaires. In *Nutritional Epidemiology*, 2nd ed.; Willett, W., Ed.; Oxford University Press: Oxford, UK, 1998.

# Using Short Dietary Questions to Develop Indicators of Dietary Behaviour for Use in Surveys Exploring Attitudinal and/or Behavioural Aspects of Dietary Choices

Alison Daly, Christina M. Pollard, Deborah A. Kerr, Colin W. Binns and Michael Phillips

**Abstract:** For countries where nutrition surveys are infrequent, there is a need to have some measure of healthful eating to plan and evaluate interventions. This study shows how it is possible to develop healthful eating indicators based on dietary guidelines from a cross sectional population survey. Adults 18 to 64 years answered questions about the type and amount of foods eaten the previous day, including fruit, vegetables, cereals, dairy, fish or meat and fluids. Scores were based on serves and types of food according to an established method. Factor analysis indicated two factors, confirmed by structural equation modeling: a recommended food healthful eating indicator (RF_HEI) and a discretionary food healthful eating indicator (DF_HEI). Both yield mean scores similar to an established dietary index validated against nutrient intake. Significant associations for the RF_HEI were education, income, ability to save, and attitude toward diet; and for the DF_HEI, gender, not living alone, living in a socially disadvantaged area, and attitude toward diet. The results confirm that short dietary questions can be used to develop healthful eating indicators against dietary recommendations. This will enable the exploration of dietary behaviours for "at risk" groups, such as those with excess weight, leading to more relevant interventions for populations.

Reprinted from *Nutrients*. Cite as: Daly, A.; Pollard, C.M.; Kerr, D.A.; Binns, C.W.; Phillips, M. Using Short Dietary Questions to Develop Indicators of Dietary Behaviour for Use in Surveys Exploring Attitudinal and/or Behavioural Aspects of Dietary Choices. *Nutrients* **2015**, *7*, 6330–6345.

## 1. Introduction

Evidence is increasing that the need to eat well as early as possible is inextricably linked to attainment and maintenance of a healthy weight and overall good health [1–4]. In 2011–2102, Australia conducted its third national nutrition survey which coincided with the release of the updated Dietary Guidelines for Australia (DGA) in 2013 [5]. The first release of results from the national nutrition survey indicate that the majority of people are not eating a diet consistent with the Dietary Guidelines [6]. Previous reviews have shown that influencing people to

411

eat well is a complex and difficult process [7,8] and that knowledge and attitudes in line with healthy eating do not necessarily translate into behaviour [9]. Many studies have provided important information about aspects of attitudes, beliefs, and behaviours surrounding good eating habits in relation to families [10,11]; socio demographics [12]; predictors of disordered eating behaviours and diet [13], and attitudes towards appearance and diet [14]. One of the difficulties in being able to conduct these necessary investigations in countries where dietary surveys are infrequent, such as Australia, is that there is not enough current information about eating choices. What is needed is an interim measure that captures important aspects of diet that can be used to investigate how people make decisions about what they eat. A recent study showed that it is possible to get an indicator of healthy eating choices using four items [15] and this study is an important step in developing measures that can be used with contextual data to provide a better picture of what drives eating choices. However such measures are limited as they cannot identify areas of diet which may be more important than others in determining problems related to overeating and poor nutrition. The study investigates whether or not it is possible to use the dietary information collected by the Nutrition Monitoring Survey Series (NMSS) to develop a measure of who is meeting dietary guidelines. The Western Australian Department of Health's NMSS commenced in July/August 1995 to provide information to assist planning interventions promoting the Australian guidelines for healthy eating. The information obtained in these surveys ranges from what people think are problems, how they see their own behaviour, skill or appearance in relation to nutrition, and what they know, believe, and do about the key components of a healthy diet, as defined by the DGA. The surveys are unique in that they collect some food consumption information, as well as knowledge, attitudes, and beliefs that accompany that behaviour. The food consumption part of the NMSS uses short dietary questions to measure consumption of key food groups [16] that have been evaluated against weighed dietary records [17,18]. The questions are used to monitor high level population based adherence to the DGA. These questions are not a measure of dietary intake nor are they a measure of nutrients; rather they are indicators of consumption of selected foods taken from the major food groups recommended for daily consumption. The underlying premise in using these questions to develop a healthful eating indicator is that it can be viewed as a latent indicator of diet quality. If the population is eating recommended serves and types of foods based on dietary guidelines, then they, by definition, must be eating a reasonable quality of diet. While imperfect, this latent assessment of diet quality can be used as a benchmark against which to assess the dietary behaviours and choices at a population level when included in surveys investigating determinants and precursors of diet. This objective of this study was to demonstrate that, with relatively few questions, a robust indicator of eating behaviour can be developed for inclusion in large-scale cross sectional surveys. These indicators have the potential to identify and add context to dietary beliefs, attitudes, and behaviours at a population level.

## 2. Experimental Section

Since 1995, about every three years, over one thousand adults aged 18 to 64 years are interviewed using Computer Assisted Telephone Interviews (CATI) and asked questions about their attitudes and beliefs about diet. The surveys are managed by the Department of Health, who grant ethics approval for the data collection Only the NMSS 2012 survey data were used to develop the healthful eating indicator as it was the most recent survey which contained dietary information across all areas of the DGA. The sample was a stratified random sample according to area of residence drawn from the most recent Electronic White Pages for Western Australia. All sample households with an address were sent a Primary Approach Letter and every household in the initial sample was called up to ten times to achieve contact. Contacted numbers were eliminated if they were not a household or if there was no person living in the household within the age range. Households with more than one adult fulfilling the requirements were asked which adult had the most recent birthday and that adult was selected for interview. No substitutes were permitted. At least ten call backs were made to achieve an interview. Interviews took place during the four weeks between mid-July and mid-August. A raw response rate of not less than 70% was required based on households contacted within the eligible age range whether or not an interview was achieved. In 2012, 1548 people, 1005 females and 543 males, aged between 18 and 64 years, were interviewed, with a response rate of 82.4% based on interviews attained divided by eligible households contacted.

### 2.1. Diet Questions

The NMSS collects information on the previous day's consumption of food groups identified by the DGA. The food groups covered include vegetable, fruit, cereals, dairy, and fish or meat. Information on fluids used are also collected. The data is self-reported and questions were about the amount and types of foods eaten the previous day. Each question contains a definition of a serve or asks for amounts in common household measures such as cups or spoons, which can be used to convert the amount to serves as defined by the DGA.

### 2.2. Sociodemographic Indicators

Indicators of sociodemographic status included sex, age, education, income, employment status, living arrangements, perceived spending power, and an area-based indication of relative socioeconomic disadvantage known as Socio-Economic Indexes for Areas (SEIFA) and developed by the Australian Bureas of Statistics [19].

## 2.3. Developing the Dietary Guideline Indicator

There are only two dietary indices that have been developed for Australia. Both were based on the 1995 National Nutrition Survey and both used a combination of the frequency foods were eaten; some consumption questions, for example fruit and vegetable consumption; and some behaviours such as whether or not meat was trimmed of fat. The first index, developed in 2007, used a relatively simple construction and had six dimensions based on the 2003 Dietary Guidelines for Australian [20]. The second index, developed in 2008, used a similar conceptual framework but had eleven components exploring more parts of the 2003 Australian Dietary Guidelines which included a measure of alcohol consumption [21]. While the NMSS does not collect information about alcohol consumption, there were more possible comparative scales with the 2008 index than with the 2007 index and for this reason it was selected as the model for the development of a NMSS healthful eating indicator (NMSS_HEI). The NMSS_HEI is based solely on consumption of key food groups the previous day. The dietary guideline index developed in 2008 (DGI_2008) used frequency as a rough indication for amount, with each frequency of consumption assumed to be at least one serve. As the NMSS collects dietary data in amounts they can be converted into serves based on the recommendations for adults aged between 18 and 64 years [22]. To accommodate the differences between frequency and consumption, and to compensate for questions used in the DGI_2008 which were not asked in the NMSS, comparable measures for the NMSS data were developed. For example, in the DGI_2008 saturated fat consumption was based on the type of milk used and whether or not meat was trimmed of fat, but the question about trimming fat from meat was not asked in the NMSS, so saturated fat consumption is made up of the type of milk, cheese, and yoghurt consumed and whether sausages and biscuits (high in saturated fat) were eaten. For type of grains, the DGI_2008 used only whole grain bread, but as there was information available for type of bread, rice, pasta, and breakfast cereals, all were used in scoring the type of grains consumption. The DGI_2008 used lean meat, fish, eggs, nuts and seeds, and legumes/beans as major sources of protein, but the only comparable measure in the NMSS were serves of meat or fish eaten the previous day. Additional foods were also differently assessed. For the NMSS_HEI when people consumed more than the recommended number of serves of a particular food group, the full score was given on the specific food component (e.g., cereals) but any serves above the recommended amount were assessed against the additional serve recommendations for each food group by age and sex [5] and scores based on compliance with these. The only exceptions to the additional food score assessments were fruit and vegetables, as the evidence base indicates that there are no known detrimental effects of consuming more than the recommended amounts of these foods [5,23]. A full description of the way in which the index was constructed is shown in Table 1. The table shows the

2013 ADG recommendation for each part of the scale with the way in which the score was assigned, what constitutes not meeting the recommendation and how derivation of the score differs from the DGI_2008.

## 2.4. Analysis

The total NMSS_HEI was the sum of the eleven individual components of the indicators described in Table 1. As with the previously developed DGI_2008, scores for each component are out of ten and as there are eleven measures, the total possible score is 110, with higher scores indicating the healthier eating. Exploratory factor analysis with confirmatory structural equation modelling (SEM) was conducted on the total NMSS_HEI to best identify the structure of the model [25]. The confirmatory SEM was conducted with the data unweighted, allowing for an estimate of comparative fit [26,27] and then the fit compared a SEM using the data weighted for the survey sample design [28]. Post estimation tests conducted on the structural equation model included the comparative fit index, the standardized root mean squared residual, the stability of the model using Wald tests, and the coefficient of determination. Means were calculated for the score components of the two indexes with 95% confidence intervals. For the mean estimates, the data were weighted using Iterative Proportional Fitting, applying a basic adjustment for the probability of selection and then fitting marginal proportional totals for age, sex, and area of residence based on the 2011 Estimated Resident Population for Western Australia. Linear regressions on the two components were conducted. Differences at $p < 0.05$ or less were considered to be significant. Stata 13.1 [29] was used for all analyses.

**Table 1.** Construction of the NMSS_HEI scale based the 2013 ADG [6] with comparison to DGI_2008 [21], NMSS 2012.

| Australian Dietary Guidelines 2013 Using Data Collected in the NMSS 2012 | Indication and Description [a,b] | Criteria for Maximum Score (10) | Criteria for Minimum Score (0) | Difference with DGI_2008 [c] |
|---|---|---|---|---|
| Enjoy a wide variety of nutritious foods | The number of different types of core foods eaten on the previous day. The following made up the variety score: vegetables; fruit; dairy and cereals | Eats four types of vegetables (4 was the median); any fruit; consumes one of milk, yoghurt or cheese; eats three types of cereal foods (breads, bread substitutes, breakfast cereals, rice or pasta) | Eats none of the foods | Used proportion of foods for each food group eaten at least once a week |
| Enjoy plenty of vegetables, including different types and colours, and legumes/beans | Serves of vegetables usually eaten. This question did not specify "yesterday" | For men aged 19–50, at least six serves; for all others at least 5 serves | Eats none | Serves of vegetables & legumes per day |
| Enjoy fruit | Serves of fruit eaten yesterday | All groups, at least 2 serves | Eats none | Serves of fruit eaten per day |
| Enjoy grain (cereal) foods | Serves of cereals eaten yesterday | Men & women aged 18, at least 7 serves; men aged 19–64, at least 6 serves; women aged 19–50, at least 6 serves; women aged 51–64, at least 4 serves. | Eats less than recommended | Frequency of consumption |
| Mostly wholegrain and/or high cereal fibre varieties | Serves of wholegrain or wholemeal cereals eaten yesterday | Full score if all types of cereals eaten yesterday were wholemeal or wholegrain | No cereal foods were wholemeal or wholegrain | Only wholemeal bread was used |
| Enjoy milk, yoghurt, cheese and/or alternatives, mostly reduced fat [d] | Serves of dairy foods used/consumed yesterday | Men & women aged 18, at least 3½; men aged 19–64 and women aged 19–50, at least 2½ serves; women aged 51–64, at least 4 serves | Used/consumed no dairy foods yesterday | Frequency of consumption of dairy foods per day |
| Enjoy lean meats and poultry, fish, eggs, tofu, nuts and seeds, and legumes/beans | Serves of meat or fish eaten yesterday [e] | Men & women aged 18, at least 2½ serves; Men aged 19–50, 3 or more serves; Women aged 19–50, 2 ½ or more serves; women aged 51–64, 2 or more serves. | Eats less than recommended | Frequency of consumption of meats and alternatives the previous day with proportion of lean. |

416

Table 1. Cont.

| Australian Dietary Guidelines 2013 Using Data Collected in the NMSS 2012 | Indication and Description [a,b] | Criteria for Maximum Score (10) | Criteria for Minimum Score (0) | Difference with DGI_2008 [c] |
|---|---|---|---|---|
| Limit intake of foods high in saturated fat | Ate full fat dairy food or sausages or biscuits | The numbers of foods eaten were converted to a score out of ten and those who ate none got a score of 10 | Ate all foods high in saturated fats | Used type of milk usually consumed as well as trimming fat from meat. |
| Drink plenty of water [f] | Litres of fluids - proportion of water to total fluids set at 66% [d] | Drank at least 8 (250) mL, cups (women) or 10 (250) mL, cups (men) of any fluid yesterday | Drank less than suggested | Used 8 cups (250 mL) |
| Limit intake of foods and drinks containing added sugars | Number of foods high in added sugar consumed yesterday including biscuits, soft drinks, crumpets, scones, muffins (cake type) and sugary breakfast cereals | No such foods eaten yesterday | Ate three types yesterday | Used frequency of consumption of cordial, fruit juice, soft drinks, jam, chocolate or confectionary |
| To achieve and maintain a healthy weight, be physically active and choose amounts of nutritious food and drinks to meet your energy needs [g] | Extra serves of any foods except fruit and vegetables consumed which were above the additional serves guidelines | No additional serves eaten | Any additional serves above upper limit | Used a combination of added sugar and extra foods. |

[a] Serves are estimated using the 2013 ADG definitions; [b] The maximum recommended serves or more is the basis for the maximum score but additional serves over recommended and more than recommended additional are then penalised under the extra serves score; [c] DGI 2008 DQI used each frequency of consumption to be a rough measure of a serve; [d] Dairy foods were weighted by fat content; [e] The only available questions on protein were about serves of meat and fish; [f] Used the cut points for fluids suggested in Educators guide for the Australian Dietary Guidelines 2013—the reference also suggests that "most" be in the form of water so 66% water was taken as an measure of "most" as there was no quantified amount suggested [24] (National Health and Medical Research Council, 2013); [g] The 2013 ADG provides an additional serves guideline for taller and more active adults and this was used to assess extra serves over and above these plus recommended.

## 3. Results

The initial NMSS_HEI score showed a wide distribution of scores that has no statistically significant departures from normality for kurtosis but is significantly negatively skewed (Figure 1). The exploratory factor analysis showed two factors, one which reflected the recommended components of the DGI, namely the variety, fruits, vegetables, grains, cereals, dairy, protein, and fluids and one that reflected the discretionary components of the total NMSS_HEI, namely fats, sugar, and additional serves.

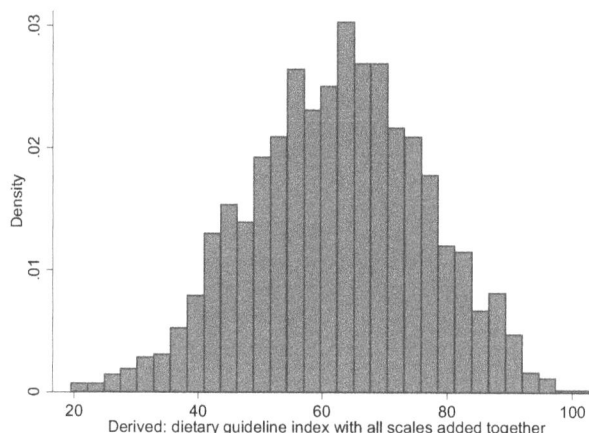

**Figure 1.** Distribution of the DGI score, NMSS 2012.

The SEM confirmed the two-component structure of the NMSS_HEI and, as with the factor analysis, one reflected the major food groups (Recommended) and the other reflected additional serves and discretionary foods (Discretionary), with each variable contribution to the components statistically significant at $p < 0.01$. Statistically significant covariance were identified for a number of variables using post estimation tests and added to the model with all covariates remaining statistically significant at $p < 0.05$ or better. The addition of the covariance associations altered the p value for the protein score and the cereal score to $p > 0.05$. The largest coefficients (contributors to the model) for the "Recommended" component were variety ($\beta = 0.62, p = 0.0001$), fruit ($\beta = 0.46, p = 0.0001$), and vegetables ($\beta = 0.37, p = 0.0001$), with protein contributing least ($\beta = 0.002$, ns). For the "Discretionary" component the contributors were sugar ($\beta = 0.74, p = 0.0001$), followed by extra serves ($\beta = 0.71, p = 0.0001$) and fat ($\beta = 0.45, p = 0.0001$). The model is a non-recursive model and post estimation tests showed it satisfied the stability condition. The raw component scores were negatively correlated but at a very low level (Spearman rho-.078 $p < 0.05$ and in the SEM covariance between the two scores failed to reach statistical significance.

For the weighted SEM, the weighted coefficient of determination (CD) was 90.4% and the CD was 91% for the unweighted SEM. The post estimation statistics for the weighted SEM (Table 2) are considered to indicate a good fit with the data [27,30]. For weighted models, no equivalent goodness of fit statistics other than the CD and the standardized root mean squared residual (SRMR) are possible because of the way in which standard errors are estimated, however both the weighted CD and the weighted SRMR are similar to the equivalent measures for the unweighted model. As the data on which the SEM are based are drawn from a cross-sectional population survey, the weighted model coefficients are the most appropriate for use and are the ones displayed in Figure 2.

**Table 2.** Post estimation statistics for the weighted SEM model, NMSS 2012.

| Fit Statistic | Value | Description |
|---|---|---|
| **Likelihood Ratio ** * | | |
| chi2_ms (33) | 51.37 | model *vs.* saturated |
| $p >$ chi2 | 0.02 | - |
| chi2_bs (55) | 1749.51 | baseline *vs.* saturated |
| $p >$ chi2 | 0 | - |
| **Population Error** | | |
| RMSEA | 0.02 | Root mean squared error of approximation |
| 90% CI, lower bound | 0.01 | - |
| 90% CI, upper bound | 0.03 | - |
| pclose | 1 | Probability RMSEA $\leqslant 0.05$ |
| **Baseline Comparison** | | |
| CFI | 0.99 | Comparative fit index |
| TLI | 0.98 | Tucker-Lewis index |
| **Size of Residuals** | | |
| SRMR | 0.02 | Standardized root mean squared residual |
| CD | 0.91 | Coefficient of determination |

* While the chi square is <0.05, the very large sample size would predict that. The chi square divided by the degrees of freedom is <3 indicating an acceptable chi square for a sample this size [26].

Even though the NMSS_HEI does not capture the whole range of foods eaten, or nutrient intake for the previous day, it does provide a comparable measure at the total component range. Table 3 shows the NMSS_HEI means and proportions meeting the recommended guidelines for the food group. Compared with the DGI_2008, on which the NMSS_HEI is based and which did an assessment of nutrients against the index, many of scales had quite similar means.

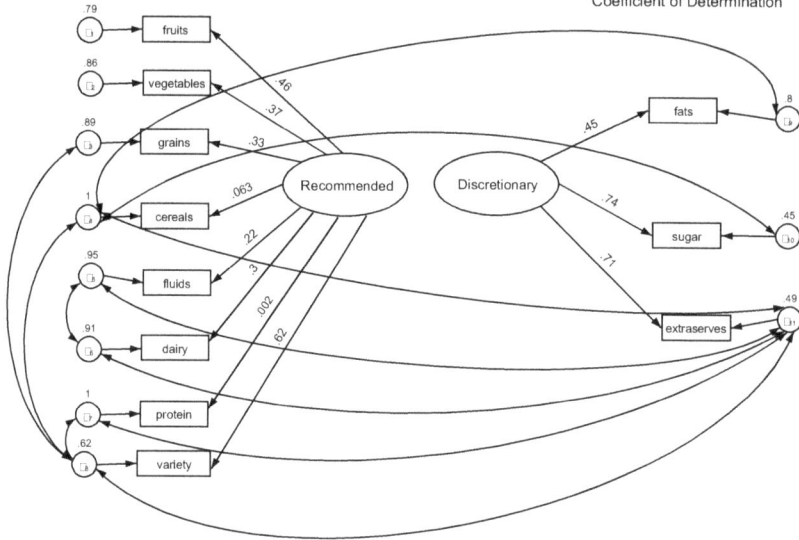

WEIGHTED MODEL
Coefficient of Determination .908
Standardized root mean squared residual .020

UNWEIGHTED MODEL
Comparative Fit Index .989
Tucker-Lewis Index .982
Coefficient of Determination .914

**Figure 2.** Model produced by structural equation modelling showing two independent components with covariance, NMSS 2012.

**Table 3.** Mean scores for each component identified by the SEM and percentage meeting the recommended dietary guideline in the 2013 ADG by sex with comparisons to the DGI_2008.

| Dietary Score Component | Males | | | Females | | |
|---|---|---|---|---|---|---|
| | RFI [1] | Diff >1 § with DGI_2008 | % Meeting RFI [2] | RFI [1] | Diff >1 § with DGI_2008 | % Meeting RFI [2] |
| Food variety | 4.96 ± 0.15 | - | 5.58 | 5.33 ± 0.10 | - | 7.00 |
| Vegetables | 4.97 ± 0.14 | - | 8.39 | 5.66 ± 0.11 | - | 14.73 |
| Fruit | 6.88 ± 0.23 | - | 58.52 | 7.74 ± 0.14 | - | 68.06 |
| Cereals | 6.78 ± 0.19 | y | 38.48 | 5.98 ± 0.13 | - | 27.50 |
| Wholemeal/grains | 4.64 ± 0.27 | y | 43.76 | 4.95 ± 0.19 | y | 47.35 |
| Protein (meat/fish) | 3.54 ± 0.19 | y | 9.48 | 3.14 ± 0.13 | y | 6.79 |
| Dairy | 5.00 ± 0.16 | - | 10.32 | 4.88 ± 0.12 | - | 11.37 |
| Fluids [3] | 6.17 ± 0.14 | - | 15.29 | 6.11 ± 0.10 | y | 23.92 |
| Fats | 7.00 ± 0.14 | y | 24.49 | 7.12 ± 0.10 | - | 29.38 |
| Sugar | 6.20 ± 0.2 | - | 46.07 | 7.12 ± 0.10 | y | 58.10 |
| Extra serves | 4.01 ± 0.22 | - | 22.22 | 4.93 ± 0.17 | y | 33.83 |

[1] Data are mean scores out of 10 weighted using raking; [2] Data are percentages meeting recommendations (score of 10) weighted using raking; § The mean score differed by more than 1 when the mean score of the NMSS_HEI was compared to the DGI_2008.

420

The largest differences were for cereals (mean scale score: DGI_2008 Males 4.2 Females 5.6; NMSS_HEI: Males 6.8 Females 6.0) and eating meats/meat alternatives (mean scale score: DGI_2008: Males 9.8 Females 9.7; NMSS_HEI: Males 3.5 Females 3.1). As the NMSS didn't ask about consumption of any meat alternatives and as forty percent of the respondents reported that they had not eaten any of the meat or fish, the difference is not unexpected. No obvious explanation exists for the difference in the cereals score unless the DGI_2008 calculation didn't include breakfast cereals which were included in the NMSS_HEI calculation. It may be that the updated 2013 ADG accounted for some of the differences in the proportions meeting guidelines with increases in the recommended serves of protein, dairy, and cereals in the later version.

Using the two components established by the SEM, a recommended food healthful eating indicator (RF_HEI) and a discretionary food healthful eating indicator (DF_HEI) were calculated by weighting each variable making up the component by the standardised coefficients generated by SEM. Table 4 shows mean scores of selected socio demographic indicators and attitudes. The groups with the highest mean scores for the RF_HEI were people who paid a lot of attention to the health aspects of diet, being retired and doing home duties; the two lowest scores were people who don't pay any attention to the health aspects of diet and being unemployed. For the DF_HEI the highest mean scores were for people living alone and people who paid a lot of attention to the health aspects of diet; the lowest scores were for people who live in the most socially disadvantaged areas and students.

After controlling for all the variables in table four, *lower* scores for the RF_HEI were significantly associated with lower education levels, having an annual household income less than $40,000, not being able to save any money and paying little or no attention to the health aspects of diet. For the DF_HEI, *lower* scores were significantly associated with being male, not living alone, living in the most socially disadvantaged areas of WA and paying little or no attention to the health aspects of diet.

For the RF_HEI attitudes toward the health aspects of a healthy diet had a linear association with the highest scores associated with paying a lot of attention to diet (Figure 3).

**Table 4.** Mean scores for RF_HEI and DF_HEI by selected socio demographics and attitude toward diet.

| Selected Descriptive Variables | RF_HEI | DF_HEI |
|---|---|---|
| **Gender** | Mean (95% CI) | Mean (95% CI) |
| Male | 44.11 (42.50, 45.73) | 16.64 (15.77, 17.50) |
| Female | 47.61 (46.46, 48.76) | 18.77 (18.10, 19.43) |
| **Age Group in Years** | | |
| 18–44 | 44.86 (43.30, 46.43) | 16.66 (15.82, 17.50) |
| 45–64 | 47.16 (46.13, 48.20) | 17.53 (16.92, 18.14) |
| **Highest Level of Education Attained** | | |
| Up to Year 12 | 42.07 (39.50, 44.64) | 18.07 (16.67, 19.47) |
| Year 12 | 43.40 (40.38, 46.43) | 17.00 (15.45, 18.54) |
| TAFE/Trade | 45.98 (44.36, 47.60) | 17.89 (17.01, 18.77) |
| Tertiary | 47.89 (46.33, 49.44) | 17.70 (16.76, 18.64) |
| **Annual Household Income** | | |
| Up to $40,000 | 46.29 (45.26, 47.32) | 17.75 (17.16, 18.34) |
| More than $40,000 | 41.39 (37.73, 45.05) | 17.15 (15.53, 18.78) |
| **Perceived Discretional Income** | | |
| Can't save | 41.88 (39.69, 44.08) | 17.10 (15.96, 18.23) |
| Can save | 47.16 (46.07, 48.26) | 17.89 (17.25, 18.53) |
| **SEIFA \*** | - | - |
| SEIFA Quintile 1 (most disadvantaged) | 43.64 (40.13, 47.15) | 14.98 (13.36, 16.59) |
| SEIFA Quintile 5 (least disadvantaged) | 46.96 (45.13, 48.78) | 18.25 (17.02, 19.48) |
| **Current Employment Status** | | |
| Employed | 46.35 (45.23, 47.48) | 17.94 (17.31, 18.57) |
| Unemployed | 38.28 (31.73, 44.84) | 17.78 (13.49, 22.07) |
| Home Duties | 48.32 (46.19, 50.45) | 17.28 (15.71, 18.85) |
| Student | 40.85 (36.12, 45.58) | 15.66 (13.09, 18.23) |
| Retired | 48.90 (46.38, 51.43) | 18.53 (16.88, 20.19) |
| Unable to work | 36.38 (29.35, 43.40) | 17.33 (13.23, 21.43) |
| **Living Arrangements** | | |
| Living with family/partner | 45.99 (44.93, 47.04) | 17.67 (17.09, 18.25) |
| Living alone | 42.30 (39.24, 45.37) | 19.41 (17.82, 21.00) |
| Other | 46.45 (40.25, 52.66) | 16.64 (13.02, 20.26) |
| **Residential Area** | - | - |
| Metropolitan Perth | 45.80 (44.58, 47.02) | 17.67 (16.98, 18.36) |
| Rest of State | 46.00 (44.33, 47.67) | 17.76 (16.88, 18.64) |
| **Country of Birth** | | |
| Australia | 45.81 (44.11, 47.52) | 17.35 (16.43, 18.27) |
| Other country | 45.87 (44.64, 47.11) | 17.86 (17.16, 18.56) |
| **Attention to Health Aspects of Diet** | | |
| Pay a lot of attention | 51.47 (50.21, 52.72) | 19.23 (18.46, 20.00) |
| Take a bit of notice | 43.17 (41.86, 44.49) | 16.68 (15.86, 17.49) |
| Don't really think much about it | 33.13 (28.93, 37.33) | 16.00 (13.98, 18.02) |

\* Comparison is in that quintile or not.

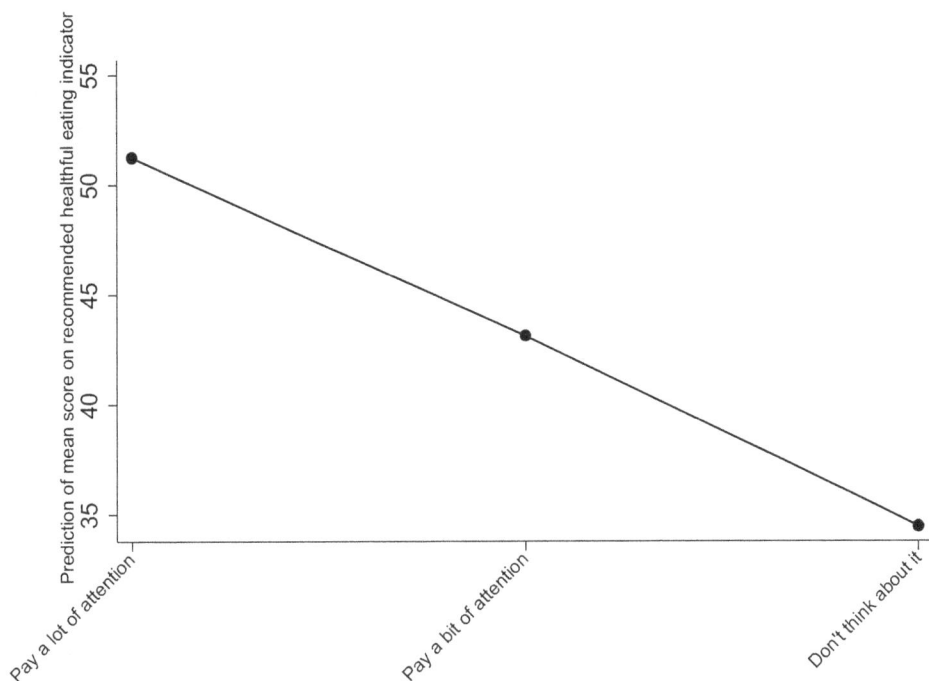

**Figure 3.** Predictive margins of attention paid to diet.

## 4. Discussion

The aim of this study was to develop a measure that could be used during years when nutrition-based dietary survey data were not available. This proved possible and, while there is no doubt that the RF_HEI and DF_HEI measures do not capture the whole range of foods eaten or have the information to make a nutrient intake assessment, they do provide a basis from which to assess how the population is doing against dietary recommendations. The fact that the initial NMSS_HEI has two independent components offers new information about how the population is approaching their diet. One way is in line with dietary recommendations about serves and types from food groups; the other is in line with dietary recommendations about discretionary foods and additional serves. This means that the same person can have a score indicating healthful eating on one component but not on the other; well on both components or well on neither component. The regression analysis showed that the predictors of eating well for each component are, for the most part, not shared, suggesting that what drives eating behaviours may stem from different influences according to the types of foods being considered. This information is intrinsically different from research, which uses cluster analysis on Australian dietary intake to identify food patterns for example, an eating pattern relatively high in fat and meat compared with an eating pattern higher in fruit and vegetables [31,32], and research using factor, cluster analyses along or ranked regression conducted on data that has not been pre-scored against any standard, such as dietary guidelines [32,33]. These methods identify eating patterns and then explore associations with health indicators [33–35], who is eating in line with particular patterns [36,37] and, more recently, other aspects such as how changes in individuals' dietary patterns affect obesity over time [36,38] and mortality [39]. The two independent components structure identified in this study using SEM suggests that there may be different attitudes and perceptions associated with each that have the potential to inform health promotion and education approaches [14,40]. Population groups such as those with excess weight can now be explored in more detail in relation to their eating choices. The healthful eating indicators as described in this study have not been explored by each of the foods and eating patterns summarised by each indicator. Breakdown of the individual indicators by foods may offer additional information about eating patterns and choices which, in turn, could lead to more precise information about population groups "at risk" due to poor diet. The ability of surveys such as the NMSS to allow the construction of a healthful eating indicator offers a rich source from which to explore important interactions between the psychosocial aspects of diet, such as attitudes, perceptions, and intentions with knowledge and behaviours associated with healthy dietary patterns in the years when detailed nutrient and dietary information with measures of related attitudes and beliefs is not available [41]. The analyses in this paper did not explore interactions or the influence of attitudes on the healthful eating indicators as the aim was to develop healthful eating indicators. To investigate these associations further studies are planned. Investigation of how closely the indicators monitor a more comprehensive measure of consumption, such as a 24 h dietary recall or a three day dietary history, would be valuable to both establish the level of congruence at the scale level and to identify any major gaps.

As with any cross-sectional survey data social desirability may determine some responses but in this case most of the responses are unlikely to be biased in this respect as the respondent would need to be aware of all of the dietary guidelines in formulating their response. In this cross-sectional survey, as in most others, [42] there was an under representation of males relative to females, suggesting a non-response bias for males. The weighting process does adjust for this and having standard errors calculated by robust methods also helps, however, the recommendation for further NMSS data collection is that a stratified random sampling method using area, gender, and age group be considered. Exploration of a more up-to-date source of telephone numbers should also be considered. It is unfortunate that the data from the six surveys could not be pooled but the different data collection methods and different questions for food eaten prohibited this. Consistency in this regard would also be beneficial.

## 5. Conclusions

It is possible to develop healthful eating indicators using validated short dietary questions for use in years when more complete nutrition data is not available. The identification of two independent indicators of healthful eating offers evidence that people approach diet in different ways. This finding suggests that fully investigating each indicator has the potential for better targeted and relevant interventions to improve diet quality in the population.

**Acknowledgments:** The Nutrition Monitoring Survey Series were funded and conducted by the Department of Health in Western Australia. Healthway, the Western Australian Health Promotion Foundation, funded Curtin University to assist the translation of research into practice through the five year "Food Law, Policy and Communications to Improve Public Health Project". Healthway awarded Alison Daly a Health Promotion Research Training Scholarship to support her training and development. The authors acknowledge the WA Department of Health who support and own the NMSS; Margaret Miller who conceived the NMSS and the people of Western Australia who have taken the time to respond.

**Author Contributions:** Alison Daly formulated the research question, designed the study, conducted the analysis and drafted the manuscript. Christina Pollard, Deborah Kerr and Colin Binns formulated the research question, designed the study, reviewed and revised the manuscript and approved it for publication. Michael Phillips formulated the research question, designed the study, provided expert statistical advice, reviewed and revised the manuscript and approved it for publication.

**Conflicts of Interest:** The authors declare no conflict of interest.

## References

1. Belin, R.J.; Greenland, P.; Allison, M.; Martin, L.; Shikany, J.M.; Larson, J.; Tinker, L.; Howard, B.V.; Lloyd-Jones, D.; van Horn, L. Diet quality and the risk of cardiovascular disease: The women's health initiative (whi). *Am. J. Clin. Nutr.* **2011**, *94*, 49–57.
2. Barker, D.J.P. The developmental origins of adult disease. *J. Am. Coll. Nutr.* **2004**, *23*, 588S–595S.
3. Barker, D.; Eriksson, J.; Forsén, T.; Osmond, C. Fetal origins of adult disease: Strength of effects and biological basis. *Int. J. Epidemiol.* **2002**, *31*, 1235–1239.
4. Vaiserman, A.M. Early-life nutritional programming of longevity. *J. Dev. Orig. Health Dis.* **2014**, *5*, 325–338.
5. National Health and Medical Research Council. *Australian Dietary Guidelines Incorporating the Australian Guide to Healthy Eating 2013*; National Health and Medical Research Council: Canberra, Australia, 2013.
6. Australian Bureau of Statistics. Australian health survey: Nutrition first results—Foods and nutrients, 2011-12. In *Cat No 4364.0.55.007*; Australian Bureau of Statistics: Canberra: Australia, 2014.

7. Brambila Macias, J.; Shankar, B.; Capacci, S.; Mazzocchi, M.; Perez-Cueto, F.J.A.; Verbeke, W.; Traill, W.B. Policy interventions to promote healthy eating: A review of what works, what does not, and what is promising. *Food Nutr. Bull.* **2011**, *32*, 365–375.

8. Buttriss, J.; Stanner, S.; McKevith, B.; Nugent, A.P.; Kelly, C.; Phillips, F.; Theobald, H.E. Successful ways to modify food choice: Lessons from the literature. *Nutr. Bull.* **2004**, *29*, 333–343.

9. Baranowski, T.; Cullen, K.W.; Baranowski, J. Psychosocial correlates of dietary intake: Advancing dietary intervention. *Ann. Rev. Nutr.* **1999**, *19*, 17–40.

10. Bergea, J.M.; Wall, M.; Larson, N.J.; Forsythd, A.; Bauere, K.W.; Neumark-Sztainer, D. Youth dietary intake and weight status: Healthful neighborhood food environments enhance the protective role of supportive family home environments. *Health Place* **2013**, *26*, 69–77.

11. Larson, N.; Laska, M.N.; Story, M.; Neumark-Sztainer, D. Predictors of fruit and vegetable intake in young adulthood. *J. Acad. Nutr. Diet.* **2012**, *112*, 1216–1222.

12. Beydoun, M.A.; Wang, Y. How do socio-economic status, perceived economic barriers and nutritional benefits affect quality of dietary intake among us adults? *Eur. J. Clin. Nutr.* **2007**, *62*, 303–313.

13. Loth, K.A.; MacLehose, R.; Bucchianeri, M.; Crow, S.; Neumark-Sztainer, D. Predictors of dieting and disordered eating behaviors from adolescence to young adulthood. *J. Adolesc. Health* **2014**, *55*, 705–712.

14. Traill, W.B.; Chambers, S.A.; Butler, L. Attitudinal and demographic determinants of diet quality and implications for policy targeting. *J. Hum. Nutr. Diet.* **2012**, *25*, 87–94.

15. Pot, G.K.; Richards, M.; Prynne, C.J.; Stephen, A.M. Development of the eating choices index (eci): A four-item index to measure healthiness of diet. *Public Health Nutr.* **2014**, *17*, 2660–2666.

16. Marks, G.C.; Webb, K.; Rutishauser, I.H.E.; Riley, M. *Monitoring Food Habits in the Australian Population Using Short Questions*; Australian Food and Nutrition Monitoring Unit, Queensland University: Queensland, Australia, 2001.

17. Riley, M.; Rutishauser, I.H.E.; Webb, K. *Comparison of Short Questions with Weighed Dietary Records*; Commonwealth Department of Health and Aged Care: Canberra, Australia, 2001.

18. Rutishauser, I.H.E.; Webb, K.; Abraham, B.; Allsopp, R. Comparison of short questions with weighed dietary records. In *Australian Food and Nutrition Monitoring Unit*; Commonwealth Department of Health and Aged Care: Canberra, Australia, 2001.

19. Australian Bureau of Statistics. *Socio-Economic Indexes for Areas (Seifa) 2011*; Australian Bureau of Statistics: Canberra, Australia, 2013.

20. Australian Institute of Health and Welfare. *Australian Diet Quality Index Project*; Cat No: PHE85. AIHW: Canberra, Australia, 2007.

21. McNaughton, S.A.; Ball, K.; Crawford, D.; Mishra, G.D. An index of diet and eating patterns is a valid measure of diet quality in an australian population. *J. Nutr.* **2008**, *138*, 86–93.

22. National Health and Medical Research Council. Australian guidelines summary dietary. In *Eat for Health*; National Health and Medical Research Council: Canberra, Australia, 2014.

23. Oyebode, O.; Gordon-Dseagu, V.; Walker, A.; Mindell, J.S. Fruit and vegetable consumption and all-cause, cancer and cvd mortality: Analysis of health survey for England data. *J. Epidemiol. Community Health* **2014**, *68*, 856–862.

24. National Health and Medical Research Council. Eat for health. In *Educators Guide*; National Health and Medical Research Council: Canberra, Australia, 2013.

25. Imamura, F.; Jacques, P.F. Invited commentary: Dietary pattern analysis. *Am. J. Epidemiol.* **2011**, *173*, 1105–1108.

26. Schreiber, J.B. Core reporting practices in structural equation modeling. *Res. Soc. Adm. Pharm* **2008**, *4*, 83–97.

27. Iacobucci, D. Everything you always wanted to know about sem (structural equations modeling) but were afraid to ask. *J. Consum. Psychol.* **2009**, *19*, 673–680.

28. Muthen, B.O.; Satorra, A. Complex sample data in structural equation modeling. *Sociol. Methodol.* **1995**, *25*, 267–316.

29. StataCorp. Stata glossary and index release 13$^{®}$. In *Statistical Software*; StataCorp LP: College Station, TX, USA, 2013.

30. Hu, F.B.; Bentler, P.M. Cut off criteria for fit indexes in covariant structure analysis: Conventional criteria *versus* new alternative. *Struct. Equ. Model.* **1999**, *6*, 1–55.

31. Grieger, J.A.; Scott, J.; Cobiac, L. Cluster analysis and food group consumption in a national sample of Australian girls. *J. Hum. Nutr. Diet.* **2012**, *25*, 75–86.

32. Moeller, S.M.; Reedy, J.; Millen, A.E.; Dixon, L.B.; Newby, P.K.; Tucker, K.L.; Krebs-Smith, S.M.; Guenther, P.M. Dietary patterns: Challenges and opportunities in dietary patterns research: An experimental biology workshop, 1 April 2006. *J. Am. Diet. Assoc.* **2007**, *107*, 1233–1239.

33. Li, W.-Q.; Park, Y.; Wu, J.W.; Goldstein, A.M.; Taylor, P.R.; Hollenbeck, A.R.; Freedman, N.D.; Abnet, C.C. Index-based dietary patterns and risk of head and neck cancer in a large prospective study. *Am. J. Clin. Nutr.* **2014**, *99*, 559–566.

34. Amini, M.; Shafaeizadeh, S.; Zare, M.; Boroujeni, H.K.; Esmaillzadeh, A. A cross-sectional study on food patterns and adiposity among individuals with abnormal glucose homeostasis. *Arch. Iran. Med.* **2012**, *15*, 131–135.

35. Xu, B.; Houston, D.; Locher, J.L.; Zizza, C. The association between healthy eating index-2005 scores and disability among older Americans. *Age Ageing* **2012**, *41*, 365–371.

36. Elstgeest, L.E.M.; Mishra, G.D.; Dobson, A.J. Transitions in living arrangements are associated with changes in dietary patterns in young women. *J. Nutr.* **2012**, *142*, 1561–1567.

37. Kant, A.K. Dietary patterns and health outcomes. *J. Am. Diet. Assoc.* **2004**, *104*, 615–635.

38. Pachucki, M.A. Food pattern analysis over time: Unhealthful eating trajectories predict obesity. *Int. J. Obes.* **2012**, *36*, 686–694.

39. Kant, A.K.; Schatzkin, A.; Graubard, B.I.; Schairer, C. A prospective study of diet quality and mortality in women. *J. Am. Med. Assoc.* **2000**, *283*, 2109–2115.

40. Lê, J.; Dallongeville, J.; Wagner, A.; Arveiler, D.; Haas, B.; Cottel, D.; Simon, C.; Dauchet, L. Attitudes toward healthy eating: A mediator of the educational level-diet relationship. *Eur. J. Clin. Nutr.* **2013**, *67*, 808–814.

41. Grunert, K.G.; Shepherd, R.; Traill, W.B.; Wold, B. Food choice, energy balance and its determinants: Views of human behaviour in economics and psychology. *Trends Food Sci. Technol.* **2012**, *28*, 132–142.

42. Galea, S.; Tracy, M. Participation rates in epidemiologic studies. *Ann. Epidemiol.* **2007**, *17*, 643–653.

# Section 6:
# Evaluation of a Dietary Intervention

# Do Overweight Adolescents Adhere to Dietary Intervention Messages? Twelve-Month Detailed Dietary Outcomes from Curtin University's Activity, Food and Attitudes Program

Kyla L. Smith, Deborah A. Kerr, Erin K. Howie and Leon M. Straker

**Abstract:** Dietary components of adolescent obesity interventions are rarely evaluated with comprehensive reporting of dietary change. The objective was to assess dietary change in overweight adolescents, including adherence to dietary intervention. The dietary intervention was part of a multi-component intervention (CAFAP) targeting the physical activity, sedentary and healthy eating behaviors of overweight adolescents ($n = 69$). CAFAP was a staggered entry, within-subject, waitlist controlled clinical trial with 12 months of follow up. Diet was assessed using three-day food records and a brief eating behavior questionnaire. Changes in dietary outcomes were assessed using linear mixed models, adjusted for underreporting. Food record data suggested reduced adherence to dietary intervention messages over time following the intervention, despite conflicting information from the brief eating behavior questionnaire. During the intervention, energy intake was stable but favorable nutrient changes occurred. During the 12 month maintenance period; self-reported eating behaviors improved, energy intake remained stable but dietary fat and saturated fat intake gradually returned to baseline levels. Discrepancies between outcomes from brief dietary assessment methods and three-day food records show differences between perceived and actual intake, highlighting the need for detailed dietary reporting. Further, adherence to dietary intervention principles reduces over time, indicating a need for better maintenance support.

Reprinted from *Nutrients*. Cite as: Smith, K.L.; Kerr, D.A.; Howie, E.K.; Straker, L.M. Do Overweight Adolescents Adhere to Dietary Intervention Messages? Twelve-Month Detailed Dietary Outcomes from Curtin University's Activity, Food and Attitudes Program. *Nutrients* **2015**, *7*, 4363–4382.

## 1. Introduction

Current rates of overweight and obesity in adolescence are concerning given the associated negative medical, psychosocial [1] and economic [2] consequences. Available evidence supports interventions with a comprehensive multi-disciplinary approach including a dietary component [3] and a family-based design with a

431

focus on food and activity behaviors and attitudes [4]. Despite recommendations suggesting a focus on lifestyle, most interventions are evaluated using only measures of weight change. Few details about the implementation and evaluation of dietary interventions have been documented [5], making it difficult to understand how weight change may be achieved. Thus, a need for timely and detailed evaluation of adolescent obesity programs has been identified [4,6,7].

Surprisingly, few adolescent intervention trials have collected and reported detailed changes in participant dietary behaviors and intake data [8]. Some studies have not reported any dietary data [9,10], have not accounted for possible underreporting [11,12] or have used dietary assessment methods that provide only limited information and are restricted in their ability to detect true dietary change [13,14]. Further, measures of adherence to dietary interventions appear to be poorly described. In adolescent studies reporting dietary outcomes, the proportion of participants adopting specific dietary targets of the intervention (*i.e.*, adherence) were not reported [11,12,14–16]. This is of particular concern as low adherence to dietary recommendations is a primary reason for poor outcomes following intervention [17]. Without adherence measures, it remains unclear how the dietary interventions create change in multi-disciplinary interventions [18].

To date, changes in diet following intervention have shown modest results, and long-term follow-up has been lacking [4]. In multi-disciplinary interventions where dietary data was collected, there have been improvements reported in some self-reported eating behaviors [15], or dietary intakes including reduction in total energy intake [14,16], absolute fat intake [12,16] and sugar intake [19]. Even these dietary findings have been limited by follow-up of less than 12 months [12,16,19] and a lack of adherence measures [12,14–16,19]. This very restricted evidence base limits the ability for future studies to replicate or compare dietary changes to determine the effectiveness of dietary interventions in overweight adolescents.

Against this background, the aim of this study was to comprehensively assess dietary change in overweight and obese adolescents for 12 months following an intervention (Curtin University's Activity, Food and Attitudes Program) to better understand dietary change in this group. The assessment included analyses of adolescent adherence to the dietary component of the intervention (including changes in the primary intervention behavioral targets), changes in selected eating behavior strategies, and a detailed analysis of dietary nutrient intake as reported in three day food records.

## 2. Experimental Section

### 2.1. Study Design

This study was a multiple cohort, staggered-entry, waitlist period controlled clinical trial conducted at three sites in Western Australia (two metropolitan areas and one regional area) [20]. Briefly, overweight adolescents were recruited and assessed three months before the eight-week intensive phase of the intervention commenced, and assessed again immediately prior to the intervention. This method was chosen because it was considered unfair to withhold services from obese adolescents in view of the lack of appropriate treatment services available [21], and the dual pre-participation assessments allowed for a within-subjects control period. The staggered start for the seven cohort groups controlled for external seasonal and public event confounders to intervention effects. Further assessments were completed at the immediate conclusion of the eight-week program and again at three months, six months and 12 months post-intervention [20]. This trial was registered on the Australian New Zealand Clinical Trials Registry (ACTRN12611001187932). Figure 1 shows the progression of participants through the 17 months of the study. Each assessment time point is represented by a box on the left of the figure. In each box, the bold number refers to the number of adolescents potentially still available for each assessment, with the number of drop outs clearly stated on the right of the figure.

### 2.2. Participants

Between January 2012 and December 2013, 69 overweight or obese adolescents aged 11–16 participated in Curtin University's Activity, Food and Attitudes Program (CAFAP). Participants were recruited via the health system, education system and from the general community and were screened by a medical practitioner for medical suitability prior to assessment. Further inclusion criteria was a BMI-for-age-and-sex above the 85th percentile [22]. Exclusion criteria included: obesity relating to an identified genetic, endocrine or metabolic disease, current treatment for psychiatric disorders or inability for parent and adolescent to attend twice weekly group sessions at a local community site. This study was approved by the Curtin University Human Ethics Research Committee (HR105/2011). Written informed assent/consent was obtained from all adolescents/parents.

### 2.3. Intervention

CAFAP was a community-based, multi-disciplinary healthy lifestyle program directed at overweight and obese adolescents and has been described in detail elsewhere [20,23]. The focus of CAFAP was increased physical activity, reduced sedentary behavior, reduced junk food intake and increased fruit and vegetable intake. The eight-week intensive phase of the intervention involved parents and adolescents and consisted of twice-weekly group sessions run by a psychologist, physiotherapist/exercise physiologist or dietitian. The intensive intervention period was followed by a tapered maintenance phase over 12 months.

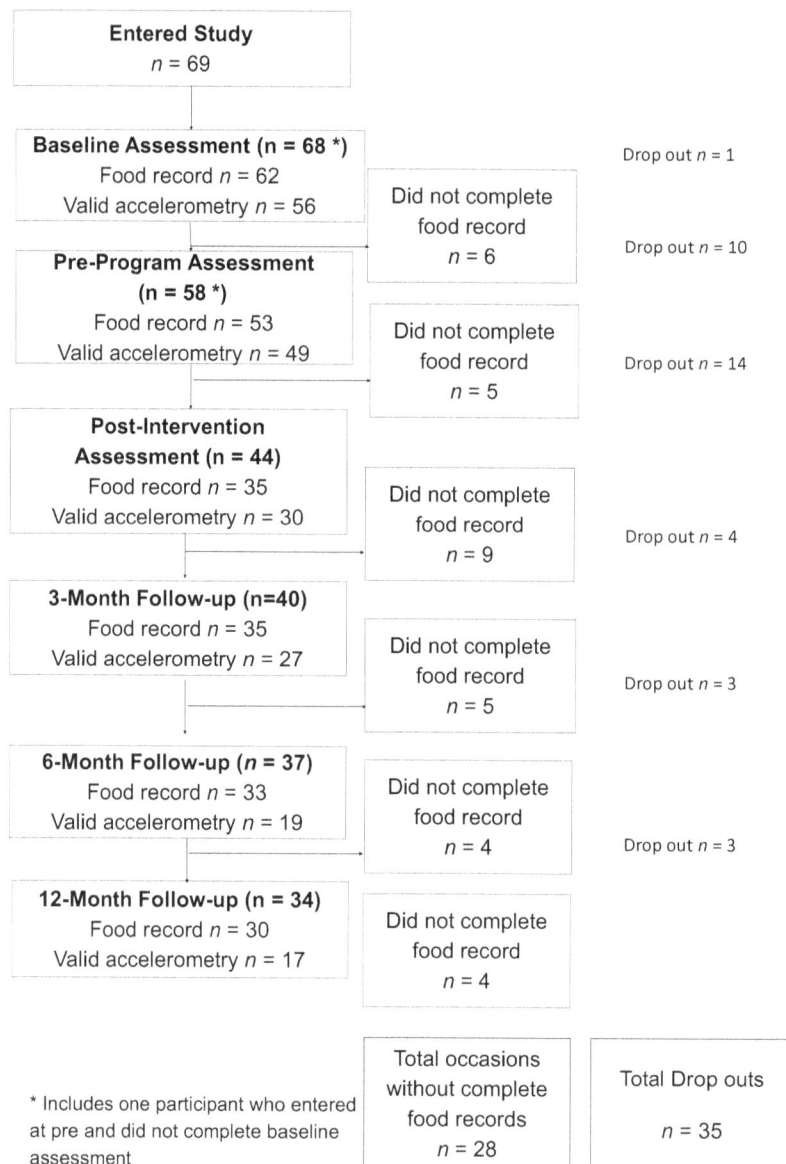

**Figure 1.** Participant numbers and food record completion during the waitlist controlled trial of Curtin University's Activity, Food, and Attitudes Program.

## 2.4. Dietary Intervention

The dietary component of the intervention was facilitated by Accredited Practising Dietitians. Delivery style was guided by self-determination theory and goal setting theory, in line with the theoretical underpinnings of the intervention [23]. The dietary component focused on food groups rather than kilojoule intakes or specific nutrients. Participants learnt skills to help them make healthy food choices and were not provided with structured meal plans as recent evidence suggests that these are not well-received by adolescents [24]. The three primary nutrition intervention messages were: Eat more fruit; eat more vegetables; eat less junk food. The term 'junk food' is used to describe 'discretionary' foods that are considered energy-dense, nutrient-poor foods [25–27]. The dietary intervention consisted of 12 group education sessions with parents and adolescents together regarding general nutrition, energy balance, food labelling, diet variety, fast food, lunch box food, portion size and recipe modification, with the key messages reinforced in each session. Parents were also given practical training in buying healthy food during a supermarket visit and both parents and adolescents were involved in cooking classes focusing on the preparation of healthy foods containing fruits and vegetables. Tailored feedback on the adolescents' diet, taken from the initial three day food record, was provided to each participant to assist with adolescent goal setting.

## 2.5. Dietary Assessment

### 2.5.1. Nutrient Intake

Three day food records were used in this study to provide comprehensive descriptive information about meal patterns and intake of foods and beverages without extensive reliance on participant memory [28]. Records were completed at all six assessment points and used to assess changes in adolescent dietary intake. Three days provides a reasonable compromise between understanding the variation in daily adolescent diets [29] and the risk of poor quality information due to excessive participant burden [30,31]. Prior to completing the food record, adolescents were given training and written instructions from the research dietitian regarding estimating portion size and household measures. The adolescents were interviewed by the research dietitian to verify the completeness of the record and to probe for any forgotten food or beverages. Figure 1 shows the number of adolescents who actually completed food records at each time point. The food records were perceived by the adolescents as a burden to complete, and thus a small financial incentive was offered for detailed records. It is commonly accepted that adolescents lack motivation to complete food records and find them tedious to complete [30], so the relatively low numbers of non-completers is a positive outcome.

Food records were analyzed using the NUTTAB 2010 and AUSNUT 2007 databases (FoodWorks Professional, Version 6, 2009; Xyris Software, Brisbane, Australia) for total energy, macronutrients and percentage contribution to energy intake, as well as intake of calcium and fiber. A food group analysis was also undertaken. Serving sizes for fruits and vegetables were derived from the Australian Guide to Healthy Eating, which specify that one serve of fruit is equivalent to 150 g and one serve of vegetables is equivalent to 75 g [27]. Servings of junk food (energy-dense, nutrient poor food) were equivalent to approximately 600 kilojoules [27]. For each participant, an average serve per day was calculated for fruits, vegetables and total junk food. The research dietitian completed all training, interviews and analysis of the food records.

### 2.5.2. Adherence to Intervention Messages

Adherence to the dietary intervention was measured by the percentage of participants who increased their intake of fruit and vegetables by at least 0.25 serves per day and reduced their intake of junk food by at least 0.5 serves per day, in line with the key dietary intervention messages. This was measured immediately post-intervention and 12 months post-intervention, using the data from three day food records. There is no accepted definition of a clinically important change in servings of key food groups, so this magnitude of change was chosen to reflect at least a 10% change in servings. This reflects the expected changes in physical activity and dietary behaviors following intervention as described in the protocol paper [20].

### 2.5.3. Eating Behaviors

A short food behavior questionnaire based on validated questionnaires used in similar cohorts [32,33] was used to assess eating behaviors likely to be related to obesity. Questions included frequency of breakfast consumption, frequency of fast food consumption, frequency of eating meals as a family and sugar sweetened beverage consumption. Participants responded to questions about eating behavior frequency using a 5 point scale: Every day, 5–6 days per week, 3–4 days per week, 1–2 days per week, rarely or never. Questions regarding perceived intake of fruit, vegetables and junk food asked for the usual number of serves consumed each day, based on standard Australian serving size descriptions [27].

### 2.6. Statistical Analysis

Data were visually inspected for potential outliers and checks completed for individual data entry errors or implausible values. Tests for normality were conducted using histograms. Descriptive statistics at each assessment point are presented as mean ± standard deviations (SD). $t$-Tests were used to compare participants who completed the program with those who dropped out. All participants who participated in at least two occasions of data collection were included in the analysis. Adherence data is presented with additional separate results for those who completed all six occasions of data collection.

There is a high likelihood of underreporting by overweight and obese adolescents with food records [34,35]. In this study, implausible food records were identified using the ratio of energy intake (EI) to total energy expenditure (TEE) as a time-varying covariate [36] in the mixed model described below. Total energy expenditure was estimated using resting energy expenditure (REE) estimation equations [37] and activity energy expenditure (AEE) based on objectively measured accelerometry [38]. Where accelerometer data was unavailable (62 of 248 occasions) TEE was estimated as 0.0149 kcal/kg/min, based on the estimation equation validated by Puyau, Adolph, Vohra, Zakeri and Butte [38]. Underreporting (EI:TEE) was used as a time-varying covariate in the analysis of the self-reported questionnaire data and the dietary intake data from the food records.

Change in eating behaviors and dietary intake analysis: Linear mixed models were used to assess within-person changes in nutrient and eating behavior outcomes at the time points following conclusion of the eight-week intervention. Models included random intercepts to account for the within-person repeated measures. Slight deviations from normality were accounted for using bootstrapped resampling to estimate standard errors with 1000 replications. Underreporting ratios were included (EI:TEE) as time-varying covariates. To account for differences in the time between assessments, the monthly rate of change during each period was compared. The rate of change was calculated for the waitlist period (baseline to pre-intervention) and compared to the rate of change in outcome variables for all assessment periods between pre-intervention and 12 months post-intervention to assess intervention effectiveness. The analysis was completed using Stata/IC 13.0 for Windows (StataCorp LP, College Station TX, USA) and results were considered statistically significant at $p < 0.05$. No adjustment was made for multiple comparisons but 95% confidence intervals and $p$-values to three decimals places are reported.

## 3. Results

Based on the number of adolescents participating at each assessment point, a total of 281 diet records were possible. However, only 248 (88.3%) diet records were completed over the 17 months of data collection and were thus available for analysis. Following the intervention, participants increased their intake of fruit and reduced their intake of junk food as measured by three day food records, but vegetable intake did not change significantly [39]. As shown in Figure 1, 25 participants dropped out of the study between baseline and post-intervention and a further eight participants did not complete food records. This is similar to the relatively high dropout rates typically reported for healthy lifestyle programs aimed at overweight young people [40]. There were no differences at baseline between completers and non-completers, as discussed in the associated primary outcomes paper [39].

## 3.1. Adherence to Intervention Messages

Data from the post-intervention food records showed 21 out of 35 participants who completed the eight week program adhered to the dietary intervention messages by increasing their fruit intake by at least 0.25 of a serve from pre-intervention levels. For vegetables, 17 out of 35 participants who completed the program increased their intake by at least 0.25 of a serve and 24 out of 35 participants reduced their junk food intake by at least 0.5 of a serve. The rate of adherence was reduced at 12 months post-intervention (see Figure 2).

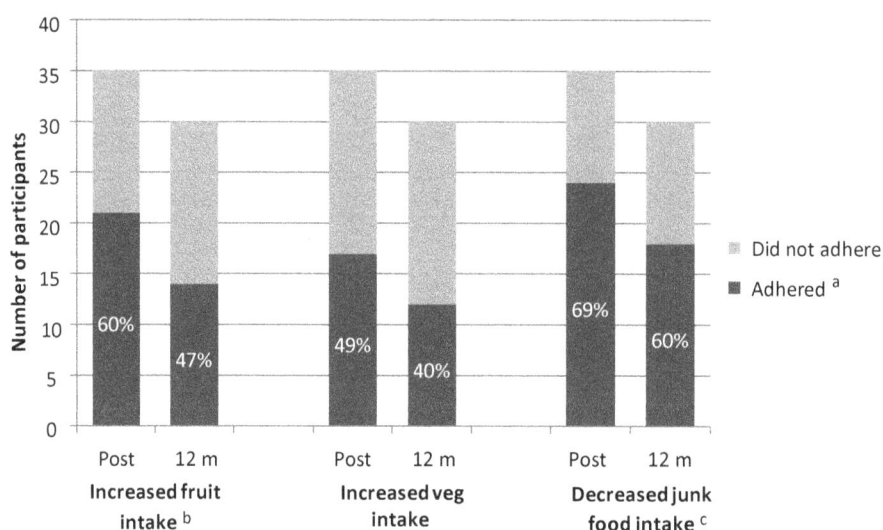

**Figure 2.** Adherence to the key CAFAP intervention messages regarding increasing intake of fruit and vegetables and decreasing intake of junk food in a group of 35 overweight adolescents. [a] Adherence data taken from three day food records; [b] An increased intake was defined as in increase in fruit or vegetable consumption by at least 0.25 servings; [c] A reduced intake was defined as a reduction in junk food consumption by at least 0.5 servings.

Of the 24 participants who had complete data at both time points, 13 adhered to the fruit message at post-intervention and 10 adhered at 12 months post-intervention. Similarly, 12 of 24 participants adhered to the vegetable message at post-intervention and 10 participants adhered at 12 months post-intervention. For junk food, 18 of 24 participants adhered by reducing their junk food intake and 14 adhered at 12 months post-intervention. Adherence to the 'reduce your junk food intake' message had the highest proportion of adherence across the measurement period, followed by 'increase your fruit intake' and lastly 'increase your vegetable intake'.

## 3.2. Eating Behaviors

The changes in self-reported eating behaviors at each time point and the monthly rate of change over each assessment period can be seen in Table 1. As expected, self-reported dietary behaviors were stable during the waitlist period (between baseline and pre-intervention). Significant improvements in frequency of breakfast consumption were reported between pre-intervention and three months post-intervention (estimated change 0.4 points, 95% CI: 0.12, 0.83). Reductions in reported fast food consumption were significantly different to pre-intervention levels at 3 months (−0.20 points, CI: −0.38, −0.02), six months (−0.24 points, CI: −0.41, −0.06) and 12 months post-intervention (−0.28 points, CI: −0.52. −0.03). Similarly, the frequency of sugar sweetened beverage consumption was significantly less than pre-intervention at six months (−0.41 points, CI: −0.71, −0.10) and 12 months post-intervention (−0.53 points, CI: −0.91, 0.15). The monthly rate of change for fast food and sugar sweetened beverage consumption did not differ from the monthly change observed during the waitlist period. Self-reported changes in fruit and vegetable consumption from the eating behavior questionnaire suggested significant increases in intake at each time point following intervention (see Table 1), although no changes were detected in reported junk food intake. The rate of change of consumption measured during the intervention period was significantly different to the waitlist period for fruit (0.17 servings per day/month, CI: 0.06, 0.28) and vegetables (0.25 servings per day/month, CI: 0.07, 0.42). Changes in the frequency of dinner consumption showed a significant monthly improvement between six and 12 months (0.04 points/month, CI: 0.01, 0.07). There were no changes detected for frequency of eating dinner as a family or eating dinner in front of the television.

## 3.3. Detailed Nutrient Intakes

The changes in nutrient intake at each time point and the monthly rate of change over each assessment period can be seen in Table 3. During the waitlist period there were no changes in energy, fat or saturated fat intake, nor any changes in the percent of energy provided by fat, saturated fat or protein. Intake of key micronutrients (zinc, calcium, iron, Vitamin C) did not change over the waitlist period. There was a reported increase in consumption of protein (69.1, SE 1.4 g/day to 74.5, SE 1.8 g/day, $p = 0.029$), and reduction in consumption of carbohydrates (202.1, SE 3.6 g/day to 188.9, SE 3.9 g/day, $p = 0.028$) and sugar (88.4, SE 3.5 g/day to 76.2, SE 3.2 g/day, $p = 0.018$) during the waitlist period. A reduction in the percent total energy provided by carbohydrates was also observed (46.6%, SE 0.6% to 44.6%, SE 0.7%, $p = 0.046$).

**Table 1.** Mean self-reported eating behavior point estimates and rates of change across intervention and follow up in a cohort of 58 overweight adolescents.

| | | Mean (SE) * | Period of Change | Mean Δ per Month (95% CI) | p-value Compared to Baseline to Pre [d] |
|---|---|---|---|---|---|
| Frequency of breakfast | Baseline | 3.0 (0.1) | | | |
| | Pre | 2.9 (0.1) | Baseline to Pre | −0.03 (−0.13, 0.08) | ref |
| | Post | 3.1 (0.1) | Pre to Post | 0.13 (−0.04, 0.29) | 0.208 |
| | 3 months | 3.4 (0.1) [a,b] | Post to 3 m | 0.07 (−0.03, 0.18) | 0.180 |
| | 6 months | 3.2 (0.2) | 3 m to 6 m | −0.05 (−0.18, 0.08) | 0.793 |
| | 12 months | 2.8 (0.2) | 6 m to 12 m | 0.07 (−0.14, −0.004) [c] | 0.475 |
| | Maintenance | | Post-12 m | −0.03 (−0.06, 0) | 0.958 |
| Frequency of fast food | Baseline | 0.6 (0.05) | | | |
| | Pre | 0.5 (0.1) | Baseline to Pre | −0.01 (−0.06, 0.04) | ref |
| | Post | 0.4 (0.1) | Pre to Post | −0.05 (−0.15, 0.06) | 0.578 |
| | 3 months | 0.3 (0.1) [a,b] | Post to 3 m | −0.03 (−0.11, 0.05) | 0.639 |
| | 6 months | 0.3 (0.1) [a,b] | 3 m to 6 m | −0.01 (−0.08, 0.05) | 0.972 |
| | 12 months | 0.3 (0.1) [a,b] | 6 m to 12 m | −0.01 (−0.05, 0.04) | 0.881 |
| | Maintenance | | | −0.01 (−0.04, 0.01) | 0.907 |
| Frequency of sweetened beverages | Baseline | 1.5 (0.1) | | | |
| | Pre | 1.3 (0.1) | Baseline to Pre | −0.04 (−0.13, 0.05) | ref |
| | Post | 1.1 (0.1) [a] | Pre to Post | −0.14 (−0.03, 0.03) | 0.353 |
| | 3 months | 1.1 (0.1) [a] | Post to 3 m | 0.01 (−0.10, 0.12) | 0.521 |
| | 6 months | 0.9 (0.1) [a,b] | 3 m to 6 m | −0.06 (−0.17, 0.07) | 0.800 |
| | 12 months | 0.8 (0.1) [a,b] | 6 m to 12 m | −0.02 (−0.09, 0.05) | 0.759 |
| | Maintenance | | Post to 12 m | −0.02 (−0.05, 0.01) | 0.741 |
| Perceived daily fruit serves | Baseline | 1.6 (0.1) | | | |
| | Pre | 1.5 (0.1) | Baseline to Pre | −0.03 (−0.10, 0.04) | ref |
| | Post | 1.9 (0.1) [a,b] | Pre to Post | 0.17 (0.06, 0.28) [c] | 0.011 |
| | 3 months | 1.8 (0.1) [b] | Post to 3 m | −0.02 (−0.10, 0.06) | 0.892 |
| | 6 months | 1.8 (0.1) [b] | 3 m to 6 m | −0.01 (−0.09, 0.06) | 0.785 |
| | 12 months | 1.9 (0.1) [b] | 6 m to 12 m | 0.01 (−0.04, 0.06) | 0.333 |
| | Maintenance | | Post to 12 m | 0 (−0.03, 0.02) | 0.476 |
| Perceived daily vegetable serves | Baseline | 2.5 (0.1) | | | |
| | Pre | 2.4 (0.1) | Baseline to Pre | −0.03 (−0.13, 0.07) | ref |
| | Post | 2.9 (0.1) [a,b] | Pre to Post | 0.25 (0.07, 0.42) [c] | 0.022 |
| | 3 months | 3.0 (0.1) [a,b] | Post to 3 m | 0.02 (−0.11, 0.15) | 0.557 |
| | 6 months | 3.1 (0.1) [a,b] | 3 m to 6 m | 0.05 (−0.08, 0.17) | 0.351 |
| | 12 months | 3.3 (0.2) [a,b] | 6 m to 12 m | 0.03 (−0.05, 0.11) | 0.348 |
| | Maintenance | | Post to 12 m | 0.03 (−0.01, 0.08) | 0.272 |
| Perceived daily junk food serves | Baseline | 1.6 (0.1) | | | |
| | Pre | 1.7 (0.1) | Baseline to Pre | 0.03 (−0.08, 0.15) | ref |
| | Post | 1.5 (0.1) | Pre to Post | −0.07 (−0.21, 0.06) | 0.331 |
| | 3 months | 1.4 (0.1) | Post to 3 m | −0.03 (−0.13, 0.07) | 0.437 |
| | 6 months | 1.5 (0.1) | 3 m to 6 m | 0.07 (−0.04, 0.19) | 0.617 |
| | 12 months | 1.6 (0.2) | 6 m to 12 m | −0.01 (−0.08, 0.06) | 0.551 |
| | Maintenance | | Post to 12 m | 0.01 (−0.03, 0.04) | 0.667 |

* SE is standard error; ref is the reference period; [a] Difference from baseline ($p < 0.05$); [b] difference from pre ($p < 0.05$); [c] significant rate of change between the two assessment points ($p < 0.05$); [d] This column identifies significant differences ($p < 0.05$) in the rate of change between the time period being measured and the waitlist control period (baseline to pre-intervention); Maintenance: The period between post-intervention and 12 months post-intervention; $n = 58$.

**Table 2.** Mean nutrient intake (point estimates) and rates of change across intervention and follow up in a cohort of 58 overweight adolescents.

| | | Mean (SE) * | Period of Change | Mean Δ per Month (95% CI) | p-value Compared to Baseline to Pre [d] |
|---|---|---|---|---|---|
| Energy (kJ) | Baseline | 6969 (46.9) | | | |
| | Pre | 6972 (50.8) | Baseline to Pre | 1.0 (−50.5, 52.4) | ref |
| | Post | 6965 (60.0) | Pre to Post | −3.2 (−86.9, 80.3) | 0.942 |
| | 3 months | 6946 (58.2) | Post to 3 m | −6.7 (−58.4, 45.0) | 0.834 |
| | 6 months | 6987 (68.2) | 3 m to 6 m | 13.9 (−43.1, 71.0) | 0.745 |
| | 12 months | 7133 (86.0) | 6 m to 12 m | 24.2 (−10.4, 58.8) | 0.473 |
| | Maintenance | | Post to 12 m | 13.9 (−2.2, 30.0) | 0.644 |
| Protein (g) | Baseline | 69.1 (1.4) | | | |
| | Pre | 74.5 (1.8) [a] | Baseline to Pre | 1.8 (0.2, 3.4) [c] | ref |
| | Post | 75.3 (2.3) [a] | Pre to Post | 0.4 (−2.7, 3.4) | 0.489 |
| | 3 months | 76.1 (2.1) [a] | Post to 3 m | 0.3 (−1.7, 2.2) | 0.213 |
| | 6 months | 76.6 (2.2) [a] | 3 m to 6 m | 0.2 (−1.7, 2.0) | 0.189 |
| | 12 months | 72.2 (2.5) [a] | 6 m to 12 m | −0.7 (−1.8, 0.4) | 0.010 |
| | Maintenance | . | Post to 12 m | −0.3 (−0.8, 0.3) | 0.015 |
| Fat (g) | Baseline | 63.4 (1.3) | | | |
| | Pre | 66.0 (1.3) | Baseline to Pre | 0.8 (−0.5, 2.2) | ref |
| | Post | 59.3 (1.6) [b] | Pre to Post | −3.3 (−5.4, −1.2) [c] | 0.005 |
| | 3 months | 62.6 (1.6) | Post to 3 m | 1.1 (−0.3, 2.5) | 0.800 |
| | 6 months | 62.8 (1.8) | 3 m to 6 m | 0.1 (−1.4, 1.5) | 0.432 |
| | 12 months | 64.7 (1.8) | 6 m to 12 m | 0.3 (−0.5, 1.1) | 0.489 |
| | Maintenance | | Post to 12m | 0.5 (0.1, 0.8) [c] | 0.568 |
| Saturated fat (g) | Baseline | 26.9 (0.8) | | | |
| | Pre | 27.5 (0.8) | Baseline to Pre | 0.2 (−0.6, 0.9) | ref |
| | Post | 23.6 (0.9) [a b] | Pre to Post | −2.0 (−3.1, −0.8) [c] | 0.011 |
| | 3 months | 25.4 (0.9) | Post to 3 m | 0.6 (−0.2, 1.4) | 0.416 |
| | 6 months | 25.8 (0.8) | 3 m to 6 m | 0.1 (−0.6, 0.9) | 0.939 |
| | 12 months | 26.5 (0.8) | 6 m to 12 m | 0.1 (−2.5, 0.4) | 0.854 |
| | Maintenance | | Post to 12 m | 0.2 (0.1, 0.4) [c] | 0.876 |
| Carbo-hydrate (g) | Baseline | 202.1 (3.6) [b] | | | |
| | Pre | 188.9 (3.9) [a] | Baseline to Pre | −4.4 (−8.3, −0.5) [c] | ref |
| | Post | 199.4 (4.8) [a] | Pre to Post | 5.2 (−1.3, 11.8) | 0.032 |
| | 3 months | 189.1 (4.0) [a b] | Post to 3 m | −3.4 (−7.6, 0.7) | 0.739 |
| | 6 months | 190.0 (5.4) [a b] | 3 m to 6 m | 0.3 (−3.8, 4.4) | 0.110 |
| | 12 months | 196.1 (4.7) [a b] | 6 m to 12 m | 1.0 (−1.1, 3.2) | 0.018 |
| | Maintenance | | Post to 12 m | −0.3 (−1.3, 0.8) | 0.048 |
| Sugar (g) | Baseline | 88.4 (3.5) | | | |
| | Pre | 76.2 (3.2) [a] | Baseline to Pre | −4.1 (−7.5, −0.7) [c] | ref |
| | Post | 83.6 (5.5) | Pre to Post | 3.7 (−2.9, 10.4) | 0.066 |
| | 3 months | 81.3 (4.1) | Post to 3 m | −0.8 (−5.3, 3.8) | 0.250 |
| | 6 months | 77.4 (4.9) | 3 m to 6 m | −1.3 (−5.3, 2.7) | 0.300 |
| | 12 months | 82.7 (4.6) | 6 m to 12 m | 0.9 (−1.2, 3.0) | 0.014 |
| | Maintenance | | Post to 12 m | −0.1 (−1.1, 1.0) | 0.027 |
| Fiber (g) | Baseline | 16.1 (0.4) | | | |
| | Pre | 15.2 (0.5) | Baseline to Pre | −0.3 (−0.7, 0.1) | ref |
| | Post | 16.8 (0.5) [b] | Pre to Post | 0.8 (0.1, 1.4) [c] | 0.017 |
| | 3 months | 16.8 (0.6) [b] | Post to 3 m | 0 (−0.5, 0.5) | 0.326 |
| | 6 months | 18.4 (0.8) [a b] | 3 m to 6 m | 0.5 (−0.03, 1.1) | 0.016 |
| | 12 months | 17.1 (0.6) [b] | 6 m to 12 m | −0.2 (−0.5, 0.1) | 0.692 |
| | Maintenance | | Post to 12 m | 0.03 (−0.1, 0.2) | 0.123 |

**Table 3.** Mean nutrient intake (point estimates) and rates of change across intervention and follow up in a cohort of 58 overweight adolescents.

| | | Mean (SE) * | Period of Change | Mean Δ per Month (95% CI) | p-value Compared to Baseline to Pre [d] |
|---|---|---|---|---|---|
| kJ from protein (%) | Baseline | 17.5 (0.3) | | | |
| | Pre | 18.4 (0.4) | Baseline to Pre | 0.3 (−0.04, 0.7) | ref |
| | Post | 19.1 (0.5) [a] | Pre to Post | 0.4 (−0.3, 1.1) | 0.869 |
| | 3 months | 19.2 (0.5) [a] | Post to 3 m | 0.02 (−0.4, 0.5) | 0.327 |
| | 6 months | 19.4 (0.5) [a] | 3 m to 6 m | 0.05 (−0.4, 0.5) | 0.364 |
| | 12 months | 18.2 (0.6) | 6 m to 12 m | −0.2 (−0.5, 0.1) | 0.022 |
| | Maintenance | | Post to 12 m | −0.1 (−0.2, 0.05) | 0.037 |
| kJ from fat (%) | Baseline | 33.1 (0.6) | | | |
| | Pre | 34.8 (0.6) | Baseline to Pre | 0.5 (−0.04, 1.1) | ref |
| | Post | 31.2 (0.8) [b] | Pre to Post | −1.7 (−2.7, −0.8) [c] | 0.001 |
| | 3 months | 33.9 (0.8) | Post to 3 m | 0.9 (0.1, 1.6) [c] | 0.471 |
| | 6 months | 33.5 (1.0) | 3 m to 6 m | −0.1 (−1.0, 0.7) | 0.212 |
| | 12 months | 34.1 (1.0) | 6 m to 12 m | 0.1 (−0.4, 0.5) | 0.224 |
| | Maintenance | | Post to 12 m | 0.2 (0.05, 0.4) [c] | 0.343 |
| kJ from sat fat (%) | Baseline | 14.0 (0.4) | | | |
| | Pre | 14.4 (0.3) | Baseline to Pre | 0.1 (−0.2, 0.4) | ref |
| | Post | 12.3 (0.4) [a b] | Pre to Post | −1.1 (−1.6, −0.5) [c] | 0.002 |
| | 3 months | 13.8 (0.5) | Post to 3 m | 0.5 (0.1, 1.0) [c] | 0.146 |
| | 6 months | 13.8 (0.4) | 3 m to 6 m | 0.02 (−0.5, 0.5) | 0.706 |
| | 12 months | 14.0 (0.4) | 6 m to 12 m | 0.03 (−0.2, 0.2) | 0.611 |
| | Maintenance | | Post to 12 m | 0.1 (0.1, 0.2) [c] | 0.902 |
| kJ from Carbo-hydrate (%) | Baseline | 46.6 (0.6) | | | |
| | Pre | 44.6 (0.7) [a] | Baseline to Pre | −0.7 (−1.3, −0.01) [c] | ref |
| | Post | 47.0 (1.0) | Pre to Post | 1.2 (−0.1, 2.5) | 0.032 |
| | 3 months | 44.0 (0.9) [a] | Post to 3 m | −1.0 (−2.0, −0.1) [c] | 0.547 |
| | 6 months | 44.3 (1.0) | 3 m to 6 m | 0.1 (−0.8, 1.0) | 0.164 |
| | 12 months | 44.7 (1.2) | 6 m to 12 m | 0.1 (−0.5, 0.6) | 0.093 |
| | Maintenance | | Post to 12 m | −0.2 (−0.5, 0.1) | 0.181 |
| Calcium (mg) | Baseline | 601.8 (22.8) | | | |
| | Pre | 598.9 (25.0) | Baseline to Pre | −1.0 (−24.9, 22.9) | ref |
| | Post | 606.2 (25.5) | Pre to Post | 3.6 (−33.5, 40.7) | 0.864 |
| | 3 months | 663.6 (30.5) | Post to 3 m | 19.1 (−6.5, 44.7) | 0.255 |
| | 6 months | 646.6 (37.9) | 3 m to 6 m | −5.7 (−35.2, 23.9) | 0.811 |
| | 12 months | 663.9 (34.0) | 6 m to 12 m | 2.9 (−13.8, 19.5) | 0.784 |
| | Maintenance | | Post to 12 m | 4.8 (−1.9, 11.5) | 0.635 |

* SE is standard error; ref is the reference period; [a] Difference from baseline (p < 0.05); [b] difference from pre (p < 0.05); [c] significant rate of change between the two assessment points (p < 0.05); [d] This column identifies significant differences (p < 0.05) in the rate of change between the time period being measured and the waitlist control period (baseline to pre-intervention); Maintenance: The period between post-intervention and 12 months post-intervention; n = 58.

Following the eight-week intervention, there was a significant reduction in point estimates of fat (66.0, SE 1.3 g/day to 59.3, SE 1.6 g/day, p = 0.002) and saturated fat consumption (27.5, SE 0.8 g/day to 23.6, SE 0.9 g/day, p = 0.001). The rate of change of fat (−3.3 g per day per month, 95%CI: −5.4, −1.2, p = 0.005) and saturated fat consumption (−2.0 g per day per month, 95%CI: −3.1, −0.8, p = 0.011) was significantly improved from the rate of change during the waitlist period. A reduction in the percentage total energy provided by fat (34.8%, SE 0.6% to 31.2%, SE 0.8%, $p \leq 0.001$) and saturated fat (14.4%, SE 0.3% to 12.3%, SE 0.4%, $p \leq 0.001$) was also observed, along with a significantly improved monthly rate of change during the intervention period compared to the waitlist period (see Table 3). There were no changes in energy, protein or sugar intake during intervention. Point estimates of fiber were significantly increased (15.2, SE 0.5 g/day to 16.8, SE 0.6 g/day, $p = 0.016$) and the monthly rate of change of fiber (0.8 g per day per month, 95%CI: 0.1, 1.4, $p = 0.017$) was significantly more than that observed during the waitlist period.

During the 12-month maintenance period nutrient intakes appeared to regress towards baseline levels (see Table 3). Point estimates of fat and saturated fat between three and 12 months post-intervention were no longer different to pre-intervention levels. The percent energy provided by macronutrients during the maintenance period was not different to pre-intervention distributions. There was a significant increase in the percent of energy provided by fat between post-intervention and three months post-intervention (31.2, SE 0.8% to 33.9 SE 0.8%, $p = 0.022$) with a significant increase in the monthly rate of change ($p = 0.002$). Total carbohydrate intake did remain lower than pre-intervention levels throughout the 12 month maintenance period and fiber intake remained significantly higher than pre-intervention levels (see Table 3). Energy, protein and sugar intake did not change during the maintenance period, nor did intakes of calcium, zinc or vitamin C.

## 4. Discussion

This study provides unique data on adherence to the dietary component of a multi-component intervention in obese adolescents and is one of the few adolescent intervention studies to consider eating behavior and dietary intake changes in the 12 month period following intervention. Further, this study used three day food records to provide detailed dietary change data for overweight adolescents. The main findings were that a large proportion of participants adhered to the key components of the dietary intervention, with modest dietary changes seen following intervention and lessening over time.

### 4.1. Adherence

More than half of the 35 participants who completed this study adhered to the key intervention messages about eating more fruit and vegetables and eating less junk food, but the percentage who adhered reduced over time. There is a lack of prior studies in overweight adolescents that incorporated any measures of adherence to dietary interventions, preventing comparisons to these results [18]. This gap in adherence measurement has begun to be addressed in this study by using data from detailed food records to measure adherence to the CAFAP dietary intervention messages. The methods used have been developed to suit the study given the lack of previous reporting of adherence in overweight adolescent interventions and the absence of guidelines regarding the best way to measure or report dietary adherence in intervention studies [41].The interpretation of the adherence levels in this study is further limited by the lack of evidence regarding what constitutes satisfactory levels of adherence. Previous studies have identified a range of 80%–120% of recommended nutrient intakes as an indicator of adherence [42]. This method was not appropriate in the current study, given that adolescents were encouraged to improve their intake rather than achieve ideal but perhaps unrealistic diet goals. Other methods from previous research measuring dichotomous variables were not applicable due to the multi-factorial nature of diet. Thus, the adherence reported in this paper relates to the proportion of participants who have adhered to the different dietary change messages. Future interventions can compare their findings to these levels of adherence and work towards a clear consensus for acceptable levels of adherence to dietary interventions based on observed changes in health status.

Behavior change as a result of the CAFAP dietary intervention was assessed by adherence to the CAFAP dietary intervention messages. It was hypothesized that targeting and improving key theoretical constructs, such as motivation and parent support, would lead to dietary behavior change [43] based on self-determination and goal setting theories [23]. However, exploratory post hoc analysis did not support this relationship. When autonomous motivation for healthy eating and perceived parental support for healthy eating were compared between those who adhered to key dietary messages and those did not adhere, there were no significant differences between those groups at either post-intervention or 12-months post-intervention. Due to the limited sample size, it was not possible to complete a full mediation analysis; however, future research should include mediation analyses of the theoretical constructs to help explain the mechanisms for successful behavior change.

## 4.2. Eating Behaviors

There were some changes in self-reported eating behaviors during the maintenance period including increased consumption of breakfast and reduced consumption of fast food and SSBs. CAFAP participants reported changes in line with prior studies of overweight adolescents, in both fast food intake [44] and SSB intake [45]. Whilst these behavior changes remained significant for CAFAP participants during the maintenance period, comparisons of sustained change are limited as no other studies have reported general eating behavior changes for at least 12 months following intervention. Thus, these findings add much-needed data to the limited evidence base around overweight adolescent eating behaviors, and provide an example of how these may change following intervention.

## 4.3. Nutrient Intakes

The modest dietary changes observed in this study, reductions in fat and saturated fat and an increase in fiber; reflect the current evidence from obesity interventions. CAFAP participants reported no changes in total energy intake compared to the waitlist control period, reflecting other recent trials where energy intake did not differ from the control comparison [14,45–48]. A recent trial demonstrated significant reductions in adolescent energy, fat and saturated fat consumption immediately post-intervention, but did not include any control group or waitlist comparison [16]. A significant reduction in adolescent total fat intake has also been previously reported, but based on a brief questionnaire not yet validated in adolescents [12]. Neither of these studies adjusted for underreporting and neither showed a reduction in percentage of total energy provided by fat as CAFAP did, which is thought to be a more reliable measure than absolute fat intake [49]. In a study of Latino adolescents, participants reported significant reductions in total sugar intake in one of two intervention groups immediately post-intervention [19], although these results may not be generalizable given both groups had received the same nutrition component of the intervention. There were no changes in reported sugar consumption following the CAFAP intervention.

Further, findings showed micronutrient levels did not change throughout the study. This suggests that CAFAP did not have a deleterious effect on nutritional intake throughout the study period. Similar results have been found in other studies with some measure of nutrient intake, with no reductions in key nutrients following intervention [16,45,50]. Calcium intake, important for growth and development, was consistently low throughout the current study (~600–650 mg), which might suggest an important potential target for future dietary interventions for adolescents.

The gradual pattern for macronutrient intake levels to regress towards baseline intake levels over the 12 month maintenance period may reflect the waning adherence to CAFAP nutrition intervention messages. This pattern was also reflected in the regression of physical activity changes [39]. The loss of changes occurred alongside the tapering maintenance support provided to adolescents, aspects of which were not well-received in the initial three months post-intervention [51]. This might suggest that future programs would benefit from more intensive support over 12 months, possibly using a mode of contact other than text messaging. Despite a loss of positive changes in macronutrient intakes during the maintenance period, these levels did not worsen from baseline levels. Future trials should monitor long-term dietary changes to understand how well dietary change is sustained, and plan maintenance support programs accordingly.

## 4.4. Dietary Assessment Methods

In this study, adolescents rated their own intake of fruits and vegetables differently using the short food behavior questionnaire compared to how they recorded their intake using a three day food record. Despite the reducing levels of adherence and modest changes in diet, as shown by the food records, the estimates of fruit and vegetable intake from the eating behavior questionnaire remained significantly increased following intervention for the entire 12 month maintenance period. For example, the food records showed no change in vegetable intake following intervention but the short questionnaire showed an increase of vegetable intake during the maintenance period of up to 0.9 serves at 12 months post-intervention. Thus, it seems that the food behavior questionnaire may have overestimated the effect of the intervention on intakes as compared to the food records, particularly for vegetables. This discrepancy may be due to a desire to report socially acceptable intakes in line with the CAFAP key messages [52], particularly given that all changes occurred after the intervention had been delivered. The wording of the questions directly reflected the nutrition intervention messages, so adolescents may have felt obliged to show they had adhered. Alternatively the participants may have truly believed that they were eating more healthfully. The differences in self-reported behaviors from questionnaire and self-reported intake from food records highlight the inherent difficulties in obtaining consistent and accurate nutrition data in this population.

## 4.5. Strengths and Limitations

The strengths of the study include the use of multiple dietary assessment measures, detailed description of obese adolescent dietary change following intervention, detailed maintenance dietary data for a further 12 months and adjustments for the impact of underreporting. The use of objective accelerometry data in the estimation of total energy expenditure provides added confidence in the adjustment for underreporting. Three day food records were used in this study to provide detailed information about consumption patterns, including timing of meals [53], without being limited by extensive reliance on memory and time available for physical assessment. Although three day food records have known limitations with potential underreporting, in this study we were able to use underreporting as a covariate to control for the effect of underreporting on the dietary outcomes, giving greater confidence in the results. Aside from the limitations associated with any assessment of self-reported diet, other limitations included a relatively small sample size. Due to recruitment difficulties and issues with retention in the study, 69 participants were included in the sample size at baseline, which is less than initially planned. There were further issues with drop outs during the study, although the attrition rate of 51% is in line with other recent pediatric weight management literature [40]. The proportionately low numbers of male participants in this study reduces the generalizability of these findings. Additional studies are needed to replicate these findings in diverse populations.

## 5. Conclusions

This is one of the first studies to report overweight and obese adolescent adherence to the dietary component of a multi-component lifestyle intervention. Findings showed that adherence rates were highest for CAFAP messages about reducing junk food. Overweight and obese adolescents who participated in CAFAP reported modest improvements in some key eating behaviors and nutrient intakes, although this differed between methods of dietary assessment. The brief eating behavior questionnaire gave a potentially more positive impression about the adolescent dietary response to intervention, and so this data should be viewed with caution. Future studies with overweight and obese adolescents should report adherence to dietary interventions and use standardized and practical methods for assessing and controlling for underreporting. These data provide evidence to support the call for more comprehensive and long-term reporting of dietary intake in obese adolescent interventions to better understand dietary changes in this group and, thus, guide the design of effective interventions.

**Acknowledgments:** This trial was funded by a Healthway Health Promotion Research Project Grant #19938. Leon Straker was supported by a National Health and Medical Research Council senior research fellowship. No funding or other input to the study was received from any pharmaceutical company. The authors would like to thank the adolescents who shared their valuable time to complete the food records.

**Author Contributions:** Kyla L. Smith reviewed the food records, conducted the dietary analysis and drafted the manuscript. Deborah A. Kerr advised on the dietary analysis. Erin K. Howie contributed to the analysis and interpretation of the results. Leon M. Straker conceived the study, and participated in its design and coordination. All authors read and approved the final manuscript.

**Conflicts of Interest:** The authors declare no conflict of interest.

## References

1. Maggio, A.B.; Martin, X.E.; Saunders Gasser, C.; Gal-Duding, C.; Beghetti, M.; Farpour-Lambert, N.J.; Chamay-Weber, C. Medical and non-medical complications among children and adolescents with excessive body weight. *BMC Pediatr.* **2014**, *14*, 232.

2. Trasande, L.; Chatterjee, S. The impact of obesity on health service utilization and costs in childhood. *Obesity* **2009**, *17*, 1749–1754.

3. Barlow, S.E. Expert committee recommendations regarding the prevention, assessment, and treatment of child and adolescent overweight and obesity: Summary report. *Pediatrics* **2007**, *120*, S164–S192.

4. Oude Luttikhuis, H.; Baur, L.; Jansen, H.; Shrewsbury, V.A.; O'Malley, C.; Stolk, R.P.; Summerbell, C.D. Interventions for treating obesity in children. *Cochrane. Database Syst. Rev.* **2009**, *1*, CD001872.

5. Collins, C.E.; Warren, J.M.; Neve, M.; McCoy, P.; Stokes, B. Systematic review of interventions in the management of overweight and obese children which include a dietary component. *Int. J. Evid. Based Healthc.* **2007**, *5*, 2–53.

6. Ho, M.; Garnett, S.P.; Baur, L.; Burrows, T.; Stewart, L.; Neve, M.; Collins, C. Effectiveness of lifestyle interventions in child obesity: Systematic review with meta-analysis. *Pediatrics* **2012**, *130*, e1647–e1671.

7. Denney-Wilson, E.; Baur, L. Adolescent obesity: Making a difference to the epidemic. *Int. J. Adolesc. Med. Health* **2007**, *19*, 235–243.

8. Collins, C.E.; Warren, J.; Neve, M.; McCoy, P.; Stokes, B.J. Measuring effectiveness of dietetic interventions in child obesity: A systematic review of randomized trials. *Arch. Pediatr. Adolesc. Med.* **2006**, *160*, 906–922.

9. Savoye, M.; Nowicka, P.; Shaw, M.; Yu, S.; Dziura, J.; Chavent, G.; O'Malley, G.; Serrecchia, J.B.; Tamborlane, W.V.; Caprio, S. Long-term results of an obesity program in an ethnically diverse pediatric population. *Pediatrics* **2011**, *127*, 402–410.

10. Steele, R.G.; Aylward, B.S.; Jensen, C.D.; Cushing, C.C.; Davis, A.M.; Bovaird, J.A. Comparison of a family-based group intervention for youths with obesity to a brief individual family intervention: A practical clinical trial of positively fit. *J. Pediatr. Psychol.* **2012**, *37*, 53–63.

11. Davis, J.N.; Kelly, L.A.; Lane, C.J.; Ventura, E.E.; Byrd-Williams, C.E.; Alexandar, K.A.; Azen, S.P.; Chou, C.P.; Spruijt-Metz, D.; Weigensberg, M.J.; *et al.* Randomized control trial to improve adiposity and insulin resistance in overweight latino adolescents. *Obesity* **2009**, *17*, 1542–1548.

12. Shaibi, G.Q.; Konopken, Y.; Hoppin, E.; Keller, C.S.; Ortega, R.; Castro, F.G. Effects of a culturally grounded community-based diabetes prevention program for obese latino adolescents. *Diabetes Educ.* **2012**, *38*, 504–512.

13. Shrewsbury, V.; O'Connor, J.; Steinbeck, K.; Stevenson, K.; Lee, A.; Hill, A.; Kohn, M.; Shah, S.; Torvaldsen, S.; Baur, L. A randomised controlled trial of a community-based healthy lifestyle program for overweight and obese adolescents: The loozit® study protocol. *BMC Public Health* **2009**, *9*, 119.

14. Janicke, D.M.; Sallinen, B.J.; Perri, M.G.; Lutes, L.D.; Huerta, M.; Silverstein, J.H.; Brumback, B. Comparison of parent-only *vs* family-based interventions for overweight children in underserved rural settings: Outcomes from project story. *Arch. Pediatr. Adolesc. Med.* **2008**, *162*, 1119–1125.

15. Nguyen, B.; Shrewsbury, V.A.; O'Connor, J.; Steinbeck, K.S.; Hill, A.J.; Shah, S.; Kohn, M.R.; Torvaldsen, S.; Baur, L.A. Two-year outcomes of an adjunctive telephone coaching and electronic contact intervention for adolescent weight-loss maintenance: The loozit randomized controlled trial. *Int. J. Obes.* **2013**, *37*, 468–472.

16. Bean, M.K.; Mazzeo, S.E.; Stern, M.; Evans, R.K.; Bryan, D.; Ning, Y.; Wickham, E.P., III; Laver, J. Six-month dietary changes in ethnically diverse, obese adolescents participating in a multidisciplinary weight management program. *Clin. Pediatr.* **2011**, *50*, 408–416.

17. Heymsfield, S.B.; Harp, J.B.; Reitman, M.L.; Beetsch, J.W.; Schoeller, D.A.; Erondu, N.; Pietrobelli, A. Why do obese patients not lose more weight when treated with low-calorie diets? A mechanistic perspective. *Am. J. Clin. Nutr.* **2007**, *85*, 346–354.

18. Ho, M.; Garnett, S.P.; Baur, L.A.; Burrows, T.; Stewart, L.; Neve, M.; Collins, C. Impact of dietary and exercise interventions on weight change and metabolic outcomes in obese children and adolescents a systematic review and meta-analysis of randomized trials. *JAMA Pediatr.* **2013**, *167*, 759–768.

19. Davis, J.N.; Tung, A.; Chak, S.S.; Ventura, E.E.; Byrd-Williams, C.E.; Alexander, K.E.; Lane, C.J.; Weigensberg, M.J.; Spruijt-Metz, D.; Goran, M.I. Aerobic and strength training reduces adiposity in overweight latina adolescents. *Med. Sci. Sports Exerc.* **2009**, *41*, 1494–1503.

20. Straker, L.M.; Smith, K.L.; Fenner, A.A.; Kerr, D.A.; McManus, A.; Davis, M.C.; Fielding, A.M.; Olds, T.S.; Hagger, M.S.; Smith, A.J.; *et al.* Rationale, design and methods for a staggered-entry, waitlist controlled clinical trial of the impact of a community-based, family-centred, multidisciplinary program focussed on activity, food and attitude habits (curtin university's activity, food and attitudes program-cafap) among overweight adolescents. *BMC Public Health* **2012**, *12*, 471.

21. Warren, J.M.; Golley, R.K.; Collins, C.E.; Okely, A.D.; Jones, R.A.; Morgan, P.J.; Perry, R.A.; Baur, L.A.; Steele, J.R.; Magarey, A.M. Randomised controlled trials in overweight children: Practicalities and realities. *Int. J. Pediatr. Obes.* **2007**, *2*, 73–85.

22. Kuczmarski, R.J.; Ogden, C.L.; Grummer-Strawn, L.M.; Flegal, K.M.; Guo, S.S.; Wei, R.; Mei, Z.; Curtin, L.R.; Roche, A.F.; Johnson, C.L. CDC growth charts: United States. *Adv. Data.* **2000**, *314*, 1–27.

23. Fenner, A.A.; Straker, L.M.; Davis, M.C.; Hagger, M.S. Theoretical underpinnings of a need-supportive intervention to address sustained healthy lifestyle changes in overweight and obese adolescents. *Psychol. Sport Exerc.* **2013**, *14*, 819–829.

24. Savoye, M.; Shaw, M.; Dziura, J.; Tamborlane, W.V.; Rose, P.; Guandalini, C.; Goldberg-Gell, R.; Burgert, T.S.; Cali, A.M.; Weiss, R.; *et al.* Effects of a weight management program on body composition and metabolic parameters in overweight children: A randomized controlled trial. *JAMA* **2007**, *297*, 2697–2704.

25. Rangan, A.M.; Randall, D.; Hector, D.J.; Gill, T.P.; Webb, K.L. Consumption of "extra" foods by australian children: Types, quantities and contribution to energy and nutrient intakes. *Eur. J. Clin. Nutr.* **2008**, *62*, 356–364.

26. Dixon, H.G.; Scully, M.L.; Wakefield, M.A.; White, V.M.; Crawford, D.A. The effects of television advertisements for junk food versus nutritious food on children's food attitudes and preferences. *Soc. Sci. Med.* **2007**, *65*, 1311–1323.

27. Johnston, L.F.; National Health and Medical Research Council. *Educator guide*; National Health and Medical Research Council: Canberra, Australia, 2013; pp. 5–6.

28. Thompson, F.E.; Subar, A.F. Dietary assessment methodology. In *Nutrition in the prevention and treatment of disease*, 2nd ed.; Coulston, A.M., Boushey, C.J., Eds.; Elsevier Academic Press: Burlington, MA, USA, 2013; pp. 5–46.

29. Livingstone, M.B.E.; Robson, P.J. Measurement of dietary intake in children. *Proc. Nutr. Soc.* **2000**, *59*, 279–293.

30. Collins, C.E.; Watson, J.; Burrows, T. Measuring dietary intake in children and adolescents in the context of overweight and obesity. *Int. J. Obesity* **2010**, *34*, 1103–1115.

31. Boushey, C.J.; Kerr, D.A.; Wright, J.; Lutes, K.D.; Ebert, D.S.; Delp, E.J. Use of technology in children's dietary assessment. *Eur. J. Clin. Nutr.* **2009**, *63*, S50–S57.

32. Martin, K.; Rosenberg, M.; Miller, M.; French, S.; McCormack, G.; Bull, F.; Giles-Corti, B.; Pratt, S. *Trends in physical activity, nutrition and body size in western australian children and adolescents: The child and adolescent physical activity and nutrition survey (capans)*; Move and Munch Final Report; The Western Australian Government: Perth, Australia, 2008.

33. Rutishauser, I.; Webb, K.; Abraham, B.; Allsopp, R. *Evaluation of short dietary questions from the 1995 national nutrition survey*; Australian Food and Nutrition Monitoring Unit, The University of Queensland: Canberra, Austrilia, 2001.

34. Singh, R.; Martin, B.R.; Hickey, Y.; Teegarden, D.; Campbell, W.W.; Craig, B.A.; Schoeller, D.A.; Kerr, D.A.; Weaver, C.M. Comparison of self-reported and measured metabolizable energy intake with total energy expenditure in overweight teens. *Am. J. Clin. Nutr.* **2009**, *89*, 1744–1750.

35. Rennie, K.L.; Coward, A.; Jebb, S.A. Estimating under-reporting of energy intake in dietary surveys using an individualised method. *Br. J. Nutr.* **2007**, *97*, 1169–1176.

36. Jennings, A.; Cassidy, A.; van Sluijs, E.M.; Griffin, S.J.; Welch, A.A. Associations between eating frequency, adiposity, diet, and activity in 9–10 year old healthy-weight and centrally obese children. *Obesity* **2012**, *20*, 1462–1468.

37. Henes, S.T.; Cummings, D.M.; Hickner, R.C.; Houmard, J.A.; Kolasa, K.M.; Lazorick, S.; Collier, D.N. Comparison of predictive equations and measured resting energy expenditure among obese youth attending a pediatric healthy weight clinic: One size does not fit all. *Nutr. Clin. Pract.* **2013**, *28*, 617–624.

38. Puyau, M.R.; Adolph, A.L.; Vohra, F.A.; Zakeri, I.; Butte, N.F. Prediction of activity energy expenditure using accelerometers in children. *Med. Sci. Sports Exerc.* **2004**, *36*, 1625–1631.

39. Straker, L.M.; Howie, E.K.; Smith, K.L.; Fenner, A.A.; Kerr, D.A.; Olds, T.S.; Abbott, R.A.; Smith, A.J. The impact of curtin university's activity, food and attitudes program on physical activity, sedentary time and fruit, vegetable and junk food consumption among overweight and obese adolescents: A waitlist controlled trial. *PLoS One* **2014**, *9*, e111954.

40. Skelton, J.A.; Beech, B.M. Attrition in paediatric weight management: A review of the literature and new directions. *Obes. Rev.* **2011**, *12*, e273–e281.

41. Vitolins, M.Z.; Rand, C.S.; Rapp, S.R.; Ribisl, P.M.; Sevick, M.A. Measuring adherence to behavioral and medical interventions. *Control. Clin. Trials* **2000**, *21*, 188S–194S.

42. Foraker, R.E.; Pennell, M.; Sprangers, P.; Vitolins, M.Z.; DeGraffinreid, C.; Paskett, E.D. Effect of a low-fat or low-carbohydrate weight-loss diet on markers of cardiovascular risk among premenopausal women: A randomized trial. *J. Womens Health* **2014**, *23*, 675–680.

43. Kristal, A.R.; Ollberding, N.J. Evaluation of nutrition interventions. In *Nutrition in the prevention and treatment of disease*, 3rd ed.; Coulston, A.M., Boushey, C.J., Ferruzzi, M.G., Eds.; Elsevier Inc.: San Diego, California, CA, USA, 2013; pp. 191–205.

44. DeBar, L.L.; Stevens, V.J.; Perrin, N.; Wu, P.; Pearson, J.; Yarborough, B.J.; Dickerson, J.; Lynch, F. A primary care-based, multicomponent lifestyle intervention for overweight adolescent females. *Pediatrics* **2012**, *129*, e611–e620.

45. Tsiros, M.D.; Sinn, N.; Brennan, L.; Coates, A.M.; Walkley, J.W.; Petkov, J.; Howe, P.R.; Buckley, J.D. Cognitive behavioral therapy improves diet and body composition in overweight and obese adolescents. *Am. J. Clin. Nutr.* **2008**, *87*, 1134–1140.

46. Davis, J.N.; Gyllenhammer, L.E.; Vanni, A.A.; Meija, M.; Tung, A.; Schroeder, E.T.; Spruijt-Metz, D.; Goran, M.I. Startup circuit training program reduces metabolic risk in latino adolescents. *Med. Sci. Sport Exer.* **2011**, *43*, 2195–2203.

47. Park, T.G.; Hong, H.R.; Lee, J.; Kang, H.S. Lifestyle plus exercise intervention improves metabolic syndrome markers without change in adiponectin in obese girls. *Ann. Nutr. Metab.* **2007**, *51*, 197–203.

48. Saelens, B.E.; Sallis, J.F.; Wilfley, D.E.; Patrick, K.; Cella, J.A.; Buchta, R. Behavioral weight control for overweight adolescents initiated in primary care. *Obes. Res.* **2002**, *10*, 22–32.

49. Hirvonen, T.; Mannisto, S.; Roos, E.; Pietinen, P. Increasing prevalence of underreporting does not necessarily distort dietary surveys. *Eur. J. Clin. Nutr.* **1997**, *51*, 297–301.

50. Ball, G.D.; Mackenzie-Rife, K.A.; Newton, M.S.; Alloway, C.A.; Slack, J.M.; Plotnikoff, R.C.; Goran, M.I. One-on-one lifestyle coaching for managing adolescent obesity: Findings from a pilot, randomized controlled trial in a real-world, clinical setting. *Paediatr. Child. Health* **2011**, *16*, 345–350.

51. Smith, K.L.; Kerr, D.A.; Fenner, A.A.; Straker, L.M. Adolescents just do not know what they want: A qualitative study to describe obese adolescents' experiences of text messaging to support behavior change maintenance post intervention. *J. Med. Internet. Res.* **2014**, *16*, e103.

52. Miller, T.; Abdel-Maksoud, M.; Crane, L.; Marcus, A.; Byers, T. Effects of social approval bias on self-reported fruit and vegetable consumption: A randomized controlled trial. *Nutr. J.* **2008**, *7*, 18.

53. Smith, K.L.; Straker, L.M.; Kerr, D.A.; Smith, A.J. Overweight adolescents eat what? And when? Analysis of consumption patterns to guide dietary message development for intervention. *J. Hum. Nutr. Diet.* **2014**, *28*, 80–93.

MDPI AG

St. Alban-Anlage 66

4052 Basel, Switzerland

Tel. +41 61 683 77 34

Fax +41 61 302 89 18

http://www.mdpi.com

*Nutrients* Editorial Office

E-mail: nutrients@mdpi.com

http://www.mdpi.com/journal/nutrients